HODGKIN'S AND NON-HODGKIN'S LYMPHOMA

Cancer Treatment and Research

Steven T. Rosen, M.D., *Series Editor*

Miller, A.B. (ed.): *Advances in Cancer Screening.* 1996. ISBN 0-7923-4019-1.
Hait , W.N. (ed.): *Drug Resistance.* 1996. ISBN 0-7923-4022-1.
Pienta, K.J. (ed.): *Diagnosis and Treatment of Genitourinary Malignancies.* 1996. ISBN 0-7923-4164-3.
Arnold, A.J. (ed.): *Endocrine Neoplasms.* 1997. ISBN 0-7923-4354-9.
Pollock, R.E. (ed.): *Surgical Oncology.* 1997. ISBN 0-7923-9900-5.
Verweij, J., Pinedo, H.M., Suit, H.D. (eds): *Soft Tissue Sarcomas: Present Achievements and Future Prospects.* 1997. ISBN 0-7923-9913-7.
Walterhouse, D.O., Cohn, S. L. (eds): *Diagnostic and Therapeutic Advances in Pediatric Oncology.* 1997. ISBN 0-7923-9978-1.
Mittal, B.B., Purdy, J.A., Ang, K.K. (eds): *Radiation Therapy.* 1998. ISBN 0-7923-9981-1.
Foon, K.A., Muss, H.B. (eds): *Biological and Hormonal Therapies of Cancer.* 1998. ISBN 0-7923-9997-8.
Ozols, R.F. (ed.): *Gynecologic Oncology.* 1998. ISBN 0-7923-8070-3.
Noskin, G. A. (ed.): *Management of Infectious Complications in Cancer Patients*1998. ISBN 0-7923-8150-5.
Bennett, C. L. (ed.): *Cancer Policy.* 1998. ISBN 0-7923-8203-X.
Benson, A. B. (ed.): *Gastrointestinal Oncology.* 1998. ISBN 0-7923-8205-6.
Tallman, M.S., Gordon, L.I. (eds): *Diagnostic and Therapeutic Advances in Hematologic Malignancies.* 1998. ISBN 0-7923-8206-4.
von Gunten, C.F. (ed.): *Palliative Care and Rehabilitation of Cancer Patients.* 1999. ISBN 0-7923-8525-X
Burt, R.K., Brush, M.M. (eds): *Advances in Allogeneic Hematopoietic Stem Cell Transplantation.* 1999. ISBN 0-7923-7714-1.
Angelos, P. (ed.): *Ethical Issues in Cancer Patient Care* 2000. ISBN 0-7923-7726-5.
Gradishar, W.J., Wood, W.C. (eds): *Advances in Breast Cancer Management.* 2000. ISBN 0-7923-7890-3.
Sparano, J. A. (ed.): *HIV & HTLV-I Associated Malignancies.* 2001. ISBN 0-7923-7220-4.
Ettinger, D. S. (ed.): *Thoracic Oncology.* 2001. ISBN 0-7923-7248-4.
Bergan, R. C. (ed.): *Cancer Chemoprevention.* 2001. ISBN 0-7923-7259-X.
Raza, A., Mundle, S.D. (eds): *Myelodysplastic Syndromes & Secondary Acute Myelogenous Leukemia* 2001. ISBN: 0-7923-7396.
Talamonti, M. S. (ed.): *Liver Directed Therapy for Primary and Metastatic Liver Tumors.* 2001. ISBN 0-7923-7523-8.
Stack, M.S., Fishman, D.A. (eds): *Ovarian Cancer.* 2001. ISBN 0-7923-7530-0.
Bashey, A., Ball, E.D. (eds): *Non-Myeloablative Allogeneic Transplantation.* 2002. ISBN 0-7923-7646-3.
Leong, S. P.L. (ed.): *Atlas of Selective Sentinel Lymphadenectomy for Melanoma, Breast Cancer and Colon Cancer.* 2002. ISBN 1-4020-7013-6.
Andersson , B., Murray D. (eds): *Clinically Relevant Resistance in Cancer Chemotherapy.* 2002. ISBN 1-4020-7200-7.
Beam, C. (ed.): *Biostatistical Applications in Cancer Research.* 2002. ISBN 1-4020-7226-0.
Brockstein, B., Masters, G. (eds): *Head and Neck Cancer.* 2003. ISBN 1-4020-7336-4.
Frank, D.A. (ed.): *Signal Transduction in Cancer.* 2003. ISBN 1-4020-7340-2.
Figlin, R. A. (ed.): *Kidney Cancer.* 2003. ISBN 1-4020-7457-3.
Kirsch, M.; Black, P. McL. (ed.): *Angiogenesis in Brain Tumors.* 2003. ISBN 1-4020-7704-1.
Keller, E.T., Chung, L.W.K. (eds): *The Biology of Skeletal Metastases.* 2004. ISBN 1-4020-7749-1.
Kumar, R. (ed.): *Molecular Targeting and Signal Transduction.* 2004. ISBN 1-4020-7822-6.
Verweij, J., Pinedo, H.M. (eds): *Targeting Treatment of Soft Tissue Sarcomas.* 2004. ISBN 1-4020-7808-0.
Finn, W.G., Peterson, L.C. (eds.): *Hematopathology in Oncology.* 2004. ISBN 1-4020-7919-2.
Farid, N. (ed.): *Molecular Basis of Thyroid Cancer.* 2004. ISBN 1-4020-8106-5.
Khleif, S. (ed.): *Tumor Immunology and Cancer Vaccines.* 2004. ISBN 1-4020-8119-7.
Balducci, L., Extermann, M. (eds): *Biological Basis of Geriatric Oncology.* 2004. ISBN
Abrey, L.E., Chamberlain, M.C., Engelhard, H.H. (eds): *Leptomeningeal Metastases.* 2005. ISBN 0-387-24198-1
Platanias, L.C. (ed.): *Cytokines and Cancer.* 2005. ISBN 0-387-24360-7.
Leong, S. P.L., Kitagawa, Y., Kitajima, M. (eds): *Selective Sentinel Lymphadenectomy for Human Solid Cancer.* 2005. ISBN 0-387-23603-1.
Small, Jr. W., Woloschak, G. (eds): *Radiation Toxicity: A Practical Guide.* 2005. ISBN 1-4020-8053-0.
Haefner, B., Dalgleish, A. (eds): *The Link Between Inflammation and Cancer.* 2006. ISBN 0-387-26282-2.
Leonard, J.P., Coleman, M. (eds): *Hodgkin's and Non-Hodgkin's Lymphoma.* 2006. ISBN 0-387-29345.

HODGKIN'S AND NON-HODGKIN'S LYMPHOMA

edited by

JOHN P. LEONARD, MD

Center for Lymphoma and Myeloma
Weill Medical College of Cornell University
New York Presbyterian Hospital
New York, NY

MORTON COLEMAN, MD

Center for Lymphoma and Myeloma
Weill Medical College of Cornell University
New York Presbyterian Hospital
New York, NY

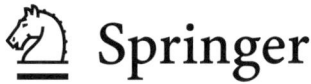 Springer

John P. Leonard, MD
Center for Lymphoma and Myeloma
Weill Medical College of Cornell University
The New York Presbyterian Hospital
New York, New York

Morton Coleman, MD
Center for Lymphoma and Myeloma
Weill Medical College of Cornell University
The New York Presbyterian Hospital
New York, New York

HODGKIN'S AND NON-HODGKIN'S LYMPHOMA

Library of Congress Control Number: 2005934592

ISBN-10: 0-387-29345-0   e-ISBN-10: 0-387-29346-9
ISBN-13: 978-0387-29345-5   e-ISBN-13: 978-0387-29346-2

Printed on acid-free paper.

Printed in the United States of America.

9 8 7 6 5 4 3 2

springer.com

CONTENTS

FOREWORD

The lymphomas are the most common malignancies where the tools of the medical oncologist serve as the principal treatment modality and can frequently result in cure of the patient. Over the past several decades, the use of chemotherapy for lymphoma has rapidly evolved to allow for improvements in efficacy as well as the reduction in some short and long term toxicities. Targeted therapies, such as unlabeled and radiolabeled monoclonal antibodies, have enhanced outcomes for patients with B and T cell malignancies. In parallel, advances in molecular biology, pathology and imaging have provided a better understanding of the pathogenesis of lymphoma to define new therapeutic strategies and have allowed for more accurate determination of prognosis to better define therapy.

In this volume, we have asked a distinguished group of lymphoma researchers to summarize the state of the art in some of the most important aspects of the disease. The result is a current review of our knowledge of the lymphomas, standard diagnostic and therapeutic approaches, as well as our views on the most promising new directions. We hope that this information provides value to anyone working in the field, for both "lymphomanics" who focus in these diseases and for those for whom dealing with lymphoma is a minor but important part of their activities.

We are grateful to many individual for their contributions to this work. Dan Muss spent many hours in formatting and editing texts, without which there would be no end result. Laura Walsh and Maureen Tobin from Springer very valiantly tried (unsuccessfully) to keep us on schedule. We are grateful to them for their patience and for the opportunity to participate in this project. A book of this nature is only as good as its contributors. We are extremely appreciative of our friends and colleagues made so many efforts in putting together this review. Our authors have provided an outstanding summary of current information, which clearly reflects an enormous effort particularly given all of their other ongoing projects and priorities. As with any of our academic efforts, this project would have been impossible without the support of our families. They constantly accept the many diversions of time and attention toward scientific and clinical activities with understanding and grace. Most importantly, we appreciate the contributions of our patients. We learn so much from them on a daily basis, as well as through their participation in research, without which there would be no progress. It is our most sincere hope that in the near future we can reach a point where all lymphoma patients can be cured.

John P. Leonard, M.D.
Morton Coleman, M.D.

CONTRIBUTING AUTHORS

Nancy L. Bartlett, MD, Associate Professor of Medicine, Washington University, Siteman Cancer Center, Division of Medical Oncology, St Louis, MO

Jesus G. Berdeja, MD, Assistant Professor of Medicine, School of Medicine, Loma Linda University, Loma Linda, CA

Ethel Cesarman, MD, PhD, Associate Professor of Pathology, Department of Pathology and Laboratory Medicine, Weill Medical College of Cornell University and The New York Presbyterian Hospital, New York, NY

Amy Chadburn, MD, Professor of Pathology and Laboratory Medicine, Department of Pathology and Laboratory Medicine, Weill Medical College of Cornell University, New York, NY Director, Immunopathology Laboratory, New York Presbyterian Hospital, NY

April Chiu, MD, Assistant Professor of Pathology, Department of Pathology and Laboratory Medicine, Weill Medical College of Cornell University, New York, NY

Morton Coleman, MD, FACP, Clinical Professor of Medicine, Weill Medical College of Cornell University, New York, NY

Andrew M. Evens, DO, MS, Instructor in Medicine and Associate Director, Hematology/Oncology Training Program, Northwestern University Feinberg School of Medicine and the Robert H. Lurie Comprehensive Cancer Center, Chicago, IL

Richard I. Fisher, MD, Samuel E. Durand Professor of Medicine, Director, Hematology-Oncology Unit , Director of Cancer Services, Strong Health, Director, James P. Wilmot Cancer Center, University of Rochester Medical Center, Rochester, NY

Ian W. Flinn, MD, PhD, Associate Professor of Oncology, Director, Lymphoma Program; Assistant Director for Clinical Research, The Sidney Kimmel Comprehensive Cancer Center at Johns Hopkins, Baltimore, MD

Jonathan W. Friedberg, MD, Associate Director, Lymphoma Clinical
Research, James P. Wilmot Cancer Center; Assistant Professor of Medicine
and Oncology, University of Rochester Medical Center, Rochester, NY

Richard R. Furman, MD, Assistant Professor, Weill Medical College of
Cornell University, Department of Medicine, Division of Hematology and
Oncology, New York, NY

John Gerecitano, MD, PhD, Memorial Sloan Kettering Cancer Center,
Department of Medicine, New York, NY

Stanley J. Goldsmith, MD, Director, Division of Nuclear Medicine, The
New York Presbyterian Hospital; Professor of Radiology and Medicine,
Weill Medical College of Cornell University, New York, NY

Lale Kostakoglu, MD, Associate Professor of Radiology at the Weill
Medical College of Cornell University, Department of Radiology, Division
of Nuclear Medicine, The New York Presbyterian Hospital, Weill Medical
College of Cornell University, New York, NY

John P. Leonard, MD, Director of the Oncology Unit, New York
Presbyterian Hospital, Assistant Professor of Medicine at the Weill Medical
College of Cornell University, Medical Director of the Center for
Lymphoma and Myeloma at NYPH-Cornell, New York, NY

Peter McLaughlin, MD, Professor of Medicine, University of Texas M.D.
Anderson Cancer Center, Department of Lymphoma/Myeloma, Houston, TX

Enrique A. Mesri, PhD, Laboratory of Viral Oncogenesis, Division
of Hematology-Oncology, Department of Medicine, Weill Medical College
of Cornell University and The New York Presbyterian Hospital, NY, NY

Sarah Montross, MD, Department of Medicine, University of California,
Los Angeles Center for Health Sciences, Los Angeles, CA

Daniel Muss, Regulatory Coordinator, Weill Medical College of Cornell
University, Department of Medicine, Division of Hematology and
Oncology, New York, NY

Owen A. O'Connor, MD, PhD, Memorial Sloan Kettering Cancer Center, Department of Medicine, Division of Hematologic Oncology, Lymphoma and Developmental Chemotherapy Services, New York, NY

Carol S. Portlock, MD, Lymphoma Service, Department of Medicine, Memorial Sloan-Kettering Cancer Center, New York, New York

Christiane Querfeld, MD, Department of Dermatology, Northwestern University Feinberg School of Medicine and the Robert H. Lurie Comprehensive Cancer Center of Northwestern University, Chicago, IL

Steven T. Rosen, MD, Division of Hematology/Oncology, Northwestern University Feinberg School of Medicine and the Robert H. Lurie Comprehensive Cancer Center of Northwestern University, Chicago, IL

Avram J. Smukler, MD, Fellow, Hematology/Oncology, Washington University, Siteman Cancer Center, Division of Medical Oncology, St. Louis, MO

David J. Straus, **MD,** Attending Physician, Lymphoma Service, Department of Medicine, Memorial Sloan-Kettering Cancer Center; Professor of Clinical Medicine, Weill Medical College of Cornell University, New York, NY

John M. Timmerman, MD, Assistant Professor of Medicine, Division of Hematology-Oncology, University of California, Los Angeles, Los Angeles, CA

Chapter 1

PATHOLOGY OF B-CELL NON-HODGKIN'S LYMPHOMAS AND MULTIPLE MYELOMA

April Chiu, MD and Amy Chadburn, MD

Department of Pathology and Laboratory Medicine, Weill Medical College of Cornell University, New York, NY

1.   INTRODUCTION

B-cell non-Hodgkin's lymphomas (B-NHLs) represent a heterogeneous group of neoplasms with respect to their clinical manifestations, histopathologic features, and biological behavior. The now widely utilized World Health Organization (WHO) classification scheme incorporates our current knowledge of the clinical and pathological features of B-cell neoplasms, and categorizes them into distinct entities (Table 1).[1,2] It is now generally accepted that B-NHLs arise from neoplastic transformation of B-cells at specific stages of differentiation, although the normal counterparts for some B-NHLs have not been clearly delineated (e.g. hairy cell leukemia). Furthermore, some entities, such as chronic lymphocytic leukemia/small lymphocytic lymphoma (CLL/SLL), appear to resemble more than one B-cell differentiation stage.   Nevertheless, a basic understanding of B-cell differentiation stages and their associated immunophenotypic characteristics facilitates accurate diagnosis and appropriate management of B-NHLs.

2.   NORMAL B-CELL DIFFERENTIATION

B-lymphocytes are a key component of humoral immunity. B-cell production is seen first in the fetal liver by 8-9 weeks of gestation; however, this role is mostly taken over by the bone marrow for the remainder of life.[3] Within the bone marrow, B-cells are derived from pluripotential lymphoid precursor cells, which sequentially progress through several stages of development. B-lymphocytes can be readily detected by flow cytometry and/or immunohistochemistry based on their expression of the pan-B cell antigens, i.e. CD19, CD20, CD22, and CD79, as well as the B-cell transcriptional factor BSAP/PAX-5. However, the pattern of expression of these antigens varies during stages of B-cell ontogeny.

Progenitor B cells are the earliest recognizable form of B-lymphocytes. They express only a limited number of surface antigens, including terminal deoxynucelotidyl transferase (TdT), HLA-DR (Ia), and CD34 (Table 2). They may also express CD79 within the cytoplasm (cCD79). They are BSAP/PAX-5 positive, and have germline (i.e. non-rearranged) immunoglobulin (Ig) genes.[4,5] These cells subsequently undergo immunoglobulin heavy chain gene rearrangement and acquire the B-cell lineage-associated antigens CD19 (surface) and CD22 (cytoplasmic; cCD22) to mature into pre-pre B cells.[6,7] They begin to synthesize cytoplasmic immunoglobulin heavy chain μ (cμ), and acquire expression of CD10 (cALLa) and CD20 to become pre-B cells.[8-10] Progenitor B cells, pre-pre-B cells, and pre-B cells are morphologically precursor B lymphoblasts, which have finely dispersed chromatin and small nucleoli.

While expression of HLA-DR and BSAP/PAX-5 is retained throughout B-cell ontogeny except for the terminal plasma cell stage,[4,5,11,12] pre-B cells begin to lose TdT, CD34, CD10, and cytoplasmic μ chain expression as they enter the immature B-cell stage. They also acquire CD21 and surface immunoglobulin M (sIgM) expression at this stage. A subset of these cells also express CD5.[13,14] They progressively increase expression of surface CD22 and IgD, and decrease sIgM expression to become resting mature (naïve) B cells.[8-10,15] From this stage on, further B-cell differentiation occurs in the peripheral lymphoid tissues (i.e. lymph nodes, spleen, and mucosa-associated lymphoid tissues [MALT]) in an antigen-dependent fashion.

Naïve B cells, which are unexposed to antigen, express HLA-DR, CD19, CD20, CD22, CD21, CD79, BSAP/PAX-5, sIgM, and sIgD; they also often express CD5 (Table 3).[16] They leave the bone marrow, circulate in the peripheral blood, and eventually migrate to the peripheral lymphoid tissue and populate the primary lymphoid follicles.[16-18] Upon exposure to antigen trapped on the cell processes of CD21(+) CD35(+) follicular dendritic cells (FDCs), the naïve B cells undergo "blast transformation", where they proliferate to become follicular B-blasts. They further differentiate into centroblasts or "large non-cleaved cells"; these are rapidly proliferating cells found predominantly within the "dark zone" of the germinal center. They transiently shed expression of sIg and the anti-apoptotic protein BCL-2, thus becoming susceptible to death through apoptosis. In addition, they regain expression of CD10 and acquire expression of the nuclear zinc-finger transcription factor BCL-6 (Fig. 1a-i). Centroblasts undergo somatic mutation of the Ig variable region genes to create more diverse antibody binding sites. As IgM has relatively low affinity for the stimulating antigen, centroblasts often also undergo immunoglobulin "class switching" by producing a higher affinity immunoglobulin, usually either IgG or IgA, during subsequent antigen exposure.[19,20] Centroblasts eventually differentiate into centrocytes, also known as small-cleaved cells due to the characteristic angulated appearance of their nuclei. Centrocytes retain the BCL-6(+) BCL-2(-) phenotype, and begin to enter a resting state. They re-express sIg of variable affinity for the inciting antigen; those with insufficient affinity die by apoptosis and are cleared by tingible body macrophages, generating a "starry-sky" pattern within the germinal center. On the other hand, centrocytes with sufficient affinity bind the antigen trapped on the FDCs and, through a complex set of interactions between with FDCs and T cells, re-express BCL-2 to escape the fate of apoptosis. These survivors subsequently turn off BCL-6 expression and, as they exit the germinal center, differentiate into memory B cells or plasma cells.[21-26] Memory B cells, which are more responsive to repeated antigen stimulation, are usually sIgM(+) but sIgD(-). They express on their surface all pan-B cell antigens (CD19, CD20, CD22 and CD79) as well as IRF4/MUM-1, and lack expression of CD5, CD10, and BCL-6. These cells can usually be seen in the marginal zone at the edge of the follicles, which is more prominent in mesenteric lymph nodes, Peyer's patches, and the spleen.[27-30] The plasma cells seen within the lymph node medulla express immunoglobulin only within the cytoplasm (cIg), usually of the IgG or IgA isotype. They express CD19 and CD79 but not other pan-B cell antigens. BSAP/PAX-5 is also down-regulated and no longer expressed by plasma cells.[4,5,11,12] They also express CD38 and CD138 (syndecan-1), but lack expression of HLA-DR, CD45, and CD56.[31-33]

3.   B-CELL NEOPLASMS

B-cell malignancies, including B-cell non-Hodgkin's lymphomas (B-NHLs) and plasma cell neoplasms, encompass many types of neoplasms in the WHO classification scheme (Table 1). For the most part, they express one or more B-cell specific antigen (i.e. CD19, CD20, CD22, CD79), the B-cell transcriptional factor BSAP/PAX-5, and either surface and/or cytoplasmic Ig. In addition, in most cases evidence of immunoglobulin gene rearrangement can be demonstrated, either by polymerase chain reaction (PCR) or Southern blot hybridization studies. Based on their primary clinical presentation, natural history, and morphologic and/or immunophenotypic resemblance to a specific stage of B-cell differentiation, B-cell neoplasms are classified into 20 distinct clinicopathological entities, the most common ten of which are discussed in this chapter. However, accurate morphologic examination and classification is highly dependent on appropriate tissue fixation, and may be severely hindered in less optimal conditions. Consequently, most pathology laboratories have become increasingly reliant upon immunophenotyping, either by flow cytometry or by immunohistochemistry, for the diagnosis and classification of lymphoid neoplasms. The basic immunophenotypic criteria of the more common types of B-NHLs are summarized in Table 4.

3.1   Precursor B-lymphoblastic leukemia/lymphoma (B-ALL/LBL)

Precursor B-lymphoblastic leukemia/lymphoma (B-ALL/LBL) is a neoplasm derived from precursor B-lymphoblasts, i.e. progenitor B cells, pre-pre-B cells, or pre-B cells. Most patients with B-ALL/LBL present with bone marrow involvement with secondary involvement of the peripheral blood; only a small number of patients initially present with disease in lymph nodes or in extra-nodal sites such as the skin.[34,35] By convention, the presence of more than 25% lymphoblasts in the bone marrow is designated as ALL, whereas the identification of one or more mass lesions, with less than 25% lymphoblasts in the marrow, establishes a diagnosis of LBL. However, as the two entities (ALL and LBL) are biologically similar, the distinction is arbitrary and of little if any clinical relevance.

Morphologically, the lymphoblasts are medium-sized with round to convoluted nuclei, finely dispersed chromatin, inconspicuous nucleoli, and a scant amount of cytoplasm (Fig. 2a and 2b). Within the lymph node, the neoplastic cells tend to exhibit a diffuse growth pattern, obliterating much of the normal nodal architecture. Frequently numerous mitotic Figures are seen, as these tumors have a high proliferation rate. Within the bone marrow the pattern of involvement by ALL/LBL is almost always diffuse and extensive.

Immunophenotypically, like their normal counterpart, the tumor cells are TdT (Fig. 2c) and HLA-DR positive. Virtually all cases express the B-cell associated markers CD19, CD79, CD22 (surface or cytoplasmic), and PAX-5.[5,34] However, B-ALL/LBLs exhibit a variety of immunophenotypic patterns with regard to CD34, CD10, CD20, and Ig (cytoplasmic or surface) expression. B-ALL/LBLs may further be separated into immunophenotypic subtypes based on these profiles, although the term "precursor B-lymphoblastic leukemia/lymphoma" encompasses all subtypes. These subtypes do not *per se* have prognostic significance, although some prognostically important cytogenetic aberrations are seen more frequently in certain immunophenotypic, i.e. differentiation, subtypes.

Representing the most immature stage of differentiation, early precursor B-ALL/LBLs are comprised of TdT, HLA-DR, CD34, CD19, cCD22, cCD79a, and BSAP/PAX-5 positive lymphoblasts.[34] However, they lack expression of CD10. This immunophenotypic profile mirrors that of the precursor B cell stage in B cell ontogeny. CD10 negative precursor B-ALL/LBLs are commonly seen in both pediatric and adult patients with chromosomal abnormalities involving the *MLL* gene at 11q23.[36,37] *MLL* gene abnormalities are particularly associated with congenital leukemias, the most common of which is the t(4;11) translocation, resulting in the fusion of *MLL* gene with *AF4* at chromosome 4q21.[34] The majority of CD10 negative B-ALL/LBLs with 11q23 rearrangements express CD15; expression of other myeloid associated antigens is also frequently found.[38-40] In the intermediate stage, or "common" B-ALL/LBLs, the malignant cells express CD10 in addition to the markers expressed by the early precursor tumors. However, they lack expression of both sIg and/or cIg expression.[41] Common B-ALL/LBLs correspond to the pre-pre-B cell stage and are the most common immunophenotypic subtype seen in both pediatric and adult patients, representing approximately 65% of the cases. Both favorable and unfavorable clinical and cytogenetic groups are seen within this immunophenotypic subtype. The pre-B-ALL/LBLs, the most differentiated subtype, resemble the pre-B cell differentiation stage in that the tumor cells express cytoplasmic μ (cμ) but lack light chain or sIg expression.[35] Most cases are TdT, HLA-DR, CD19, CD22, BSAP/PAX-5, and CD10 positive, and show heterogeneous CD20 expression. However, the tumor cells are generally CD34 negative. The t(1;19)(q23;p13) translocation is seen in approximately 20% of the cases of pre-B-ALL/LBLs, where the *E2A* gene at 19p13.3 fuses with *PBX* at 1q23, creating a potent transcriptional factor.[34] Patients with this translocation tend to present with high-risk clinical features, such as high blast counts in the peripheral blood and central nervous system involvement.[42] They also tend to respond poorly to standard chemotherapeutic regimens and but may respond favorably to more intensive regimens.[43,44]

Usually B-ALL/LBLs do not express surface immunoglobulin (sIg); however, sIg expression can be seen rare cases.[45-48] These so-called "mature" B-ALL/LBLs appear to behave like the other subtypes of B-ALL/LBL clinically.

A variety of other cytogenetic abnormalities are commonly seen in B-ALL/LBL. These can be divided into two prognostic groups--favorable and unfavorable. B-ALL/LBLs which are hyperdiploid (i.e. greater than 51 chromosomes) are associated with a good prognosis, as are those with the t(12;21)(p13;q22) translocation (TEL-AML1; ETV6-AML1). The latter tend to be CD20 negative, but often express the myeloid associated antigen CD13.[49-51] B-ALL/LBLs with unfavorable prognosis include those with translocations involving *BCR/ABL* [t(9;22)(q34;q11.2)], *AF4/MLL* [t(4;11)(q21;q23)] or *MLL* with other partner chromosomes [t(v;11)(v;q23)], and *E2A/PBX1* [t(1;19)(q23;p13)]. However, as mentioned previously, patients with the latter cytogenetic abnormality may respond to more intensive therapy.

3.2   Mature B-Cell Neoplasms

Mature B-cell neoplasms encompass neoplasms derived from tumor cells that have differentiated beyond the precursor B, pre-pre-B, and pre-B cell stages in B cell ontogeny. These are clonal proliferations of B cells at various stages of maturation, ranging from naïve B cells to plasma cells. According to the WHO classification, these mature B-cell neoplasms may be grouped based on their major clinical presentation: predominately disseminated lymphoma/leukemias, primary extranodal lymphomas, and predominantly nodal lymphomas.[52,53] These neoplasms may also be grouped according to their biologic behavior: indolent, aggressive, and highly aggressive.[54]   Clinically,   most   predominately   disseminated lymphoma/leukemias and primarily extranodal lymphomas tend to be indolent neoplasms, whereas primarily nodal lymphomas may be clinically indolent or aggressive. The majority of the indolent B cell lymphomas are composed of small, relatively bland-appearing lymphocytes, with or without plasma cell differentiation. Some examples of indolent B-cell lymphomas include chronic lymphocytic leukemia/small lymphocytic lymphomas, follicular lymphoma, and marginal zone lymphoma. Although they are biologically indolent, they also tend to be resistant to standard therapy and are considered incurable in most instances. While theoretically subtypes of indolent lymphoma possess distinct morphologic features that facilitate in their classification, in practicality the tumor cells may be morphologically indistinguishable from one another, particularly when the tissue is poorly preserved. However, these morphologically similar, and often clinically similar, lesions can usually be categorized into to separate entities based on their characteristic antigen expression profiles as determined by immunophenotypic studies (Table 4). On the other hand, in some instances, additional analyses such as molecular and/or cytogenetic studies are necessary to classify these neoplasms. The aggressive/highly aggressive lymphomas represent a heterogeneous group of neoplasms both in terms of their morphology and clinical course. Two examples of aggressive/highly aggressive B cell lymphomas are diffuse large B-cell lymphoma and Burkitt lymphoma. Even within a diagnostic subtype, e.g. diffuse large B-cell lymphoma, the tumor cells may exhibit significant morphologic and clinical heterogeneity. However, efforts attempting to divide these neoplasms into smaller, more biologically specific groups, particularly with the advent of DNA microarray technology, are ongoing and may possibly delineate additional clinically and biologically relevant genetic and immunophenotypic characteristics of these neoplasms.[55]

3.3   B-cell chronic lymphocytic leukemia/small lymphocytic lymphoma

B-chronic lymphocytic leukemia/small lymphocytic lymphoma (B-CLL/SLL), the prototype of predominately disseminated lymphoma/leukemias, is the most common adult leukemia in North America and Western Europe.[56] This neoplastic process tends to occur in older adults (>50 years of age) with a male to female ratio of 2:1. Most patients with B-CLL/SLLs present with bone marrow and peripheral blood involvement, where the absolute lymphocyte count is frequently >10 x 10^9/L. In addition, the tumor cells typically disseminate widely with frequent involvement of liver, spleen, lymph nodes, and a variety of extranodal sites. Some patients may also have a small amount of monoclonal protein in the serum. Rare aleukemic cases, i.e. those without bone marrow and/or peripheral blood involvement, do occur, in which the designation of B-SLL is used. However, as in the case of B-ALL/LBL, the tumor cells in B-CLL and B-SLL are biologically similar. Like most other predominately disseminated lymphoma/leukemias, B-CLL/SLLs are clinically indolent but not usually curable with available therapy.

The neoplastic cells are small in size (i.e. their nuclei are similar in size to an erythrocyte) with round nuclei, clumped chromatin, and scanty cytoplasm (Fig. 3a). Some cases also show plasmacytoid differentiation. The mitotic rate is usually very low. B-chronic lymphocytic leukemia/small lymphocytic lymphoma diffusely involves lymph nodes, however, usually a vaguely nodular pattern is seen (Fig. 3b). This vague nodularity is due to the presence of collections of cells containing increased numbers of prolymphocytes and paraimmunoblasts known as pseudofollicles or proliferation centers. Prolymphocytes and paraimmunoblasts are intermediate to large cells with single to multiple nucleoli and are proliferating malignant cells.

In the bone marrow, the pattern of involvement may be nodular, interstitial, diffuse, or a combination of the three. Pseudofollicles are generally less apparent in the bone marrow than in the lymph nodes, although they can occasionally be seen. In the cases of nodular involvement, the neoplastic lymphoid aggregates tend to be randomly distributed in the interstitial area of the marrow without a predilection for the paratrabecular regions. The patterns of bone marrow involvement by B-CLL/SLL have a prognostic significance: nodular and interstitial patterns (i.e. the tumor cells form distinct aggregates or are admixed with hematopoietic elements, respectively) are seen in early disease, whereas a diffuse pattern of infiltration (i.e. complete effacement of the marrow space by sheets of tumor cells) signifies more advanced disease and worse prognosis.[57,58]

The peripheral blood is usually involved by B-CLL/SLL and most patients have an absolute lymphocytosis. The B-CLL/SLL cells in the peripheral blood are morphologically similar to those seen in the tissues; i.e. they are small and round with scant cytoplasm and clumped chromatin. Prolymphocytes usually constitute less than 10% of the circulating malignant lymphoid cells. Increased numbers of prolymphocytes (more than 10% but less than 55%) are seen in association with p53 abnormalities and trisomy 12, and warrant the diagnosis of CLL with increased prolymphocytes (CLL/PL).[59]

Immunophenotypically, the neoplastic cells express the pan-B cell antigens CD19, CD20 (weak), CD22 (very weak or absent) and CD79a, as well as BSAP/PAX-5; they also faintly express monotypic surface immunoglobulin (usually kappa) and either sIgM alone, or sIgM and sIgD simultaneously. In addition, they express both the T-cell antigen CD5 and the activation marker CD23 (Fig. 4), and usually faintly express the adhesion molecule CD11c. These neoplastic cells lack expression of CD10 and/or BCL-6, markers typically expressed by follicular lymphomas. They also lack expression of BCL-1 (cyclin-D1), thus separating B-CLL/SLL from mantle cell lymphoma, a B-cell neoplasm which is also CD5 positive but generally CD23 negative. Lastly, B-CLL/SLLs usually lack FMC7 expression, in contrast to most other types of indolent B-cell lymphoma.[60,61]

B-CLL/SLLs have been regarded in the past as a neoplasm arising from recirculating CD5+ CD23+ IgM+ IgD+ naïve B cells that are normally found in the peripheral blood, primary follicles, and mantle cell zones of secondary follicles; these B cells have an unmutated variable region of the immunoglobulin gene (IgV).[17,62] However, recently a second category of B-CLL/SLL containing somatic mutations in IgV has emerged; these cases are thought to arise from memory B cells based on gene expression profiling studies.[63] Although the mutated cases more frequently have an "atypical" appearance (i.e. irregular nuclear contours), in general the mutated and unmutated cases of B-CLL/SLL are morphologically very similar. There are, however, definite differences between the mutated and unmutated cases in terms of clinical behavior, i.e. those with a mutated Ig V region tend to be associated with a more indolent clinical course, whereas those without the mutations tend to have more aggressive clinical behavior.[64] Since most laboratories lack the resources to sequence the IgV region, two "surrogate" phenotypic markers have been identified that correlate with IgV mutational status--CD38, a regulator of activation and proliferation, and ZAP-70, a protein kinase normally expressed by T cells.[65] Cases of B-CLL/SLL without somatic mutations, i.e. of naïve B-cells, are more frequently CD38 and ZAP-70 positive, are associated with higher stage of disease at presentation as well as shorter survival, and are less responsive to chemotherapy.[66] On the other hand, cases with mutated IgV less frequently express CD38 or ZAP-70, and are associated with a more indolent clinical course and longer survival. Of the two markers, ZAP-70 is felt to be more sensitive and specific, predicting IgV mutational status in 93% of patients, in comparison to CD38 which correlates with mutation status in only 67-77% of cases.[67] Furthermore, ZAP-70 expression does not change over time, while CD38 expression may change during the course of the disease.[67,68,69] In addition, ZAP-70 can be detected by either flow cytometry and by immunohistochemistry in routine formalin fixed tissue sections (Fig. 5); CD38 immunoreactivity, although reliably detected by flow cytometry, is often faint and highly variable in paraffin tissue sections based on fixation.[65,67,68,70-72]

Other important prognostic indicators include the proliferation-associated antigen Ki-67 (MIB-1) and p53. Typically only a small number of CLL/SLL cells are Ki-67 positive;[73] however, cases of chemotherapy resistant CLL/SLL have a higher percentage of Ki-67 positive cells in the peripheral blood.[74] Expression of the p53 in B-CLL/SLLs also confers worse outcome, with a shorter treatment free interval, poorer response to therapy, and decreased survival time.[75]

Transformation to high-grade lymphoma occurs not infrequently in patients with B-CLL/SLLs.[76] The most common type of B-CLL/SLL transformation is prolymphocytic transformation, seen in 15% of patients, in which an increased proportion of prolymphocytes is seen. The next most frequent type of transformation is "Richter's syndrome", seen in 3-10% of the cases. Morphologically these transformations are usually diffuse large cell lymphomas (Fig. 6), although cases resembling Hodgkin lymphoma may also occur. Other types of B-CLL/SLL transformation are rare; these include blastic, plasmacytoid, and paraimmunoblastic transformations. In most patients, when transformation occurs, the prognosis worsens and death ensues within a short period of time.

4.   MANTLE CELL LYMPHOMA

Although mantle cell lymphoma (MCL) is classified as an indolent lymphoma since its survival is measured in years rather than months, the median survival is still significantly less than the other indolent lymphoid neoplasms.[77] Patients with MCL are usually elderly, male, and present with nodal disease. However, peripheral blood involvement can be seen in about 25% of cases.[78] The most common extranodal site of involvement is the gastrointestinal tract, which is present in approximately 30% of the cases. When the neoplastic infiltrate in the gastrointestinal tract results in multiple polypoid mucosal lesions, it is called "lymphomatoid polyposis". In addition, the bone marrow and spleen are also frequently involved.

The cell of origin is postulated to be the CD5+ CD23- unstimulated B cells of the inner mantle zone, although the precise cell type has not been definitively determined. The neoplastic cells are generally small to medium in size with variably irregular nuclear contours and a scant amount of cytoplasm. Scattered epithelioid histiocytes are also frequently seen, giving rise to a pseudo- "starry-sky" appearance (Fig. 7). Mantle cell lymphoma can be morphologically difficult to distinguish from CLL/SLL, follicular lymphoma, and marginal zone lymphoma both architecturally and cytologically (Fig. 8). However, immunophenotypically, MCL in most instances can be separated from these other entities. Mantle cell lymphomas are positive for the pan-B cell antigens CD19, CD20, CD22, BSAP/PAX-5 and CD79a. They express high density ("bright") monoclonal surface immunoglobulin, usually sIgM alone or simultaneously sIgM and sIgD. The neoplastic cells are CD5 positive, a feature not seen in follicular lymphoma and present only in a small fraction of marginal zone lymphomas. In contrast to CLL/SLL, which is also CD5 positive, most cases of MCL lack expression of CD23 (Fig. 9) but express FMC-7.[79,80] Furthermore, MCL cells lack expression of CD10 and BCL-6, markers typically expressed by follicular lymphoma cells.[81-84] The tumor cells are also usually CD43 positive[85] and are often associated with loose, ill-defined CD21 or CD35 positive follicular dendritic cell meshworks.[86] In contrast to other sIg positive mature B cell neoplasms, which usually show immunoglobulin light chain kappa restriction, MCL cells more often express the lambda immunoglobulin light chain determinant.[80]

Mantle cell lymphomas characteristically carry the cytogenetic translocation t(11;14)(q13;q32), in which the *BCL1 (PRAD1, CCND1)* gene on 11q13 is juxtaposed with the Ig heavy chain gene locus on 14q32; this results in overexpression of the BCL-1 (CYCLIN D1) protein which can be detected by immunostaining in the nuclei of the tumor cells in formalin fixed paraffin tissue sections (Fig. 10).[87-89] Expression of BCL-1 is relatively unique to MCLs, as it is not detected in most other subtypes of B-cell neoplasia with the exception of hairy cell leukemia[90,91] and some cases of multiple myeloma.[92] Thus, inclusion of BCL-1 in the immunohistochemistry panel can prove extremely valuable distinguishing MCLs from other indolent lymphomas, such as B-CLL/SLL, follicular lymphomas, and marginal zone lymphomas.

The median survival of patients with MCL is 3 to 5 years. However, in the event of abnormalities/structural alterations involving other cell cycle proteins, such as p53, p16, and p18, the median survival decreases to approximately 18 months.[93-95] Overexpression of p53, p21, p16, all of which can be detected in paraffin tissue sections by immunohistochemical staining, is associated with more aggressive disease and a poorer prognosis.[93,94] In addition, a high proliferation rate, which can be demonstrated by Ki-67 immunostaining, also confers an adverse prognosis.[96,97]

Histologic transformation to a large cell lymphoma does not occur with MCL. However, morphologic variants exist.[98] The most common of these is the blastic/blastoid variants, in which the tumor cells either resemble lymphoblasts with dispersed chromatin, or are pleomorphic with cleaved nuclei and at times prominent nucleoli. The blastic/blastoid variant of MCL is associated with high mitotic rate and a more aggressive disease course.

5.   FOLLICULAR LYMPHOMA

Follicular lymphoma (FL) is the most common type of low grade non-Hodgkin's lymphoma in the western world.[99] Although primarily a nodal lymphoma, FLs are characterized by widespread disease at presentation, including frequent involvement of the bone marrow. The affected patients are generally older adults. Follicular lymphomas are associated with an initially indolent disease course; however, transformation to a large cell lymphoma, generally diffuse, occurs in 25-35% of the cases.[100] In these cases, the patients usually rapidly deteriorate clinically and die as the tumor is generally refractory to treatment.[101]

Typical cases of FL are characterized by a predominantly follicular growth pattern (Fig. 11). The neoplastic cells, centrocytes and centroblasts (Fig. 12), are thought to arise from germinal center B cells. Follicular lymphomas are graded based on the number of centroblasts present in 40x high-power microscopic field (hpf). Grade 1 FLs have 0-5 centroblasts/hpf, grade 2 cases have 6-15 centroblasts/hpf, and grade 3 cases have >15 centroblasts/hpf.

Immunophenotypically, the neoplastic cells express the pan-B cell antigens CD19, CD20, CD22, BSAP/PAX-5 and CD79a. They usually express sIg (IgM with or without IgD, IgG or IgA); however, a few cases lack sIg expression.[102] The tumors cells also usually express the follicle center cell-associated antigens CD10 and BCL-6 (Fig. 13).[84,103] In contrast to B-CLL/SLL and MCL, FL tumor cells are usually CD5 and CD43 negative; only rare cases of grade 3 FLs are CD43 positive.[85,104,105] When a follicular growth pattern is present, the neoplastic follicles are associated with CD21 positive follicular dendritic cell (FDC) meshworks. The FDC meshworks are usually relatively intact around the periphery but are often centrally fragmented.[106,107] The tumor cells, in general, express the anti-apoptotic protein BCL-2 (Fig. 13); this is in sharp contrast to normal germinal center B cells, which normally turn off BCL-2 expression (Fig. 1h). Thus, overexpression of the BCL-2 protein distinguishes neoplastic follicles from reactive ones. The abnormal expression of the BCL-2 protein is due to the t(14;18) translocation where the *BCL-2* gene on chromosome 18 is juxtaposed to the *IgH* gene chromosome 14. Consequently, *BCL-2* gene transcription comes under the control of the immunoglobulin heavy chain gene promoter, resulting in overexpression of the BCL-2 protein and conferring upon the tumor cells a survival advantage. The incidence of BCL-2 expression tends to vary according to the cytologic grade, ranging from nearly 100% in grade 1, greater than 80% in grade 2, and 70% of grade 3 FL.[108] Approximately 15% of FLs lack a t(14;18) translocation but bear other cytogenetic abnormalities.[109-111]

Primary cutaneous FL is currently a distinct variant of FL in the WHO classification scheme. In contrast to FLs with nodal presentation, primary cutaneous FLs frequently lack BCL-2 overexpression and lack the t(14;18) rearrangement.[112,113] They are frequently localized to the head and neck region or trunk, treatable by local therapy, and associated with an even more indolent clinical behavior compared to conventional FLs. The biological relationship between primary cutaneous FLs and those with nodal presentation remained to be elucidated.

6.   MARGINAL ZONE LYMPHOMA

Marginal zone lymphoma (MZL) was recognized as a distinct subtype of B-NHLs in the REAL and WHO classification schemes. Marginal zone lymphomas are divided into three subtypes: nodal MZL, extra-nodal MZL of mucosa-associated lymphoid tissue ("MALT" lymphoma), and splenic MZL (SMZL) / splenic lymphoma with villous lymphocytes (SLVL). These neoplasms, for the most part, are morphologically and immunophenotypically similar. The neoplastic cells, small to medium in size, are postulated to be derived from the marginal B-cell compartment of the secondary lymphoid tissue, representing post-germinal center B cells.[114] The cellular composition of these lymphomas shows considerable variation, however; the neoplastic cells may exhibit centrocytic, monocytoid (clear cells with moderate amount of pale cytoplasm), immunoblastic, centroblastic, and/or plasmacytic differentiation (Fig. 14).[114-116] In all types of MZL, "follicular colonization," where residual reactive germinal centers are invaded by neoplastic cells, may be present.[114]

Immunophenotypically, MZL cells express pan B-cell associated antigens, such as CD20 and CD79a. In cases with plasmacytic differentiation, the tumor cells may express monotypic cytoplasmic immunoglobulin (Fig. 15). The neoplastic cells in general lack expression of CD5, CD10, CD23, BCL-1, and BCL-6. The cells are FMC7 positive and sometimes CD43 positive; however, SMZLs are usually CD43 negative.[85,104,117,118] These immunophenotypic findings help facilitate the recognition of MZLs. However, there is not a marker that clearly demonstrates the marginal zone cell origin of the neoplastic cells. Thus, the immunoarchitectural features of the specimen are often crucial in reaching the diagnosis of MZL. Immunostaining for CD21 and CD35 often shows the presence of follicular dendritic cell (FDC) meshworks with extensive fragmentation at the edges, "broken-down" by the infiltrating neoplastic MZL cells (Fig. 16a), a pattern unlike that seen in FLs (i.e. intact edges; Fig. 13b). The neoplastic MZL cells, which are usually BCL-2 positive, may extensively infiltrate among the BCL-2 negative residual benign germinal center cells (Fig. 16b), simulating the BCL-2 positive follicles seen in FLs. However, the MZL cells lack immunoreactivity for both CD10 and BCL-6; the serpiginous areas of CD10/BCL6 negative staining are not seen in either reactive follicles or FL follicles.[81,108,119]

Despite their morphologic and immunophenotypic similarities, SMZLs, nodal MZLs, and MALT lymphomas differ in terms of their clinical presentation and behavior, and thus are best considered separate clinicopathologic entities.

6.1   Splenic marginal zone lymphoma

Splenic marginal zone lymphoma (SMZL) is a rare neoplasm, representing less than 1% of lymphoid neoplasms.[120] The tumor involves the spleen, splenic hilar lymph nodes, bone marrow, and peripheral blood. Most patients are over 50 years of age who present with splenomegaly, autoimmune thrombocytopenia or anemia, and/or peripheral blood villous lymphocytes. In the spleen, the neoplastic cells involve both the white and red pulp (Fig. 17). Within the white pulp, the neoplastic cells surround or replace the germinal centers, often with effacement of the mantle cell zone, and infiltrate the marginal zone. In the red pulp, the tumor cells form nodules and sheets, and infiltrate the sinuses.[121,122] In the peripheral blood, the circulating neoplastic cells usually have relatively abundant cytoplasm and polar villous projections.

Immunophenotypically the neoplastic cells, aside from the aforementioned markers, express surface IgM and IgD.[123-126] Splenic marginal zone lymphomas in general lack expression of CD43; in contrast, this antigen is occasionally expressed by nodal or extranodal MZLs.[85] Due to clinical splenomegaly and the frequent prominent red pulp infiltration seen on routine morphologic examination, hairy cell leukemia is an important diagnostic consideration. However, the tumor cells in SMZL lack expression of the hairy cell leukemia-associated markers CD25, CD11c, CD103, HC-2, and TRAP.[125,127]

Although a small number of cases of SMZL progress to large cell lymphoma, in contrast to CLL/SLL and MCL, this progression is not usually associated with p53 mutation or overexpression, but rather with a higher proliferation rate as indicated by Ki-67 expression.[128] However, the small number of patients with transformed SMZL/SLVL in which p53 mutations have been identified have significantly worse survival.[129]

6.2   Nodal marginal zone lymphoma

Nodal MZLs are also rare, comprising less than 2% of lymphoid neoplasms.[99] Patients with nodal MZLs present with peripheral lymphadenopathy, and occasionally bone marrow and peripheral blood involvement.

Within the lymph node a variety of growth patterns may be seen. These include parafollicular, perisinusoidal, nodular, and diffuse patterns of infiltration. As in other types of MZLs, the neoplastic cells may assume a variety of morphologic appearances. Nodal MZL with a prominent monocytoid B-cells component has been described and classified as monotyoid B-cell lymphoma of the lymph node in the past.[130-132]

Nodal MZLs are generally immunophenotypically similar to other types of MZLs. In contrast to SMZLs, however, nodal MZL cells usually express surface immunoglobulin IgM, IgG, or IgA, and are usually IgD negative. However, some IgD positive cases have been reported.[123]

6.3 Extra-nodal marginal zone lymphoma of mucosa-associated lymphoid tissue (MALT)

Extra-nodal marginal zone lymphoma of mucosa-associated lymphoid tissue (MALT lymphoma) is an indolent B-cell neoplasm virtually always presenting in extranodal sites. These neoplasms comprise 7-8% of all B-cell lymphomas[99] and up to 50% of primary gastric lymphomas.[133,134] Although frequently diagnosed in the stomach, MALT lymphomas also occur in other sites, such as the orbit,[135] salivary glands,[136] and skin.[137] Many cases of MALT lymphoma appear to be associated with chronic inflammatory conditions, such as *Helicobacter pylori* (*H. pylori*) infection which is frequently seen in association with gastric MALT lymphomas[138,139] and *Chlamydia psittaci* infection in ocular MALT lymphomas.[135,140] Furthermore, patients with autoimmune diseases, such as Sjogren's syndrome[141,142] and Hashimoto's thyroiditis,[143,144] are also at an increased risk for MALT lymphoma.

The tumor cells often arise in the marginal zone of the reactive follicles in mucosa-associated lymphoid tissue and extend into the interfollicular areas. In epithelial tissues, the tumor cells may extend into the epithelium, forming lymphoepithelial lesions—a feature characteristic, but not diagnostic, of MALT lymphomas (Fig. 18).[145,146]

Immunophenotypically, MALT lymphomas are similar to nodal MZL with respect to surface immunoglobulin heavy chain expression, i.e. IgM, IgA, or IgG. They do not generally express IgD.[123] In contrast to splenic MZL, many cases of MALT lymphoma are CD43 positive. The malignant cells are otherwise immunophenotypically similar to other types of MZLs. They may also express CD21 and CD35. MALT lymphomas generally lack expression of CD5; however, occasional CD5 positive cases have been reported. These have been reported to be associated with a clinically aggressive course and tendency for dissemination.[147-149] As in other types of MZLs, infiltration of FDC meshworks by CD10 negative, BCL-6 negative, BCL-2 positive neoplastic cells is frequently seen in MALT lymphomas. In addition, the characteristic lymphoepithelial lesions can be accentuated by immunostaining for cytokeratin and B cell markers (Fig. 18). In gastric MALT, identification of *H. pylori*, which can be facilitated by immunostaining for the organism, may direct treatment, since some cases of gastric MALT lymphoma can be cured by antibiotic therapy.[150,151]

A variety of cytogenetic aberrations have been described in MALT lymphoma. The t(11;18)(q21;q21) translocation is detected in 14% of MALT lymphomas of all sites, but is more common in gastric (24%) and pulmonary (53%) MALT lymphomas, and is least common in ocular (3%) and salivary gland (2%) lesions.[152] In this translocation, the *API2* gene on chromosome 11 is fused to the *MALT1* gene on chromosome 18 to produce a chimeric *API2-MALT1* fusion transcript.[153] MALT lymphomas confined to the stomach (Stage IE) with t(11;18) do not respond to *H. pylori* eradication.[154,155] The recently described t(14;18)(q32;q21) translocation is detected in 11% of MALT lymphomas overall but is seen more frequently in ocular (24%), skin (14%), and salivary gland (12%) cases.[152] In addition, these cases frequently harbor additional cytogenetic abnormalities.[156]

The t(1;14)(q22;q23) translocation is encountered in <2% of MALT lymphomas of all sites, but is more commonly seen in the intestine (13%) and the lung (7%).[152] This involves translocation of *BCL10*, a tumor suppressor gene, to the *IgH* locus at 14q32, resulting in overexpression of the BCL-10 protein in the nucleus.[157] BCL-10 may also be expressed in gastric MALT lymphomas with t(11;18) but without t(1;14); the expression of BCL-10 in these cases is associated with higher stage disease.[158] Numeric chromosomal aberrations such as trisomy 3 and trisomy 18 are also commonly encountered in MALT lymphomas.[159]

7.   HAIRY CELL LEUKEMIA

Hairy cell leukemia (HCL) is a rare type of lymphoid neoplasm with leukemic presentation, accounting for 2% of all leukemias.[160,161] The median age at diagnosis is 55 years, with a male to female ratio of 4-5:1.[162,163] Most patients present with splenomegaly and pancytopenia. Monocytopenia is also nearly always present in untreated patients.[164] The leukemic cells typically infiltrate the splenic red pulp; peripheral blood and bone marrow are also usually involved at presentation. The tumor may also be seen infrequently in the liver, lymph nodes, and skin.[161,163] The cell of origin is unknown, but is thought to be derived from a B-cell of a post-germinal center stage of differentiation.

Morphologically, the neoplastic cells are medium in size and bland-appearing (Fig. 19a). They have oval or indented (bean-shaped) nuclei and relatively abundant cytoplasm with circumferential "hairy" cytoplasmic projections.

Immunophenotypically, HCL cells are CD19, CD20, CD22, CD79a positive B cells which express relatively bright monotypic surface immunoglobulin (IgM, IgMD, IgG or IgA). They are CD5, CD10 and CD23 negative, but brightly express CD11c, CD25, CD103, HC-2 and FMC7.[125,127,165] They also are tartrate resistant acid phosphatase (TRAP), DBA.44, and CD25 positive by immunohistochemical staining (Fig. 19b-d). As most patients with HCL have a "dry-tap" on bone marrow aspirate, the concomitant expression of these three latter markers are extremely helpful in making the diagnosis on paraffin-embedded sections.[166,167]

8.   BURKITT LYMPHOMA

Burkitt lymphoma (BL) is highly aggressive, frequently involving extranodal sites, peripheral blood, and bone marrow at presentation.[168,169] BL may be seen in an endemic form occurring in equatorial Africa and New Guinea, arise sporadically throughout the world, or be associated with human immunodeficiency virus (HIV) infection. The abdomen is involved in the majority of sporadic BLs,[170,171] while involvement of the jaws, orbit, and other head and neck structures is seen more often in the endemic form.[168,172] In BL arising in the setting of HIV infection, the neoplastic infiltrate more often presents in lymph nodes and the bone marrow. The postulated cell of origin is thought to be the B-blast from early in the germinal center reaction.

The neoplastic infiltrate is composed of monotonous medium-sized lymphoid cells. These cells have round nuclei, multiple nucleoli, and relatively abundant basophilic cytoplasm. A large number of tingible body macrophages (macrophages containing phagocytic debris) is usually present, imparting a starry-sky pattern (Fig. 20a). Numerous mitotic Figures are present, reflecting the extremely high growth fraction of the tumor cells.

The tumor cells express CD19, CD20, CD22, CD79a, CD10, BCL-6, and sIgM; they lack expression of CD5, CD23, and BCL-2. [27,108,173-175] Many of the cases are CD43 positive.[108,176] The majority of the endemic cases are CD21 positive, the receptor for both C3d and the Epstein-Barr virus (EBV).[177] Nearly 100% of the cells are Ki-67 positive (Fig. 20b).[53,175,178]

Virtually all endemic cases, 25-40% of the immunodeficiency associated cases, and a variable number of the sporadic cases are associated with the Epstein Barr virus.[179-184] All cases have a translocation involving the *MYC* gene at chromosome 8 and an immunoglobulin gene, either the heavy chain (on chromosome 14) or a light chain (kappa on chromosome 2 or lambda on chromosome 22).[184-186]

9.   DIFFUSE LARGE B-CELL LYMPHOMA

Diffuse large B-cell lymphoma (DLBCL) accounts for 30-40% of adult NHLs in the western countries. These clinically aggressive tumors may present in lymph nodes or in extra-nodal sites.[53,187] A variety of extranodal sites may be involved, including the gastrointestinal tract, bone, skin, central nervous system, liver, and spleen. Presentation in the bone marrow and/or peripheral blood, however, is rare.[188] DLBCLs can occur in patients of all ages, including children.[99,120,189] Most cases arise de novo; however, some cases represent transformation from a previous low-grade lymphoma, e.g. B-CLL/SLL, FL, MZL.

Diffuse large B-cell lymphomas have a diffuse growth pattern, obliterating the normal architecture of the involved lymph node or extranodal site. However, DLBCLs are heterogeneous with regards to cellular morphology (Fig. 21a-f). In most cases the neoplastic large lymphoid cells resemble centroblasts (large non-cleaved cells) or immunoblasts (large lymphoid cells with a single, centrally-placed nucleoli). They may also appear multilobated, Reed-Sternberg cell-like, and/or anaplastic (i.e. cells with bizarre pleomorphic nuclei). Another morphologic variant is T cell/histiocyte rich B cell lymphoma, where the neoplastic B cells account for only 10% or less of the malignant cell population.[190-192] There are also distinct forms of DLBCL, including mediastinal (thymic) large B-cell lymphoma, intravascular large B cell lymphoma, and primary effusion lymphoma (PEL). The latter two lymphomas are extremely rare; in addition, PEL occurs primarily in HIV-positive individuals.[193] Mediastinal large B-cell lymphoma is thought to arise from thymic B cells, and is clinically, immunophenotypically, and genetically distinct from other DLBCLs.[194-196]

Diffuse large B-cell lymphomas usually express the pan-B cell antigens, such as CD19, CD20, CD22, BSAP/PAX-5, and CD79a. However, some cases may lack expression of one or more of these antigens.[176,188,197] The cells may express surface and/or cytoplasmic Ig; the latter is usually seen in cases that exhibit plasmacytic differentiation.[198,199] Some cases may also express CD30.[198,199] Approximately 30% and 80% of the cases express CD10 and BCL-6, respectively. BCL-2 is positive in approximately 50% of the cases express. CD138 expression is only rarely seen. Expression of IRF4/MUM1 is frequently found. Approximately one-third of cases express CD43, including a number of those that lack expression of all pan-B cell antigens. In these "CD43 only" cases, it is important to perform additional studies, including immunoglobulin and T cell receptor chain gene rearrangement analyses to determine the cell lineage, since CD43 can be expressed by myeloid tumors as well as by T and B cell neoplasms.

Occasional cases of DLBCLs are CD5 positive. These may arise either de novo or represent transformed cases of CLL/SLL or MCL; a transformed case of MCL usually expresses BCL-1,[200] while many of the transformed CLL/SLL cases retain CD23 expression.[201,202] De novo CD5 positive DLBCLs are associated with a more aggressive clinical course and decreased survival.[203,204] Other adverse prognostic indicators include BCL-2 and/or p53 overexpression.[205,206] Recent gene profiling studies have identified two categories of DLBCLs according to patterns of gene expression: germinal center cell-like and activated B cell-like.[55] Patients with the former type had a better overall survival than the latter. CD10 and BCL-6 are two markers commonly associated with germinal center B cell-like DLBCLs, whereas IRF4/MUM1 expression is associated with the activated B-cell type (Fig. 22).[207]

10.   PLASMA CELL NEOPLASM

The broad diagnostic category of plasma cell neoplasm (PCN) includes many clinicopathological entities according to the WHO classification scheme: plasma cell myeloma (including the variants non-secretory myeloma, smoldering myeloma, indolent myeloma, and plasma cell leukemia), plasmacytoma (solitary or extramedullary type), immunoglobulin deposition diseases (primary amyloidosis, systemic light/heavy chain deposition disease), osteosclerotic myeloma (POEMS syndrome), and heavy chain disease (gamma, mu, and alpha).[208] The most common type of PCN, however, is plasma cell myeloma.

Plasma cell myeloma (i.e. multiple myeloma) usually presents as a multifocal bone marrow neoplasm, although solitary bone or extramedullary (i.e. tissue) presentation may be seen. Peripheral blood and/or lymph node involvement is only rarely present. The incidence of plasma cell myeloma is higher in blacks than whites, and tends to increase with advancing age.[209] The afflicted patients have one or more of a myriad of clinical manifestations of the disease process, including serum or urine "M" (monoclonal) protein, pathologic fractures, bone pain, hypercalcemia, anemia, recurrent infections, and renal failure in addition to having neoplastic plasma cells.[208,210] The diagnosis is based on a constellation of clinical, radiologic and pathologic findings. In general, a diagnosis of plasma cell myeloma can be made when at least two of the following criteria are met: marrow plasmacytosis, lytic bone lesions, monoclonal protein (M component) in the serum or urine, plasmacytoma on tissue biopsy, and reduced production of normal immunoglobulins.[208]

Bone marrows involved by plasma cell myeloma show an excess number of plasma cells. These plasma cells often form large aggregates and sheets, in contrast to normal plasma cells that tend to be scattered or form small clusters around vessels. The myeloma plasma cells may have variable morphologic appearances (Fig. 23), including mature forms indistinguishable from normal plasma cells ("clock-face" chromatin without nucleoli, perinuclear hof, eccentric nucleoli), immature forms with more dispersed chromatin and prominent eosinophilic nucleoli, and those with "plasmablastic" features such as high nuclear to cytoplasmic ratio, prominent nucleoli, and blastic nuclei. The latter morphologic appearance has been associated with a poor prognosis.[211,212] These different morphologic variations may be seen together in a single patient and even in the same biopsy.

The neoplastic plasma cells, like their normal counterpart, lack surface expression of most antigens, including sIg. However, they express cIg that is monotypic, mostly commonly IgG and less commonly IgA.[213] Expression of the other Ig isotypes, i.e. IgD, IgM, and IgE, is rare. Regardless the isotype, the M component in most cases is secreted as a whole Ig molecule, complete with heavy and light chain. However, in about 15% of cases only immunoglobulin light chains are produced ("Bence-Jones" myeloma). Most myeloma plasma cells lack expression the B-cell markers CD20 and CD22; however, they express cCD79a. CD20 expression is detected in 20% of the cases of plasma cell myeloma; these malignant plasma cells are usually small in size and contain t(11;14) (Fig. 24).[214] Patients with CD20-positive plasma cell myeloma may benefit from anti-CD20 monoclonal antibody therapy. Although normal plasma cells are CD19 positive and express the B-cell transcription factor PAX-5, neoplastic plasma cells are negative for both.[215] As the PAX-5 gene is a regulator of CD19 transcription, the lack of PAX-5 expression may be responsible for the lack of CD19 expression by the myeloma cells.[32,215,216] Myeloma plasma cells express CD38, CD138 (syndecan-1), and sometimes CD56 (N-CAM). As CD56 is not expressed by normal plasma cells, CD56 expression by plasma cells is indicative of their malignant nature.[32,217,218] In addition, CD56 expression is frequently associated with lytic bone lesions in myeloma patients.[217] Myeloma plasma cells, like normal plasma cells, often express non-hematopoeitic antigens, such as epithelial membrane antigen (EMA).[219,220] Although most patients with multiple myeloma have low plasma cell proliferation activity, those whose neoplastic plasma cells exhibit higher proliferation rate, as measured by Ki-67 immunostaining, have more rapid clinical progression and shorter survival.[221] Specifically, the presence of more than 8% Ki-67 positive plasma cells is associated with a poor prognosis.[222,223]

Multiple cytogenetic abnormalities have been identified in plasma cell myeloma. Gains in chromosomes 3, 5, 7, 9, 11, 15, and 19, and losses in chromosomes 8, 13, 14, X, are most common.[32,208] Structural abnormalities involving the p53 gene on chromosome 17, identified in up to 25% of cases, are associated with a poorer prognosis.[224] Structural abnormalities involving chromosome 11, such as t(11;14) translocation or trisomy 11, are also common, which result in overexpression of BCL-1 (CYCLIN D1). BCL-1 overexpression has been associated with a more favorable prognosis with prolonged survival following autologous transplantation.[225] The t(4;14) translocation, detected in approximately 20% of the myeloma cases, results in over-expression of FGFR-3 (fibroblast growth factor receptor 3), which has been found to contribute to disease progression.[226]

Table 1. World Health Organization (WHO) Classification of B-Cell Neoplasms

Precursor B-cell neoplasm
Precursor B lymphoblastic leukemia/lymphoma

Mature B-cell neoplasms
Chronic lymphocytic leukemia/small lymphocytic lymphoma
B-cell prolymphocytic leukemia
Lymphoplasmacytic lymphoma
Splenic marginal zone lymphoma
Hairy cell leukemia
Plasma cell myeloma
Solitary plasmacytoma of bone
Extraosseus plasmacytoma
Extranodal marginal zone B-cell lymphoma of mucosa-associated lymphoid tissue (MALT lymphoma)
Nodal marginal zone lymphoma
Follicular lymphoma
Mantle cell lymphoma
Diffuse large B-cell lymphoma
Mediastinal (thymic) large B-cell lymphoma
Intravascular large B-cell lymphoma
Primary effusion lymphoma
Burkitt lymphoma/leukemia

Table 2. B-Cell Differentiation: Immunophenotypic Profiles of Normal B Lymphoblasts

	Progenitor B	Pre-Pre-B	Pre-B
TdT	+	+	+
CD19	-	+	+
CD20	-	See below	+
CD22	-	Cytoplasmic	Cytoplasmic
CD79	See below	+	+
BSAP/PAX-5	+	+	+
CD10	-	+	+
HLA-DR	+	+	+
CD34	+	+	See below
Miscellaneous	May be cCD79a+	sCD20 in later stage	May be CD34+; cytoplasmic m+

* Modified from Chadburn A. and Narayanan S: Lymphoid malignancies: Immunophenotypic analysis. Adv Clin Chem 2003;37:293-353, with permission.

Table 3. Immunophenotype of Benign B-Cells*

	Naïve	Centroblast	Centrocyte	Memory	Plasma Cell
CD19	+	+	+	+	+
CD20	+	+	+	+	-
CD22	-	+	+	+	-
BSAP/ PAX-5	+	+	+	+	-
CD10	-	+	+	-	+
BCL2	+	-	-	+	+
BCL6	-	+	+	-	-
CD38	-	-	-	-	+
CD138	-	-	-	-	+
sIg	Usually MD	-	+	M, not D	-
cIg	-	-	-	-/+	+
Miscellaneous	Some CD5+	Ki67+, undergo IgH class switching			IgG>IgA; others rare

* Limited immunophenotypic profile
**Modified from Chadburn A. and Narayanan S: Lymphoid malignancies:
Immunophenotypic analysis. Adv Clin Chem 2003;37:293-353, with permission.

Table 4. Immunophenotypic Features B-Cell Neoplasms

Neoplasm	PAX-5	CD19	CD20	CD22	CD79a	CD5	CD10	CD11c	CD23	CD43	BCL1	BCL2	BCL6	FMC7	Other useful markers
Precursor B-lymphoblastic lymphoma/leukemia	+	+	-/+	+ (c or s)	+	-	+/-	-	-	+/-	-	+	-	*	TdT+; CD34+; sIg-
B-chronic lymphocytic leukemia /small lymphocytic lymphoma	+	+	wk+	wk+	+	+	-	+/-	+	+	-	+	-	-	Faint sIgM(D)+
Mantle cell lymphoma	+	+	+	+	+	+	-	-	-	+	+	+	-	+	Bright sIgMD+
Follicular lymphoma	+	+	+	+	+	-	+/-[1]	-	+/-	-	-	+/-[2]	+	+	CD21[3]
Marginal zone B-cell lymphoma (nodal, extranodal)	+	+	+	+	+	-/+	-	+/-	+/-	+/-	-	+	-	+	IgD-; cIg+ with plasma cell differentiation; CD214
Splenic marginal zone lymphoma	+	+	+	+	+	-	-	+/- +/-	+/- +/-	-	-	+	-	+	IgD+; cIg+ with plasma cell differentiation
Hairy cell leukemia	+	+	+	+	+	-	-	+	-	-	-/+	+	-	+	CD25+,CD103+, TRAP+, DBA.44+
Plasma cell myeloma	-	-	-/+	-	+(c)	-	-	-	-	+	-/+	+	-	*	CD138+, cIg + (usu. G or A), many CD56+
Diffuse large B-cell lymphoma	+	+	+	+	+	-/+ -/+	-/+	*	-/+ +/-	+/-	-	+/- -/+	-/+	*	
Burkitt lymphoma	+	+	+	+	+	-	+	*	+/-	+/-	-	-	+	*	Ki-67 ~100%

C: cytoplasmic; s: surface; *: Insufficient data; 1: about on third of the cases are negative; 2: higher grade follicular lymphomas tend to be negative; 3: CD21 staining highlights expanded follicular dendric cell meshworks with intact edges but disrupted centers; 4: CD21 staining highlights follicular dendric cell meshworks with disrupted edges

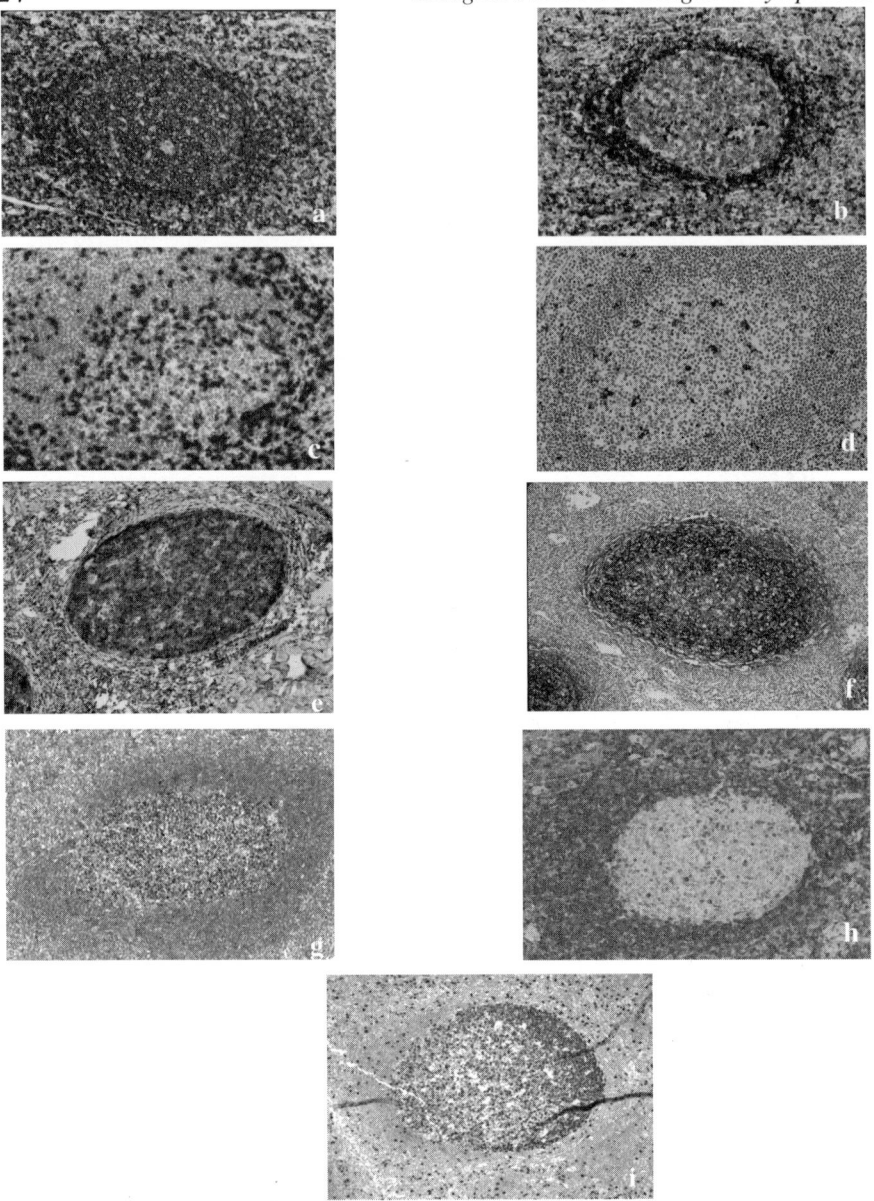

Figure 1. Immunophenotype and immunoarchitecture of a reactive follicle. a. CD20 (B cells), b. CD79a (B cells), c. CD2 (T cells), d. CD68 (macrophages), e. CD10 (follicle center B cells), f. CD21 (follicular dendritic cells), g. BCL6 (follicle center B cells and a subset of T cells), h. BCL2 (an anti-apoptotic protein not normally expressed by follicle center B cells), i. Ki67 (proliferation marker; immunoperoxidase, 64 x original magnification); a-h from Chadburn A and Narayanan S: Lymphoid malignancies: Immunophenotypic analysis. Adv Clin Chem 2003;37:293-353, with permission.

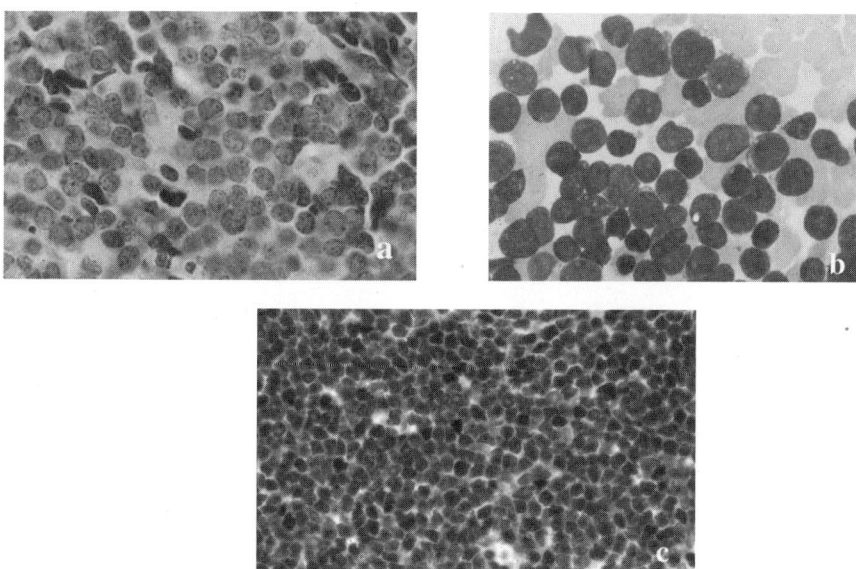

Figure 2. Precursor B-lymphoblastic leukemia/lymphoma (B-ALL/LBL). a. The blasts have finely dispersed chromatin, small nucleoli and a scant amount of cytoplasm. Scattered mitotic figures are present (hematoxylin and eosin 100x original magnification). b. In the peripheral blood blasts with finely dispersed chromatin and scant cytoplasm are seen; the white blood cell count is often elevated (Wright-Geimsa 100x original magnification). c. Immunostaining for TdT shows intranuclear positivity (immunoperoxidase 40x original magnification).

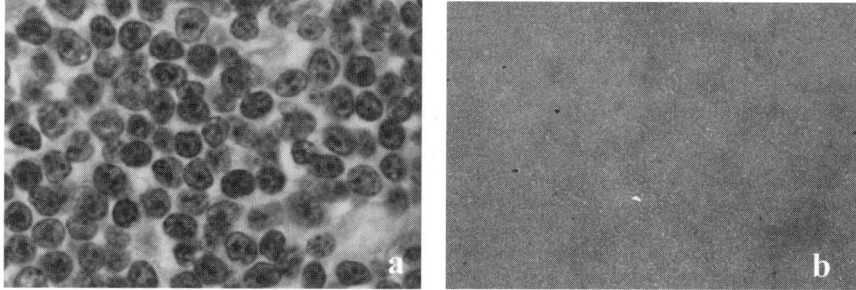

Figure 3. B-chronic lymphocytic leukemia/small lymphocytic lymphoma (B-CLL/SLL). a. The cells are small, with a round nucleus, clumped chromatin and only a small amount of cytoplasm (hematoxylin and eosin, 100x original magnification). b. CLL/SLL is a diffuse infiltrate, but often has a vaguely nodular appearance due to the presence of proliferations centers (hematoxylin and eosin, 2x original magnification).

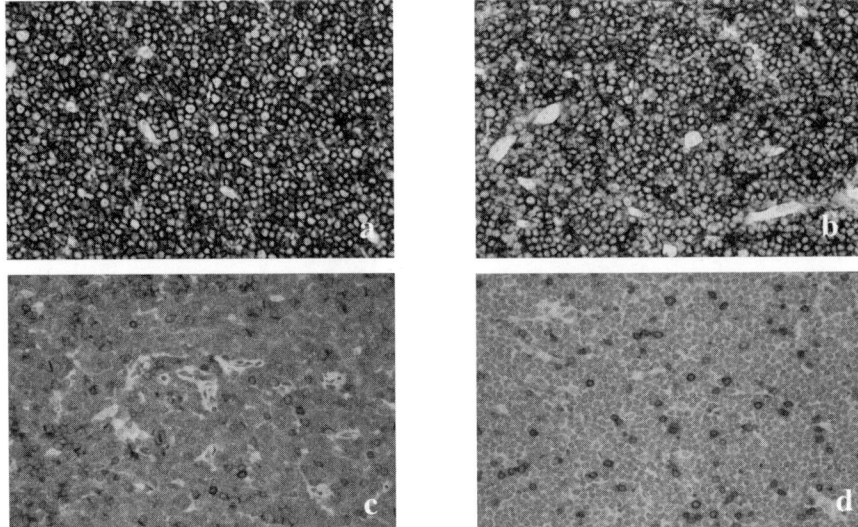

Figure 4. Immunophenotyping of B-chronic lymphocytic leukemia/small lymphocytic lymphoma (B-CLL/SLL) in formalin fixed paraffin embedded tissue sections: a. CD20, b. CD23, c. CD5, d. CD3 (immunoperoxidase 64x original magnification). Immunostaining shows that the tumor cells are CD20, CD23 and CD5 positive. Note that there are two populations of CD5 positive cells: the bright CD5 positive cells that correspond to the benign CD3 positive T cells, whereas the faint CD5 positive cells correspond to malignant B cells (from Chadburn A and Narayanan S: Lymphoid malignancies: Immunophenotypic analysis. Adv Clin Chem 2003;37:293-353, with permission).

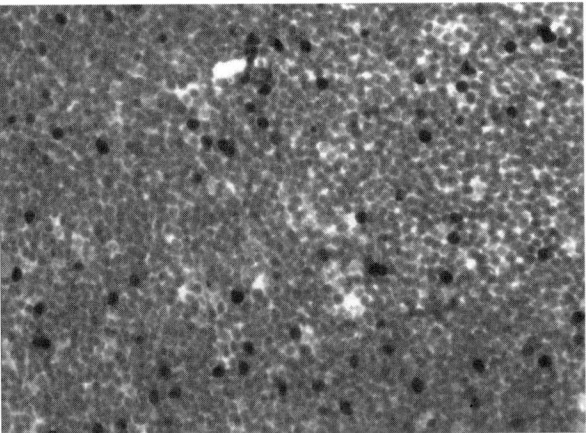

Figure 5. Immunostaining for the prognostic marker ZAP-70 shows two populations of cells in this case of B-CLL/SLL: the bright positive benign T cells and the faint positive malignant B cells. ZAP-70 expression in B-CLL/SLL correlates with the presence (ZAP-70 negative) or absence (ZAP-70 positive) somatic mutations in the variable region of the immunoglobulin gene (immunoperoxidase staining of a formalin fixed cell clot specimen 40x original magnification).

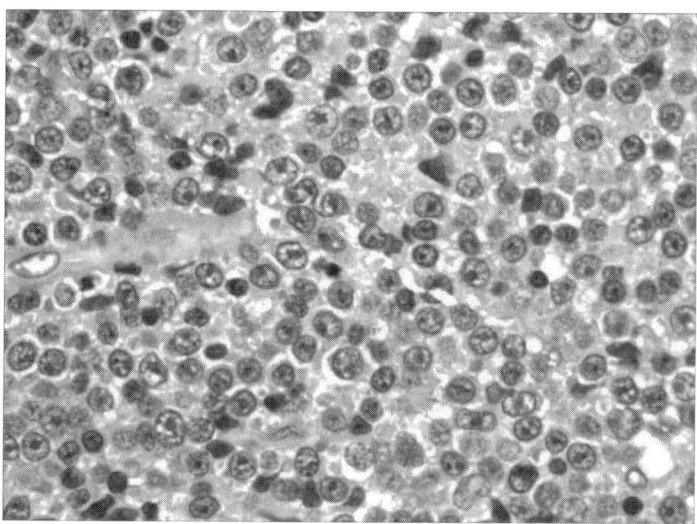

Figure 6. Transformation of B-CLL/SLL. Large cell transformation of B-CLL/SLL occurs in approximately 3-10% of cases. These tumor cells are larger than CLL/SLL cells and have prominent nucleoli (hematoxylin and eosin 40x original magnification).

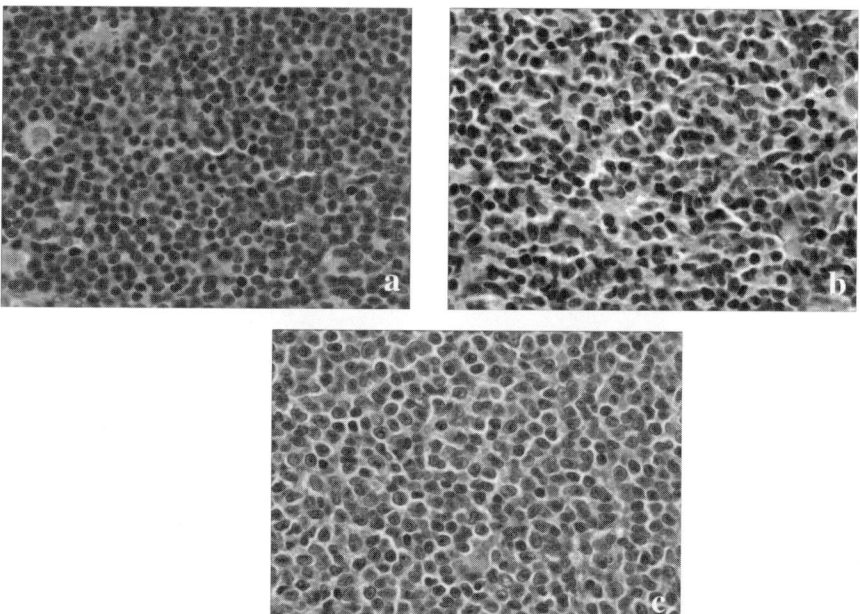

Figure 7. Mantle cell lymphoma: a-c. different cytologic appearances. Note the epitheliod histiocytes, best seen in "a" (hematoxylin and eosin, 40x original magnification).

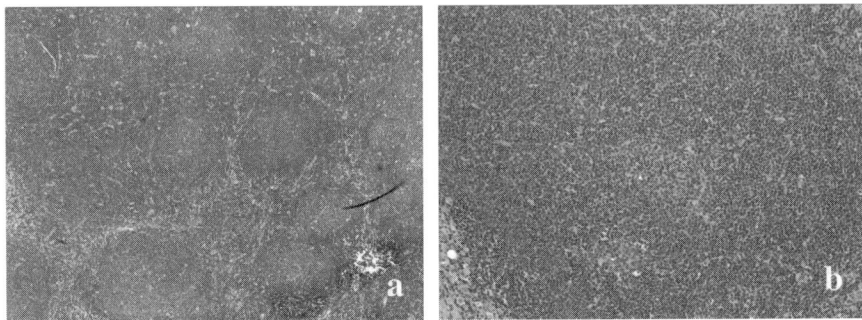

Figure 8. Mantle cell lymphoma can exhibit a diffuse, nodular (a) or mantle zone (b) pattern (hematoxylin and eosin; 4x and 10x original magnification).

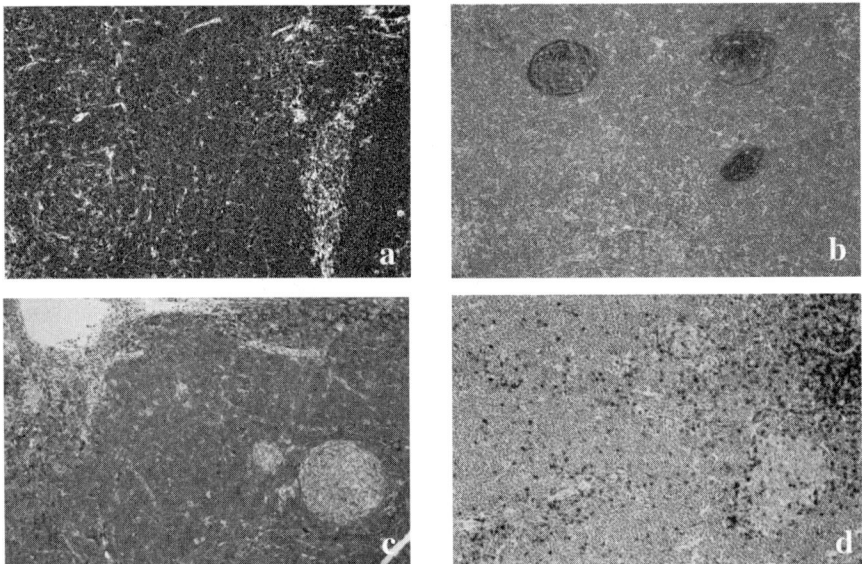

Figure 9. Immunophenotyping of mantle cell lymphoma in formalin fixed paraffin embedded tissue sections: a. CD20, b. CD23, c. CD5, d. CD3 (immunoperoxidase 20x original magnification). In contrast to B-CLL/SLL, mantle cell lymphoma cells are CD20, positive and CD5 positive, but lack expression of CD23. Immunostaining for CD23 highlights the uninvolved follicles, also seen as negative areas in the CD5 immunostained section (from Chadburn A and Narayanan S: Lymphoid malignancies: Immunophenotypic analysis. Adv Clin Chem 2003;37:293-353, with permission).

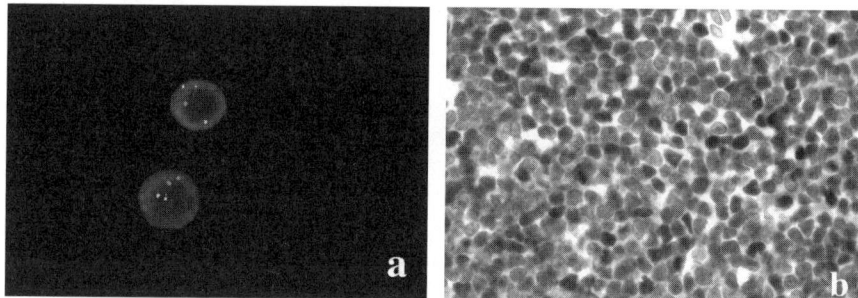

Figure 10. Mantle cell lymphoma: a. FISH analysis shows the presence of t(11;14) (yellow dots; immunofluorescent staining 100x original magnification). b. Immunostaining shows overexpression of cyclinD1 within the nucleus of the tumor cells (immunoperxoidase 40x original magnification).

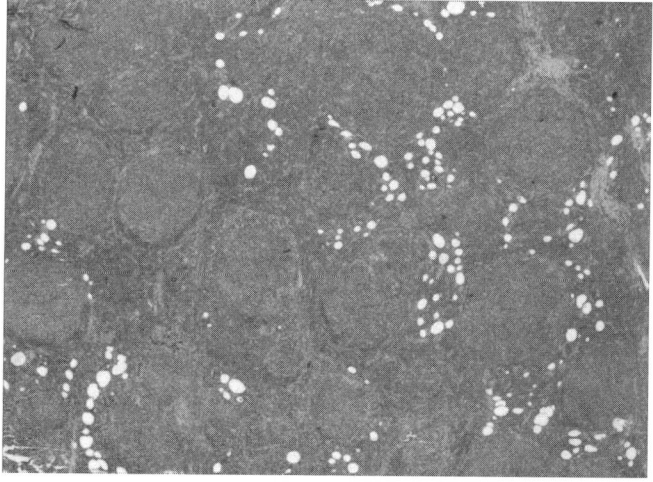

Figure 11. Typical cases of follicular lymphoma are characterized by a predominantly follicular growth pattern (hematoxylin and eosin 4x original magnification).

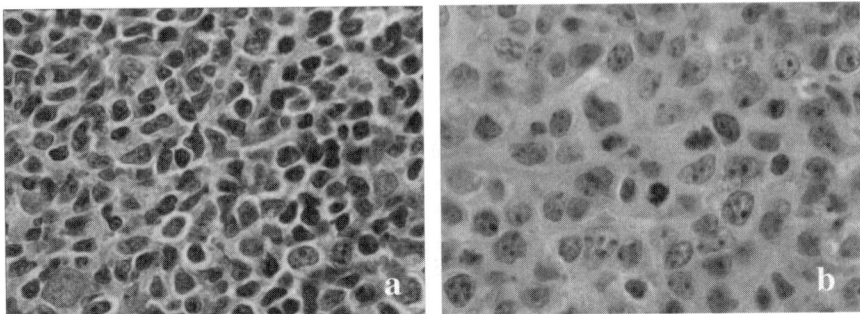

Figure 12. Follicular lymphoma: a. Centrocytes and b. centroblasts (hematoxylin and eosin 60x original magnification). The relative proportion of these cells determines the cytologic grade.

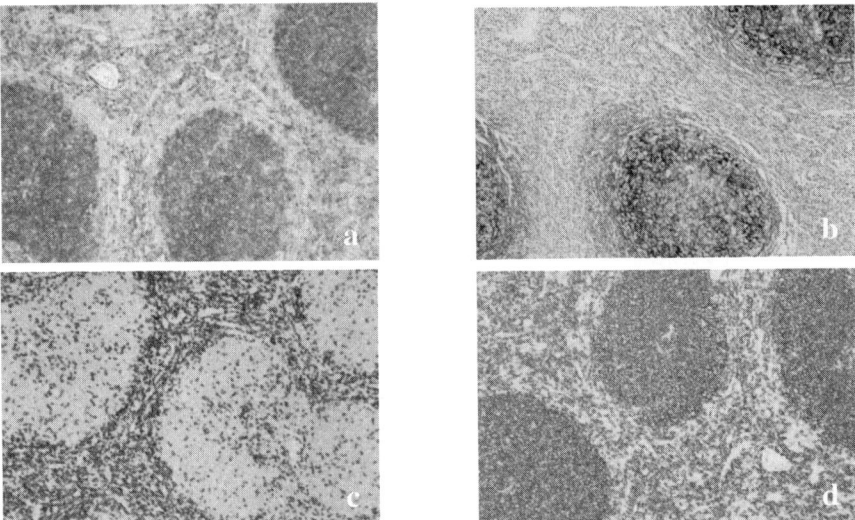

Figure 13. Immunophenotyping of follicular lymphoma in formalin fixed paraffin embedded tissue sections: a. CD10, b. CD21, c, CD3, d. BCL2. In this case the follicle center cells, as in normal follicles, are CD10 positive (a). Note that there are increased numbers of CD10 follicle center cells in the interfollicular area. The structure of the CD21 positive follicular dendritic cell meshwork (b) is intact at the edges. In contrast to reactive follicles where only scattered CD3 positive (c), BCL2 positive cells are present, both the CD3 positive T cells and the malignant follicle center cells are BCL2 positive (d). In reactive follicles the follicle center cells are BCL2 negative (immunoperoxidase 10x original magnification); from Chadburn A and Narayanan S: Lymphoid malignancies: Immunophenotypic analysis. Adv Clin Chem 2003;37:293-353, with permission).

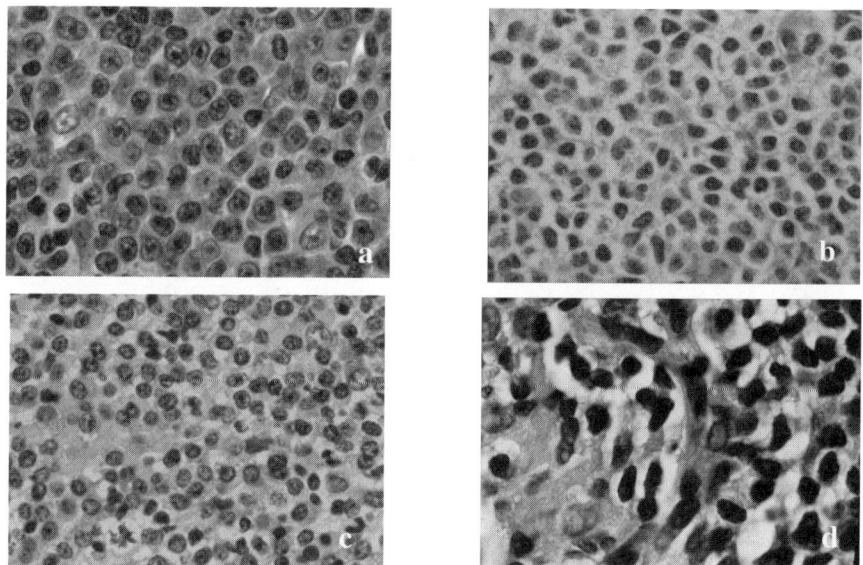

Figure 14. Marginal zone lymphoma: some of the different cytologic appearances (hematoxylin and eosin; a-c 60x and d 100x original magnification).

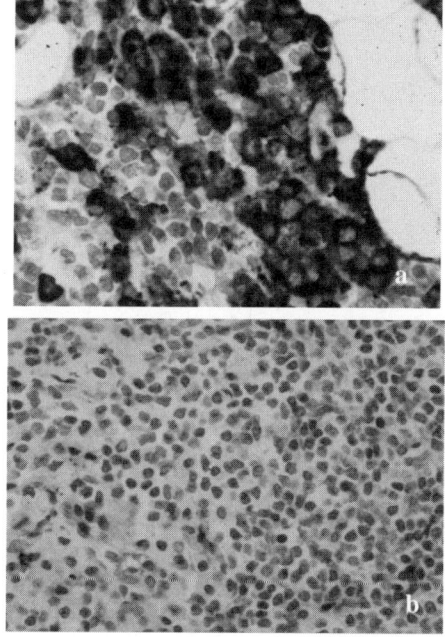

Figure 15. Marginal zone lymphoma: immunostaining for cytoplasmic kappa (a) and lambda (b). In cases with plasmacytic differentiation, the tumor cells may exhibit monotypic immunoglobulin expression within the cytoplasm (immunoperoxidase 20x original magnification).

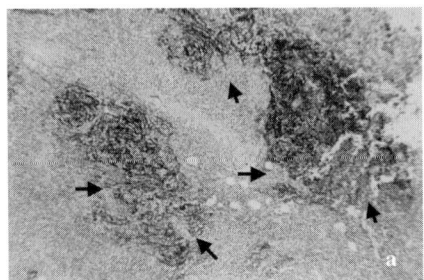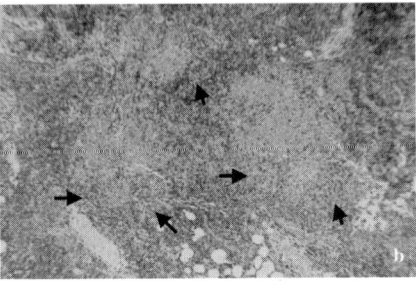

Figure 16. Marginal zone lymphoma. The immunoarchitectural features are often crucial in reaching the diagnosis. Immunostaining for CD21 (a) shows follicular dendritic cell meshworks with extensive fragmentation at the edges (arrows); (b) these areas of fragmentation are "broken-down" by infiltrating BCL2 positive neoplastic marginal zone cells (arrows; immunoperoxidase staining 4x original magnification).

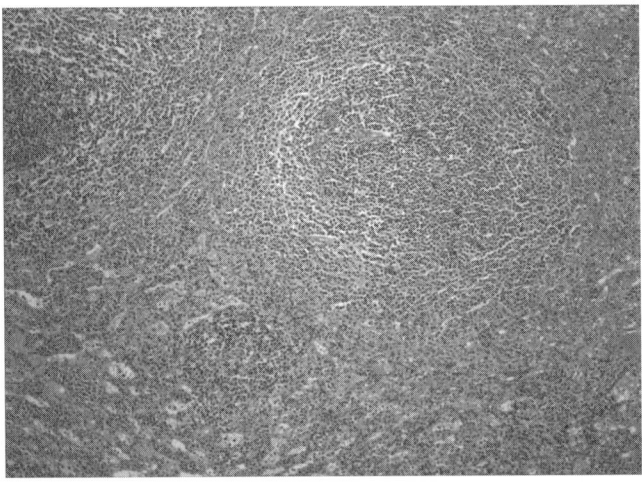

Figure 17. Splenic marginal zone lymphoma: The white pulp is prominent and clusters of malignant cells are seen in the red pulp (hematoxylin and eosin 4x original magnification).

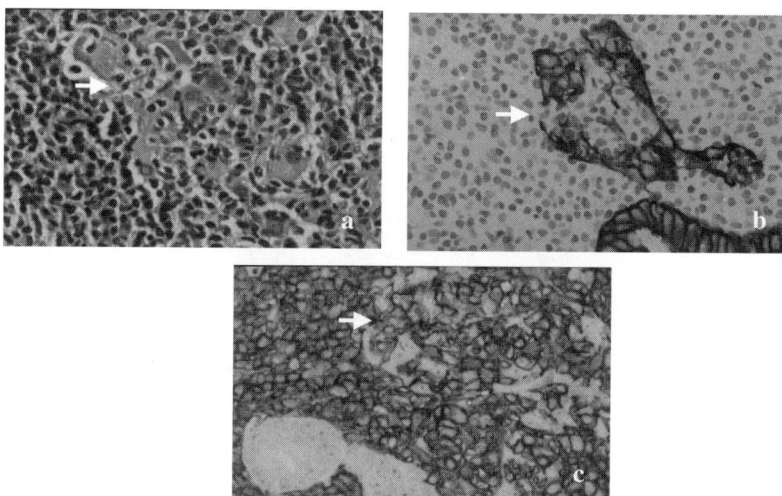

Figure 18. Extra-nodal marginal zone lymphoma of mucosa-associated lymphoid tissue (MALT lymphoma): The tumor cells extend in the epithelium (arrows) forming lymphoepithelial lesions (a; hematoxylin and eosin 60x original magnification) which are highlighted by immunostaining for cytokeratin (b) and CD20 (b, c immunoperoxidase 60x original magnification). From Chadburn A and Narayanan S: Lymphoid malignancies: Immunophenotypic analysis. Adv Clin Chem 2003;37:293-353, with permission.

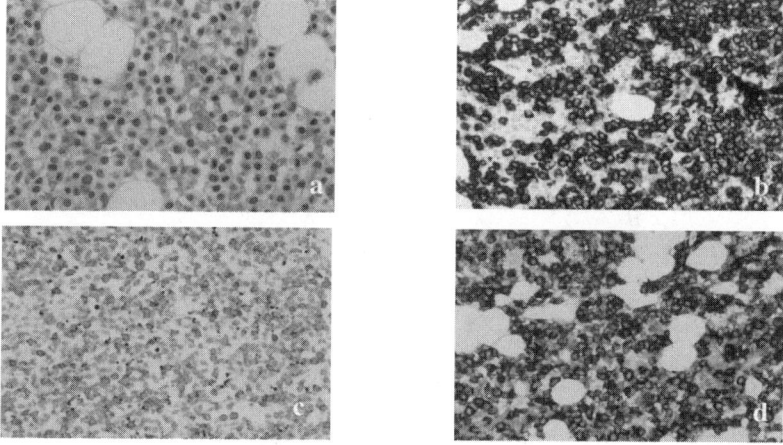

Figure 19. Hairy cell leukemia: The neoplastic cells are medium in size and have relatively abundant cytoplasm (a; hematoxylin and eosin 40x original magnification). As most patients with hairy cell leukemia have a "dry-tap" on bone marrow aspiration, immunostaining in paraffin tissue sections for CD20 (b), tartrate resistant acid phosphatase (TRAP, c) and CD25 (d) is helpful in identifying this malignant process (b-d immunoperoxidase 40x original magnification) (a-c from Chadburn A and Narayanan S: Lymphoid malignancies: Immunophenotypic analysis. Adv Clin Chem 2003;37:293-353, with permission).

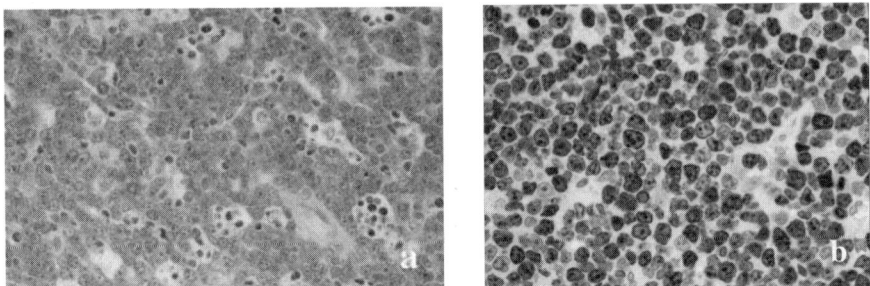

Figure 20. Burkitt lymphoma: The neoplastic cells are medium in size with round nuclei. They are associated with a large number of tingible body macrophages that impart a "starry-sky" appearance (a; hematoxylin and eosin 40x original magnification). Nearly all of the cells are positive for Ki-67, indicating the high proliferation rate (b; immunoperoxidase 60x original magnification).

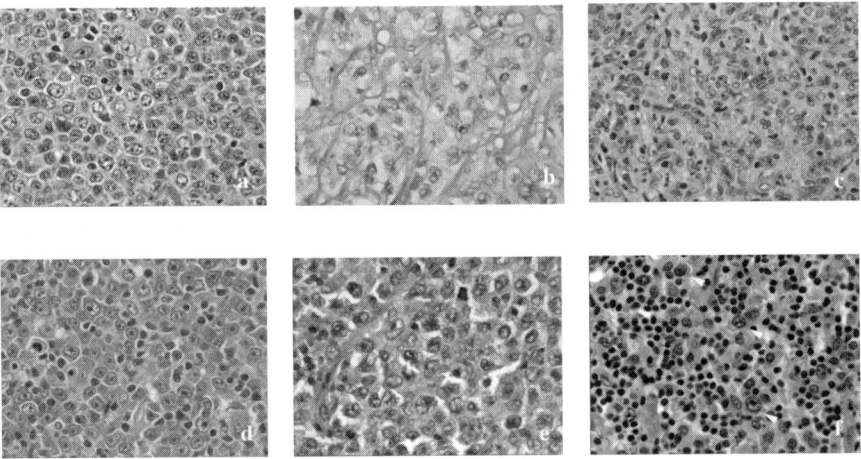

Figure 21. Diffuse large cell lymphoma: Diffuse large cell lymphoma is morphologically heterogeneous. Note in "f", a T cell rich diffuse large B cell lymphoma, the small number of scattered malignant cells is highlighted by the arrows (a-f; hematoxylin and eosin 40x original magnification).

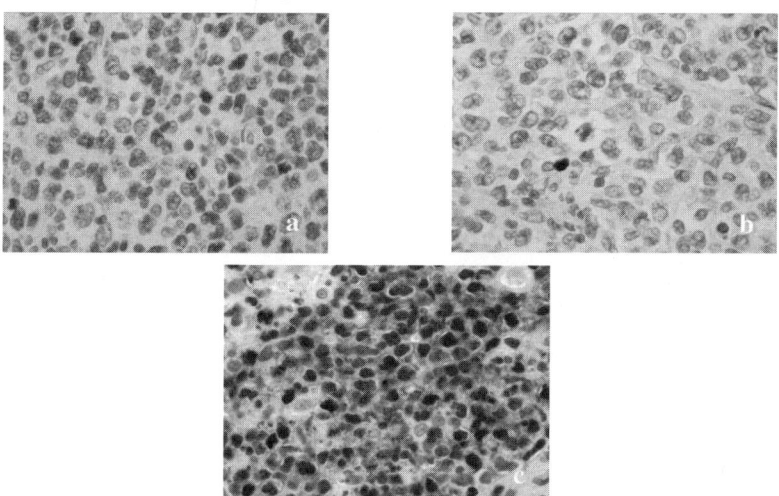

Figure 22. Prognostic markers in diffuse large cell lymphoma based on genetic microarray studies include the follicle center cell associated markers, BCL6 (a) and CD10 (b) and interferon regulatory factor-4 / multiple myeloma-1 (IFR4/MUM1; c). IFR4/MUM1 expression is associated with the activated B-cell phenotype (a-c; immunoperoxidase 40x original magnification).

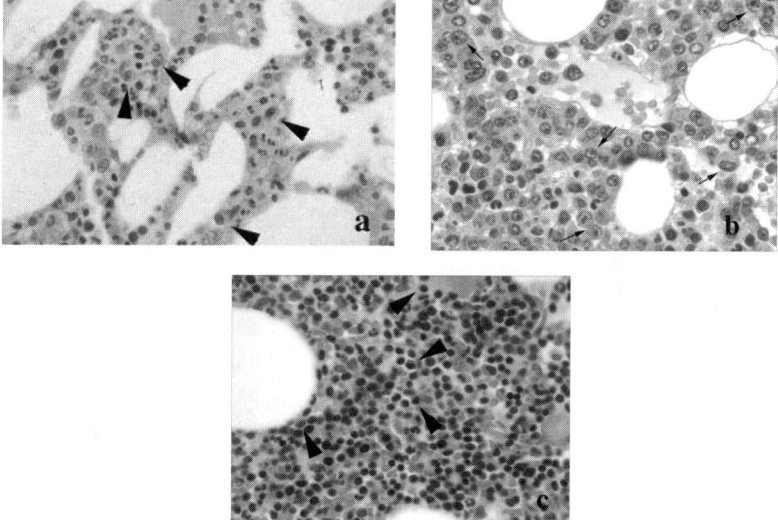

Figure 23. Multiple myeloma: The malignant plasma cells are morphologically variable ranging from those that are relatively normal in appearance (a; hematoxylin and eosin stained, Bouin's fixation, 40x original magnification) to those with more dispersed chromatin and nucleoli (b; hematoxylin and eosin stained, Bouin's fixation, 40x original magnification). With formalin fixation, the plasma cells may be difficult to distinguish from erythroid precursors (c; formalin fixation, 40x original magnification).

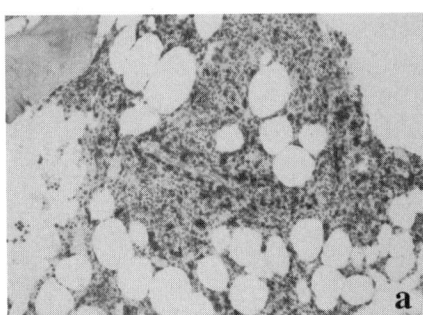
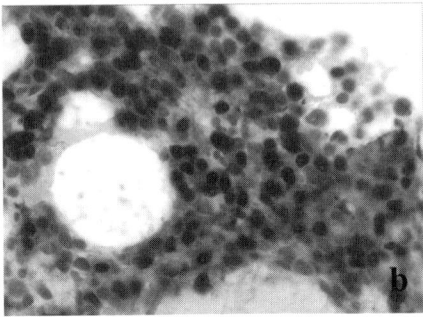

Figure 24. Multiple myeloma: CD20 expression is detected in 20% of cases of plasma cell myeloma (a; immunoperoxidase staining 20x original magnification) and are associated with t(11;14) and cyclinD1 expression (b; CD138 (red) and cyclinD1 (brown) double immunostaining; immunoalkaline phosphatase (red) and immunoperoxidase (brown), 40x original magnification).

11.   REFERENCES

1. Jaffe, E.S., Harris, N.L., Stein, H., Vardiman, J.W., (eds.)."World Health Organization Classification of Tumours. Pathology and Genetics of Tumours of Haematopoietic and Lymphoid Tissues." IARC Press, Lyon, 2001.

2. Harris NL, Jaffe ES, Stein H *et al*. A revised European-American classification of lymphoid neoplasms: a proposal from the International Lymphoma Study Group. *Blood.* 1994;84:1361-1392.

3. Gathings WE, Lawton AR, Cooper MD. Immunofluorescent studies of the development of pre-B cells, B lymphocytes and immunoglobulin isotype diversity in humans. *Eur J Immunol.* 1977;7:804-810.

4. Falini B, Mason DY. Proteins encoded by genes involved in chromosomal alterations in lymphoma and leukemia: clinical value of their detection by immunocytochemistry. *Blood.* 2002;99:409-426.

5. Torlakovic E, Torlakovic G, Nguyen PL *et al*. The value of anti-pax-5 immunostaining in routinely fixed and paraffin-embedded sections: a novel pan pre-B and B-cell marker. *Am J Surg Pathol.* 2002;26:1343-1350.

6. Korsmeyer SJ, Hieter PA, Ravetch JV *et al*. Developmental hierarchy of immunoglobulin gene rearrangements in human leukemic pre-B-cells. *Proc Natl Acad Sci U S A.* 1981;78:7096-7100.

7. Expression of cytoplasmic CD22 in B-cell ontogeny. *In* "Leukocyte Typing III: White Cell Differentiation Antigens."(McMichael A.J., Beverley P.C.L., Cobbold S. *et al.*, eds.)474-476. Oxford University Press, Oxford, 1987.

8. Anderson KC, Bates MP, Slaughenhoupt BL *et al*. Expression of human B cell-associated antigens on leukemias and lymphomas: a model of human B cell differentiation. *Blood*. 1984;63:1424-1433.

9. Foon KA, Todd RF, III. Immunologic classification of leukemia and lymphoma. *Blood*. 1986;68:1-31.

10. Nadler LM, Korsmeyer SJ, Anderson KC *et al*. B cell origin of non-T cell acute lymphoblastic leukemia. A model for discrete stages of neoplastic and normal pre-B cell differentiation. *J Clin Invest*. 1984;74:332-340.

11. Krenacs L, Himmelmann AW, Quintanilla-Martinez L *et al*. Transcription factor B-cell-specific activator protein (BSAP) is differentially expressed in B cells and in subsets of B-cell lymphomas. *Blood*. 1998;92:1308-1316.

12. Klein B, Tarte K, Jourdan M *et al*. Survival and proliferation factors of normal and malignant plasma cells. *Int J Hematol*. 2003;78:106-113.

13. Delves PJ, Roitt IM. The immune system. First of two parts. *N Engl J Med*. 2000;343:37-49.

14. Knowles DM. Immunophenotypic markers. *In* "Neoplastic Hematopathology."(Knowles D.M., ed.)93-226. Lippincott Williams & Wilkins, Philadelphia, 2001.

15. Mason DY, van Noesel CJ, Cordell JL *et al*. The B29 and mb-1 polypeptides are differentially expressed during human B cell differentiation. *Eur J Immunol*. 1992;22:2753-2756.

16. Kipps TJ. The CD5 B cell. *Adv Immunol*. 1989;47:117-185.

17. Inghirami G, Foitl DR, Sabichi A *et al*. Autoantibody-associated cross-reactive idiotype-bearing human B lymphocytes: distribution and characterization, including Ig VH gene and CD5 antigen expression. *Blood*. 1991;78:1503-1515.

18. MacLennan IC, Gulbranson-Judge A, Toellner KM *et al*. The changing preference of T and B cells for partners as T-dependent antibody responses develop. *Immunol Rev*. 1997;156:53-66.

19. Kraal G, Hardy RR, Gallatin WM *et al*. Antigen-induced changes in B cell subsets in lymph nodes: analysis by dual fluorescence flow cytofluorometry. *Eur J Immunol*. 1986;16:829-834.

20. Kraal G, Weissman IL, Butcher EC. Germinal centre B cells: antigen specificity and changes in heavy chain class expression. *Nature*. 1982;298:377-379.

21. Cattoretti G, Chang CC, Cechova K *et al*. BCL-6 protein is expressed in germinal-center B cells. *Blood*. 1995;86:45-53.

22. Hanna MG. An autoradiographic study of the germinal center in spleen white pulp during early intervals of the immune response. *Lab Invest*. 1964;13:95-104.

23. Liu YJ, Mason DY, Johnson GD *et al*. Germinal center cells express bcl-2 protein after activation by signals which prevent their entry into apoptosis. *Eur J Immunol*. 1991;21:1905-1910.

24. MacLennan IC. Germinal centers. *Annu Rev Immunol*. 1994;12:117-139.

25. Pittaluga S, Ayoubi TA, Wlodarska I *et al*. BCL-6 expression in reactive lymphoid tissue and in B-cell non-Hodgkin's lymphomas. *J Pathol*. 1996;179:145-150.

26. Liu YJ, Zhang J, Lane PJ *et al*. Sites of specific B cell activation in primary and secondary responses to T cell-dependent and T cell-independent antigens. *Eur J Immunol*. 1991;21:2951-2962.

27. Dogan A, Bagdi E, Munson P *et al*. CD10 and BCL-6 expression in paraffin sections of normal lymphoid tissue and B-cell lymphomas. *Am J Surg Pathol*. 2000;24:846-852.

28. Spencer J, Finn T, Pulford KA *et al*. The human gut contains a novel population of B lymphocytes which resemble marginal zone cells. *Clin Exp Immunol*. 1985;62:607-612.

29. van den Oord JJ, Wolf-Peeters C, Desmet VJ. The marginal zone in the human reactive lymph node. *Am J Clin Pathol*. 1986;86:475-479.

30. van Krieken JH, von Schilling C, Kluin PM *et al.* Splenic marginal zone lymphocytes and related cells in the lymph node: a morphologic and immunohistochemical study. *Hum Pathol.* 1989;20:320-325.

31. Barker HF, Hamilton MS, Ball J *et al.* Expression of adhesion molecules LFA-3 and N-CAM on normal and malignant human plasma cells. *Br J Haematol.* 1992;81:331-335.

32. Harada H, Kawano MM, Huang N *et al.* Phenotypic difference of normal plasma cells from mature myeloma cells. *Blood.* 1993;81:2658-2663.

33. Ridley RC, Xiao H, Hata H *et al.* Expression of syndecan regulates human myeloma plasma cell adhesion to type I collagen. *Blood.* 1993;81:767-774.

34. Brunning RD, Borowitz MJ, Matutes E et al. Precursor lymphoblastic leukaemia/lymphoblastic lymphoma (precursor B-cell acute lymphoblastic leukaemia). *In* "Pathology and Genetics of Tumours of Haematopoietic and Lymphoid Tissues."(Jaffe E.S., Harris N.L., Stein H. *et al.*, eds.)111-114. IARC Press, Lyon, 2001.

35. Knowles DM. Lymphoblastic lymphoma. *In* "Neoplastic Hematopathology."(Knowles D.M., ed.)915-951. Lippincott Williams & Wilkins, Philadelphia, 2001.

36. Ludwig WD, Rieder H, Bartram CR *et al.* Immunophenotypic and genotypic features, clinical characteristics, and treatment outcome of adult pro-B acute lymphoblastic leukemia: results of the German multicenter trials GMALL 03/87 and 04/89. *Blood.* 1998;92:1898-1909.

37. Johansson B, Moorman AV, Haas OA *et al.* Hematologic malignancies with t(4;11)(q21;q23)--a cytogenetic, morphologic, immunophenotypic and clinical study of 183 cases. European 11q23 Workshop participants. *Leukemia.* 1998;12:779-787.

38. Parkin JL, Arthur DC, Abramson CS *et al.* Acute leukemia associated with the t(4;11) chromosome rearrangement: ultrastructural and immunologic characteristics. *Blood.* 1982;60:1321-1331.

39. Schardt C, Ottmann OG, Hoelzer D *et al.* Acute lymphoblastic leukemia with the (4;11) translocation: combined cytogenetic, immunological and molecular genetic analyses. *Leukemia.* 1992;6:370-374.

40. Ludwig WD, Bartram CR, Harbott J *et al.* Phenotypic and genotypic heterogeneity in infant acute leukemia. I. Acute lymphoblastic leukemia. *Leukemia.* 1989;3:431-439.

41. Acute Lymphoblastic Lymphoma *In* "Bone Marrow Pathology"(Foucar K., ed.)485-514. ASCP Press, Chicago, 2001.

42. Faderl S, Kantarjian HM, Talpaz M *et al.* Clinical significance of cytogenetic abnormalities in adult acute lymphoblastic leukemia. *Blood.* 1998;91:3995-4019.

43. Crist WM, Carroll AJ, Shuster JJ *et al.* Poor prognosis of children with pre-B acute lymphoblastic leukemia is associated with the t(1;19)(q23;p13): a Pediatric Oncology Group study. *Blood.* 1990;76:117-122.

44. Lampert F, Harbott J, Ritterbach J *et al.* Karyotypes in acute childhood leukemias may lose prognostic significance with more intensive and specific chemotherapy. *Cancer Genet Cytogenet.* 1991;54:277-279.

45. Vasef MA, Brynes RK, Murata-Collins JL *et al.* Surface immunoglobulin light chain-positive acute lymphoblastic leukemia of FAB L1 or L2 type: a report of 6 cases in adults. *Am J Clin Pathol.* 1998;110:143-149.

46. Li S, Lew G. Is B-lineage acute lymphoblastic leukemia with a mature phenotype and l1 morphology a precursor B-lymphoblastic leukemia/lymphoma or Burkitt leukemia/lymphoma? *Arch Pathol Lab Med.* 2003;127:1340-1344.

47. Talmant P, Berger R, Robillard N *et al.* Childhood B-cell acute lymphoblastic leukemia with FAB-L1 morphology and a t(9;11) translocation involving the MLL gene. *Hematol Cell Ther.* 1996;38:265-268.

48. Tsao L, Draoua HY, Osunkwo I *et al.* Mature B-cell acute lymphoblastic leukemia with t(9;11) translocation: a distinct subset of B-cell acute lymphoblastic leukemia. *Mod Pathol.* 2004;17:832-839.

49. Alessandri AJ, Reid GS, Bader SA *et al.* ETV6 (TEL)-AML1 pre-B acute lymphoblastic leukaemia cells are associated with a distinct antigen-presenting phenotype. *Br J Haematol.* 2002;116:266-272.

50. Rubnitz JE, Camitta BM, Mahmoud H *et al.* Childhood acute lymphoblastic leukemia with the MLL-ENL fusion and t(11;19)(q23;p13.3) translocation. *J Clin Oncol.* 1999;17:191-196.

51. De Zen L, Orfao A, Cazzaniga G *et al.* Quantitative multiparametric immunophenotyping in acute lymphoblastic leukemia: correlation with specific genotype. I. ETV6/AML1 ALLs identification. *Leukemia.* 2000;14:1225-1231.

52. Harris NL. Mature B-cell neoplasms: Introduction. *In* "World Health Organization Classification of Tumours. Pathology and Genetics of Tumours of Haematopoietic and Lymphoid Tissues."(Jaffe E.S., Harris N.L., Stein H. *et al.*, eds.) IARC Press, Lyon, 2001.

53. Harris NL, Jaffe ES, Diebold J *et al.* World Health Organization classification of neoplastic diseases of the hematopoietic and lymphoid tissues: report of the Clinical Advisory Committee meeting-Airlie House, Virginia, November 1997. *J Clin Oncol.* 1999;17:3835-3849.

54. Harris NL, Jaffe ES, Stein H *et al.* A revised European-American classification of lymphoid neoplasms: a proposal from the International Lymphoma Study Group [see comments]. *Blood.* 1994;84:1361-1392.

55. Alizadeh AA, Eisen MB, Davis RE *et al.* Distinct types of diffuse large B-cell lymphoma identified by gene expression profiling. *Nature.* 2000;403:503-511.

56. Muller-Hermelink HK, Catovsky D, Monrserrat E et al. Chronic lymphocytic leukaemia/small lymphocytic lymphoma. *In* "Pathology and Genetics of Tumours of Haematopoietic and Lymphoid Tissues."(Jaffe E.S., Harris N.L., Stein H. *et al.*, eds.)127-130. IARC Press, Lyon, 2001.

57. Rozman C, Hernandez-Nieto L, Montserrat E *et al.* Prognostic significance of bone-marrow patterns in chronic lymphocytic leukaemia. *Br J Haematol.* 1981;47:529-537.

58. Geisler C, Ralfkiaer E, Hansen MM *et al.* The bone marrow histological pattern has independent prognostic value in early stage chronic lymphocytic leukaemia. *Br J Haematol.* 1986;62:47-54.

59. Matutes E, Oscier D, Garcia-Marco J *et al.* Trisomy 12 defines a group of CLL with atypical morphology: correlation between cytogenetic, clinical and laboratory features in 544 patients. *Br J Haematol.* 1996;92:382-388.

60. Foucar K. Chronic lymphoid leukemias and lymphoproliferative disorders. *Mod Pathol.* 1999;12:141-150.

61. Matutes E, Polliack A. Morphological and immunophenotypic features of chronic lymphocytic leukemia. *Rev Clin Exp Hematol.* 2000;4:22-47.

62. MacLennan IC, Liu YJ, Oldfield S *et al.* The evolution of B-cell clones. *Curr Top Microbiol Immunol.* 1990;159:37-63.

63. Klein U, Tu Y, Stolovitzky GA *et al.* Gene expression profiling of B cell chronic lymphocytic leukemia reveals a homogeneous phenotype related to memory B cells. *J Exp Med.* 2001;194:1625-1638.

64. Hamblin TJ, Davis Z, Gardiner A *et al.* Unmutated Ig V(H) genes are associated with a more aggressive form of chronic lymphocytic leukemia. *Blood.* 1999;94:1848-1854.

65. Crespo M, Bosch F, Villamor N *et al.* ZAP-70 expression as a surrogate for immunoglobulin-variable-region mutations in chronic lymphocytic leukemia. *N Engl J Med.* 2003;348:1764-1775.

66. Damle RN, Wasil T, Fais F *et al.* Ig V gene mutation status and CD38 expression as novel prognostic indicators in chronic lymphocytic leukemia. *Blood.* 1999;94:1840-1847.

67. Wiestner A, Rosenwald A, Barry TS *et al.* ZAP-70 expression identifies a chronic lymphocytic leukemia subtype with unmutated immunoglobulin genes, inferior clinical outcome, and distinct gene expression profile. *Blood.* 2003;101:4944-4951.

68. Hamblin TJ, Orchard JA, Ibbotson RE *et al.* CD38 expression and immunoglobulin variable region mutations are independent prognostic variables in chronic lymphocytic leukemia, but CD38 expression may vary during the course of the disease. *Blood.* 2002;99:1023-1029.

69. Thunberg U, Johnson A, Roos G *et al.* CD38 expression is a poor predictor for VH gene mutational status and prognosis in chronic lymphocytic leukemia. *Blood.* 2001;97:1892-1894.

70. Durig J, Nuckel H, Cremer M *et al.* ZAP-70 expression is a prognostic factor in chronic lymphocytic leukemia. *Leukemia.* 2003;17:2426-2434.

71. Del Poeta G, Maurillo L, Venditti A *et al.* Clinical significance of CD38 expression in chronic lymphocytic leukemia. *Blood.* 2001;98:2633-2639.

72. Orchard JA, Ibbotson RE, Davis Z *et al.* ZAP-70 expression and prognosis in chronic lymphocytic leukaemia. *Lancet.* 2004;363:105-111.

73. de Melo N, Matutes E, Cordone I *et al.* Expression of Ki-67 nuclear antigen in B and T cell lymphoproliferative disorders. *J Clin Pathol.* 1992;45:660-663.

74. Astsaturov IA, Samoilova RS, Iakhnina EI *et al.* The relevance of cytological studies and Ki-67 reactivity to the clinical course of chronic lymphocytic leukemia. *Leuk Lymphoma.* 1997;26:337-342.

75. Cordone I, Masi S, Mauro FR *et al.* p53 expression in B-cell chronic lymphocytic leukemia: a marker of disease progression and poor prognosis. *Blood.* 1998;91:4342-4349.

76. Foucar K. B-cell chronic lymphocytic and prolymphocytic leukemia. *In* "Neoplastic Hematopathology."(Knowles D.M., ed.)1505-1529. Lippincott Williams & Wilkins, Philadelphia, 2001.

77. Swerdlow SH, Berger F, Isaacson PG et al. Mantle cell lymphoma. *In* "Pathology and Genetics of Tumours of Haematopoietic and Lymphoid Tissues."(Jaffe E.S., Harris N.L., Stein H. *et al.*, eds.)168-170. IARC Press, Lyon, 2001.

78. Gu J, Huh YO, Jiang F *et al.* Evaluation of peripheral blood involvement of mantle cell lymphoma by fluorescence in situ hybridization in comparison with immunophenotypic and morphologic findings. *Mod Pathol.* 2004;17:553-560.

79. Dorfman DM, Pinkus GS. Distinction between small lymphocytic and mantle cell lymphoma by immunoreactivity for CD23. *Mod Pathol.* 1994;7:326-331.

80. Kilo MN, Dorfman DM. The utility of flow cytometric immunophenotypic analysis in the distinction of small lymphocytic lymphoma/chronic lymphocytic leukemia from mantle cell lymphoma. *Am J Clin Pathol.* 1996;105:451-457.

81. Xu Y, McKenna RW, Kroft SH. Assessment of CD10 in the diagnosis of small B-cell lymphomas: a multiparameter flow cytometric study. *Am J Clin Pathol.* 2002;117:291-300.

82. Zukerberg LR, Medeiros LJ, Ferry JA *et al.* Diffuse low-grade B-cell lymphomas. Four clinically distinct subtypes defined by a combination of morphologic and immunophenotypic features. *Am J Clin Pathol.* 1993;100:373-385.

83. Falini B, Fizzotti M, Pileri S *et al.* Bcl-6 protein expression in normal and neoplastic lymphoid tissues. *Ann Oncol.* 1997;8 Suppl 2:101-104.

84. Raible MD, Hsi ED, Alkan S. Bcl-6 protein expression by follicle center lymphomas. A marker for differentiating follicle center lymphomas from other low-grade lymphoproliferative disorders. *Am J Clin Pathol.* 1999;112:101-107.

85. Lai R, Weiss LM, Chang KL *et al.* Frequency of CD43 expression in non-Hodgkin lymphoma. A survey of 742 cases and further characterization of rare CD43+ follicular lymphomas. *Am J Clin Pathol.* 1999;111:488-494.

86. Swerdlow SH. Small B-cell lymphomas of the lymph nodes and spleen: practical insights to diagnosis and pathogenesis. *Mod Pathol.* 1999;12:125-140.

87. de Boer CJ, Schuuring E, Dreef E *et al.* Cyclin D1 protein analysis in the diagnosis of mantle cell lymphoma. *Blood.* 1995;86:2715-2723.

88. Swerdlow SH, Yang WI, Zukerberg LR *et al.* Expression of cyclin D1 protein in centrocytic/mantle cell lymphomas with and without rearrangement of the BCL1/cyclin D1 gene. *Hum Pathol.* 1995;26:999-1004.

89. Zukerberg LR, Yang WI, Arnold A *et al.* Cyclin D1 expression in non-Hodgkin's lymphomas. Detection by immunohistochemistry. *Am J Clin Pathol.* 1995;103:756-760.

90. de Boer CJ, Kluin-Nelemans JC, Dreef E *et al.* Involvement of the CCND1 gene in hairy cell leukemia. *Ann Oncol.* 1996;7:251-256.

91. Bosch F, Campo E, Jares P *et al.* Increased expression of the PRAD-1/CCND1 gene in hairy cell leukaemia. *Br J Haematol.* 1995;91:1025-1030.

92. Pruneri G, Fabris S, Baldini L *et al.* Immunohistochemical analysis of cyclin D1 shows deregulated expression in multiple myeloma with the t(11;14). *Am J Pathol.* 2000;156:1505-1513.

93. Hernandez L, Fest T, Cazorla M *et al.* p53 gene mutations and protein overexpression are associated with aggressive variants of mantle cell lymphomas. *Blood.* 1996;87:3351-3359.

94. Pinyol M, Hernandez L, Cazorla M *et al.* Deletions and loss of expression of p16INK4a and p21Waf1 genes are associated with aggressive variants of mantle cell lymphomas. *Blood.* 1997;89:272-280.

95. Williams ME, Whitefield M, Swerdlow SH. Analysis of the cyclin-dependent kinase inhibitors p18 and p19 in mantle-cell lymphoma and chronic lymphocytic leukemia. *Ann Oncol.* 1997;8 Suppl 2:71-73.

96. Argatoff LH, Connors JM, Klasa RJ *et al.* Mantle cell lymphoma: a clinicopathologic study of 80 cases. *Blood.* 1997;89:2067-2078.

97. Swerdlow SH, Habeshaw JA, Murray LJ *et al.* Centrocytic lymphoma: a distinct clinicopathologic and immunologic entity. A multiparameter study of 18 cases at diagnosis and relapse. *Am J Pathol.* 1983;113:181-197.

98. Ott G, Kalla J, Hanke A *et al.* The cytomorphological spectrum of mantle cell lymphoma is reflected by distinct biological features. *Leuk Lymphoma.* 1998;32:55-63.

99. The Non-Hodgkin's Lymphoma Classification Project. A Clinical Evaluation of the International Lymphoma Study Group Classification of Non-Hodgkin's Lymphoma. *Blood.* 1997;89:3909-3918.

100. Horning SJ, Rosenberg SA. The natural history of initially untreated low-grade non-Hodgkin's lymphomas. *N Engl J Med.* 1984;311:1471-1475.

101. Gallagher CJ, Gregory WM, Jones AE *et al.* Follicular lymphoma: prognostic factors for response and survival. *J Clin Oncol.* 1986;4:1470-1480.

102. Ngan B, Warnke A, Cleary ML. Variability of immunoglobulin expression in follicular lymphoma. An immunohistologic and molecular genetic study. *Am J Pathol.* 1989;135:1139-1144.

103. Kaufmann O, Flath B, Spath-Schwalbe E *et al.* Immunohistochemical detection of CD10 with monoclonal antibody 56C6 on paraffin sections. *Am J Clin Pathol.* 1999;111:117-122.

104. de Leon ED, Alkan S, Huang JC *et al.* Usefulness of an immunohistochemical panel in paraffin-embedded tissues for the differentiation of B-cell non-Hodgkin's lymphomas of small lymphocytes. *Mod Pathol.* 1998;11:1046-1051.

105. Dorfman DM, Shahsafaei A. Usefulness of a new CD5 antibody for the diagnosis of T-cell and B-cell lymphoproliferative disorders in paraffin sections. *Mod Pathol.* 1997;10:859-863.

106. Scoazec JY, Berger F, Magaud JP *et al.* The dendritic reticulum cell pattern in B cell lymphomas of the small cleaved, mixed, and large cell types: an immunohistochemical study of 48 cases. *Hum Pathol.* 1989;20:124-131.

107. de Leval L, Harris NL, Longtine J *et al.* Cutaneous b-cell lymphomas of follicular and marginal zone types: use of Bcl-6, CD10, Bcl-2, and CD21 in differential diagnosis and classification. *Am J Surg Pathol.* 2001;25:732-741.

108. Lai R, Arber DA, Chang KL *et al.* Frequency of bcl-2 expression in non-Hodgkin's lymphoma: a study of 778 cases with comparison of marginal zone lymphoma and monocytoid B-cell hyperplasia. *Mod Pathol.* 1998;11:864-869.

109. Horsman DE, Gascoyne RD, Coupland RW *et al.* Comparison of cytogenetic analysis, southern analysis, and polymerase chain reaction for the detection of t(14; 18) in follicular lymphoma. *Am J Clin Pathol.* 1995;103:472-478.

110. Knutsen T. Cytogenetic mechanisms in the pathogenesis and progression of follicular lymphoma. *Cancer Surv.* 1997;30:163-192.

111. Horsman DE, Okamoto I, Ludkovski O *et al.* Follicular lymphoma lacking the t(14;18)(q32;q21): identification of two disease subtypes. *Br J Haematol.* 2003;120:424-433.

112. Bergman R, Kurtin PJ, Gibson LE *et al.* Clinicopathologic, immunophenotypic, and molecular characterization of primary cutaneous follicular B-cell lymphoma. *Arch Dermatol.* 2001;137:432-439.

113. Yang B, Tubbs RR, Finn W *et al.* Clinicopathologic reassessment of primary cutaneous B-cell lymphomas with immunophenotypic and molecular genetic characterization. *Am J Surg Pathol.* 2000;24:694-702.

114. Maes B, Wolf-Peeters C. Marginal zone cell lymphoma--an update on recent advances. *Histopathology.* 2002;40:117-126.

115. Ortiz-Hidalgo C, Wright DH. The morphological spectrum of monocytoid B-cell lymphoma and its relationship to lymphomas of mucosa-associated lymphoid tissue. *Histopathology.* 1992;21:555-561.

116. Nizze H, Cogliatti SB, von Schilling C *et al.* Monocytoid B-cell lymphoma: morphological variants and relationship to low-grade B-cell lymphoma of the mucosa-associated lymphoid tissue. *Histopathology.* 1991;18:403-414.

117. Garcia DP, Rooney MT, Ahmad E *et al.* Diagnostic usefulness of CD23 and FMC-7 antigen expression patterns in B-cell lymphoma classification. *Am J Clin Pathol.* 2001;115:258-265.

118. Kurtin PJ, Hobday KS, Ziesmer S *et al.* Demonstration of distinct antigenic profiles of small B-cell lymphomas by paraffin section immunohistochemistry. *Am J Clin Pathol.* 1999;112:319-329.

119. Flenghi L, Bigerna B, Fizzotti M *et al.* Monoclonal antibodies PG-B6a and PG-B6p recognize, respectively, a highly conserved and a formol-resistant epitope on the human BCL-6 protein amino-terminal region. *Am J Pathol.* 1996;148:1543-1555.

120. Armitage JO, Weisenburger DD. New approach to classifying non-Hodgkin's lymphomas: clinical features of the major histologic subtypes. Non-Hodgkin's Lymphoma Classification Project. *J Clin Oncol.* 1998;16:2780-2795.

121. Hammer RD, Glick AD, Greer JP *et al.* Splenic marginal zone lymphoma. A distinct B-cell neoplasm. *Am J Surg Pathol.* 1996;20:613-626.

122. Isaacson PG, Piris MA, Catovksy D et al. Splenic marginal zone lymphoma. *In* "Pathology and Genetics of Tumours of Haematopoietic and Lymphoid Tissues."(Jaffe E.S., Harris N.L., Stein H. *et al.*, eds.)135-137. IARC Press, Lyon, 2001.

123. Campo E, Miquel R, Krenacs L *et al.* Primary nodal marginal zone lymphomas of splenic and MALT type. *Am J Surg Pathol.* 1999;23:59-68.

124. Isaacson PG, Matutes E, Burke M *et al*. The histopathology of splenic lymphoma with villous lymphocytes. *Blood*. 1994;84:3828-3834.

125. Matutes E, Morilla R, Owusu-Ankomah K *et al*. The immunophenotype of splenic lymphoma with villous lymphocytes and its relevance to the differential diagnosis with other B-cell disorders. *Blood*. 1994;83:1558-1562.

126. Mollejo M, Lloret E, Menarguez J *et al*. Lymph node involvement by splenic marginal zone lymphoma: morphological and immunohistochemical features. *Am J Surg Pathol*. 1997;21:772-780.

127. Matutes E, Morilla R, Owusu-Ankomah K *et al*. The immunophenotype of hairy cell leukemia (HCL). Proposal for a scoring system to distinguish HCL from B-cell disorders with hairy or villous lymphocytes. *Leuk Lymphoma*. 1994;14 Suppl 1:57-61.

128. Camacho FI, Mollejo M, Mateo MS *et al*. Progression to large B-cell lymphoma in splenic marginal zone lymphoma: a description of a series of 12 cases. *Am J Surg Pathol*. 2001;25:1268-1276.

129. Gruszka-Westwood AM, Hamoudi RA, Matutes E *et al*. p53 abnormalities in splenic lymphoma with villous lymphocytes. *Blood*. 2001;97:3552-3558.

130. Sheibani K, Sohn CC, Burke JS *et al*. Monocytoid B-cell lymphoma. A novel B-cell neoplasm. *Am J Pathol*. 1986;124:310-318.

131. Piris MA, Rivas C, Morente M *et al*. Monocytoid B-cell lymphoma, a tumour related to the marginal zone. *Histopathology*. 1988;12:383-392.

132. Cousar JB, McGinn DL, Glick AD *et al*. Report of an unusual lymphoma arising from parafollicular B-lymphocytes (PBLs) or so-called "monocytoid" lymphocytes. *Am J Clin Pathol*. 1987;87:121-128.

133. Doglioni C, Wotherspoon AC, Moschini A *et al*. High incidence of primary gastric lymphoma in northeastern Italy. *Lancet*. 1992;339:834-835.

134. Radaszkiewicz T, Dragosics B, Bauer P. Gastrointestinal malignant lymphomas of the mucosa-associated lymphoid tissue: factors relevant to prognosis. *Gastroenterology*. 1992;102:1628-1638.

135. White WL, Ferry JA, Harris NL *et al*. Ocular adnexal lymphoma. A clinicopathologic study with identification of lymphomas of mucosa-associated lymphoid tissue type. *Ophthalmology*. 1995;102:1994-2006.

136. Hsi ED, Zukerberg LR, Schnitzer B *et al*. Development of extrasalivary gland lymphoma in myoepithelial sialadenitis. *Mod Pathol*. 1995;8:817-824.

137. Bailey EM, Ferry JA, Harris NL *et al*. Marginal zone lymphoma (low-grade B-cell lymphoma of mucosa-associated lymphoid tissue type) of skin and subcutaneous tissue: a study of 15 patients. *Am J Surg Pathol*. 1996;20:1011-1023.

138. Eidt S, Stolte M, Fischer R. Helicobacter pylori gastritis and primary gastric non-Hodgkin's lymphomas. *J Clin Pathol*. 1994;47:436-439.

139. Wotherspoon AC, Ortiz-Hidalgo C, Falzon MR *et al*. Helicobacter pylori-associated gastritis and primary B-cell gastric lymphoma. *Lancet*. 1991;338:1175-1176.

140. Ferreri AJM, Guidoboni M, Ponzoni M *et al*. Evidence for an Association Between Chlamydia psittaci and Ocular Adnexal Lymphomas. *J Natl Cancer Inst*. 2004;96:586-594.

141. Royer B, Cazals-Hatem D, Sibilia J *et al*. Lymphomas in patients with Sjogren's syndrome are marginal zone B-cell neoplasms, arise in diverse extranodal and nodal sites, and are not associated with viruses. *Blood*. 1997;90:766-775.

142. Kassan SS, Thomas TL, Moutsopoulos HM *et al*. Increased risk of lymphoma in sicca syndrome. *Ann Intern Med*. 1978;89:888-892.

143. Kato I, Tajima K, Suchi T *et al*. Chronic thyroiditis as a risk factor of B-cell lymphoma in the thyroid gland. *Jpn J Cancer Res*. 1985;76:1085-1090.

144. Holm LE, Blomgren H, Lowhagen T. Cancer risks in patients with chronic lymphocytic thyroiditis. *N Engl J Med*. 1985;312:601-604.

145. Isaacson PG, Spencer J. Malignant lymphoma of mucosa-associated lymphoid tissue. *Histopathology.* 1987;11:445-462.

146. Isaacson PG, Muller-Hermelink HK, Piris MA et al. Extranodal marginal zone B-cell lymphoma of mucosa-associated lymphoid tissue (MALT lymphoma). *In* "Pathology and Genetics of Tumours of Haematopoietic and Lymphoid Tissues."(Jaffe E.S., Harris N.L., Stein H. *et al.*, eds.)**157-160**. IARC Press, Lyon, 2001.

147. Ballesteros E, Osborne BM, Matsushima AY. CD5+ low-grade marginal zone B-cell lymphomas with localized presentation. *Am J Surg Pathol.* 1998;22:201-207.

148. Ferry JA, Yang WI, Zukerberg LR *et al.* CD5+ extranodal marginal zone B-cell (MALT) lymphoma. A low grade neoplasm with a propensity for bone marrow involvement and relapse. *Am J Clin Pathol.* 1996;105:31-37.

149. Wenzel C, Dieckmann K, Fiebiger W *et al.* CD5 expression in a lymphoma of the mucosa-associated lymphoid tissue (MALT)-type as a marker for early dissemination and aggressive clinical behaviour. *Leuk Lymphoma.* 2001;42:823-829.

150. Chen LT, Lin JT, Shyu RY *et al.* Prospective study of Helicobacter pylori eradication therapy in stage I(E) high-grade mucosa-associated lymphoid tissue lymphoma of the stomach. *J Clin Oncol.* 2001;19:4245-4251.

151. Wotherspoon AC, Doglioni C, Diss TC *et al.* Regression of primary low-grade B-cell gastric lymphoma of mucosa-associated lymphoid tissue type after eradication of Helicobacter pylori. *Lancet.* 1993;342:575-577.

152. Streubel B, Simonitsch-Klupp I, Mullauer L *et al.* Variable frequencies of MALT lymphoma-associated genetic aberrations in MALT lymphomas of different sites. *Leukemia.* 2004;18:1722-1726.

153. Dierlamm J, Baens M, Wlodarska I *et al.* The Apoptosis Inhibitor Gene API2 and a Novel 18q Gene, MLT, Are Recurrently Rearranged in the t(11;18)(q21;q21) Associated With Mucosa-Associated Lymphoid Tissue Lymphomas. *Blood.* 1999;93:3601-3609.

154. Liu H, Ye H, Ruskone-Fourmestraux A *et al.* T(11;18) is a marker for all stage gastric MALT lymphomas that will not respond to H. pylori eradication. *Gastroenterology.* 2002;122:1286-1294.

155. Liu H, Ruskon-Fourmestraux A, Lavergne-Slove A *et al.* Resistance of t(11;18) positive gastric mucosa-associated lymphoid tissue lymphoma to Helicobacter pylori eradication therapy. *Lancet.* 2001;357:39-40.

156. Streubel B, Lamprecht A, Dierlamm J *et al.* T(14;18)(q32;q21) involving IGH and MALT1 is a frequent chromosomal aberration in MALT lymphoma. *Blood.* 2003;101:2335-2339.

157. Willis TG, Jadayel DM, Du MQ *et al.* Bcl10 is involved in t(1;14)(p22;q32) of MALT B cell lymphoma and mutated in multiple tumor types. *Cell.* 1999;96:35-45.

158. Liu H, Ye H, Dogan A *et al.* T(11;18)(q21;q21) is associated with advanced mucosa-associated lymphoid tissue lymphoma that expresses nuclear BCL10. *Blood.* 2001;98:1182-1187.

159. Remstein ED, Kurtin PJ, James CD *et al.* Mucosa-Associated Lymphoid Tissue Lymphomas with t(11;18)(q21;q21) and Mucosa-Associated Lymphoid Tissue Lymphomas with Aneuploidy Develop Along Different Pathogenetic Pathways. *Am J Pathol.* 2002;161:63-71.

160. Bernstein L, Newton P, Ross RK. Epidemiology of hairy cell leukemia in Los Angeles County. *Cancer Res.* 1990;50:3605-3609.

161. Frassoldati A, Lamparelli T, Federico M *et al.* Hairy cell leukemia: a clinical review based on 725 cases of the Italian Cooperative Group (ICGHCL). Italian Cooperative Group for Hairy Cell Leukemia. *Leuk Lymphoma.* 1994;13:307-316.

162. Flandrin G, Sigaux F, Sebahoun G *et al.* Hairy cell leukemia: clinical presentation and follow-up of 211 patients. *Semin Oncol.* 1984;11:458-471.

163. Bouroncle BA. Leukemic reticuloendotheliosis (hairy cell leukemia). *Blood.* 1979;53:412-436.

164. Seshadri RS, Brown EJ, Zipursky A. Leukemic reticuloendotheliosis. A failure of monocyte production. *N Engl J Med.* 1976;295:181-184.

165. Ahmad E, Garcia D, Davis BH. Clinical utility of CD23 and FMC7 antigen coexistent expression in B-cell lymphoproliferative disorder subclassification. *Cytometry.* 2002;50:1-7.

166. Salomon-Nguyen F, Valensi F, Troussard X *et al.* The value of the monoclonal antibody, DBA44, in the diagnosis of B-lymphoid disorders. *Leuk Res.* 1996;20:909-913.

167. Yaziji H, Janckila AJ, Lear SC *et al.* Immunohistochemical detection of tartrate-resistant acid phosphatase in non-hematopoietic human tissues. *Am J Clin Pathol.* 1995;104:397-402.

168. Burkitt D, A sarcoma involving the jaws in African children. *Br J Surg.* 1958;46:218-223.

169. Soussain C, Patte C, Ostronoff M *et al.* Small noncleaved cell lymphoma and leukemia in adults. A retrospective study of 65 adults treated with the LMB pediatric protocols. *Blood.* 1995;85:664-674.

170. Levine PH, Kamaraju LS, Connelly RR *et al.* The American Burkitt's Lymphoma Registry: eight years' experience. *Cancer.* 1982;49:1016-1022.

171. Philip T, Lenoir GM, Bryon PA *et al.* Burkitt-type lymphoma in France among non-Hodgkin malignant lymphomas in Caucasian children. *Br J Cancer.* 1982;45:670-678.

172. Diebold J, Jaffe ES, Raphael M et al. Burkitt lymphoma. *In* "Pathology and Genetics of Tumours of Haematopoietic and Lymphoid Tissues."(Jaffe E.S., Harris N.L., Stein H. *et al.*, eds.)181-184. IARC Press, Lyon, 2001.

173. Braziel RM, Arber DA, Slovak ML *et al.* The Burkitt-like lymphomas: a Southwest Oncology Group study delineating phenotypic, genotypic, and clinical features. *Blood.* 2001;97:3713-3720.

174. Hui PK, Feller AC, Lennert K. High-grade non-Hodgkin's lymphoma of B-cell type. I. Histopathology. *Histopathology.* 1988;12:127-143.

175. Spina D, Leoncini L, Megha T *et al.* Cellular kinetic and phenotypic heterogeneity in and among Burkitt's and Burkitt-like lymphomas. *J Pathol.* 1997;182:145-150.

176. Chadburn A, Knowles DM. Paraffin-resistant antigens detectable by antibodies L26 and polyclonal CD3 predict the B- or T-cell lineage of 95% of diffuse aggressive non-Hodgkin's lymphomas. *Am J Clin Pathol.* 1994;102:284-291.

177. Fingeroth JD, Weis JJ, Tedder TF *et al.* Epstein-Barr virus receptor of human B lymphocytes is the C3d receptor CR2. *Proc Natl Acad Sci U S A.* 1984;81:4510-4514.

178. Harris NL, Jaffe ES, Stein H *et al.* A revised European-American classification of lymphoid neoplasms: a proposal from the International Lymphoma Study Group [see comments]. *Blood.* 1994;84:1361-1392.

179. Hamilton-Dutoit SJ, Raphael M, Audouin J *et al.* In situ demonstration of Epstein-Barr virus small RNAs (EBER 1) in acquired immunodeficiency syndrome-related lymphomas: correlation with tumor morphology and primary site. *Blood.* 1993;82:619-624.

180. Knowles DM. Immunodeficiency-associated lymphoproliferative disorders. *Mod Pathol.* 1999;12:200-217.

181. Prevot S, Hamilton-Dutoit S, Audouin J *et al.* Analysis of African Burkitt's and high-grade B cell non-Burkitt's lymphoma for Epstein-Barr virus genomes using in situ hybridization. *Br J Haematol.* 1992;80:27-32.

182. Tao Q, Robertson KD, Manns A *et al.* Epstein-Barr virus (EBV) in endemic Burkitt's lymphoma: molecular analysis of primary tumor tissue. *Blood.* 1998;91:1373-1381.

183. Anwar N, Kingma DW, Bloch AR *et al.* The investigation of Epstein-Barr viral sequences in 41 cases of Burkitt's lymphoma from Egypt: epidemiologic correlations. *Cancer.* 1995;76:1245-1252.

184. Gutierrez MI, Bhatia K, Barriga F *et al.* Molecular epidemiology of Burkitt's lymphoma from South America: differences in breakpoint location and Epstein-Barr virus association from tumors in other world regions. *Blood.* 1992;79:3261-3266.

185. Zech L, Haglund U, Nilsson K *et al.* Characteristic chromosomal abnormalities in biopsies and lymphoid-cell lines from patients with Burkitt and non-Burkitt lymphomas. *Int J Cancer.* 1976;17:47-56.

186. Bernheim A, Berger R, Lenoir G. Cytogenetic studies on African Burkitt's lymphoma cell lines: t(8;14), t(2;8) and t(8;22) translocations. *Cancer Genet Cytogenet.* 1981;3:307-315.

187. Harris NL, Jaffe ES, Stein H *et al.* A revised European-American classification of lymphoid neoplasms: a proposal from the International Lymphoma Study Group [see comments]. *Blood.* 1994;84:1361-1392.

188. Gatter KC, Warnke A. Diffuse large B-cell lymphoma. *In* "Pathology and Genetics of Tumours of Haematopoietic and Lymphoid Tissues."(Jaffe E.S., Harris N.L., Stein H. *et al.*, eds.)**171-176**. IARC Press, Lyon, 2001.

189. Armitage JO, Dick FR, Corder MP. Diffuse histiocytic lymphoma after histologic conversion: a poor prognostic variant. *Cancer Treat Rep.* 1981;65:413-418.

190. Delabie J, Vandenberghe E, Kennes C *et al.* Histiocyte-rich B-cell lymphoma. A distinct clinicopathologic entity possibly related to lymphocyte predominant Hodgkin's disease, paragranuloma subtype. *Am J Surg Pathol.* 1992;16:37-48.

191. Ramsay AD, Smith WJ, Isaacson PG. T-cell-rich B-cell lymphoma. *Am J Surg Pathol.* 1988;12:433-443.

192. Wang J, Sun NC, Chen YY *et al.* T-Cell/Histiocyte-Rich Large B-Cell Lymphoma Displays a Heterogeneity Similar to Diffuse Large B-Cell Lymphoma: A Clinicopathologic, Immunohistochemical, and Molecular Study of 30 Cases. *Appl Immunohistochem Mol Morphol.* 2005;13:109-115.

193. Nador RG, Cesarman E, Chadburn A *et al.* Primary effusion lymphoma: a distinct clinicopathologic entity associated with the Kaposi's sarcoma-associated herpes virus. *Blood.* 1996;88:645-656.

194. Banks PM, Warnke RA. Mediastinal (thymic) large B-cell lymphoma. *In* "World Health Organization Classification of Tumours. Patholoy and Genetics of Tumours of Haematopoietic and Lymphopid Tissues."(Jaffe E.S., Harris N.L., Stein H. *et al.*, eds.)**175-176**. IARC Press., Lyon, 2001.

195. Kirn D, Mauch P, Shaffer K *et al.* Large-cell and immunoblastic lymphoma of the mediastinum: prognostic features and treatment outcome in 57 patients. *J Clin Oncol.* 1993;11:1336-1343.

196. Moller P, Lammler B, Eberlein-Gonska M *et al.* Primary mediastinal clear cell lymphoma of B-cell type. *Virchows Arch A Pathol Anat Histopathol.* 1986;409:79-92.

197. Kennedy GA, Cull G, Gill D *et al.* Identification of tumours with the CD43 only phenotype during the investigation of suspected lymphoma: a heterogeneous group not necessarily of T cell origin. *Pathology.* 2002;34:46-50.

198. Doggett RS, Wood GS, Horning S *et al.* The immunologic characterization of 95 nodal and extranodal diffuse large cell lymphomas in 89 patients. *Am J Pathol.* 1984;115:245-252.

199. Stein H, Lennert K, Feller AC *et al.* Immunohistological analysis of human lymphoma: correlation of histological and immunological categories. *Adv Cancer Res.* 1984;42:67-147.

200. Bernard M, Gressin R, Lefrere F *et al.* Blastic variant of mantle cell lymphoma: a rare but highly aggressive subtype. *Leukemia.* 2001;15:1785-1791.

201. Dunphy CH, Wheaton SE, Perkins SL. CD23 expression in transformed small lymphocytic lymphomas/chronic lymphocytic leukemias and blastic transformations of mantle cell lymphoma. *Mod Pathol.* 1997;10:818-822.

202. Kroft SH, Dawson DB, McKenna RW. Large cell lymphoma transformation of chronic lymphocytic leukemia/small lymphocytic lymphoma. A flow cytometric analysis of seven cases. *Am J Clin Pathol.* 2001;115:385-395.

203. Yamaguchi M, Seto M, Okamoto M *et al.* De novo CD5+ diffuse large B-cell lymphoma: a clinicopathologic study of 109 patients. *Blood.* 2002;99:815-821.

204. Harada S, Suzuki R, Uehira K *et al.* Molecular and immunological dissection of diffuse large B cell lymphoma: CD5+, and CD5- with CD10+ groups may constitute clinically relevant subtypes. *Leukemia.* 1999;13:1441-1447.

205. Barrans SL, Carter I, Owen RG *et al.* Germinal center phenotype and bcl-2 expression combined with the International Prognostic Index improves patient risk stratification in diffuse large B-cell lymphoma. *Blood.* 2002;99:1136-1143.

206. Kramer MH, Hermans J, Parker J *et al.* Clinical significance of bcl2 and p53 protein expression in diffuse large B-cell lymphoma: a population-based study. *J Clin Oncol.* 1996;14:2131-2138.

207. Hans CP, Weisenburger DD, Greiner TC *et al.* Confirmation of the molecular classification of diffuse large B-cell lymphoma by immunohistochemistry using a tissue microarray. *Blood.* 2004;103:275-282.

208. Grogan TM, Van Camp B, Kyle RA et al. Plasma cell neoplasms. *In* "Pathology and Genetics of Tumours of Haematopoietic and Lymphoid Tissues."(Jaffe E.S., Harris N.L., Stein H. *et al.*, eds.)142-156. IARC Press, Lyon, 2001.

209. Young JL, Jr., Percy CL, Asire AJ *et al.* Cancer incidence and mortality in the United States, 1973-77. *Natl Cancer Inst Monogr.* 1981;1-187.

210. Grogan TM, Spier C. B-cell immunoproliferative disorders, including multiple myeloma and amyloidosis. *In* "Neoplastic Hematopathology"1557-1587. Lippincott Williams & Wilkins, Philadelphia, 2001.

211. Bartl R, Frisch B, Burkhardt R *et al.* Bone marrow histology in myeloma: its importance in diagnosis, prognosis, classification and staging. *Br J Haematol.* 1982;51:361-375.

212. Greipp PR, Leong T, Bennett JM *et al.* Plasmablastic morphology--an independent prognostic factor with clinical and laboratory correlates: Eastern Cooperative Oncology Group (ECOG) myeloma trial E9486 report by the ECOG Myeloma Laboratory Group. *Blood.* 1998;91:2501-2507.

213. Kronland R, Grogan T, Spier C *et al.* Immunotopographic assessment of lymphoid and plasma cell malignancies in the bone marrow. *Hum Pathol.* 1985;16:1247-1254.

214. Robillard N, Avet-Loiseau H, Garand R *et al.* CD20 is associated with a small mature plasma cell morphology and t(11;14) in multiple myeloma. *Blood.* 2003;102:1070-1071.

215. Mahmoud MS, Huang N, Nobuyoshi M *et al.* Altered expression of Pax-5 gene in human myeloma cells. *Blood.* 1996;87:4311-4315.

216. Lima M, Teixeira MA, Fonseca S *et al.* Immunophenotypic aberrations, DNA content, and cell cycle analysis of plasma cells in patients with myeloma and monoclonal gammopathies. *Blood Cells Mol Dis.* 2000;26:634-645.

217. Ely SA, Knowles DM. Expression of CD56/neural cell adhesion molecule correlates with the presence of lytic bone lesions in multiple myeloma and distinguishes myeloma from monoclonal gammopathy of undetermined significance and lymphomas with plasmacytoid differentiation. *Am J Pathol.* 2002;160:1293-1299.

218. Van Camp B, Durie BG, Spier C *et al.* Plasma cells in multiple myeloma express a natural killer cell- associated antigen: CD56 (NKH-1; Leu-19). *Blood.* 1990;76:377-382.

219. Beschorner R, Horny HP, Petruch UR *et al.* Frequent expression of haemopoietic and non-haemopoietic antigens by reactive plasma cells: an

immunohistochemical study using formalin-fixed, paraffin-embedded tissue. *Histol Histopathol.* 1999;14:805-812.

220. Pileri S, Poggi S, Baglioni P *et al.* Histology and immunohistology of bone marrow biopsy in multiple myeloma. *Eur J Haematol Suppl.* 1989;51:52-59.

221. Knowles DM. B-cell immunoproliferative disorders. *In* "Neoplastic Hematopathology."(Knowles D.M., ed.) Lippincott Williams & Wilkins, Philadelphia, 2001.

222. Alexandrakis MG, Passam FH, Kyriakou DS *et al.* Ki-67 proliferation index: correlation with prognostic parameters and outcome in multiple myeloma. *Am J Clin Oncol.* 2004;27:8-13.

223. Garcia-Sanz R, Gonzalez-Fraile MI, Mateo G *et al.* Proliferative activity of plasma cells is the most relevant prognostic factor in elderly multiple myeloma patients. *Int J Cancer.* 2004;112:884-889.

224. Drach J, Ackermann J, Fritz E *et al.* Presence of a p53 gene deletion in patients with multiple myeloma predicts for short survival after conventional-dose chemotherapy. *Blood.* 1998;92:802-809.

225. Soverini S, Cavo M, Cellini C *et al.* Cyclin D1 overexpression is a favorable prognostic variable for newly diagnosed multiple myeloma patients treated with high-dose chemotherapy and single or double autologous transplantation. *Blood.* 2003;102:1588-1594.

226. Chesi M, Brents LA, Ely SA *et al.* Activated fibroblast growth factor receptor 3 is an oncogene that contributes to tumor progression in multiple myeloma. *Blood.* 2001;97:729-736.

Chapter 2

PATHOGENESIS OF VIRAL LYMPHOMAS

Ethel Cesarman, MD, PhD,* Enrique A. Mesri, PhD+

*Department of Pathology and Laboratory Medicine, and +Laboratory of Viral Oncogenesis, Division of Hematology-Oncology, Department of Medicine, Weill Medical College of Cornell University and The New York Presbyterian Hospital, New York, NY

1.   INTRODUCTION

Epstein-Barr virus (EBV), Kaposi's sarcoma herpesvirus (KSHV), also called Human Herpesvirus 8 (HHV-8), and human T-cell lymphotrophic virus (HTLV-1) are viruses that are well documented to be causally associated with lymphoid neoplasia in humans. Other viruses have also been proposed to be involved in lymphomagenesis, but their role may be indirect, or the association is not well established. Current knowledge suggests that EBV, KSHV and HTLV-1 contribute to lymphomagenesis by subverting the host-cell molecular signaling machinery to deregulate cell growth and survival. It appears that de-regulation of the NF-κB pathway is a common strategy used by these three viruses to promote cell survival, thereby playing a critical role in tumorigenesis. The understanding of the mechanisms of viral carcinogenesis could lead to the identification of novel therapeutic targets and to the development of rationally designed therapies. In this chapter, the basic information and recent developments that have contributed to our understanding of viral lymphomagenesis, and its possible therapeutic implications are reviewed.

The first observation that a viral infection could lead to the development of leukemia was made in 1907 (Ellerman and Bang, 1908). Since this time, many associations between viruses and leukemia/ lymphoma have been proposed but only a few firmly demonstrated. Nowadays, in order to consider that a viral entity is causally associated with a human cancer, it must fulfill the criteria of four so-called Koch-like postulates (Zur Hauzen 1999): 1) Solid epidemiologic evidence that the virus represents a risk factor for the development of the tumor; 2) Consistent presence or persistence of the viral genome in the tumor cells; 3) Proven oncogenic effects of viral infection or transfection of viral genes to cells; and 4) Demonstration that the malignant phenotype of tumor cells depends on functions conferred by the viral genomes. Based on these rigorous criteria only three human viruses are clearly directly associated with lymphoid neoplasia: Epstein-Barr virus (EBV) or human herpesvirus 4 (HHV-4), Kaposi's sarcoma herpesvirus (KSHV) or human herpesvirus 8 (HHV-8), and human T-cell lymphotropic virus 1 (HTLV-1).

Although the prevalence of lymphomagenic viruses in the normal population is quite high (as high as 94% for EBV), only a small number of infected immunocompetent people ever develop the virus-induced malignancy and do so only after a long latency period. This observation reflects the multistep nature of oncogenesis, with the viral infection representing only one of these steps. In the following sections, the current understanding and recent developments concerning the pathobiology of EBV, KSHV, and HTLV-1 and their role in lymphomagenesis are reviewed. We also briefly review the evidence implicating hepatitis C virus (HCV) in the development of lymphomas.

2.   EPSTEIN-BARR VIRUS (EBV)

2.1   Epstein-Barr Virus and Lymphomagenesis

The association of EBV with several specific lymphoid malignancies is quite consistent, indicating an etiopathogenic role in their development. EBV infection is practically ubiquitous in healthy adults, so it has been difficult to establish the exact role of this virus in lymphomagenesis. Nevertheless, extensive epidemiologic and experimental data support the notion that EBV is an oncogenic virus. EBV can infect and transform normal human B-cells in vitro, resulting in their "immortalization" and leading to continuously growing lymphoblastoid cell lines (LCLs) (Rickinson and Kieff, 1996). In addition, loss of EBV episomes from transformed lymphoma cell lines results in loss of tumorigenicity.

2.2   Patterns of Epstein-Barr Virus Latency

EBV establishes a lifelong infection in the vast majority of immunocompetent individuals without causing any disease. Recent studies based on careful analysis of expression patterns in different tissues from EBV-infected immunocompetent individuals led to the description of five different transcription programs that are used to establish and maintain EBV infection (Figure 1); reviewed by (Thorley-Lawson, 2001; Thorley-Lawson and Gross, 2004). Some of the same transcriptional programs are recapitulated in lymphomas and lymphoproliferative disease. Therefore, describing the patterns of latency is critical to understand the role of EBV genes in lymphomagenesis.

When EBV first infects a naïve B cell, a transient "growth program" is established, where EBV expresses EBNA 1-6, as well as LMP1, LMP2A and LMP2B. These proteins force the infected cells to become proliferating B cell blasts, probably allowing EBV infection to be propagated. In vitro generated LCLs have this growth program indefinitely. However, since many of these proteins are antigenic, this state is very transient in immunocompetent individuals. As soon as an immune response is established, most of the cells with this program are eliminated, or otherwise switch to a "default program" of EBV expression, where only EBNA1, LMP1 and LMP2A are expressed. This stage is also temporary because LMP1 and LMP2A mimick CD40 and antigen receptor signaling, thereby inducing the B cells in peripheral lymphoid organs to behave like germinal center B cells and differentiate into resting memory B cells (Babcock et al., 2000; Laichalk et al., 2002). These infected cells in turn switch to a "latency program" where no viral genes are expressed, allowing lifetime persistence of EBV. Dividing peripheral blood infected memory B cells express only EBNA1, which is not immunogenic but allows the EBV episome to segregate and be propagated in dividing cells.

Three different patterns of EBV expression have been described in infected cells in lymphoproliferative disorders, Latency I, II or III, illustrated in Figure 1 (Kieff, 1996; Rickinson and Kieff, 1996) . Latency III corresponds to the "growth program" and involves the unrestricted expression of all 9 latent genes including six EBV-encoded nuclear antigens (EBNA1-6) (Kieff, 1996) and three latent membrane proteins (LMP1, LMP2A, and LMP2B). In Latency I, EBNA1 is the major viral protein produced. Latency II corresponds to the "default program", and consists of expression of EBNA1 and varying amounts of the three LMP proteins.

Because EBNA proteins are immunogenic, with the exception of EBNA1, an important feature of Latency III is the recognition and elimination of the EBV-infected cells by the immune system. Therefore, lymphomas with unrestricted EBV latency are generally only encountered in immunodeficient individuals. In contrast, most lymphomas in immunocompetent hosts will have Latency I or II, because down-regulation of the immunogenic EBNA proteins is an important mechanism of immune evasion by EBV (Rickinson and Kieff, 1996).

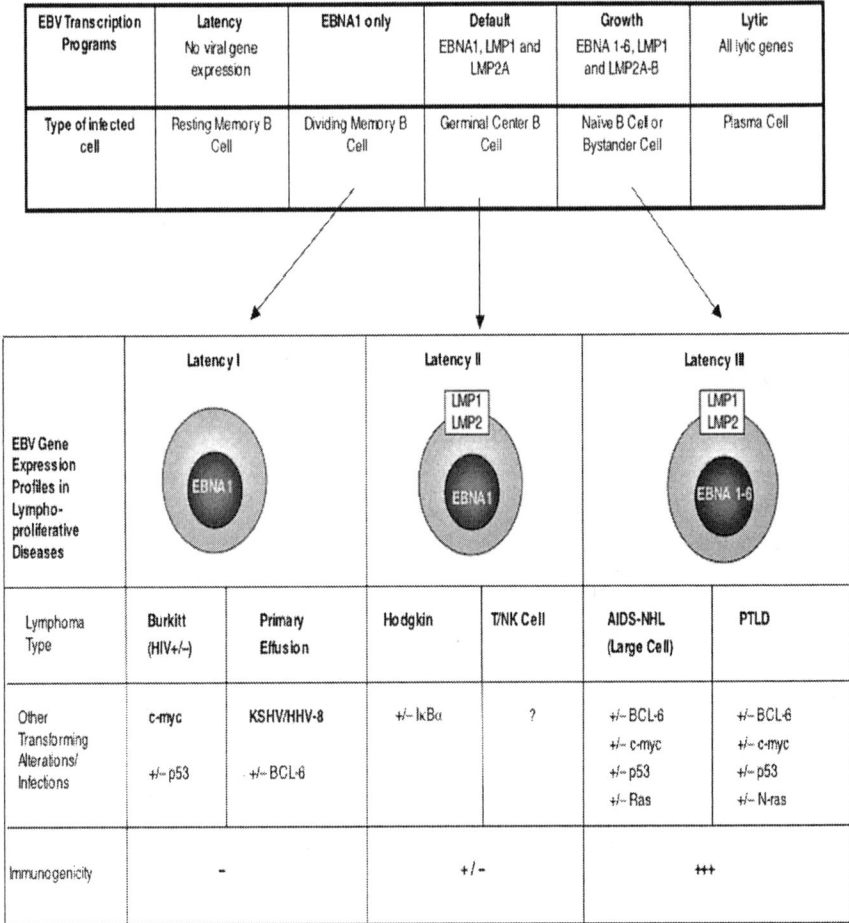

Figure 1. Patterns of EBV gene expression in malignant lymphomas. The relevant EBV genes that are expressed in various EBV-associated lymphoproliferative disorders are illustrated, and compared to latency patterns observed in infected normal individuals (top). The transforming EBV gene LMP1 is expressed in latencies II and III, and the highly immunogenic EBNAs only in Latency III. Cellular genetic alteration and/or viral co-infection known to occur in these lesions are listed as other transforming alterations/infections.

2.3 Role of EBV Latently Expressed Genes in Maintenance and Determination of the Transformed Phenotype

Although it is clear that EBV can transform B-cells, its role in the maintenance of the transformed state is still unknown. When episomal EBV was eliminated from LCL cells by hydroxyurea treatment, they ceased to proliferate (Chodosh et al., 1998). Additionally, loss of the EBV genome from the BL cell line Akata results in loss of the malignant phenotype, although Akata is a Latency I cell line and does not express the major EBV transforming genes, LMP1 and EBNA2 (Shimizu et al., 1994). Two studies showed that re-establishment of Latency I in EBV-negative Akata cells restores tumorigenicity (Komano et al., 1998; Ruf et al., 1999). An increased resistance to apoptosis accompanies this effect, perhaps due to a decrease in c-myc and increase in Bcl-2 protein levels. This restored tumorigenicity is not simply due to expression of the EBNA1 protein, because both studies showed that enforced expression of EBNA1 in EBV-negative Akata cells does not restore tumorigenicity or apoptosis resistance. Therefore, a restricted latency pattern of gene expression is also important for malignancy, although the precise mechanism is unknown.

2.4 Molecular Mechanisms of EBV Mediated Transformation

The specific pattern of expression of EBV latent genes is associated with specific lymphoma subtypes. In some cases EBV gene expression can be linked specific molecular and oncogenic phenotypes of the lymphoid malignancies. Lymphomas such as Burkitt's lymphoma (BL) with Latency I only express EBNA1. Although EBNA1 transgenic mice have an increased incidence of lymphomas (Wilson et al., 1996), the role of EBNA1 in tumorigenesis is unclear. There is evidence that infection of B cells with EBV lacking EBNA1 can lead to the development of LCLs that are tumorigenic in mice, but this process is much less efficient than with wild type EBV (Humme et al., 2003). In general it is thought that EBNA1 is not a major oncogene of KSHV. Lymphomas with Latency I bear cellular oncogenic alterations, such as translocations involving the c-myc oncogene characteristic of Burkitt's lymphomas (BLs), and these are probably essential because EBNA1 is insufficient to drive cellular proliferation. Of the EBV proteins expressed in Latency III, EBNA2 and LMP1 are essential for transformation by EBV in vitro. EBNA2 is thought to represent a

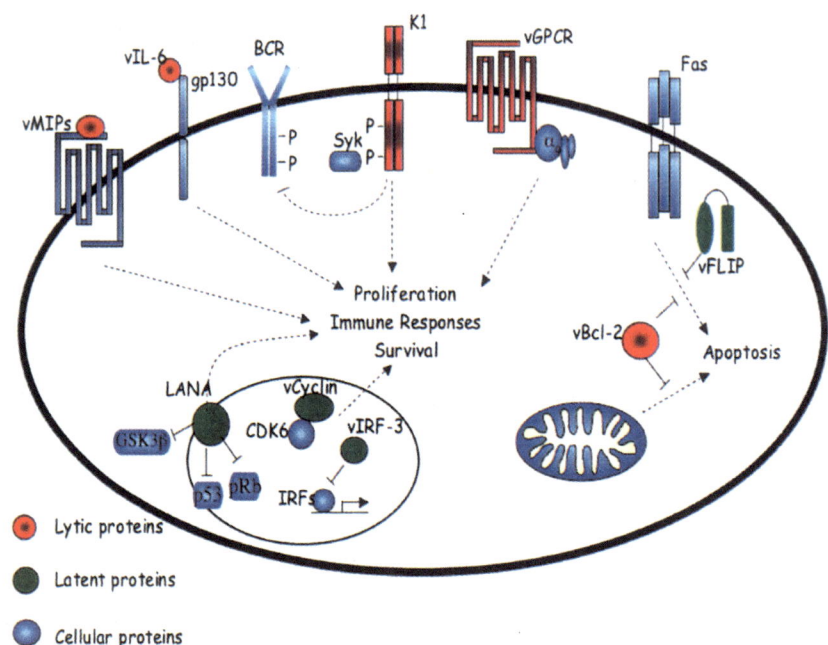

Figure 2. Representative KSHV-encoded proteins that can affect cellular proliferation, survival, differentiation and/or angiogenesis. KSHV contains several open reading frames encoding homologues to cellular proteins involved in vital proliferative and survival functions. Among these are: 1) secreted autocrine/paracrine factors (vIL-6 and vMIPs); 2) transmembrane signaling molecules (vGPCR and K1); 3) transcriptional regulators (vIRFs and LANA); 4) a cell cycle regulator (vCYC); 5) tumor suppressor gene-binding activity (LANA) and 5) apoptosis inhibitors (vBCL-2 and vFLIP). Those genes clearly demonstrated to be expressed in latently-infected cells of Kaposi's sarcoma are illustrated in green ovals.

constitutively active member of the Notch signaling pathway (Grossman et al., 1994; Hsieh and Hayward, 1995). The LMP1 protein is transforming and tumorigenic in vitro (Wang et al., 1985), and in vivo. Transgenic mice expressing LMP1 under the control of immunoglobulin gene regulatory elements develop B-cell lymphomas (Kulwichit et al., 1998). LMP1 functions as a constitutively active CD40 receptor, a member of the TNF (tumor necrosis factor)-receptor family. LMP1 aggregates in the membrane as its cytoplasmic tail interacts with TNF receptor-associated factors

(TRAFs) and TNFR-1-associated death domain protein (TRADD), leading to activation of nuclear factor (NF-κB) and the c-Jun amino-terminal kinase (JNK) (Eliopoulos et al., 1999; Kieser et al., 1997; Kilger et al., 1998), a kinase cascade activated by inflammatory cytokines and involved in bcr-abl leukemogenesis (Dickens et al., 1997).

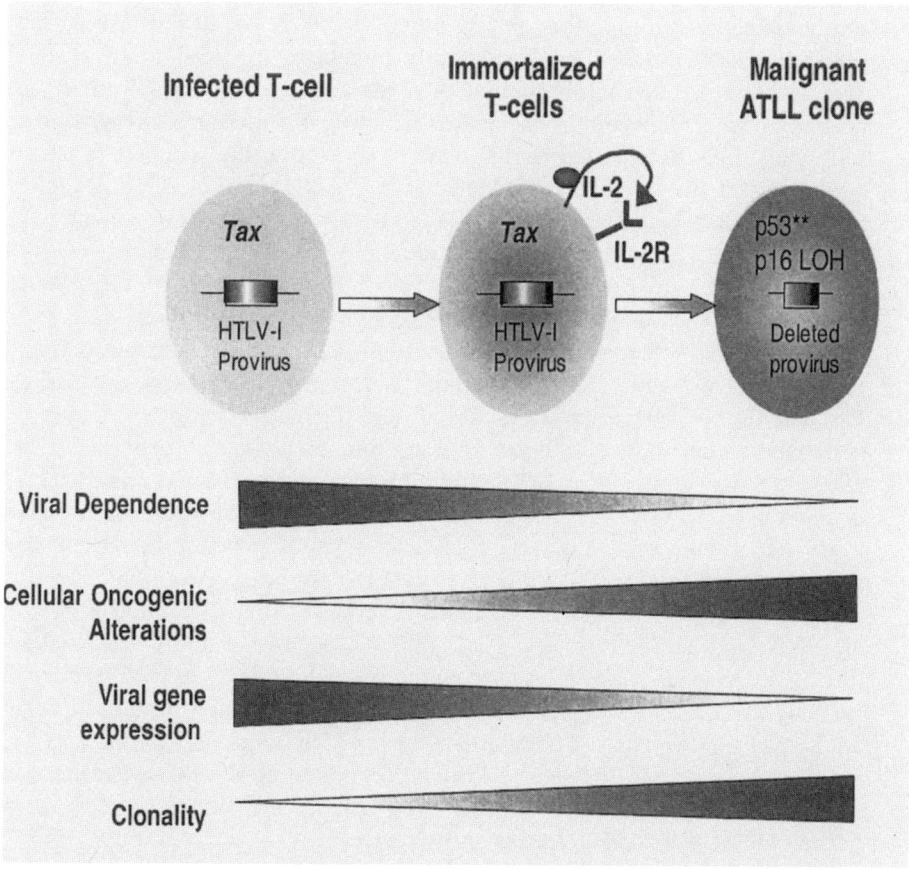

Figure 3. Stages of human T-cell leukemia virus –1 mediated lymphomagenesis: role of Tax. A polyclonal population of HTLV-1 de novo infected cells express the transactivator Tax. Transactivation by Tax of cellular genes involved in T cell proliferation and survival, such as simultaneous expression of IL-2 and IL-2 receptor, creating an autocrine loop, leads to a polyclonal population of immortalized T cells. Immortalized T cells accumulate further oncogenic mutations because Tax induces genetic instability. In ATLL malignant clones, proviruses are heavily deleted, there is frequently no viral gene expression, and there are cytogenetic abnormalities and oncogenic alterations such as p53 inactivation and p16/CDKN2 loss of heterozygosity (LOH). With permission from Lippincott Williams & Wilkins.

2.5   LMP-1 and NF-κB

NF-κB is an important transcription factor, the activation of which appears to be a subverted by the three lymphomagenic viruses discussed in this chapter (Figure 4). NF-κB can be activated, depending on the cell type, by treatment with phorbol esters, tumor necrosis factor (TNF), antigen receptor ligation, inflammatory cytokines, bacterial endotoxin, stress responses and viral infection, among other stimuli. Some of these signals, in particular those induced by TNF family members, can lead to survival or apoptosis, which are mainly mediated by the activation of the NF-κB or the death pathways respectively. Receptors of the TNF superfamily relay signals following ligand-mediated trimerization by recruiting adapter proteins containing death domains (TRADD, RIP, FADD) and/or TNF receptor-associated factor (TRAF) domains (TRAF1-6). Signaling leading to apoptosis is mediated by a death-inducing signaling complex (DISC) containing TRADD-FADD-caspase-8. In contrast, the TRADD-TRAF-RIP-IKK cascade leads to activation of NF-κB signaling and survival. Activation of NF-κB leads to expression of a variety of cellular genes related to B-cell proliferation and malignancy, including IL-6, ICAM-1, LFA-3, CD40, EBI3, Fas, and TRAF1 (Devergne et al., 1998), and the matrix metalloproteinase-9, which may contribute to tumor invasion and metastasis (Yoshizaki et al., 1998). Association of LMP1 with TRAF-1 and TRAF-3, as well as activation of NF-κB, have been demonstrated to occur in vivo in EBV-associated lymphomas expressing LMP1, suggesting that this is indeed a relevant pathobiologic pathway in EBV-related lymphomagenesis (Liebowitz, 1998). While LMP1 binds several TRAFs, only TRAF3 (Xie et al., 2004) and TRAF 6 (Luftig et al., 2003) have been found to be involved in LMP1 signaling. The relevance of the NF-κB pathway in EBV-mediated lymphomagenesis has been supported by studies in which inhibition using an IκB phosphorylation-deficient mutants which sequesters NF-κB in the cytoplasm, rendering it inactive (Cahir-McFarland et al., 2000; Feuillard et al., 2000), or a pharmacological inhibitor called Bay11-7082 (Cahir-McFarland et al., 2004), (Keller and Cesarman, manuscript in preparation). These studies have shown that elimination of NF-κB activity induces apoptosis of EBV-infected lymphoma cell lines, indicating that this is an essential pathway that is induced by viral oncoproteins.

2.6   Epstein-Barr virus-associated lymphomas

Burkitt's Lymphoma
Epstein-Barr virus is invariably present in African (endemic) BL, but is found only in a minority of sporadic cases. Most of our understanding of

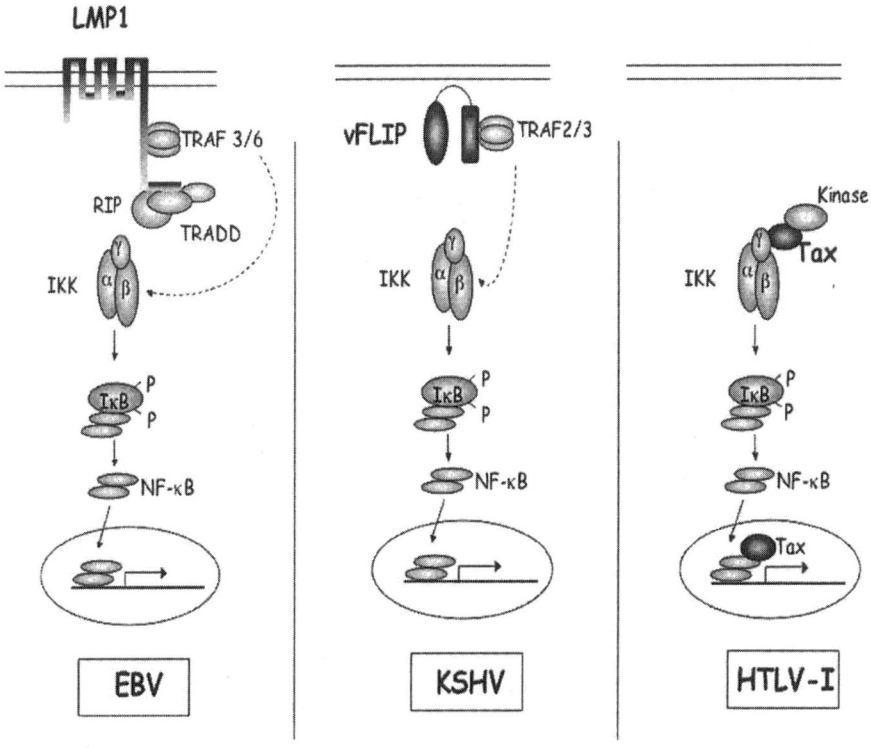

Figure 4. Viral proteins can activate NF-κB. Transforming proteins of EBV, KSHV and HTLV-1 include LMP-1, vFLIP and Tax, respectively. These three proteins share the ability to activate the NF-κB pathway. While all three have been shown to activate this pathway through canonical and non-cannonical mechanisms, only the canonical pathway is shown. This pathway involves activation of the IKK complex by the corresponding viral protein with subsequent phosphorylation of IκBα that leads to its degradation. This results in the release of Rel proteins, which are translocated to the nucleus and dimerize to form different NF-κB complexes that bind to specific sequences to activate the transcription of multiple genes.

EBV gene expression was originally derived from the study of BL cell lines; however, in vivo expression has also been examined in endemic BL tissue biopsies (Tao et al., 1998a). EBV-positive BLs have EBNA1, and usually LMP2A, transcripts, in the absence of lytic transcripts or other latent transcripts. Translocation of c-myc into one of the immunoglobulin loci is considered by some to be a prerequisite for classification of a lymphoma as

BL or atypical BL. The most common translocation is a t(8;14), involving the c-myc and immunoglobulin heavy chain genes, but in 10% of the cases it can involve c-myc and one of the light chain genes. It is thought that this translocation leads to deregulated expression of the c-myc gene. Mutations of the c-myc locus also occur in Burkitt lymphoma, and these may also lead to abnormal expression.

2.7   Post-Transplantation Lymphoproliferative Disorder

Post-transplantation lymphoproliferative disorders (PTLDs) develop in the setting of iatrogenic immunosuppression following solid organ transplantation (SOT) or allogeneic bone marrow transplantation (BMT). The incidence of these lesions varies based on the type of organ transplanted as well as on the type and amount of immunosuppression employed. In these immunosuppressed patients morphology does not accurately predict clinical course. In some SOT recipients a lesion may regress completely following a reduction in immunosuppression, while morphologically similar lesion(s) in other patients may progress despite aggressive clinical intervention resulting in the patient's demise. Furthermore, institution of the correct therapy in patients with PTLD is crucial since a reduction in immunosuppression can potentially result in organ loss while chemotherapy can lead to life-threatening infection in an already immunosuppressed individual. Although in some studies specific molecular events correlate well with biologic aggressiveness of the lesions, in other studies these findings could not be confirmed. It may be that differences in the type of organ transplanted, the immunosuppressive regimens as well as host/donor factors influence the pathogenesis and biologic behavior of PTLDs. In contrast to SOT PTLDs, patients who develop PTLDs following allogeneic BMT usually have an aggressive, frequently fatal, clinical course. As with other immunodeficiency-related lymphoproliferative disorders, the development of PTLDs in both SOT and BMT recipients is highly associated with EBV infection. Furthermore, the relative incidence of these lesions is higher in patients who are EBV negative at the time of transplantation.

The overall incidence of PTLD after SOT is ~1.5%, but varies from 0.3 to 12.5% depending on the organ transplanted and the immunosuppressive regimen, with a higher incidence in children than adults. Studies of PTLDs occurring in SOT recipients (primarily heart, kidney and lung recipients) have shown that most of these lesions can be separated into three categories based on morphologic and molecular genetic criteria. These categories correlate with the biologic behavior of the lesions. Because of the special clinical setting, i.e. that of iatrogenic immunosuppression that can be modulated, a unique classification scheme was originally developed by Nalesnik, et al. (Nalesnik et al., 1988), to describe the clinical course and outcome of SOT PTLD patients, and subsequently modified by Knowles, et al. (Knowles et al., 1995). This classification divides cases into three major categories: (1) Plasmacytic hyperplasia (PH) lesions show retention of the overall architecture of the tissue. Genotypically these lesions in general are polyclonal based on Ig rearrangement studies, or have small monoclonal/oligoclonal populations. The majority of cases are EBV positive. These lesions do not contain structural alterations of known oncogenes or tumor suppressor genes. Furthermore, examination of EBV antigen expression shows that these lesions express LMP1 and in some instances EBNA2 indicating they exhibit either the latency type II or III pattern of EBV gene expression. (2) Polymorphic PTLD lesions histologically show destruction of the underlying architecture and are composed of a heterogeneous (polymorphic) cell population. At the genetic level these lesions are monoclonal based both on immunoglobulin studies and the presence of clonal EBV. Polymorphic PTLDs lack structural alterations in oncogenes and tumor suppressor genes except for the presence of *BCL6* gene mutations, which have been identified in approximately half of the cases studied (Cesarman et al., 1998). Lesions containing the wild-type configuration of the *BCL6* gene regress following a reduction in immunosuppression, while those lesions containing *BCL6* gene mutations exhibit more aggressive behavior requiring clinical intervention. Polymorphic PTLDs, like the PHs, exhibit the latency type II or III pattern of EBV gene expression, although expression of specific EBV genes at the cellular level is very heterogeneous. Type II and III latency include expression of the transforming but immunogenic LMP and EBNA viral proteins, suggesting that reconstitution of an immune response in the host is more likely to result in elimination of these infected cells. (3) Monomorphic PTLD (malignant lymphoma/multiple myeloma) lesions are composed of cytologically malignant cells and should be classified according to the WHO classification. They are monoclonal based both on Ig and EBV studies. Additionally they contain structural alterations in oncogenes and tumor suppressor genes frequently involved in lymphomagenesis such as *P53* and *MYC* (Knowles et al., 1995). In contrast to the other solid organ PTLDs these lesions often exhibit the latency type I pattern of EBV gene expression, suggesting that they are less dependent on EBV and that they may no longer be recognized by the immune system even after immune reconstitution.

PTLDs occurring in allogeneic BMT recipients are biologically distinct from those occurring in SOT recipients. BMT PTLDs are of donor origin, often have an explosive clinical presentation and are frequently fatal. Furthermore, BMT PTLDs tend to occur in the first six months following transplantation, since the level of anti-EBV cytotoxic T cell precursors only returns to normal approximately 6 months after transplantation. In comparison to SOT PTLDs, the incidence of BMT PTLDs is relatively low (cumulative incidence of 1% at ten years). As with SOT PTLDs, the vast majority of BMT PTLD cases are associated with EBV infection. Morphologically, BMT PTLDs consist of lesions exhibiting the histologic features of plasmacytic hyperplasia and polymorphic PTLD as seen in SOT recipients (Shapiro et al., 1988). However, none of the PTLDs studied from 27 allogeneic BMT recipients showed the morphologic features of monomorphic PTLD (Chadburn et al., 2000), although other investigators have identified such lesions (Abed et al., 2004). While morphology correlates with clinical outcome, B cell clonality status does not correlate with morphology nor with clinical outcome, based on PCR analysis of the early onset PTLDs (Chadburn et al., 2000). Specifically, patients with both monoclonal/oligoclonal as well as those with polyclonal PTLDs died of PTLD. In contrast to SOT PTLDs, examination of the BMT PTLDs for *BCL6* mutations did not identify any correlation of this genetic alteration with patient outcome (Chadburn et al., 2001). All BMT PTLDs in this study exhibited EBV latency patterns type II or III (expressed LMP-1 with or without EBNA2), indicating that these lesions are EBV driven (Chadburn et al., 2000). The clinical outcome of BMT PTLD patients is largely related to the number and competence of EBV-specific cytotoxic T cells rather than to intrinsic differences in BMT PTLD subtypes.

2.8   AIDS-related non-Hodgkin's lymphomas

The incidence of non-Hodgkin lymphomas (NHL) in HIV positive individuals is estimated to be between 4 and 10%, but the incidence of at least some subsets appears to be decreasing with combination antiretroviral therapy. The incidence of Hodgkin lymphoma is somewhat increased in HIV-infected individuals, but it is not considered to be an AIDS-defining condition. The pathogenesis of NHL in the context AIDS is complex and thought to be related to disrupted immune surveillance, chronic antigenic stimulation, genetic alterations, cytokine dysregulation and herpes virus infection (Carbone, 2003; Gaidano et al., 1998; Knowles, 2001). Although HIV-related lymphomas are almost always of B cell origin, they are morphologically diverse. Several subtypes are similar to lymphomas occurring in immunocompetent patients, while others preferentially develop in the context of AIDS. HIV-related lymphomas can be classified by morphology (as in the WHO classification), and/or by primary site of presentation (i.e. systemic, primary central nervous system, body cavity)(Knowles, 2001; Raphael et al., 2001). Viral associations in HIV-related lymphomas are summarized in Table 1.

Table 1. Correlation of morphology and viral infection IN HIV-related lymphomas

Virus	BL	CB	IB	EL	Poly	PCNSL
EBV	25-75%	20-40%	80%	87%	40%	100%
LMP-1+	0%	Rare	65%	Rare	ND	90%
KSHV	0%	0%	15%	100%	ND	0%
HIV-1	0%	0%	0%	0%	0%	0%

BL, Burkitt and Burkitt-like lymphoma; CB, centroblastic diffuse large B-cell lymphoma; IB, Immunoblastic diffuse large B-cell lymphoma; PEL, primary effusion lymphoma; Poly, Polymorphic B-cell lymphoma (PTLD-like); PCNSL, Primary CNS lymphoma.

2.9 Lymphomas Also Occurring in Immunocompetent Patients

HIV-related Burkitt lymphomas (BL) include cases exhibiting the features of classical BL (described above), those showing plasmacytoid differentiation and those exhibiting features of atypical Burkitt/Burkitt-like lymphoma. In terms of EBV infection, AIDS-related BL resembles sporadic BL, with 25 to 75% of cases reported to be positive. Diffuse large B-cell lymphoma (DLBCL) can be divided into centroblastic (CB) and immunoblastic (IB) categories. While these morphologically and immunophenotypically resemble lesions found in immunocompetend individuals, the frequent association with EBV is almost exclusive of immunodefficient patients. The IB type is more frequently associated with EBV infection, and patients with these lymphomas are usually significantly immunosuppressed with low CD4 counts (median <100 x10^6/L) and approximately one-third have been previously diagnosed with an AIDS-defining illness. This degree of immune dysfunction allows EBV to be the driving proliferative force, with expression of the oncogenic but also immunogenic LMP and EBNA proteins. In addition, while DLBCL express adhesion molecules that are important for immune recognition, BLs do not.

These observations suggest that defective EBV immunity is involved in the pathogenesis of DLBCLs (Kersten et al., 1998).

2.10   Lymphomas Occurring Primarily in HIV-Positive Patients

Primary central nervous system lymphomas (PCNSL) differ from systemic DLBCLs, with the majority of cases exhibiting IB morphology and EBV-positivity. According to one study, PCNSL can be divided into two categories-those with immunoblastic features, which express LMP-1 in conjunction with BCL-2 but no BCL-6 expression, and those with a large, noncleaved cell morphology, which do not express LMP-1 or BCL-2, but express BCL-6 (Larocca et al., 1998). Another type of lymphoma described in the context of HIN infection is the plasmablastic lymphoma of the oral cavity. It has features similar to IB lymphomas, but are less heterogeneous and polymorphic. Approximately 50% of cases are associated with EBV infection. Polymorphic B-cell lymphomas (PTLD-like) are extremely rare lesions but morphologically resemble polymorphic PTLDs. The last category of lymphoma predominantly occurring in HIV-positive patients is primary effusion lymphoma. The latter, while positive for EBV, also contain KSHV, and will be discussed in the following section.

2.11   T/NATURAL KILLER CELL LYMPHOMAS

The angiocentric (nasal and nasal-type) T/natural killer (T/NK)-cell lymphomas are invariably associated with EBV infection (Jaffe et al., 1999). These have a high prevalence in Asia, but cases from other countries have also shown an association with EBV (Elenitoba-Johnson et al., 1998). Studies on cell lines indicate that T/NK cell lymphomas have a Latency II (Kanegane et al., 1998; Tsuchiyama et al., 1998). Although EBV has also been reported to be present in peripheral T-cell lymphomas, it has been shown to be preferentially localized in B-cells rather than the neoplastic T cells (Ho et al., 1998).

2.12   Hodgkin's Disease

Classical Hodgkin's disease (HD) has been found to be associated with EBV infection in approximately 40% of cases in Western countries and more frequently in developing countries and in younger patients (Harris,

1998). HD results from a monoclonal expansion of B-cells containing somatic hypermutations of the immunoglobulin genes. These mutations may be "crippling", resulting in lack of antigen-receptor expression. Therefore, the Hodgkin's-Reed-Sternberg (HRS) cells are derived from germinal B-cells destined to undergo apoptosis, but were protected by some transforming event, such as EBV (Kuppers and Rajewsky, 1998). In HD, EBV establishes Latency II within HRS cells, with expression of LMP-1 and LMP2, which are subdominant targets for CTL recognition. HRS cells in EBV-associated HD do express MHC class I molecules, as well as the transporter-associated molecules TAP1 and TAP2, necessary for a CTL response (Lee et al., 1998c). This raises the possibility of developing immunotherapy for the treatment of EBV-positive HD.

2.13 Novel therapeutic approaches targeting EBV

Conventional chemotherapy has been used with variable success for the treatment of EBV-associated lymphomas, and addition of Rituxan has improved the outcome is some of these. However, newer approaches to specifically target EBV hold promise of more effectiveness with less toxicity. One approach for the treatment of EBV associated malignancies has been immunotherapy, either by developing vaccines, performing adoptive transfer of EBV-specific cytotoxic T cells or manipulating the EBV-infected cells to express immunogenic antigens. Most PT-LPDs have EBV Latency III, with expression of immunogenic EBNAs. Therefore, PT-LPDs are often sensitive to immune-restoration therapy. In the solid-organ transplant setting, this may sometimes be achieved by withdrawal or reduction of immunosuppressive agents. PT-LPDs occurring following allogeneic bone marrow transplantation are ideal candidates for adoptive immunotherapy. Unselected populations of peripheral blood lymphocytes from the donor, containing EBV-specific T cells, have been used (Heslop et al., 1994; Papadopoulos et al., 1994). However, this treatment led to complications that arose from the presence of alloreactive T cells in the infusions. Subsequently, preparations of EBV-specific T-cell lines from donor lymphocytes have been generated (Orentas et al., 1998) and used successfully in the prophylaxis and treatment of PT-LPDs in bone marrow transplant recipients (Rooney et al., 1998). More efficient and faster methods for the production of EBV-specific CTLs are being developed, such as the use of EBV-loaded dendritic cells (Wheatley et al., 1998; Gottschalk et al., 2003; Bollard et al., 2004).

Manipulation of antigen presentation has also been explored. The lack of immune recognition of EBV-associated BLs is secondary to inefficient processing of class I-restricted cytotoxic T-lymphocyte (CTL) epitopes because of a loss of peptide transporters (TAP) and major histocompatibility expression (Masucci and Klein, 1991). CD40 engagement has been reported to upregulate TAP-1 and HLA class I expression in BL cells, allowing recognition by virus-specific CTLs (Khanna et al., 1997). Therefore, treatment with CD40 ligand has been proposed as a potential approach to allow the use of immunotherapy for the treatment of EBV-related BLs.

Several approaches have been evaluated to manipulate latently infected tumor cells to express viral antigens. Expression of the Latency I EBNA1 transcript, and repression of Latency III transcripts in Burkitt's lymphomas is thought to result from differences in CpG methylation of the relevant promoters (Tao et al., 1998b). Therefore, it may be possible to induce changes in the methylation status of the EBV promoters, resulting in the induction of expression of immunogenic Latency III proteins followed by anti-tumor immune response. One recent study reported that in a clinical trial with 5-azacitidine, reversal of dense CpG methylation in tumor tissues was obtained, suggesting that his effect can be achieved in patients (Chan et al., 2004). Novel therapies EBV-associated lymphomas have also been proposed based on intentional induction of the lytic form of EBV infection combined with treatment with antiviral agents, for example the nucleoside analogue ganciclovir (GCV). GCV is only active in the presence of virally encoded kinases, which are expressed only during the lytic form of infection, and convert GCV into its active, cytotoxic form. Two drugs were reported to induce lytic EBV infection in EBV-transformed B cells: gemcitabine and doxorubicin (but not 5-azacytidine, cis-platinum, or 5-fluorouracil). The combination of gemcitabine or doxorubicin and GCV was significantly more effective for the inhibition of EBV-driven lymphoproliferative disease in SCID mice than chemotherapy alone, suggesting that the addition of GCV to either gemcitabine- or doxorubicin-containing chemotherapy regimens may enhance the therapeutic efficacy of these drugs for EBV-driven lymphoproliferative disease (Feng et al., 2004). A recent study evaluated a different approach to combine and antiviral effect with modulation of EBV gene expression. Azidothymidine (AZT) was found to induce apoptosis in early passage EBV positive BL (Kurokawa et al., 2005). This effect was found to be due to NF-κB inhibition, followed by upregulation of EBV gene expression including viral thymidine kinase (vTK) and apoptosis. Phosphorylation, as well as apoptosis, was markedly enhanced in the presence of hydroxyurea so AZT in combination with hydroxyurea may represent an inexpensive, targeted regimen for endemic BL.

Specific targeting of cellular pathways involved in viral lymphomagenesis are also being explored for therapeutic application. Inhibition of NF-κB by pharmacological inhibitors leads to apoptosis of

EBV infected tumor cells in vitro (Cahir-McFarland et al., 2004), (Keller and Cesarman, manuscript in preparation). As this transcription factor is activated by LMP-1 and LMP-2A, it is possible that signals stemming from expression of these viral proteins are involved in survival of infected tumor cells, and these two viral proteins may represent future virus-specific therapeutic targets.

3. KAPOSI'S SARCOMA-ASSOCIATED HERPESVIRUS (KSHV)

3.1 Kaposi's sarcoma-associated herpesvirus and lymphomagenesis

Kaposi's sarcoma-associated herpesvirus is found invariably in Kaposi's sarcoma, and compelling evidence suggests that it is an etiologic agent for this disease (Boshoff and Weiss, 1998). KSHV is also present in several lymphoproliferative disorders that include primary effusion lymphoma (PEL), multicentric Castleman's disease (MCD) and MCD-associated plasmablastic lymphoma.

Primary effusion lymphomas are a subset of malignant lymphomas that possess distinctive and unusual clinicopathologic features, including their presentation as lymphomatous effusions in body cavities, therefore being initially called body-cavity-based lymphomas (Cesarman et al., 1995a; Nador et al., 1996). Although they are more common in HIV-positive males, PELs also occur in HIV-negative men and women (Nador et al., 1995; Said et al., 1996). PELs contain many KSHV genomes, ranging between 40 to 80 copies per cell. The presence of KSHV in this subset of lymphomas allowed the development of cell lines that have been used as a tool for its propagation, and for serologic assays (Arvanitakis et al., 1996; Boshoff et al., 1998; Cesarman et al., 1995b; Renne et al., 1996). Purified virus from PEL cell lines has been used to demonstrate its ability to infect B-cells (Mesri et al., 1996) and endothelial cells (Cannon et al., 2000; Flore et al., 1998; Moses et al., 1999).

Because some KSHV-negative lymphomas, such as BL, can involve body cavities as lymphomatous effusions, and KSHV-positive lymphomas can present as solid-tissue masses, diagnostic criteria for PEL have been proposed (Cesarman and Knowles, 1999; Nador et al., 1996). These criteria include immunoblastic-anaplastic large-cell morphology, null-cell phenotype (including the lack of B cell-associated antigen and immunoglobulin expression in most cases), and B-cell genotype. The expression of

CD138/Syndecan-1 (Gaidano et al., 1997) and hypermutation of the immunoglobulin genes (Matolcsy et al., 1998) suggest that PELs are at a preterminal stage of B-cell differentiation. This assumption was more recently confirmed by gene expression profiling of PEL (Jenner et al., 2003; Klein et al., 2003), where PEL resembled plasma cells, and had a profile between multiple myeloma and EBV-associated immunoblastic lymphoma.

Lymphomas containing KSHV can also present as solid tissue masses, similar to other AIDS-related non-Hodgkin's lymphomas. While some of these lymphomas subsequently develop an effusion, others apparently do not. They usually present as solid extranodal lymphomas and are diagnosed as diffuse large cell, immunoblastic, or anaplastic large cell lymphomas, in which the presence of KSHV in practically all the lymphoma cells could be demonstrated by immunohistochemistry or molecular techniques (Carbone et al., 2005; Chadburn et al., 2004; Deloose et al., 2005; Engels et al., 2003). Most of these are immunoblastic in appearance, have a high mitotic rate and variable amounts off apoptotic debris. These lymphomas appear to fall in the spectrum of PEL, as they usually lack expression of B cell antigens and immunoglobulin, they have a similar morphology, and they are frequently co-infected with EBV.

Plasmablastic lymphomas, associated with multicentric Castleman's disease, have also been described in HIV positive patients (Dupin et al., 2000). While these plasmablastic lymphomas are KSHV positive, they differ from PEL in a number of ways. Plasmablastic lymphomas are EBV negative, do not contain mutations in the Ig genes, and are thought to arise from naive IgM lambda-expressing B cells rather than terminally differentiated B cells (Du et al., 2001). In addition, KSHV has been documented in germinotropic lymphoproliferative disorders in HIV-negative patients (Du et al., 2002), suggesting that this virus is present in a heterogenous but distinct group of lymphoproliferative diseases, and may be more common than previously thought.

3.2   Molecular oncogenesis of primary effusion lymphomas

The almost invariable presence of KSHV in PELs suggests that it is necessary for their development. However, PELs are rare tumors, even in populations with high KSHV seroprevalence, accounting for about 3% of AIDS-related lymphomas and 0.4% of all AIDS unrelated diffuse large cell NHLs (Carbone et al., 1996). Therefore, it is evident that KSHV infection represents only one of several events involved in the development of PEL. Another co-factor appears to be EBV, because most PELs contain both viral genomes. The majority of PELs in vivo, as well as in culture, are latently infected with both viruses, but there is a small proportion of cells in which EBV and/or KSHV productive infection takes place. Analysis of the pattern of EBV gene expression in PELs revealed that only EBNA1 was expressed, corresponding to Latency I (Horenstein et al., 1997; Szekely et al., 1998). In addition, PELs lack structural alterations in most cellular-transforming genes frequently involved in lymphomagenesis, with the possible exception of mutation in the regulatory region of Bcl-6 (Carbone et al., 1998; Nador et al., 1996). These observations suggest that KSHV plays a transforming role in PELs. In addition, expression of single latent KSHV gene, vFLIP, is completely essential for PEL cell survival [(Guasparri et al., 2004); see below].

Molecular mechanisms of Kaposi sarcoma-associated herpesvirus-induced lymphomagenesis

The majority of primary effusion lymphomas are latently infected by KSHV. Latency allows the virus to remain in the infected cell, ensuring that the cell survives and is not recognized as infected by the host immune system. Upon initial infection, KSHV produces viral proteins that inhibit innate antiviral responses, and subsequently during latency it produces a protein that ensures maintenance of viral DNA in the form of extrachromosomal circles, called episomes, in dividing cells. It also produces proteins during latency that promote survival of the infected cells. Since promotion of cell survival is a main feature of cancer, it is not surprising that KSHV is associated with malignancies.

3.3   Latent viral proteins

Six major KSHV proteins have been confirmed to be produced in latently-infected lymphoma cells. They are called LANA-1, vCyclin (vCYC), vFLIP, vIL-6, LANA-2 (or vIRF-3). Other proteins have also been reported to be expressed during latency (like K15 and the Kaposins), but this data is either controversial or not confirmed at the protein level. Many of these genes bear potential to participate in lymphomagenesis and the maintenance of the malignant phenotype by affecting cellular survival, and/or proliferation. Their function is illustrated in Figure 2, and can be summarized as follows:

LANA-1: This protein, essential for episome maintenance, has been shown to have the ability to transform cells. LANA-1 has the ability to affect several pathways that are involved in tumorigenesis: it can bind and inactivate the retinoblastoma (Rb) protein (Radkov et al., 2000), and similarly bind and inactivate p53 (Friborg et al., 1999). LANA-1 can also bind and inactivate GSK3β, leading to activation of the β-catenin pathway involved in solid tumors (Fujimuro and Hayward, 2004). It has also been show to have transcriptional effects on a variety of genes.

LANA-2 (vIRF-3): This protein was shown to potently inhibit p53 in reporter assays (Rivas et al., 2001), and thus may be involved in deregulation of apoptosis. Although LANA-2 is not a DNA-binding protein, it is recruited to the interferon promoters via its interaction with cellular IRF-3 and IRF-7, and stimulates their transcriptional activity (Lubyova et al., 2004).

vIL-6: This is sometimes considered to be a lytic gene because its expression is increased upon lytic reactivation. However, it is expressed by a variable but significant proportion of latently-infected PEL cells. Considering the fact that this protein can be secreted, it may affect other tumor cells that don't express it, and play a role in their proliferation. vIL-6 differs from cellular IL-6 in that it is selectively glycosylated and can bind the gp130 receptor in the absence of the high affinity IL-6 receptor to activate IL-6-responsive genes and promote B-cell survival (Molden et al., 1997; Moore et al., 1996; Nicholas et al., 1997).

vCYC: This protein is a functional cyclin that can associate with CDK6 and induce phosphorylation of retinoblastoma (Rb) protein and overcome Rb-mediated cell-cycle arrest (Godden-Kent et al., 1997; Li et al., 1997). vCYC differs from the cellular cyclin D in its ability to induce degradation of the CDK inhibitor p27Kip when complexed with CDK6 (Ellis et al., 1999; Mann et al., 1999). Therefore, vCYC is likely to modulate cell cycle in PEL cells, avoiding normal regulatory checkpoints. Transgenic mice with vCYC develop lymphomas, but only in the absence of p53, and a model has been proposed whereby vCYC induces genome instability and that loss of p53 subsequently allows expansion of tumorigenic clones (Verschuren et al., 2004; Verschuren et al., 2002).

vFLIP (K13): This protein is homologous to cFLIP, that is an inhibitor of the pro-apoptotic molecule FLICE/Caspase-8 (Thome et al., 1997). vFLIP can activate NF-κB though both the classical and alternative pathways (Chaudhary et al., 1999; Matta and Chaudhary, 2004), and through this mechanism induce expression of anti-apoptotic genes and protect cells from Fas-induced cell death in vitro and in vivo (Djerbi et al., 1999; Guasparri et al., 2004). vFLIP protects PEL cells from spontaneous apoptosis and is the first viral protein shown to be essential for tumor cell survival in vitro and in vivo (Guasparri et al., 2004, Godfrey et al., 2005).

3.4   Lytic viral proteins

Although mostly latent genes are expressed in PELs, some lytic genes are expressed to some extent in a minority of cells, and several of these have oncogenic potential. In addition, patterns of KSHV gene expression in de novo infection and during initial steps of lymphomagenesis are not known. These lytic genes encode for some functionally interesting proteins. The viral interferon regulatory factor 1 (K9, vIRF-1) (Li et al., 1998), the viral G protein-coupled receptor (ORF 74, vGPCR) (Bais et al., 1998), and ORF K1 (Lee et al., 1998b), can transform rodent cells and/or cause tumors in animal models. Three transmembrane proteins are potentially important in PEL lymphomagenesis because they can trigger signaling cascades relevant for B- and T-cell growth. These are:

vGPCR: This is a constitutively active G protein-coupled receptor able to trigger the mitogen-activated protein (MAP) kinase signaling cascades and induce secretion of vascular endothelial growth factor (VEGF) (Bais et al., 1998). MAP kinase cascades such as those triggered by vGPCR are activated by inflammatory cytokines and mitogens. VEGF is an angiogenic and vascular permeability factor that could contribute to the effusion phenotype (Aoki and Tosato, 1999). In PEL cells, vGPCR can activate a variety of signaling cascades activating the transcription factors AP-1, NF-κB, CREB and NFAT (Cannon et al., 2003; Cannon and Cesarman, 2004).

K1: This protein has an ITAM motif that can activate cytoplasmic tyrosine kinases and mimic signaling by the B-cell antigen receptor (Lee et al., 1998a). K15 contains a variable number of transmembrane regions and cytoplasmic SH2 and SH3 domains. K1 can activate the MAP kinase and NF-κB signaling pathways and have potential antiapoptotic functions (Brinkmann et al., 2003; Sharp et al., 2002). K15 has also been shown to activate the Akt and Src kinases (Prakash et al., 2005; Tomlinson and Damania, 2004). Therefore, like vGPCR it appears to have very broad signaling capabilities.

K15: This open reading frame encodes a protein with complex splicing and multiple transmembrane motifs, structurally resembling EBV LMP-2A. It has SH2 and SH3 motifs, and also a TRAF binding motif, and can also activate signaling cascades that include NF-κB and MAP kinase (Brinkmann et al., 2003). Also like EBV LMP-2A, K15 can inhibit B cell receptor signaling (Choi et al., 2000). K15 protein has been found to be present in most latently infected cells by one study (Sharp et al., 2002), but the RNA expression data is controversial, most studies arguing for lytic expression. K15 has been proposed to have anti-apoptotic functions (Sharp et al., 2002).

Other interesting molecules that expressed during lytic replication and have a potential role in PEL pathogenesis are:

vIRF1: this protein can inhibit interferon-induced transcriptional activation (Li et al., 1998; Zimring et al., 1998).

vBCL-2 (ORF16): This protein is homologous to cellular BCL-2, which is involved a cellular oncogene involved in the development of follicular lymphomas. vBCL-2 can block apoptosis as efficiently as cellular Bcl-2, Bcl-xL, or the EBV Bcl-2 homologue, BHRF1 (Cheng et al., 1997). Interestingly, the KSHV Bcl-2 cannot homodimerize nor heterodimerize with other Bcl-2 family members, suggesting that it may have evolved to escape any negative regulatory effects of the cellular Bax and Bak proteins.

3.5   Therapeutic approaches for KSHV-associated lymphomas

Survival of PEL patients with conventional chemotherapy is dismal, so it is important to develop novel therapeutic approaches. A promising cellular target is the transcription factor NF-κB, that is constitutively active in PEL cells, and pharmacologic inhibition with Bay 11-7082 leads to tumor cell apoptosis (Keller et al., 2000). In addition, in a mouse model of PEL, treatment with Bay 11-7082 results in improved survival and cures in some mice (Keller et al., manuscript in preparation). While this particular inhibitor is not being pursued with therapeutic intent, other compounds such as the proteosomal inhibitor Bortezomib (Velcade) affect NF-κB, and may be useful for the treatment of PEL. A promising new approach, that also targets the NF-κB pathway, is the combination of AZT and IFN-alpha. This approach has been proven effective in one reported patient with PEL and has the advantage of using available and clinically approved agents (Ghosh et al., 2003).

While cellular targets, such as NF-κB have the advantage that they are being developed at a rapid pace for other diseases, in particular other cancers and inflammation, viral targets would have the added advantage of specificity and low toxicity. KSHV encodes several genes that can activate NF-κB, but only vFLIP is largely responsible for the constitutive NF-κB activity in PEL cells. Elimination of vFLIP results in marked reduction of NF-κB, decreased in expression of NF-κB-regulated genes and cellular apoptosis (Guasparri et al., 2004). Therefore, vFLIP functions as a viral oncogene is KSHV lymphomagenesis, and is a promising therapeutic target.

4. HUMAN T-CELL LYMPHOTROPIC VIRUS-1 (HTLV-1)

4.1 Human T-cell Lymphotropic Virus-1 and Adult T-cell Leukemia/Lymphoma

Human T-cell lymphotropic virus-1, the first described human lymphotropic retrovirus (Poiesz et al., 1980), is the etiologic agent for adult T-cell leukemia/lymphoma (ATLL). This is an often aggressive malignancy of mature CD4+ lymphocytes. Four clinical subtypes of ATLL are recognized: acute, chronic, lymphomatous, and smoldering. The typical acute form of ATLL is characterized clinically by generalized lymph node, peripheral blood, and skin involvement by pleomorphic tumor cells with hyperlobated nuclei, lytic bone lesions, hypercalcemia, rapidly progressive clinical course, and relatively short survival (Watanabe et al., 1992). The nature of the T-cell tropism of HTLV-I is still unsolved. The receptor for HTLV-I was recently identified as the glucose transporter 1 (GLUT1), which is expressed in a wide variety of cells. Therefore, it is likely that HTLV-1 infects T cell preferentially not only by the presence of GLUT1, but also by the ability of the virus to interact with the intracellular host machinery and lead to a successful infection. Cumulative evidence points to HTLV-1 as the causal agent of ATLL (Cann and Chen, 1996; Dalgleish, 1998) : 1) seroepidemiologic studies show a close association between ATLL and HTLV-1 infection; 2) throughout malignant progression ATLL cell clonality or oligoclonality correlates with the clonality or oligoclonality of retroviral insertion; 3) HTLV-1 can transform T cells in vitro resulting in immortalized cell lines; and 4) HLTV-1 can induce cancers in animal models.

4.2 Human T-cell lymphotropic virus-1 mediated oncogenesis

Human T-cell lymphotropic virus-1 seems to play a role in the early steps of ATLL malignant progression and not necessarily in the maintenance of the transformed phenotype (Cann and Chen, 1996), because ATLL tumor cells lack expression of HTLV-1 genes (Reitz et al., 1983) and carry viral genomes that tend to be heavily deleted (Yoshida et al., 1985; Yoshida et al., 1984). ATLL tumor cells do have oncogenic alterations in p53 (Cesarman et al., 1992; Pise-Masison et al., 1998b) and CDKN2/p16 tumor suppressor genes (Uchida et al., 1998) and chromosomal aberrations (Fukuhara et al., 1983; Maruyama et al., 1990), the complexity of which correlates with tumor aggressiveness (Sanada et al., 1985). Therefore, oncogenesis of ATLL seems to involve an HTLV-1-dependent step in which transformation of T cells results in a polyclonal population of proliferating immortalized T cells, with subsequent acquisition of new oncogenic genetic alterations, clonal expansion, and progression to full malignancy and HTVL-1 independence (Cann and Chen, 1996) (Fig. 3). In contrast to other animal retroviruses that transform cells by transduction of oncogenes or activation of oncogenes adjacent to insertion sites, HTLV-1 transforms T cells by a rather complex mechanism that is mediated by its transactivator protein Tax (Cann and Chen, 1996; Felber et al., 1985; Flint and Shenk, 1997; Hiscott et al., 1995). Evidence supporting an oncogenic role for Tax stems from its ability to induce T-cell immortalization (Grassmann et al., 1992; Grassmann et al., 1989) and mesenchymal tumors in transgenic mice (Hinrichs et al., 1987; Nerenberg et al., 1987). Transgenic mice in which the expression of Tax was specifically targeted to T cells developed a large granular T-cell lymphocytic leukemia (Grossman et al., 1995).

4.3   Tax Mediated Transactivation and Human T-cell Leukemia Virus-1 Oncogenesis

Although HTLV-1 Tax is not generally able to directly interact with DNA (Cann and Chen, 1996; Lenzmeier et al., 1998), it is able to exert powerful biologic responses by increasing the activity of transcription factors that are able to transactivate both the HTLV-1 LTR and genes involved in T-cell proliferation (Felber et al., 1985; Flint and Shenk, 1997; Hiscott et al., 1995). Tax can interact with members of the NF-κB family of transcription factors (Cann and Chen, 1996; Flint and Shenk, 1997; Leung and Nabel, 1988; Ruben et al., 1988), its physiological IκB inhibitors (Nicot et al., 1998; Petropoulos and Hiscott, 1998), and its activating kinases (Geleziunas et al., 1998), leading to increased transcription from NF-κB responsive promoters. NF-κB can activate transcription of many genes related to T-cell proliferation and growth such as c-rel, c-myc, and both IL-2 and IL-2 receptor. Simultaneous activation of IL-2 and its receptor can lead to IL-2-independent proliferation of T cells expressing Tax (Iwanaga et al., 1999). Although not all HTLV-1 transformed cells express IL-2, the creation of an IL-2 autocrine loop by Tax may be important in the early stages of malignant progression (Cann and Chen, 1996) (Fig. 3). Additionally, expression SHP-1, a physiologic inhibitor of the IL-2/Jak/Stat signaling pathway is repressed in HTLV-1-transformed cells (Migone et al., 1998). Another group of transcription factors activated by Tax is the cAMP Responsive Element Binding proteins (CREB/ATF-1), a family of bZIP transcription factors (Bantignies et al., 1996; Flint and Shenk, 1997; Yin et al., 1995). Although CREB is normally modulated by protein kinase A (PKA) activity, recent studies suggest that Tax can activate the CREB-mediated transcription in a PKA-independent manner (Gachon et al., 1998). Tax also regulates the activity of many other transcription factors by affecting their interaction with the general transcriptional-coactivator CREB-binding protein (CBP/p300) (Flint and Shenk, 1997; Harrod et al., 1998; Kwok et al., 1996). The importance of the CREB-regulating activity of Tax in transformation is stressed by a study showing that although the NF-κB transactivating activity may be dispensable in a model of Tax transformation, CREB activity is not (Rosin et al., 1998). The potential of Tax for oncogenesis is further stressed by its ability to promote cell cycle entry by CDK activation (Neuveut et al., 1998; Schmitt et al., 1998; Sieburg et al., 2004) and to impair activity of the p53 tumor suppressor gene (Mahieux et al., 2000; Mulloy et al., 1998; Pise-Masison et al., 1998a). The consequence of de-regulating cell-cycle checkpoints, and inhibiting cell-cycle arrest and apoptosis in response to genotoxic stress, is genetic instability. Indeed, it was found that Tax expression increases the mutation rate in the cellular genome (Miyake et al., 1999), and therefore its likelihood of acquiring oncogenic alterations.

4.4   NF-κB Activation by Tax Plays a Central Role in HTLV-I Mediated Oncogenesis

It appears that HTLV-1 has evolved multiple strategies to subvert the NF-κB pathway, a major regulator of T-cell survival, activation, differentiation and proliferation (Yoshida, 2001). The canonical pathway of NF-κB involves IKK mediated IκB phosphorylation which leads to its degradation with release of NF-κB (Rel family) members that can translocate to the nucleus and activate transcription. A non-canonical pathway of NF-κB activation has more recently been described, which involves proteolytic cleavage of the Rel family member p100 to yield the active subunit, p52. It is regulated by the NF-κB inducing kinase NIK, which can regulate IKKalpha. HTLV-1 Tax can activate NF-κB both through the canonical or classical and the non-cannonical or alternative pathways. HTLV-I Tax can physically interact with IKKgamma and activate phosphorylation and degradation of IKKalpha and IKKbeta, thus activating NF-κB through the canonical pathway (Harhaj and Sun, 1999; Sun and Ballard, 1999). In addition, HTLV-I transformed cells consistently express p52 indicating that the non-cannonical NF-κB pathway is constitutively activated. Indeed, it was found that HTLV-1 Tax is able to stimulate p100 processing into p52 by bridging the interaction between p100 and IKKalpha (Xiao et al., 2001). The multiple roles that NF-κB could play in T-cell tumorigenesis, in addition to the multiple strategies devised by HTLV-I to subvert it, indicate that this pathway is critical for HTLV-1 mediated lymphomagenesis and therefore, it could be an attractive therapeutic target. Bay 11-7082, an NF-κB inhibitor that acts by inhibiting IκBα degradation, was shown to induce apoptosis of HTLV-1 infected T-cells but not uninfected T-cells or PMBC (Mori et al., 2002). Moreover, Bay 11-7082 efficiently suppressed ATLL tumor growth in a new model in immunodeficient NOD/SCID gamma-null (NOG) mice (Dewan et al., 2003). These data demonstrated the involvement of the NF-κB pathway in HTLV-1 tumorigenesis and point to NF-κB as an attractive target for therapy that can be inhibited to achieve selective cytotoxicity in HTLV-1-associated ATLL tumors

4.5   Hepatitis C Virus

Mounting epidemiological and experimental evidence suggests a role for hepatitis C virus (HCV) infection in the development of B cell lymphomas and mixed cryoglobulinemia. Over 50 studies epidemiologic are published evaluating the frequency of HCV infection in patients with lymphoma. The relative risk of B-cell NHL among HCV-positive individuals versus HCV-negative individuals appears to range from 2 to 4, although not all studies have reported a positive association between HCV and lymphoma, and geographical differences seem to be important [reviewed in(Negri et al., 2004)].. A recent multi-center case-control study showed positive associations with specific lymphoma typed, namely follicular, marginal zone and mucosa-associated lymphoid tissue (MALT) non-Hodgkin's lymphomas (Engels et al., 2004). One study found HCV-RNA in 37% of the lymphoma tissue samples, but this high incidence has not been confirmed by others and remains controversial (Paydas et al., 2004). However the possibility that on occasion lymphomas can contain the HCV genome is suggested by the report of a single B cell lymphoma cell line containing the replicating viral genome(Sung et al., 2003). In this cell line, genetic instability was observed and a hit-and-run mechanism has been proposed (Machida et al., 2004). However, most evidence suggests an indirect role resulting from antigenic stimulation; lymphomas in patients with HCV express a limited number of immunoglobulin sequences, suggesting an antigenic drive, and some lymphomas have been identified that actually express an antigen receptor that recognizes HCV (Weng and Levy, 2003). Treatment of HCV infection with antiviral agents (ribavirin plus interferon alph) has resulted in regression of a significant proportion of low-grade lymphomas in these patients (Hermine et al., 2002; Saadoun et al., 2005), strongly implicating antigen stimulation in the maintenance of the tumor.

Conclusions

EBV, KSHV and HTLV-1 are associated with specific subsets of malignant lymphomas, and accumulated evidence indicates that they play an etiopathogenic role in their development. Although these viruses differ in many respects, they all carry genes that subvert the host molecular machinery to deregulate cell growth and immortalize infected lymphoid cells, setting the stage for further genetic alterations to take place so that the cells will progress to full malignancy. However, their ability to transform cells and to lead to lymphomagenesis is highly dependent on host factors. Understanding the oncogenic and immunologic mechanisms involved in the pathobiology of virus-associated lymphomas is important for the development of targeted therapeutic and preventive approaches.

5.   ACKNOWLEDGEMENTS

Supported in part by the National Institutes of Health Grants CA68939, CA103646 and a Leukemia and Lymphoma Society Translational Research grant to EC and CA95718 to EAM.

6.   REFERENCES

1. Abed, N., Casper, J. T., Camitta, B. M., Margolis, D., Trost, B., Orentas, R., and Chang, C. C. (2004). Evaluation of histogenesis of B-lymphocytes in pediatric EBV-related post-transplant lymphoproliferative disorders. Bone Marrow Transplant *33*, 321-327.
2. Aoki, Y., and Tosato, G. (1999). Role of Vascular Endothelial Growth Factor/Vascular Permeability Factor in the Pathogenesis of Kaposi's Sarcoma-Associated Herpesvirus-Infected Primary Effusion Lymphomas. Blood *94*, 4247-4254.
3. Arvanitakis, L., Mesri, E. A., Nador, R., Said, J. W., Asch, A. S., Knowles, D. M., and Cesarman, E. (1996). Establishment and characterization of a primary effusion (body cavity-based) lymphoma cell line (BC-3) harboring Kaposi's sarcoma-associated herpesvirus (KSHV/HHV-8) in the absence of Epstin-Barr virus. Blood *88*, 2648-2654.
4. Babcock, G. J., Hochberg, D., and Thorley-Lawson, A. D. (2000). The expression pattern of Epstein-Barr virus latent genes in vivo is dependent upon the differentiation stage of the infected B cell. Immunity *13*, 497-506.
5. Bais, C., Santomasso, B., Coso, O., Arvanitakis, L., Geras Raaka, E., Gutkind, J. S., Asch, A. S., Cesarman, E., Gershengorn, M. C., and Mesri, E. (1998). G-protein-coupled receptor of Kaposi's sarcoma-associated herpesvirus is a viral oncogene and angiogenesis activator. Nature *391*, 86-89.
6. Bantignies, F., Rousset, R., Desbois, C., and Jalinot, P. (1996). Genetic characterization of transactivation of the human T-cell leukemia virus type 1 promoter: Binding of Tax to Tax-responsive element 1 is mediated by the cyclic AMP-responsive members of the CREB/ATF family of transcription factors. Mol Cell Biol *16*, 2174-2182.
7. Bollard CM, Straathof KC, Huls MH, Leen A, Lacuesta K, Davis A, Gottschalk S, Brenner MK, Heslop HE, Rooney CM (2004). The generation and characterization of LMP2-specific CTLs for use as adoptive transfer from patients with relapsed EBV-positive Hodgkin disease. J Immunother. 27:317-27.
8. Boshoff, C., Gao, S. J., Healy, L. E., Matthews, S., Thomas, A. J., Coignet, L., Warnke, R. A., Strauchen, J. A., Matutes, E., Kamel, O. W., *et al.* (1998). Establishing a KSHV+ cell line (BCP-1) from peripheral blood and characterizing its growth in Nod/SCID mice. Blood *91*, 1671-1679.
9. Boshoff, C., and Weiss, R. A. (1998). Kaposi's sarcoma-associated herpesvirus. Adv Cancer Res *75*, 57-86.
10. Brinkmann, M. M., Glenn, M., Rainbow, L., Kieser, A., Henke-Gendo, C., and Schulz, T. F. (2003). Activation of mitogen-activated protein kinase and NF-kappaB pathways by a Kaposi's sarcoma-associated herpesvirus K15 membrane protein. J Virol *77*, 9346-9358.
11. Cahir-McFarland, E. D., Carter, K., Rosenwald, A., Giltnane, J. M., Henrickson, S. E., Staudt, L. M., and Kieff, E. (2004). Role of NF-kappa B in cell survival and transcription of latent membrane protein 1-expressing or Epstein-Barr virus latency III-infected cells. J Virol *78*, 4108-4119.
12. Cahir-McFarland, E. D., Davidson, D. M., Schauer, S. L., Duong, J., and Kieff, E. (2000). NF-kappa B inhibition causes spontaneous apoptosis in Epstein-Barr virus-transformed lymphoblastoid cells. Proc Natl Acad Sci U S A *97*, 6055-6060.

13. Cann, A. J., and Chen, I. S. Y. (1996). Human T-cell leukemia virus types I and II. In Fields Virology, B. N. Fields, D. M. Knipe, and P. M. Howley, eds. (Philadelphia, Lippincott-Raven), pp. 1849-1880.
14. Cannon, J. S., Ciufo, D., Hawkins, A. L., Griffin, C. A., Borowitz, M. J., Hayward, G. S., and Ambinder, R. F. (2000). A new primary effusion lymphoma-derived cell line yields a highly infectious Kaposi's sarcoma herpesvirus-containing supernatant. J Virol *74*, 10187-10193.
15. Cannon, M., Philpott, N. J., and Cesarman, E. (2003). The Kaposi's sarcoma-associated herpesvirus G protein-coupled receptor has broad signaling effects in primary effusion lymphoma cells. J Virol *77*, 57-67.
16. Cannon, M. L., and Cesarman, E. (2004). The KSHV G protein-coupled receptor signals via multiple pathways to induce transcription factor activation in primary effusion lymphoma cells. Oncogene *23*, 514-523.
17. Carbone, A. (2003). Emerging pathways in the development of AIDS-related lymphomas. Lancet Oncol *4*, 22-29.
18. Carbone, A., Gaidano, G., Gloghini, A., Larocca, L. M., Capello, D., Canzonieri, V., Antinori, A., Tirelli, U., Falini, B., and Dalla-Favera, R. (1998). Differential expression of BCL-6, CD138/syndecan-1, and Epstein-Barr virus-encoded latent membrane protein-1 identifies distinct histogenetic subsets of acquired immunodeficiency syndrome-related non-Hodgkin's lymphomas. Blood *91*, 747-755.
19. Carbone, A., Gloghini, A., Vaccher, E., Cerri, M., Gaidano, G., Dalla-Favera, R., and Tirelli, U. (2005). Kaposi's sarcoma-associated herpesvirus/human herpesvirus type 8-positive solid lymphomas: a tissue-based variant of primary effusion lymphoma. J Mol Diagn *7*, 17-27.
20. Carbone, A., Gloghini, A., Vaccher, E., Zagonel, V., Pastore, C., Dalla Palma, P., Branz, F., Saglio, G., Volpe, R., Tirelli, U., and Gaidano, G. (1996). Kaposi's sarcoma-associated herpesvirus DNA sequences in AIDS-related and AIDS-unrelated lymphomatous effusions. Br J Haematol *94*, 533-543.
21. Cesarman, E., Chadburn, A., Inghirami, G., Gaidano, G., and Knowles, D. M. (1992). Structural and functional analysis of oncogenes and tumor suppressor genes in adult T-cell leukemia/lymphoma shows frequent p53 mutations. Blood *80*, 3205-3216.
22. Cesarman, E., Chadburn, A., Liu, Y. F., Migliazza, A., Dalla-Favera, R., and Knowles, D. M. (1998). BCL-6 gene mutations in posttransplantation lymphoproliferative disorders predict response to therapy and clinical outcome. Blood *92*, 2294-2302.
23. Cesarman, E., Chang, Y., Moore, P. S., Said, J. W., and Knowles, D. M. (1995a). Kaposi's Sarcoma-associated Herpesvirus-like DNA sequences in AIDS-related body cavity-based lymphomas. N Eng J Med *332*, 1186-1191.
24. Cesarman, E., and Knowles, D. M. (1999). The role of Kaposi's sarcoma-associated herpesvirus (KSHV/HHV-8) in lymphoproliferative diseases. Semin Cancer Biol *9*, 165-174.
25. Cesarman, E., Moore, P. S., Rao, P., Inghirami, G., Knowles, D. M., and Chang, Y. (1995b). In vitro establishment and characterization of two acquired immunodeficiency syndrome-related lymphoma cell lines (BC-1 and BC-2) containing Kaposi's sarcoma-associated herpesvirus-like (KSHV) DNA sequences. Blood *86*, 2708-2714.
26. Chadburn, A., Hyjek, E., Frizzera, G., Schulman, H., Pan, L., Cesarman, E., and Knowles, D. M. (2000). Post-transplantation lymphoproliferative disorders (PT-LPDs) in bone marrow and solid organ transplant recipients differ. Blood *96 suppl 1*, 505a.

27. Chadburn, A., Hyjek, E., Mathew, S., Cesarman, E., Said, J., and Knowles, D. M. (2004). KSHV-positive solid lymphomas represent an extra-cavitary variant of primary effusion lymphoma. Am J Surg Pathol *28*, 1401-1416.

28. Chadburn, A., Hyjek, E., Pan, L., Liu, Y. F., Frizzera, G., Schulman, H., Cesarman, E., and Knowles, D. M. (2001). Bcl-6 gene mutations in bone marrow transplantation (BMT). Mod Pathol *14*, 167A.

29. Chan, A. T., Tao, Q., Robertson, K. D., Flinn, I. W., Mann, R. B., Klencke, B., Kwan, W. H., Leung, T. W., Johnson, P. J., and Ambinder, R. F. (2004). Azacitidine induces demethylation of the Epstein-Barr virus genome in tumors. J Clin Oncol *22*, 1373-1381.

30. Chaudhary, P. M., Jasmin, A., Eby, M. T., and Hood, L. (1999). Modulation of the NF-kappa B pathway by virally encoded death effector domains-containing proteins. Oncogene *14*, 5738-5746.

31. Cheng, E. H. Y., Nicholas, J., Bellows, D. S., Hayward, G. S., Guo, H. G., Reitz, M. S., and Hardwick, J. M. (1997). A Bcl-2 homolog encoded by Kaposi sarcoma-associated virus, human herpesvirus 8, inhibits apoptosis but does not heterodimerize with Bax or Bak. Proc Natl Acad Sci USA *94*, 690-694.

32. Chodosh, J., Holder, V. P., Gan, Y. J., Belgaumi, A., Sample, J., and Sixbey, J. W. (1998). Eradication of latent Epstein-Barr virus by hydroxyurea alters the growth-transformed cell phenotype. J Infect Dis *177*, 1194-1201.

33. Choi, J. K., Lee, B. S., Shim, S. N., Li, M., and Jung, J. U. (2000). Identification of the novel K15 gene at the rightmost end of the Kaposi's sarcoma-associated herpesvirus genome. J Virol *74*, 436-446.

34. Dalgleish, A. G. (1998). Human T-Ccell lymphotropic virus type 1 - Infections and pathogenesis. Current Opinion in Infectious Diseases *11*, 195-199.

35. Deloose, S. T., Smit, L. A., Pals, F. T., Kersten, M. J., van Noesel, C. J., and Pals, S. T. (2005). High incidence of Kaposi sarcoma-associated herpesvirus infection in HIV-related solid immunoblastic/plasmablastic diffuse large B-cell lymphoma. Leukemia *19*, 851-855.

36. Devergne, O., McFarland, E. C., Mosialos, G., Izumi, K. M., Ware, C. F., and Kieff, E. (1998). Role of the TRAF binding site and NF-kappaB activation in Epstein-Barr virus latent membrane protein 1-induced cell gene expression. J Virol *72*, 7900-7908.

37. Dewan, M. Z., Terashima, K., Taruishi, M., Hasegawa, H., Ito, M., Tanaka, Y., Mori, N., Sata, T., Koyanagi, Y., Maeda, M., *et al.* (2003). Rapid tumor formation of human T-cell leukemia virus type 1-infected cell lines in novel NOD-SCID/gammac(null) mice: suppression by an inhibitor against NF-kappaB. J Virol *77*, 5286-5294.

38. Dickens, M., Rogers, J. S., Cavanagh, J., Raitano, A., Xia, Z., Halpern, J. R., Greenberg, M. E., Sawyers, C. L., and Davis, R. J. (1997). A cytoplasmic inhibitor of the JNK signal transduction pathway. Science *277*, 693-696.

39. Djerbi, M., Screpanti, V., Catrina, A. I., Bogen, B., Biberfeld, P., and Grandien, A. (1999). The inhibitor of death receptor signaling, FLICE-inhibitory protein defines a new class of tumor progression factors [see comments]. J Exp Med *190*, 1025-1032.

40. Du, M. Q., Diss, T. C., Liu, H., Ye, H., Hamoudi, R. A., Cabecadas, J., Dong, H. Y., Harris, N. L., Chan, J. K., Rees, J. W., *et al.* (2002). KSHV- and EBV-associated germinotropic lymphoproliferative disorder. Blood *100*, 3415-3418.

41. Du, M. Q., Liu, H., Diss, T. C., Ye, H., Hamoudi, R. A., Dupin, N., Meignin, V., Oksenhendler, E., Boshoff, C., and Isaacson, P. G. (2001). Kaposi sarcoma-associated herpesvirus infects monotypic (IgM lambda) but polyclonal naive B cells in Castleman disease and associated lymphoproliferative disorders. Blood *97*, 2130-2136.

42. Dupin, N., Diss, T. L., Kellam, P., Tulliez, M., Du, M. Q., Sicard, D., Weiss, R. A., Isaacson, P. G., and Boshoff, C. (2000). HHV-8 is associated with a plasmablastic variant of Castleman disease that is linked to HHV-8-positive plasmablastic lymphoma. Blood *95*, 1406-1412.

43. Elenitoba-Johnson, K. S., Zarate-Osorno, A., Meneses, A., Krenacs, L., Kingma, D. W., Raffeld, M., and Jaffe, E. S. (1998). Cytotoxic granular protein expression, Epstein-Barr virus strain type, and latent membrane protein-1 oncogene deletions in nasal T- lymphocyte/natural killer cell lymphomas from Mexico. Mod Pathol *11*, 754-761.

44. Eliopoulos, A. G., Blake, S. M., Floettmann, J. E., Rowe, M., and Young, L. S. (1999). Epstein-Barr virus-encoded latent membrane protein 1 activates the JNK pathway through its extreme C terminus via a mechanism involving TRADD and TRAF2. Journal of Virology *73*, 1023-1035.

45. Ellerman, V., and Bang, O. (1908). Experimentelle Leukamie bei Huhnern. Zentalbl Bakteriol Alet I *46*, 595-597.

46. Ellis, M., Chew, Y. P., Fallis, L., Freddersdorf, S., Boshoff, C., Weiss, R. A., Lu, X., and Mittnacht, S. (1999). Degradation of p27(Kip) cdk inhibitor triggered by Kaposi's sarcoma virus cyclin-cdk6 complex [In Process Citation]. Embo J *18*, 644-653.

47. Engels, E. A., Chatterjee, N., Cerhan, J. R., Davis, S., Cozen, W., Severson, R. K., Whitby, D., Colt, J. S., and Hartge, P. (2004). Hepatitis C virus infection and non-Hodgkin lymphoma: results of the NCI-SEER multi-center case-control study. Int J Cancer *111*, 76-80.

48. Engels, E. A., Pittaluga, S., Whitby, D., Rabkin, C., Aoki, Y., Jaffe, E. S., and Goedert, J. J. (2003). Immunoblastic lymphoma in persons with AIDS-associated Kaposi's sarcoma: a role for Kaposi's sarcoma-associated herpesvirus. Mod Pathol *16*, 424-429.

49. Felber, B. K., Paskalis, H., Kleinman-Ewing, C., Wong-Staal, F., and Pavlakis, G. N. (1985). The pX protein of HTLV-I is a transcriptional activator of its long terminal repeats. Science *229*, 675-679.

50. Feng, W. H., Hong, G., Delecluse, H. J., and Kenney, S. C. (2004). Lytic induction therapy for Epstein-Barr virus-positive B-cell lymphomas. J Virol *78*, 1893-1902.

51. Feuillard, J., Schuhmacher, M., Kohanna, S., Asso-Bonnet, M., Ledeur, F., Joubert-Caron, R., Bissieres, P., Polack, A., Bornkamm, G. W., and Raphael, M. (2000). Inducible loss of NF-kappaB activity is associated with apoptosis and Bcl-2 down-regulation in Epstein-Barr virus-transformed B lymphocytes. Blood *95*, 2068-2075.

52. Flint, J., and Shenk, T. (1997). Viral transactivating proteins. Annual Review of Genetics *31*, 177-212.

53. Flore, O., Rafii, S., Ely, S., O'Leary, J. J., Hyjek, E. M., and Cesarman, E. (1998). Transformation of primary human endothelial cells by Kaposi's sarcoma-associated herpesvirus. Nature *394*, 588-592.

54. Friborg, J., Jr., Kong, W., Hottiger, M. O., and Nabel, G. J. (1999). p53 inhibition by the LANA protein of KSHV protects against cell death. Nature *402*, 889-894.

55. Fujimuro, M., and Hayward, S. D. (2004). Manipulation of glycogen-synthase kinase-3 activity in KSHV-associated cancers. J Mol Med.

56. Fukuhara, S., Hinuma, Y., Gotoh, Y. I., and Uchino, H. (1983). Chromosome aberrations in T lymphocytes carrying adult T-cell leukemia-associated antigens (ATLA) from healthy adults. Blood *61*, 205-207.

57. Gachon, F., Peleraux, A., Thebault, S., Dick, J., Lemasson, I., Devaux, C., and Mesnard, J. M. (1998). CREB-2, a cellular CRE-dependent transcription

repressor, functions in association with Tax as an activator of the human T-cell leukemia virus type 1 promoter. J Virol *72*, 8332-8337.

58. Gaidano, G., Carbone, A., and Dalla-Favera, R. (1998). Genetic basis of acquired immunodeficiency syndrome-related lymphomagenesis. J Natl Cancer Inst Monogr, 95-100.

59. Gaidano, G., Gloghini, A., Gattei, V., Rossi, M. F., Cilia, A. M., Godeas, C., Degan, M., Perin, T., Canzonieri, V., Aldinucci, D., *et al.* (1997). Association of Kaposi's sarcoma-associated herpesvirus-positive primary effusion lymphoma with expression of the CD138/syndecan-1 antigen. Blood *90*, 4894-4900.

60. Geleziunas, R., Ferrell, S., Lin, X., Mu, Y., Cunningham, E. T., Jr., Grant, M., Connelly, M. A., Hambor, J. E., Marcu, K. B., and Greene, W. C. (1998). Human T-cell leukemia virus type 1 Tax induction of NF-kappaB involves activation of the IkappaB kinase alpha (IKKalpha) and IKKbeta cellular kinases. Mol Cell Biol *18*, 5157-5165.

61. Ghosh, S. K., Wood, C., Boise, L. H., Mian, A. M., Deyev, V. V., Feuer, G., Toomey, N. L., Shank, N. C., Cabral, L., Barber, G. N., *et al.* (2003). Potentiation of TRAIL-induced apoptosis in primary effusion lymphoma through azidothymidine-mediated inhibition of NF-kappa B. Blood *101*, 2321-2327.

62. Godden-Kent, D., Talbot, S. J., Boshoff, C., Chang, Y., Moore, P., Weiss, R. A., and Mittnacht, S. (1997). The cyclin encoded by Kaposi's sarcoma-associated herpesvirus stimulates cdk6 to phosphorylate the retinoblastoma protein and histone H1. J Virol *71*, 4193-4198.

63. Godfrey A, Anderson J, Papanastasiou A, Takeuchi Y, Boshoff C. (2005). Related Articles,LinksInhibiting primary effusion lymphoma by lentiviral vectors encoding short hairpin RNA. Blood 105:2510-8.

64. Gottschalk S, Edwards OL, Sili U, Huls MH, Goltsova T, Davis AR, Heslop HE, Rooney CM (2003). Generating CTLs against the subdominant Epstein-Barr virus LMP1 antigen for the adoptive immunotherapy of EBV-associated malignancies.

65. Blood 101:1905-12

66. Grassmann, R., Berchtold, S., Radant, I., Alt, M., Fleckenstein, B., Sodroski, J. G., Haseltine, W. A., and Ramstedt, U. (1992). Role of human T-cell leukemia virus type 1 X region proteins in immortalization of primary human lymphocytes in culture. J Virol *66*, 4570-4575.

67. Grassmann, R., Dengler, C., Muller-Fleckenstein, I., Fleckenstein, B., McGuire, K., Dokhelar, M. C., Sodroski, J. G., and Haseltine, W. A. (1989). Transformation to continuous growth of primary human T lymphocytes by human T-cell leukemia virus type I X-region genes transduced by a Herpesvirus saimiri vector. Proc Natl Acad Sci U S A *86*, 3351-3355.

68. Grossman, S. R., Johannsen, E., Tong, X., Yalamanchili, R., and Kieff, E. (1994). The Epstein-Barr virus nuclear antigen 2 transactivator is directed to response elements by the J kappa recombination signal binding protein. Proc Natl Acad Sci U S A *91*, 7568-7572.

69. Grossman, W. J., Kimata, J. T., Wong, F. H., Zutter, M., Ley, T. J., and Ratner, L. (1995). Development of leukemia in mice transgenic for the tax gene of human T-cell leukemia virus type I. Proc Natl Acad Sci U S A *92*, 1057-1061.

70. Guasparri, I., Keller, S. A., and Cesarman, E. (2004). KSHV vFLIP Is Essential for the Survival of Infected Lymphoma Cells. J Exp Med *199*, 993-1003.

71. Harhaj, E. W., and Sun, S. C. (1999). IKKgamma serves as a docking subunit of the IkappaB kinase (IKK) and mediates interaction of IKK with the human T-cell leukemia virus Tax protein. J Biol Chem *274*, 22911-22914.

72. Harris, N. L. (1998). The many faces of Hodgkin's disease around the world: what have we learned from its pathology? Ann Oncol *9*, S45-56.
73. Harrod, R., Tang, Y., Nicot, C., Lu, H. S., Vassilev, A., Nakatani, Y., and Giam, C. Z. (1998). An exposed KID-like domain in human T-cell lymphotropic virus type 1 Tax is responsible for the recruitment of coactivators CBP/p300. Mol Cell Biol *18*, 5052-5061.
74. Hermine, O., Lefrere, F., Bronowicki, J. P., Mariette, X., Jondeau, K., Eclache-Saudreau, V., Delmas, B., Valensi, F., Cacoub, P., Brechot, C., *et al.* (2002). Regression of splenic lymphoma with villous lymphocytes after treatment of hepatitis C virus infection. N Engl J Med *347*, 89-94.
75. Heslop, H. E., Brenner, M. K., and Rooney, C. M. (1994). Donor T cells to treat EBV-associated lymphoma [letter; comment]. N Engl J Med *331*, 679-680.
76. Hinrichs, S. H., Nerenberg, M., Reynolds, R. K., Khoury, G., and Jay, G. (1987). A transgenic mouse model for human neurofibromatosis. Science *237*, 1340-1343.
77. Hiscott, J., Petropoulos, L., and Lacoste, J. (1995). Molecular interactions between HTLV-1 Tax protein and the NF-kappa B/kappa B transcription complex. Virology *214*, 3-11.
78. Ho, J. W., Ho, F. C., Chan, A. C., Liang, R. H., and Srivastava, G. (1998). Frequent detection of Epstein-Barr virus-infected B cells in peripheral T-cell lymphomas. J Pathol *185*, 79-85.
79. Horenstein, M. G., Nador, R. G., Chadburn, A., Hyjek, E. M., Inghirami, G., Knowles, D. M., and Cesarman, E. (1997). Epstein-Barr virus latent gene expression in primary effusion lymphomas containing Kaposi's sarcoma-associated herpesvirus human herpesvirus-8. Blood *90*, 1186-1191.
80. Hsieh, J. J., and Hayward, S. D. (1995). Masking of the CBF1/RBPJ kappa transcriptional repression domain by Epstein-Barr virus EBNA2. Science *268*, 560-563.
81. Humme S, Reisbach G, Feederle R, Delecluse HJ, Bousset K, Hammerschmidt W, Schepers A (2003). The EBV nuclear antigen 1 (EBNA1) enhances B cell immortalization several thousandfold. Proc Natl Acad Sci U S A. 100:10989-94.
82. Iwanaga, Y., Tsukahara, T., Ohashi, T., Tanaka, Y., Arai, M., Nakamura, M., Ohtani, K., Koya, Y., Kannagi, M., Yamamoto, N., and Fujii, M. (1999). Human T-cell leukemia virus type 1 tax protein abrogates interleukin-2 dependence in a mouse T-cell line. J Virol *73*, 1271-1277.
83. Jaffe, E. S., Krenacs, L., Kumar, S., Kingma, D. W., and Raffeld, M. (1999). Extranodal peripheral T-cell and NK-cell neoplasms. Am J Clin Pathol *111*, S46-55.
84. Jenner, R. G., Maillard, K., Cattini, N., Weiss, R. A., Boshoff, C., Wooster, R., and Kellam, P. (2003). Kaposi's sarcoma-associated herpesvirus-infected primary effusion lymphoma has a plasma cell gene expression profile. Proc Natl Acad Sci U S A *100*, 10399-10404.
85. Kanegane, H., Yachie, A., Miyawaki, T., and Tosato, G. (1998). EBV-NK cells interactions and lymphoproliferative disorders. Leuk Lymphoma *29*, 491-498.
86. Keller, S. A., Dunne, C. E., Schattner, E. J., and Cesarman, E. (2000). Inhibition of NF-kB induces apoptosis of KSHV-infected primary effusion lymphoma cells. Blood *96*, 830a.
87. Kersten, M. J., Van Gorp, J., Pals, S. T., Boon, F., and Van Oers, M. H. (1998). Expression of Epstein-Barr virus latent genes and adhesion molecules in AIDS-related non-Hodgkin's lymphomas: correlation with histology and CD4-cell number. Leuk Lymphoma *30*, 515-524.

88. Khanna, R., Cooper, L., Kienzle, N., Moss, D. J., Burrows, S. R., and Khanna, K. K. (1997). Engagement of CD40 antigen with soluble CD40 ligand up-regulates peptide transporter expression and restores endogenous processing function in Burkitt's lymphoma cells. J Immunol *159*, 5782-5785.

89. Kieff, E. (1996). Epstein-Barr virus and its replication. In Virology, B. N. Fields, D. M. Knipe, and P. M. Howley, eds. (Philadelphia, Lippincott-Raven Publishers), pp. 2343-2396.

90. Kieser, A., Kilger, E., Gires, O., Ueffing, M., Kolch, W., and Hammerschmidt, W. (1997). Epstein-barr-virus latent membrane protein-1 triggers ap-1 activity via the c-jun n-terminal kinase cascade. Embo Journal *16*, 6478-6485.

91. Kilger, E., Kieser, A., Baumann, M., and Hammerschmidt, W. (1998). Epstein-Barr virus-mediated B-cell proliferation is dependent upon latent membrane protein 1, which simulates an activated CD40 receptor. EMBO Journal *17*, 1700-1709.

92. Klein, U., Gloghini, A., Gaidano, G., Chadburn, A., Cesarman, E., Dalla-Favera, R., and Carbone, A. (2003). Gene expression profile analysis of AIDS-related primary effusion lymphoma (PEL) suggests a plasmablastic derivation and identifies PEL-specific transcripts. Blood *101*, 4115-4121.

93. Knowles, D. M. (2001). Neoplastic Hematopathology, Second edn (Baltimore, Williams and Wilkins).

94. Knowles, D. M., Cesarman, E., Chadburn, A., Frizzera, G., Chen, J., Rose, E. A., and Michler, R. E. (1995). Correlative morphologic and molecular genetic analysis demonstrates three distinct categories of posttransplantation lymphoproliferative disorders. Blood *85*, 552-565.

95. Komano, J., Sugiura, M., and Takada, K. (1998). Epstein-Barr virus contributes to the malignant phenotype and to apoptosis resistance in Burkitt's lymphoma cell line Akata. J Virol *72*, 9150-9156.

96. Kulwichit, W., Edwards, R. H., Davenport, E. M., Baskar, J. F., Godfrey, V., and Raab-Traub, N. (1998). Expression of the Epstein-Barr virus latent membrane protein 1 induces B cell lymphoma in transgenic mice. Proc Natl Acad Sci U S A *95*, 11963-11968.

97. Kuppers, R., and Rajewsky, K. (1998). The origin of Hodgkin and Reed/Sternberg cells in Hodgkin's disease. Annu Rev Immunol *16*, 471-493.

98. Kurokawa, M., Ghosh, S. K., Ramos, J. C., Mian, A. M., Toomey, N. L., Cabral, L., Whitby, D., Barber, G. N., Dittmer, D. P., and Harrington Jr, W. J. (2005). Azidothymidine inhibits NF-{kappa}B and induces Epstein-Barr virus gene expression in Burkitt lymphoma. Blood.

99. Kwok, R. P., Laurance, M. E., Lundblad, J. R., Goldman, P. S., Shih, H., Connor, L. M., Marriott, S. J., and Goodman, R. H. (1996). Control of cAMP-regulated enhancers by the viral transactivator Tax through CREB and the co-activator CBP. Nature *380*, 642-646.

100. Laichalk, L. L., Hochberg, D., Babcock, G. J., Freeman, R. B., and Thorley-Lawson, D. A. (2002). The dispersal of mucosal memory B cells: evidence from persistent EBV infection. Immunity *16*, 745-754.

101. Larocca, L. M., Capello, D., Rinelli, A., Nori, S., Antinori, A., Gloghini, A., Cingolani, A., Migliazza, A., Saglio, G., Cammilleri-Broet, S., et al. (1998). The molecular and phenotypic profile of primary central nervous system lymphoma identifies distinct categories of the disease and is consistent with histogenetic derivation from germinal center-related B cells. Blood *92*, 1011-1019.

102. Lee, H., Guo, J., Li, M., Choi, J. K., DeMaria, M., Rosenzweig, M., and Jung, J. U. (1998a). Identification of an immunoreceptor tyrosine-based activation

motif of K1 transforming protein of Kaposi's sarcoma-associated herpesvirus. Mol Cell Biol *18*, 5219-5228.

103. Lee, H., Veazey, R., Williams, K., Li, M., Guo, J., Neipel, F., Fleckenstein, B., Lackner, A., Desrosiers, R. C., and Jung, J. U. (1998b). Deregulation of cell growth by the K1 gene of Kaposi's sarcoma-associated herpesvirus. Nature Medicine *4*, 435-440.

104. Lee, S. P., Constandinou, C. M., Thomas, W. A., Croom-Carter, D., Blake, N. W., Murray, P. G., Crocker, J., and Rickinson, A. B. (1998c). Antigen presenting phenotype of Hodgkin Reed-Sternberg cells: analysis of the HLA class I processing pathway and the effects of interleukin-10 on epstein-barr virus-specific cytotoxic T-cell recognition. Blood *92*, 1020-1030.

105. Lenzmeier, B. A., Giebler, H. A., and Nyborg, J. K. (1998). Human T-cell leukemia virus type 1 Tax requires direct access to DNA for recruitment of CREB binding protein to the viral promoter. Mol Cell Biol *18*, 721-731.

106. Leung, K., and Nabel, G. J. (1988). HTLV-1 transactivator induces interleukin-2 receptor expression through an NF-kappa B-like factor. Nature *333*, 776-778.

107. Li, M., Lee, H., Guo, J., Neipel, F., Fleckenstein, B., Ozato, K., and Jung, J. U. (1998). Kaposi's sarcoma-associated herpesvirus viral interferon regulatory factor. Journal of Virology *1998*, 5433-5440.

108. Li, M., Lee, H., Yoon, D.-W., Albrecht, J.-C., Fleckenstein, B., and Jung, J. (1997). Kaposi's sarcoma-associated herpesvirus encodes a functional cyclin. Journal of Virology *71*, 1984-1991.

109. Liebowitz, D. (1998). Epstein-Barr virus and a cellular signaling pathway in lymphomas from immunosuppressed patients. N Engl J Med *338*, 1413-1421.

110. Lubyova, B., Kellum, M. J., Frisancho, A. J., and Pitha, P. M. (2004). Kaposi's sarcoma-associated herpesvirus-encoded vIRF-3 stimulates the transcriptional activity of cellular IRF-3 and IRF-7. J Biol Chem *279*, 7643-7654.

111. Luftig, M., Prinarakis, E., Yasui, T., Tsichritzis, T., Cahir-McFarland, E., Inoue, J., Nakano, H., Mak, T. W., Yeh, W. C., Li, X., *et al.* (2003). Epstein-Barr virus latent membrane protein 1 activation of NF-kappaB through IRAK1 and TRAF6. Proc Natl Acad Sci U S A *100*, 15595-15600.

112. Machida, K., Cheng, K. T., Sung, V. M., Shimodaira, S., Lindsay, K. L., Levine, A. M., Lai, M. Y., and Lai, M. M. (2004). Hepatitis C virus induces a mutator phenotype: enhanced mutations of immunoglobulin and protooncogenes. Proc Natl Acad Sci U S A *101*, 4262-4267.

113. Mahieux, R., Pise-Masison, C. A., Lambert, P. F., Nicot, C., De Marchis, L., Gessain, A., Green, P., Hall, W., and Brady, J. N. (2000). Differences in the ability of human T-cell lymphotropic virus type 1 (HTLV-1) and HTLV-2 tax to inhibit p53 function. J Virol *74*, 6866-6874.

114. Mann, D. J., Child, E. S., Swanton, C., Laman, H., and Jones, N. (1999). Modulation of p27Kip1 levels by the cyclin encoded by Kaposi's sarcoma-associated herpesvirus. EMBO Journal *18*, 654-663.

115. Maruyama, K., Fukushima, T., Kawamura, K., and Mochizuki, S. (1990). Chromosome and gene rearrangements in immortalized human lymphocytes infected with human T-lymphotropic virus type I. Cancer Res *50*, 5697S-5702S.

116. Masucci, M. G., and Klein, E. (1991). Cell phenotype dependent expression of MHC class I antigens in Burkitt's lymphoma cell lines. Semin Cancer Biol *2*, 63-71.

117. Matolcsy, A., Nador, R. G., Cesarman, E., and Knowles, D. M. (1998). Immunoglobulin VH gene mutational analysis suggests that primary effusion lymphomas derive from different stages of B cell maturation. American Journal of Pathology *153*, 1609-1614.

118. Matta, H., and Chaudhary, P. M. (2004). Activation of alternative NF-kappa B pathway by human herpes virus 8-encoded Fas-associated death domain-like IL-1 beta-converting enzyme inhibitory protein (vFLIP). Proc Natl Acad Sci U S A *101*, 9399-9404.

119. Mesri, E. A., Cesarman, E., Arvanitakis, L., Rafii, S., Moore, M. A. S., Posnett, D. N., Knowles, D. M., and Asch, A. S. (1996). Human herpesvirus-8/Kaposi's sarcoma-associated herpesvirus is a new transmissible virus that infects B cells. Journal of Experimental Medicine *183*, 2385-2390.

120. Migone, T. S., Cacalano, N. A., Taylor, N., Yi, T., Waldmann, T. A., and Johnston, J. A. (1998). Recruitment of SH2-containing protein tyrosine phosphatase SHP-1 to the interleukin 2 receptor; loss of SHP-1 expression in human T-lymphotropic virus type I-transformed T cells. Proc Natl Acad Sci U S A *95*, 3845-3850.

121. Miyake, H., Suzuki, T., Hirai, H., and Yoshida, M. (1999). Trans-activator Tax of human T-cell leukemia virus type 1 enhances mutation frequency of the cellular genome. Virology *253*, 155-161.

122. Molden, J., Chang, Y., You, Y., Moore, P. S., and Goldsmith, M. A. (1997). A Kaposi's sarcoma-associated herpesvirus-encoded cytokine homolog (vIL-6) activates signaling through the shared gp130 receptor subunit. J Biol Chem *272*, 19625-19631.

123. Moore, P. S., Boschoff, C., Weiss, R. A., and Chang, Y. (1996). Molecular mimicry of human cytokine and cytokine response pathway genes by KSHV. Science *274*, 1739-1744.

124. Mori, N., Yamada, Y., Ikeda, S., Yamasaki, Y., Tsukasaki, K., Tanaka, Y., Tomonaga, M., Yamamoto, N., and Fujii, M. (2002). Bay 11-7082 inhibits transcription factor NF-kappaB and induces apoptosis of HTLV-I-infected T-cell lines and primary adult T-cell leukemia cells. Blood *100*, 1828-1834.

125. Moses, A. V., Fish, K. N., Ruhl, R., Smith, P. P., Strussenberg, J. G., Zhu, L., Chandran, B., and Nelson, J. A. (1999). Long-term infection and transformation of dermal microvascular endothelial cells by human herpesvirus 8. J Virol *73*, 6892-6902.

126. Mulloy, J. C., Kislyakova, T., Cereseto, A., Casareto, L., LoMonico, A., Fullen, J., Lorenzi, M. V., Cara, A., Nicot, C., Giam, C., and Franchini, G. (1998). Human T-cell lymphotropic/leukemia virus type 1 Tax abrogates p53- induced cell cycle arrest and apoptosis through its CREB/ATF functional domain. J Virol *72*, 8852-8860.

127. Nador, R. G., Cesarman, E., Chadburn, A., Dawson, D. B., Ansari, M. Q., Said, J., and Knowles, D. M. (1996). Primary effusion lymphoma: a distinct clinicopathologic entity associated with the Kaposi's sarcoma-associated herpesvirus. Blood *88*, 645-656.

128. Nador, R. G., Cesarman, E., Knowles, D. M., and Said, J. W. (1995). Herpes-like DNA sequences in a body-cavity-based lymphoma in an HIV-negative patient (Letter to the Editor). New England Journal of Medicine *333*, 943.

129. Nalesnik, M. A., Jaffe, R., Starzl, T. E., Demetris, A. J., Porter, K., Burnham, J. A., Makowka, L., Ho, M., and Locker, J. (1988). The pathology of posttransplant lymphoproliferative disorders occurring in the setting of cyclosporine A-prednisone immunosuppression. Am J Pathol *133*, 173-192.

130. Negri, E., Little, D., Boiocchi, M., La Vecchia, C., and Franceschi, S. (2004). B-cell non-Hodgkin's lymphoma and hepatitis C virus infection: a systematic review. Int J Cancer *111*, 1-8.

131. Nerenberg, M., Hinrichs, S. H., Reynolds, R. K., Khoury, G., and Jay, G. (1987). The tat gene of human T-lymphotropic virus type 1 induces mesenchymal tumors in transgenic mice. Science *237*, 1324-1329.

132. Neuveut, C., Low, K. G., Maldarelli, F., Schmitt, I., Majone, F., Grassmann, R., and Jeang, K. T. (1998). Human t-cell leukemia virus type 1 tax and cell cycle progression - role of cyclin d-cdk and p110rb. Molecular & Cellular Biology *18*, 3620-3632.

133. Nicholas, J., Ruvolo, V. R., Burns, W. H., Sandford, G., Wan, X. Y., Ciufo, D., Hendrickson, S. B., Guo, H. G., Hayward, G. S., and Reitz, M. S. (1997). Kaposi's sarcoma-associated human herpesvirus-8 encodes homologues of macrophage inflammatory protein-1 and interleukin-6. Nature Med *3*, 287-292.

134. Nicot, C., Tie, F., and Giam, C. Z. (1998). Cytoplasmic forms of human T-cell leukemia virus type 1 Tax induce NF- kappaB activation. J Virol *72*, 6777-6784.

135. Orentas, R. J., Lemas, M. V., Mullin, M. J., Colombani, P. M., Schwarz, K., and Ambinder, R. (1998). Feasibility of cellular adoptive immunotherapy for Epstein-Barr virus- associated lymphomas using haploidentical donors. J Hematother *7*, 257-261.

136. Papadopoulos, E. B., Ladanyi, M., Emanuel, D., Mackinnon, S., Boulad, F., Carabasi, M. H., Castro-Malaspina, H., Childs, B. H., Gillio, A. P., Small, T. N., and et al. (1994). Infusions of donor leukocytes to treat Epstein-Barr virus-associated lymphoproliferative disorders after allogeneic bone marrow transplantation [see comments]. N Engl J Med *330*, 1185-1191.

137. Paydas, S., Ergin, M., Tanriverdi, K., Yavuz, S., Disel, U., Kilic, N. B., Erdogan, S., Sahin, B., Tuncer, I., and Burgut, R. (2004). Detection of hepatitis C virus RNA in paraffin-embedded tissues from patients with non-Hodgkin's lymphoma. Am J Hematol *76*, 252-257.

138. Petropoulos, L., and Hiscott, J. (1998). Association between HTLV-1 Tax and I kappa B alpha is dependent on the I kappa B alpha phosphorylation state. Virology *252*, 189-199.

139. Pise-Masison, C. A., Choi, K. S., Radonovich, M., Dittmer, J., Kim, S. J., and Brady, J. N. (1998a). Inhibition of p53 transactivation function by the human T-cell lymphotropic virus type 1 Tax protein. J Virol *72*, 1165-1170.

140. Pise-Masison, C. A., Radonovich, M., Sakaguchi, K., Appella, E., and Brady, J. N. (1998b). Phosphorylation of p53: a novel pathway for p53 inactivation in human T- cell lymphotropic virus type 1-transformed cells. J Virol *72*, 6348-6355.

141. Poiesz, B. J., Ruscetti, F. W., Gazdar, A. F., Bunn, P. A., Minna, J. D., and Gallo, R. C. (1980). Detection and isolation of type C retrovirus particles from fresh and cultured lymphocytes of a patient with cutaneous T-cell lymphoma. Proc Natl Acad Sci U S A *77*, 7415-7419.

142. Prakash, O., Swamy, O. R., Peng, X., Tang, Z. Y., Li, L., Larson, J. E., Cohen, J. C., Gill, J., Farr, G., Wang, S., and Samaniego, F. (2005). Activation of Src kinase Lyn by the Kaposi sarcoma-associated herpesvirus K1 protein: implications for lymphomagenesis. Blood *105*, 3987-3994.

143. Radkov, S. A., Kellam, P., and Boshoff, C. (2000). The latent nuclear antigen of kaposi sarcoma-associated herpesvirus targets the retinoblastoma-E2F pathway and with the oncogene hras transforms primary rat cells. Nat Med *6*, 1121-1127.

144. Raphael, M., Borisch, B., and E.S., J. (2001). Lymphomas associated with infection by the human immune deficiency virus (HIV). In World Health organization Classification of Tumors, Tumors of Haematopoietic and Lymphoid Tissues., E. S. Jaffe, N. L. Harris, H. Stein, and J. W. Vardiman, eds. (Lyon, France, IARC Press), pp. 260-263.

145. Reitz, M. S., Jr., Popovic, M., Haynes, B. F., Clark, S. C., and Gallo, R. C. (1983). Relatedness by nucleic acid hybridization of new isolates of human T-

cell leukemia-lymphoma virus (HTLV) and demonstration of provirus in uncultured leukemic blood cells. Virology *126*, 688-672.

146. Renne, R., Zhong, W., Herndier, B., McGrath, M., Abbey, N., Kedes, D., and Ganem, D. (1996). Lytic growth of Kaposi's sarcoma-associated herpesvirus (human herpesvirus 8) in culture. Nature Med *2*, 342-346.

147. Rickinson, A. B., and Kieff, E. (1996). Epstein-Barr virus. In Virology, B. N. Fields, D. M. Knipe, and P. M. Howley, eds. (Philadelphia, Lippincott-Raven Publishers), pp. 2397-2446.

148. Rivas, C., Thlick, A. E., Parravicini, C., Moore, P. S., and Chang, Y. (2001). Kaposi's sarcoma-associated herpesvirus LANA2 is a B-cell-specific latent viral protein that inhibits p53. J Virol *75*, 429-438.

149. Rooney, C. M., Smith, C. A., Ng, C. Y., Loftin, S. K., Sixbey, J. W., Gan, Y., Srivastava, D. K., Bowman, L. C., Krance, R. A., Brenner, M. K., and Heslop, H. E. (1998). Infusion of cytotoxic T cells for the prevention and treatment of Epstein-Barr virus-induced lymphoma in allogeneic transplant recipients. Blood *92*, 1549-1555.

150. Rosin, O., Koch, C., Schmitt, I., Semmes, O. J., Jeang, K. T., and Grassmann, R. (1998). A human T-cell leukemia virus Tax variant incapable of activating NF- kappaB retains its immortalizing potential for primary T-lymphocytes. J Biol Chem *273*, 6698-6703.

151. Ruben, S., Poteat, H., Tan, T. H., Kawakami, K., Roeder, R., Haseltine, W., and Rosen, C. A. (1988). Cellular transcription factors and regulation of IL-2 receptor gene expression by HTLV-I tax gene product. Science *241*, 89-92.

152. Ruf, I. K., Rhyne, P. W., Yang, H., Borza, C. M., Hutt-Fletcher, L. M., Cleveland, J. L., and Sample, J. T. (1999). Epstein-barr virus regulates c-MYC, apoptosis, and tumorigenicity in burkitt lymphoma [In Process Citation]. Mol Cell Biol *19*, 1651-1660.

153. Saadoun, D., Suarez, F., Lefrere, F., Valensi, F., Mariette, X., Aouba, A., Besson, C., Varet, B., Troussard, X., Cacoub, P., and Hermine, O. (2005). Splenic lymphoma with villous lymphocytes, associated with type II cryoglobulinemia and HCV infection: a new entity? Blood *105*, 74-76.

154. Said, J. W., Tasaka, T., Takeuchi, T., Asou, H., de Vos, S., Cesarman, E., Knowles, D. M., and Koeffler, H. P. (1996). Primary effusion lymphoma in women: Report of two cases of Kaposi's sarcoma-herpes virus-associated effusion-based lymphoma in human immunodeficiency virus-negative women. Blood *88*, 3124-3128.

155. Sanada, I., Tanaka, R., Kumagai, E., Tsuda, H., Nishimura, H., Yamaguchi, K., Kawano, F., Fujiwara, H., and Takatsuki, K. (1985). Chromosomal aberrations in adult T cell leukemia: relationship to the clinical severity. Blood *65*, 649-654.

156. Schmitt, I., Rosin, O., Rohwer, P., Gossen, M., and Grassmann, R. (1998). Stimulation of cyclin-dependent kinase activity and G1- to S-phase transition in human lymphocytes by the human T-cell leukemia/lymphotropic virus type 1 Tax protein. J Virol *72*, 633-640.

157. Shapiro, R. S., McClain, K., Frizzera, G., Gajl-Peczalska, K. J., Kersey, J. H., Blazar, B. R., Arthur, D. C., Patton, D. F., Greenberg, J. S., Burke, B., and et al. (1988). Epstein-Barr virus associated B cell lymphoproliferative disorders following bone marrow transplantation. Blood *71*, 1234-1243.

158. Sharp, T. V., Wang, H. W., Koumi, A., Hollyman, D., Endo, Y., Ye, H., Du, M. Q., and Boshoff, C. (2002). K15 protein of Kaposi's sarcoma-associated herpesvirus is latently expressed and binds to HAX-1, a protein with antiapoptotic function. J Virol *76*, 802-816.

159. Shimizu, N., Tanabe-Tochikura, A., Kuroiwa, Y., and Takada, K. (1994). Isolation of Epstein-Barr virus (EBV)-negative cell clones from the EBV-positive Burkitt's lymphoma (BL) line Akata: malignant phenotypes of BL cells are dependent on EBV. J Virol *68*, 6069-6073.

160. Sieburg, M., Tripp, A., Ma, J. W., and Feuer, G. (2004). Human T-cell leukemia virus type 1 (HTLV-1) and HTLV-2 tax oncoproteins modulate cell cycle progression and apoptosis. J Virol *78*, 10399-10409.

161. Sun, S. C., and Ballard, D. W. (1999). Persistent activation of NF-kappaB by the tax transforming protein of HTLV-1: hijacking cellular IkappaB kinases. Oncogene *18*, 6948-6958.

162. Sung, V. M., Shimodaira, S., Doughty, A. L., Picchio, G. R., Can, H., Yen, T. S., Lindsay, K. L., Levine, A. M., and Lai, M. M. (2003). Establishment of B-cell lymphoma cell lines persistently infected with hepatitis C virus in vivo and in vitro: the apoptotic effects of virus infection. J Virol *77*, 2134-2146.

163. Szekely, L., Chen, F., Teramoto, N., Ehlin-Henriksson, B., Pokrovskaja, K., Szeles, A., Manneborg-Sandlund, A., Lowbeer, M., Lennette, E. T., and Klein, G. (1998). Restricted expression of Epstein-Barr virus (EBV)-encoded, growth transformation-associated antigens in an EBV- and human herpesvirus type 8-carrying body cavity lymphoma line. General Virology *79*, 1445-1452.

164. Tao, Q., Robertson, K. D., Manns, A., Hildesheim, A., and Ambinder, R. F. (1998a). Epstein-Barr virus (EBV) in endemic Burkitt's lymphoma: molecular analysis of primary tumor tissue [published erratum appears in Blood 1998 Apr 15;91(8):3091]. Blood *91*, 1373-1381.

165. Tao, Q., Robertson, K. D., Manns, A., Hildesheim, A., and Ambinder, R. F. (1998b). The Epstein-Barr virus major latent promoter Qp is constitutively active, hypomethylated, and methylation sensitive. J Virol *72*, 7075-7083.

166. Thome, M., Schneider, P., Hofmann, K., Fickenscher, H., Meinl, E., Neipel, F., Mattmann, C., Burns, K., Bodmer, J. L., Schroter, M., *et al.* (1997). Viral FLICE-inhibitory proteins (FLIPs) prevent apoptosis induced by death receptors. Nature *386*, 517-521.

167. Thorley-Lawson, D. A. (2001). Epstein-Barr virus: exploiting the immune system. Nat Rev Immunol *1*, 75-82.

168. Thorley-Lawson, D. A., and Gross, A. (2004). Persistence of the Epstein-Barr virus and the origins of associated lymphomas. N Engl J Med *350*, 1328-1337.

169. Tomlinson, C. C., and Damania, B. (2004). The K1 protein of Kaposi's sarcoma-associated herpesvirus activates the Akt signaling pathway. J Virol *78*, 1918-1927.

170. Tsuchiyama, J., Yoshino, T., Mori, M., Kondoh, E., Oka, T., Akagi, T., Hiraki, A., Nakayama, H., Shibuya, A., Ma, Y., *et al.* (1998). Characterization of a novel human natural killer-cell line (NK-YS) established from natural killer cell lymphoma/leukemia associated with Epstein-Barr virus infection. Blood *92*, 1374-1383.

171. Uchida, T., Kinoshita, T., Murate, T., Saito, H., and Hotta, T. (1998). CDKN2 (MTS1/p16INK4A) gene alterations in adult T-cell leukemia/lymphoma. Leuk Lymphoma *29*, 27-35.

172. Verschuren, E. W., Hodgson, J. G., Gray, J. W., Kogan, S., Jones, N., and Evan, G. I. (2004). The role of p53 in suppression of KSHV cyclin-induced lymphomagenesis. Cancer Res *64*, 581-589.

173. Verschuren, E. W., Klefstrom, J., Evan, G. I., and Jones, N. (2002). The oncogenic potential of Kaposi's sarcoma-associated herpesvirus cyclin is exposed by p53 loss in vitro and in vivo. Cancer Cell *2*, 229-241.

174. Wang, D., Liebowitz, D., and Kieff, E. (1985). An EBV membrane protein expressed in immortalized lymphocytes transforms established rodent cells. Cell *43*, 831-840.
175. Watanabe, S., Mukai, K., and Shimoyama, M. (1992). Adult T cell leukemia/lymphoma. In Neoplastic Hematopathology, D. Knowles, ed. (Baltimore, Williams & Wilkins), pp. 1281-1294.
176. Weng, W. K., and Levy, S. (2003). Hepatitis C virus (HCV) and lymphomagenesis. Leuk Lymphoma *44*, 1113-1120.
177. Wheatley, G. H., 3rd, McKinnon, K. P., Iacobucci, M., Mahon, S., Gelber, C., and Lyerly, H. K. (1998). Dendritic cells improve the generation of Epstein-Barr virus-specific cytotoxic T lymphocytes for the treatment of posttransplantation lymphoma. Surgery *124*, 171-176.
178. Wilson, J. B., Bell, J. L., and Levine, A. J. (1996). Expression of Epstein-Barr virus nuclear antigen-1 induces B cell neoplasia in transgenic mice. Embo J *15*, 3117-3126.
179. Xiao, G., Cvijic, M. E., Fong, A., Harhaj, E. W., Uhlik, M. T., Waterfield, M., and Sun, S. C. (2001). Retroviral oncoprotein Tax induces processing of NF-kappaB2/p100 in T cells: evidence for the involvement of IKKalpha. Embo J *20*, 6805-6815.
180. Xie, P., Hostager, B. S., and Bishop, G. A. (2004). Requirement for TRAF3 in signaling by LMP1 but not CD40 in B lymphocytes. J Exp Med *199*, 661-671.
181. Yin, M. J., Paulssen, E., Seeler, J., and Gaynor, R. B. (1995). Chimeric proteins composed of Jun and CREB define domains required for interaction with the human T-cell leukemia virus type 1 Tax protein. J Virol *69*, 6209-6218.
182. Yoshida, M. (2001). Multiple viral strategies of HTLV-1 for dysregulation of cell growth control. Annu Rev Immunol *19*, 475-496.
183. Yoshida, M., Hattori, S., and Seiki, M. (1985). Molecular biology of human T-cell leukemia virus associated with adult T-cell leukemia. Curr Top Microbiol Immunol *115*, 157-175.
184. Yoshida, M., Seiki, M., Yamaguchi, K., and Takatsuki, K. (1984). Monoclonal integration of human T-cell leukemia provirus in all primary tumors of adult T-cell leukemia suggests causative role of human T-cell leukemia virus in the disease. Proc Natl Acad Sci U S A *81*, 2534-2537.
185. Yoshizaki, T., Sato, H., Furukawa, M., and Pagano, J. S. (1998). The expression of matrix metalloproteinase 9 is enhanced by Epstein- Barr virus latent membrane protein 1. Proc Natl Acad Sci U S A *95*, 3621-3626.
186. Zimring, J. C., Goodbourn, S., and Offermann, M. K. (1998). Human herpesvirus 8 encodes an interferon regulatory factor (IRF) homolog that represses IRF-1-mediated transcription. J Virol *72*, 701-707.

Chapter 3

THE INDOLENT B-CELL LYMPHOMAS

Peter McLaughlin, MD

University of Texas M.D. Anderson Cancer Center, Department of Lymphoma/Myeloma, 1515 Holcombe Blvd., Box 429, Houston, TX 77030

1.   INTRODUCTION

The indolent B-cell lymphomas account for about one third of all lymphomas in the Western world. The follicular lymphomas are the largest and most easily recognized category of indolent lymphoma, representing about one quarter of lymphomas in the Western world.[1-3] The incidence of follicular lymphoma is markedly lower in Asia than in the West, for unclear reasons.[4] Other well-defined indolent lymphomas (and their approximate percentage incidence) are: small lymphocytic lymphoma (6%); nodal marginal zone B-cell lymphoma (1-2%); extranodal marginal zone B-cell lymphoma of mucosa-associated lymphoid tissue, or MALT (5-7%); splenic marginal zone B-cell lymphoma, and the variant splenic lymphoma with villous lymphocytes (< 1%); and lymphoplasmacytic lymphoma (1%).

Many general concepts about the indolent lymphomas derive most clearly from experience with follicular lymphoma. In this chapter, distinctive features of the other indolent lymphomas[5] will be mentioned, but the review will focus mainly on follicular lymphoma data.

The indolent lymphomas occur most commonly in the sixth and seventh decades of life. Females are affected as often as males, in contrast to most other categories of lymphoma in which there is a male preponderance. Most patients with indolent lymphoma have advanced stage disease at the time of diagnosis. Relatively few have constitutional symptoms or poor performance status at diagnosis, even though many have fairly bulky disease (Table 1).

2.   PATHOLOGY/BIOLOGY

INDOLENT BUT NOT BENIGN

The classification of the malignant lymphomas is based on our evolving understanding of the biology of these diseases. A detailed description of the pathology of the indolent lymphomas is beyond the scope of this chapter. However, noteworthy examples of how biological insights relate to patient management deserve to be mentioned.

Formerly, many of the entities now classified as marginal zone B-cell lymphomas of mucosa-associated lymphoid tissue (MALT) were regarded as "pseudolymphoma", i.e., it was arguable whether they were malignancies. For many of these lymphomas, it is now clear that there is an immune-stimulating event early in the pathogenesis of the process. The best understood example of this is the relationship between *Helicobacter pylori* and gastric MALT lymphoma. *H. pylori* infection is associated with peptic ulcer disease, gastric carcinoma, and gastric MALT lymphoma. Not all strains of *H. pylori* carry the same risk to promote malignancy; strains that express the CagA protein are most worrisome.[6] Since *H. pylori* exposure is widespread but the development of malignancy is uncommon, the *H. pylori* infection is felt to be an early but not the only step in pathogenesis of the malignancy. Eradication of the *H. pylori* infection with antibiotic therapy can lead to regression of the lymphoma.[7]

Other infections that may be linked to the development of MALT lymphoma include *Borrelia burgdorferi* with cutaneous MALT lymphoma[8], and *Chlamydia psittaci* with conjunctival MALT lymphoma.[9] Additional intriguing relationships include the linkage of Hashimoto's thyroiditis with thyroid MALT lymphoma, and Sjogren's syndrome with parotid MALT lymphoma.

Although antibiotic management can sometimes lead to regression of MALT lymphoma, the MALT lymphomas are not benign inflammatory conditions. Cytogenetic and molecular genetic abnormalities have been identified for many of these lymphomas[10,11], and these diseases have the potential for local spread, distant dissemination, and late relapse.

Normal reactive T-cells have been suspected for many years to play a role in the evolution of follicular lymphoma.[12] The immune response of the host is regarded as a key factor in the known tendency for these diseases sometimes to wax and wane. Consequently, these diseases are considered to be prime candidates for therapeutic approaches with vaccines. Recent gene expression profile data has suggested that the molecular signatures most clearly associated with prognosis (survival) in follicular lymphoma are ones that derive not so much from the malignant B-cell population as from the background T-cell and macrophage populations.[13]

Other gene expression profile observations have provided better understanding of the clinical and morphological spectrum that is displayed in follicular lymphoma and in the process of transformation to aggressive diffuse large B-cell lymphoma (DLBCL).[14-16] Genes that have been shown to be dysregulated in more aggressive or transformed follicular lymphoma include the oncogene c-myc, and several genes that are related to cell cycle control and increased metabolism. At the DLBCL end of this spectrum, it is becoming clear that DLBCL can be subdivided; one common and favorable profile is that of the "germinal center B-cell" type of DLBCL.[17] This subset of DLBCL is clearly of germinal center B-cell origin, with expression of surface CD10 and expression of Bcl-6, hallmarks of follicular lymphoma as well.

These observations indicate that the boundaries between benign/malignant and indolent/aggressive are being defined more clearly. Hopefully, this expanding biological and molecular knowledge will lead not just to a better understanding of the disease process, but also to new ways to intervene therapeutically.

The bcl-2 story is another one that ties the biological understanding of these diseases to patient management.[18] In the Western world, most follicular lymphomas (about 85%) have bcl-2 gene rearrangement, with breakpoints most commonly occurring at the MBR or mcr loci. There are other bcl-2 breakpoint loci as well[19], but a fraction of follicular lymphoma cases appear not to have bcl-2 gene rearrangement[20,21] and in many of these cases, there are other molecular genetic events involved in the genesis of the disease.[22]

Molecular observations about bcl-2 have led to strategies that are already utilized in the clinic. The polymerase chain reaction (PCR) provides a way to monitor most follicular lymphoma patients for the presence of cells with bcl-2 gene rearrangement; this approach has provided a sensitive measure of subclinical residual disease.[23,24] At another level, bcl-2 insights have provided therapeutic opportunities; antisense oligonucleotide molecules and other approaches have been developed to address the resistance to therapy that is conferred by overexpression of Bcl-2.[25]

3. NATURAL HISTORY

The initial pace of indolent lymphoma is usually slow, and there can be spontaneous fluctuations of node size. With a variety of treatments, partial or complete response is common. But relapse is virtually inevitable, usually within 3-4 years with some of the better reported therapies, and even sooner with many therapies. Response to salvage therapy is frequent, but second and subsequent remissions are typically of steadily shorter durations. Ultimately these diseases are usually fatal, and lymphoma is usually the primary cause or a contributing cause of death. The median survival in large series of patients ranges from 7-10+ years.

Transformation or histologic evolution is a common development; it is recognized during the clinical course of about half of patients, and some autopsy series show transformation in over 90% of patients. There can be discordant disease even at the time of initial presentation so a clinically suspicious finding such as an atypical site or a particularly bulky or rapidly changing mass (classically in the abdomen) should prompt consideration of a biopsy of that site. More commonly, transformation is a later event, at the time of relapse. Repeat biopsy at the time of relapse is always warranted. Transformation is usually an ominous development, particularly if it occurs during therapy, or shortly thereafter.

The apparent incurability of the indolent lymphoma and the apparent lack of improvement in results in the latter part of the twentieth century[26] (mainly with alkylating agent therapy) have fostered a variety of patient management strategies. Immediate therapy is clearly not always necessary. Numerous studies have shown that selected patients can be observed for months or occasionally years without intevention[27-29], particularly grade 1 follicular lymphoma and small lymphocytic lymphoma[30]. Some clinicians approach these diseases with a pessimism that borders on nihilism, and advocate just palliative therapy. Many others advocate innovative approaches, which range from biological approaches, to utilization of newer classes of chemotherapeutic agents, to high-dose therapy with stem cell support. Prime opportunities exist for these patients to participate in clinical trials.

Notably, truisms about indolent lymphoma sometimes do not hold true. Although often disseminated at presentation, some patients are diagnosed with early stage disease. Although usually indolent, the disease can be fulminant and rapidly life-threatening. And, although usually incurable, encouraging data exist to suggest that treatment results have improved over the last 25 years[31], and that sometimes therapy can be curative.[32,33]

4.   DIAGNOSTIC EVALUATION

The diagnostic evaluation for lymphoma patients must start with a biopsy that is adequate to classify the lymphoma. The availability of increasingly sophisticated molecular diagnostic techniques makes it tempting to think that definitive information can routinely be gotten from minimal tissue. The opposite is true. To perform some of the most sophisticated analyses, it is more important than ever to obtain adequate unfixed tissue for processing. For initial classification of lymphoma, the temptation to rely on just a fine needle aspirate should be avoided; the limitations of that technique have recently been emphasized in the literature.[34]

4.1   Staging: Beyond the Ann Arbor staging system

The staging evaluation serves both to profile the patient's prognostic features and to plan appropriate initial therapy. At the simplest level, the Ann Arbor Staging System for Hodgkin's disease is a tool to help decide if radiation therapy is appropriate (stage I-II and possibly III) or not (stage IV and many stage III cases). Since the Ann Arbor staging system was designed for Hodgkin's disease, it is not surprising that other systems have been explored in aggressive lymphoma and indolent lymphoma, leading to the development of prognostic indices which perform better than the Ann Arbor system. However, in both the International Prognostic Index (IPI), developed for aggressive lymphoma[35], and the Follicular Lymphoma International Prognostic Index (FLIPI)[36], the crucial importance of defining the anatomic distribution of disease as outlined in the Ann Arbor staging system is still a key factor.

The IPI, although developed for patients with aggressive lymphoma, has established utility for patients with indolent lymphoma[37]. But for indolent lymphoma, a drawback of the IPI is that very few patients are identified in the highest risk category. Consequently, if the model is to be used to select innovative or more intensive treatment programs for high-risk patients, the IPI has limitations for indolent lymphoma patients, since so few patients would be profiled as high risk. The recently described FLIPI identifies a more substantial fraction of patients with high-risk disease. The five simple clinical features that make up the FLIPI are: age ($\geq$ 60 years adverse); stage (III-IV adverse); LDH (any elevation adverse); hemoglobin (<12 gm% adverse); and number of nodal sites ($\geq$ 5 adverse). Nodal sites are counted as illustrated in Figure 1. Patients with 0-1 adverse features (36% of patients) have a 90% 5-year survival with standard therapy; those with 2 factors (37% of patients) have a 78% 5-year survival; and those with $\geq$ 3 factors (27% of patients) have only a 53% 5-year survival.

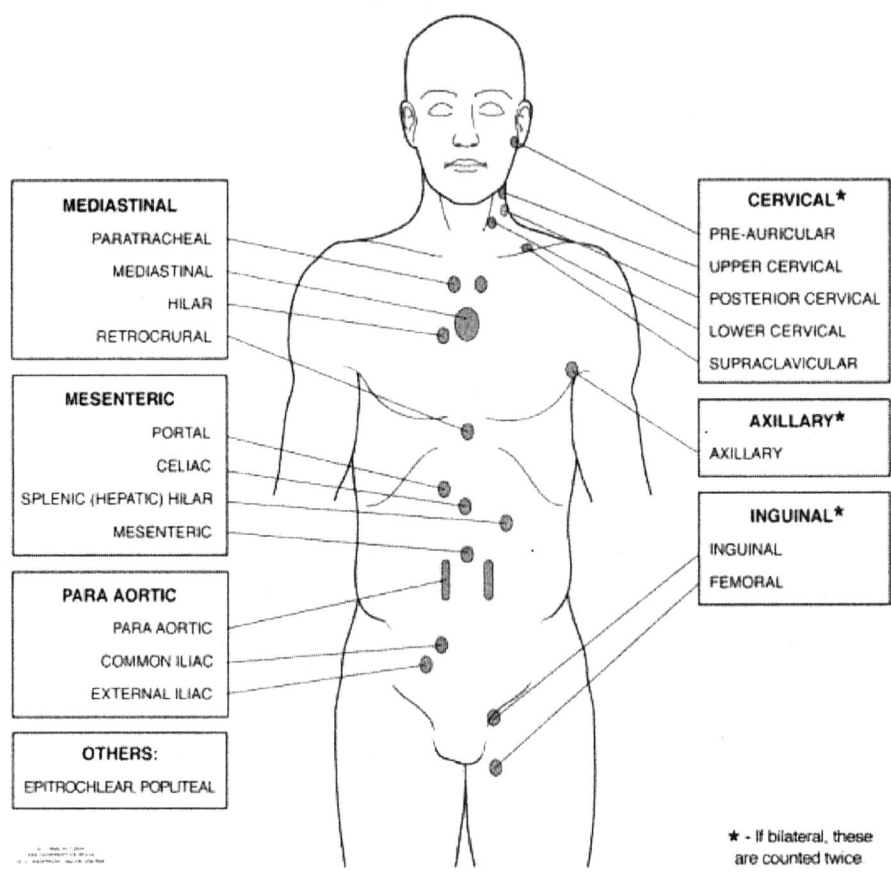

MEDIASTINAL
PARATRACHEAL
MEDIASTINAL
HILAR
RETROCRURAL

MESENTERIC
PORTAL
CELIAC
SPLENIC (HEPATIC) HILAR
MESENTERIC

PARA AORTIC
PARA AORTIC
COMMON ILIAC
EXTERNAL ILIAC

OTHERS:
EPITROCHLEAR, POPLITEAL

CERVICAL*
PRE-AURICULAR
UPPER CERVICAL
POSTERIOR CERVICAL
LOWER CERVICAL
SUPRACLAVICULAR

AXILLARY*
AXILLARY

INGUINAL*
INGUINAL
FEMORAL

★ - If bilateral, these
are counted twice.

Figure 1. Nodal Sites as Analyzed in the FLIPI.

The validity of the IPI and FLIPI models is compelling. They were both derived from very large multiinstitutional databases, and long-term survival data was available for the patients included in these models. Necessarily, the IPI and the FLIPI do not incorporate diagnostic tools that were not widely available 15-20 years ago. Among useful newer tests that are not incorporated into the FLIPI, two examples are the serum $\beta 2$ microglobulin level and PCR testing for bcl-2 gene rearrangement.

4.1.1 β2 Microglobulin

In the report describing the FLIPI, several parameters in the univariate analysis had significant correlations with survival, including serum albumin, erythrocyte sedimentation rate, and β2 microglobulin. The β2 microglobulin (B2M) data is of particular interest because of the vast amount of data that corroborates its prognostic utility in Hodgkin's disease[38], aggressive lymphoma[39], indolent lymphoma[40], and a number of other hematological malignancies. Moreover, its biology is of interest: β2m is a non-covalently bound component of the MHC class I molecule; its shedding may be an indicator of immune dysregulation and potential tumor escape from host defenses.

4.1.2 bcl-2

In the West, up to 85% of patients with follicular lymphoma have bcl-2 gene rearrangement as a genetic hallmark of their disease. When the involved lymphoid tissue has bcl-2 gene rearrangement, subclinical evidence of cells with this rearrangement is detectable in essentially all patients when either the blood or bone marrow is tested by PCR techniques. This biological insight provides: (1) a humbling bit of evidence that these diseases are almost always disseminated at the time of initial diagnosis, even when we think they are localized; and (2) a stringent measure of treatment response, since at least some current therapies are able to induce "molecular remission", whereby the bone marrow and/or blood can revert from positive to negative.

The PCR technique has limitations that call into question its suitability, at least yet, for widespread standard use. First, the methodology is not standardized.[41] For instance, different primers and different numbers of amplification cycles are utilized at different laboratories. Second, PCR techniques are in evolution; in particular, a transition is occurring at many centers from qualitative to real-time and quantitative techniques.[42] Third, cells with bcl-2 gene rearrangement can be detected in normal individuals, which calls into question whether a positive tests always indicates the presence of cells with malignant potential.[43] Fourth, a positive test does not necessarily mean that relapse is imminent.[44-46] Despite these limitations, there is a substantial body of evidence in the literature that PCR data for bcl-2 can provide clinically useful information (Table 2).[47-49] In some trials, PCR data has been used to drive treatment decisions.[50] But, as with virtually all topics pertaining to indolent lymphomas, there is confounding or contradictory evidence as well.

4.1.3   Bone Marrow Biopsy

While a unilateral bone marrow biopsy is felt by many to suffice for the staging of patients with indolent lymphoma, it is still our routine to perform bilateral bone marrow biopsies. If only a unilateral bone marrow is done, and if it is negative, there should be consideration of checking the contralateral side if it would influence the management decision.

4.1.4   Imaging

Standard imaging still includes the plain chest x-ray, and a CT scan of the abdomen and pelvis. In most cases, CT scanning of the chest and the head and neck are also useful baseline assessments.

Increasingly, PET scanning is a consideration for patients with malignant lymphoma. In indolent lymphoma, the PET scan findings can be more subtle than in aggressive lymphoma or Hodgkin's disease. Thus, depending on the quality and the reader of the study, there may be variability of the interpretation, including the potential for false negative or otherwise misleading results. However, where available, PET scanning is likely to become an increasingly useful adjunct to the standard staging assessment of patients with indolent lymphoma. [51,52]

4.1.5   Other tests

In MALT lymphomas originating in sites other than the stomach, upper endoscopy might be considered if it would change the management. A fairly high yield has been seen at our center; about one third of non-gastric MALT lymphomas were found to have GI tract involvement on screening upper GI endoscopy.[53]

The rarity of central nervous system (CNS) involvement in indolent lymphoma makes spinal fluid assessment unnecessary, unless there are CNS symptoms.

5. MANAGEMENT

5.1   Stage I-II

Only about 15% of patients with follicular lymphoma are detected with early stage (stage I-II) disease. Involved field radiation therapy may be curative for about 40% of such patients.[33, 54-56]

The addition of chemotherapy to radiation appears to increase the fraction of patients with prolonged disease-free survival, up to 70% at 5-10 years in one large single-center prospective trial.[57] Other trials have explored the incorporation of chemotherapy along with radiation therapy in localized indolent lymphoma, with variable results; this may be partly explained by small numbers of patients, inconsistent or marginal chemotherapy, and other issues. A randomized trial addressing the role of chemotherapy in conjunction with involved field radiation therapy in this setting is underway. To date, there is no trial that addresses the potential role of rituximab in the stage I-II setting.

The potential for cure in stage I-II follicular lymphoma represents an argument to forego consideration of the "watch and wait" approach in these patients. However, given the indolent nature of the disease, some investigators have elected to observe stage I-II patients without intervention.[58,59] While this approach is feasible, the radiotherapy and chemotherapy-radiotherapy literature indicates that transdiaphragmatic and out-of-field relapse is common, while in-field relapse is infrequent.[56] If the "watch and wait" approach is taken, and if the disease disseminates, the opportunity for definitive therapy may be lost. Overall, the current data favor intervention in the setting of stage I-II follicular lymphoma, because there appears to be a legitimate chance for cure of a fraction of these patients.

5.2   Stage III

In the most widely used current prognostic models (IPI and FLIPI), patients with stage III disease are lumped together with stage IV patients in the category of advanced stage disease. Consistent with this view, most investigators have approached stage III-IV disease with chemotherapy only. However, there have been a number of trials that have explored the role of radiation therapy in stage III disease.[60,61] This approach, which involves total lymphoid radiation utilizing sequential (usually three) fields, has been shown to be feasible and effective. Remissions and even molecular remissions are attainable. A combined modality approach utilizing CHOP-Bleo and sequential radiation therapy in a "sandwich" technique has also been shown to be capable of inducing durable remissions.[62] However, it is arguable whether combined chemotherapy-radiotherapy in the stage III situation has added substantially to the results that might be attained with radiation therapy alone.

While total lymphoid radiation is infrequently employed at this time, the efficacy of this approach should not be forgotten. Important advances are being made in our utilization of radioimmunotherapy; this approach may deserve consideration as a logical successor to conventional external beam radiation therapy.

5.3   Advanced Stage (Stage III-IV)

The systemic therapy of patients with advanced stage indolent lymphoma is considered by some to be an area that is mired in confusion and controversy. Rather, the wide range of attractive options should be regarded as an opportunity to tailor therapy to a patient's particular needs, or, better still, as a strong motive to encourage patients to participate in clinical trials, which is a recommended approach in the NCCN guidelines.[63]

5.4   Chemotherapy

Chemotherapy is the most straightforward systemic therapy approach. Combination programs are prevalent and effective, but it is still unresolved whether combination chemotherapy is always superior to single alkylating agent therapy. A recent CALGB trial suggested that single agent cyclophosphamide is as effective as CHOP-Bleo for patients with grade 1 follicular lymphoma, but that the combination is probably warranted for patients with grade 2 follicular lymphoma.[64] Another ongoing controversy is whether to include doxorubicin or not. Some trials suggest an advantage for the inclusion of doxorubicin[65] while others do not.[66] Meta-analyses have suggested that biological therapy with interferon is most effective in the context of doxorubicin-containing combinations.[67,68] In the era of rituximab therapy, the R-CHOP regimen has been widely adopted.[69] Alternatives to alkylators or anthracyclines exist, notably the purine nucleoside analogs, which have been utilized as single agents[70,71] and in combinations, notably fludarabine-mitoxantrone (FN) combinations.[72-75] In a recent retrospective comparison, the SWOG concluded that FN was no better than CHOP, but it was no worse.[76] A recent randomized trial from Italy concluded that FN may be superior to CHOP in some respects, including molecular response rate, complete remission rate, and patient tolerance.[75]

In a review of the stage IV follicular lymphoma experience at M.D. Anderson over the past 25 years[31], stepwise improvements have been observed in both survival and failure-free survival (Table 4), most notably following the incorporation of biological therapies (first IFN and then rituximab) along with chemotherapy.

5.5 Interferon

Interferon represented the first immunotherapeutic agent to be used widely in the treatment of lymphoma, although BCG and other agents had been explored prior to interferon. Interferon has been utilized concurrently with chemotherapy and as a maintenance strategy following chemotherapy. In both settings, it has been shown, often [67,68, 77,78] but not always[79], to be beneficial in terms of failure-free survival. Moreover, a survival benefit has been observed in some studies when interferon has been incorporated with chemotherapy.[77,78] However, tolerance of interferon has been an issue, even though quality of life studies have indicated a net benefit with the use of interferon.[80]

Despite its established efficacy, the net impact of interferon has been judged to be only modest, and interferon is falling into disuse. It would be of interest if the benefits of IFN could be attained with less arduous strategies, for instance through the increased expression of interferon-inducible genes with CpG oligonucleotide therapy.[81]

5.6 Rituximab

After its approval for use as a single agent in the management of recurrent indolent lymphoma[82,83], rituximab has rapidly been incorporated along with chemotherapy in the front-line management of B-cell lymphoma and other B-cell disorders.

Rituximab has been used as a single agent in the front-line setting, and it has established efficacy.[84-87] Programs that utilize extended or maintenance therapy with rituximab have resulted in more durable remissions than with a single four-week treatment course.

Rituximab has been used widely in conjunction with chemotherapy, partly because of non-overlapping toxicities, but also because there is in vitro evidence that rituximab sensitizes some B-cell lymphoma cell lines to the cytotoxic effects of a number of chemotherapeutic agents.[88,89] In clinical trials with a variety of chemotherapy regimens, there has been a consistent pattern of superior response rates and failure-free survival rates when rituximab is used in conjunction with chemotherapy.[90-92] Table 3 illustrates preliminary results (median follow-up 32 months) of a recent randomized trial conducted at M.D. Anderson Cancer Center, in which concurrent R-FND was compared to sequential FND followed by rituximab.[90] In both arms of the trial, IFN maintenance therapy was given. Molecular response is attained more frequently and rapidly with R-FND, and failure-free survival appears to be superior with R-FND.

Emerging data also indicates that rituximab can prolong the duration of remission when used after chemotherapy.[93]

5.7   Radioimmunotherapy

Extensive marrow infiltration with lymphoma is a contraindication to the use of radioimmunotherapy. However, involvement by indolent lymphoma in the marrow is often focal, even at presentation, so a large fraction of advanced stage indolent lymphoma patients might be candidates for radioimmunotherapy. Only one small trial of this approach has been conducted, but results of that trial are very impressive.[94] Further experience with radioimmunotherapy in the front-line setting, either by itself or following chemotherapy[95,96], is an appropriate subject for further clinical trials.

5.8   Vaccines

Vaccine approaches in indolent lymphoma have evolved slowly but steadily. The renewed interest in the role of T-cells in the genesis of follicular lymphoma[13] might serve to stimulate greater participation in trials exploring this approach. Measurable stimulation of the patients' immune response has been demonstrated with vaccine approaches, and strategies to enhance the immune response are being tested.[97,98] Preparing a vaccine involves the procurement of tissue. While the vaccine is being prepared, several ongoing trials are utilizing standard chemotherapy approaches, with subsequent patient vaccination after completing several courses of chemotherapy. The ultimate role of vaccine strategies, and other approaches to augment the patient's T-cell response,[99] remains to be established.

5.9   Autologous Stem Cell Transplantation

While most experience with transplant is in the setting of relapse, several trials have explored transplant as a consolidation strategy in first remission. Phase II trials have shown impressively durable remissions with this approach.[100, 101]   Recently reported results from two European multi-center trials have been encouraging, with more durable remissions reported for patients who receive high dose therapy and autologous stem cell transplant in first remission.[102,103]

6.   MANAGEMENT OF RELAPSE

Relapse and histologic evolution are virtually inevitable in indolent lymphoma. Response to salvage therapy is common, even when the same therapy has been used repeatedly. However, typically the response rate is lower, and the second or subsequent remissions are of progressively shorter duration than with the initial therapy.[104]

Numerous treatment options exist for recurrent indolent lymphoma. Alkylating agents are no longer the only or even the best option. Notable successes have been achieved with chemotherapy (e.g., the nucleoside analogs)[70], biological therapy (e.g., rituximab)[81,82], and transplantation strategies (viz., allogeneic[32] and "mini-allo" transplant strategies).[105] Given the many possibilities, some long-view thinking is appropriate. If the patient is reasonably young and has an HLA-identical sibling, an allogeneic transplant strategy can be a consideration even at first relapse, since it is a potentially curative option. If the long-term plan might include autologous transplant, it might be prudent to limit the exposure to agents that impair stem cell harvesting, such as the nucleoside analogs.[106] Algorithms that loosely outline a stepwise management plan have been proposed[63], but ultimately treatment decisions must be individualized.

6.1   Chemotherapy

The nucleoside analogs, particularly fludarabine, are important agents in the management of patients with recurrent indolent lymphoma.[70,72,73] Support for the use of fludarabine in combination with a DNA-damaging agent such as cyclophosphamide is provided by cellular pharmacology evidence that fludarabine impairs the DNA-repair process, thereby augmenting the therapeutic impact of the alkylator.[107]

Many other chemotherapy combinations have been developed which utilize agents other than those in the CHOP regimen, such as ESHAP.[108] In the rituximab era, the monoclonal antibody is often incorporated into the program, as in the recently described R-GEMOX regimen.[109]

In recent years, new agents are developed with consideration of the presumed biological pathway that will be affected. For instance, bortezomib works at least in part by targeting the NF-Kβ pathway. Since that pathway appears to be dysregulated in the "activated B-cell" category of DLBCL[110], it might be predicted that bortezomib would be most promising in this category of DLBCL. However, to date, clinical trials indicate that bortezomib's most impressive impact may be against mantle cell lymphoma,[111] and possibly also indolent lymphoma.[112] Expectations based on cell biology must be tested with an open mind in clinical trials.

Other recent agents of interest (and their putative major mechanism of action) include: Bryostatin C (protein kinase C inhibitor); flavopiridol (cyclin dependant kinase inhibitor); CCI-779 (mammalian target of rapamycin, or mTOR, inhibitor); and tumor necrosis factor-related apoptosis-inducing ligand, or TRAIL (Fas-associated death domain protein signaling agent).

6.2   Targeted Therapy

Development of the anti-CD20 monoclonal antibody rituximab represented a landmark in the evolution of biological therapies. Other cell surface antigens had been targeted before CD20, notably the immunoglobulin idiotype, but CD20 has proven to be a highly suitable target, by virtue of its expression on virtually all mature B-cells, its relative lack of modulation or shedding from the cell surface, its sufficiently dense expression on most B-cell malignancies, and its absence on stem cells which results in only a temporary impact on the patient's normal B-cells.

HLA-DR is another target against which antibodies have been developed and tested in clinical trials.[113] CD22 and CD19 are other pan-B-cell antigens against which monoclonal antibodies have been developed; these surface antigens internalize, so these therapeutic antibodies can be utilized either as the "naked" antiibody [114] or linked to toxins and utilized as delivery systems.[115, 116]

Toxins can be linked to other agents besides antibodies. The immunotoxin denileukin diftitox is a fusion product that delivers the catalytic domain of diptheria toxin, but in which the receptor-binding domain of native diptheria toxin is replaced by sequences encoding the interleukin-2 (IL-2) gene. It targets cells that express the high-affinity IL-2 receptor (CD25), which includes cutaneous T-cell lymphoma and also some B-cell lymphomas.[117]

Antibodies against CD20 and other antigens have also been linked to radioisotopes and developed as radioimmunotherapy (RIT) agents. Following pioneering radioimmunotherapy work[118] with Lym-1 and other antibodies, RIT agents targeting CD20 have been developed, and are commercially available.[119,120] The delineation of the best time to utilize these agents is still a matter of clinical investigation; most experience to date has been in the setting of relapse rather than in front-line therapy. A particularly promising setting for RIT may be in the context of myeloablative therapy with subsequent stem cell transplantation.[121] While the logistics involved in the RIT approach make teamwork and planning crucial and somewhat daunting, RIT represents an important expansion of our therapeutic armamentarium.

6.3   Combination Biological Therapy

Immunotherapeutic agents have been used in various combinations. The experience with rituximab in conjunction with standard chemotherapeutic approaches in front-line therapy has been addressed earlier. The use of rituximab in conjunction with other biological agents has also been explored. Examples include combinations with other monoclonal antibodies such as anti-CD22,[122] with cytokines such as interferon-alfa, IL-2, GM-CSF, G-CSF, or IL-12,[123-126] and with other agents such as CpG oligonucleotides[81] or bcl-2 antisense oligonucleotides.[127]

6.4   Other Biological Therapy Approaches

Vaccine approaches have to date been explored most extensively in the setting of relapse. There is justifiable interest in exploring vaccines in less extensively treated patients, since the host immune response can be impaired following extensive chemotherapy.

In addition to its use with rituximab, bcl-2 antisense oligonucleotide therapy can be effective by itself.[25] Moreover, since overexpression of Bcl-2 confers resistance to chemotherapy in many malignancies, this approach also has the potential to enhance the efficacy of numerous chemotherapeutic agents.

6.5   Stem Cell Transplantation

The majority of the transplant experience has been with autologous transplant strategies, in the setting of relapse.[47,128]   Durable remissions can be attained, and this strategy appears to be more effective than many standard treatment approaches. However, long-term follow-up indicates that these patients are not cured, and there have been reports of late adverse effects, notably myelodysplasia. Importantly, the risk for myelodysplasia may not be attributable solely to the transplant strategy; the preceding chemotherapy exposure is likely a major contributor to the risk of myelodysplasia in these patients.[129]

The limited experience with conventional allogeneic transplant in indolent lymphoma is very encouraging.[32,130]   This approach can result in long-term disease-free survival, and even potential cure, in up to 40% of patients. However, standard allogeneic transplant is a high-risk approach, with a treatment related mortality rate approaching 30-40%. The advent of non-myeloablative allogeneic transplant strategies appears to represent a major step forward, with only about a 10% treatment related mortality rate.[105]   Early experience with this approach suggests that the potential for long-term disease control is preserved with this approach, so it can be expected that "mini-allo" strategies will be increasingly utilized in the future, even in older patients.

7.   DISTINCTIVE ASPECTS OF NON-FOLLICULAR INDOLENT B-CELL LYMPHOMAS

Treatment generalizations about all indolent lymphomas are often extrapolated from experience with follicular lymphoma. It is important to recognize key distinguishing features of other distinct indolent B-cell lymphomas.

The morphologic and phenotypic distinction of these entities from follicular lymphoma is not difficult. The follicular architecture is absent. CD10 is typically expressed in follicular lymphomas, but not in the other indolent B-cell lymphomas. CD5 and CD23 are typically expressed in small lymphocytic lymphoma, but not in the marginal zone lymphomas. Plasmacytoid features are characteristic for lymphoplasmacytic lymphoma.

7.1   Small Lymphocytic Lymphoma

In the WHO classification[1], SLL is grouped together with chronic lymphocytic leukemia (CLL). The clinical feature that distinguishes between CLL and SLL is, of course, the presence of the threshold number of circulating lymphocytes in CLL, and their absence in SLL. The biological features that control this homing are not yet clearly delineated.

Important advances have taken place in the biological understanding of CLL. The mutation status of the immunoglobulin heavy-chain variable-region (IgV_H) gene correlates with outcome in CLL. Patients with mutated IgV_H genes typically have slow progression of disease and long survival. Conversely, patients with unmutated IgV_H genes have more aggressive disease with anticipated shorter survival.[131] Gene microarray studies in CLL corroborate the importance of the IgV_H gene mutation status.[132] The CLL B-cells of many patients with unmutated IgV_H genes express ZAP-70, a signaling molecule that is normally expressed in T-cells.[133] These biological observations for CLL are presumably also applicable to SLL.

Gene expression profile observations are also emerging in SLL. Distinctive patterns are seen which permit discrimination among several lymphomas of small lymphocytes: SLL; mantle cell lymphoma; and splenic marginal zone B-cell lymphoma.[134] Genes associated with cell adhesion, angiogenesis, and inhibition of apoptosis are up-regulated in SLL.

SLL is a B-cell lymphoma, with consistent CD20 expression. However, the density of CD20 expression is substantially less in SLL than in many other categories of B-cell lymphoma.[135] This may partly explain the observed lower response rate of SLL to rituximab therapy than is seen with follicular lymphoma.[82] In the front-line setting, patients with SLL have been reported to respond nicely to standard doses of rituximab.[136] But in general, single agent therapy with rituximab at standard doses has been disappointing in SLL. Rituximab has been more successfully incorporated into CLL therapy using alternative approaches, including higher doses, the use of cytokines to increase surface CD20 expression of the CLL cells[137], and especially the development of combination programs with rituximab and chemotherapy, such as FCR or PCR.[138, 139]

While most therapeutic approaches for CLL would be expected to be effective in SLL as well, there may be some exceptions. The anti-CD52 monoclonal antibody alemtuzumab is an effective agent for CLL.[140] But it is most effective in clearing the peripheral blood and bone marrow, with less impressive results in controlling nodal disease. This "compartment" effect suggests that the node- and tissue-based presentation of SLL may not be so amenable to therapy with alemtuzumab.

7.2   Lymphoplasmacyic Lymphoma

Lymphoplasmacytic lymphoma is a rare disease, but it is a famous entity because it includes the clinical syndrome of Waldenstrom's macroglobulinemia, with its characteristic IgM serum paraprotein and the associated clinical features.[141]

Rearrangement of the PAX-5 gene in association with t(9;14) is a common finding in patients with lymphoplasmacytic lymphoma.[142]

Hepatitis C exposure has been linked to several categories of lymphoma.[143] Its association with type II mixed cryoglobulinemia and lymphoplasmacytoid lymphoma is particularly notable.[144]

Lymphoplasmacytic lymphoma is usually indolent. Plasmapheresis is needed if there are features of the hyperviscosity syndrome. Numerous chemotherapy strategies can be effective, including programs with nucleoside analogs.[145] Some treatment strategies that are effective in multiple myeloma have shown promising results in Waldenstrom's macroglobulinemia, including thalidomide and bortezomib.

7.3   Marginal Zone Lymphoma

Three entities are defined as marginal zone lymphomas.[146-150] Although they all typically have the same phenotype (B-cell, but CD10 negative, CD5 negative, and CD23 negative), they have distinctly different clinical and biological features.

Extranodal Marginal Zone Lymphoma of Mucosa-Associated Lymphoid Tissue (MALT)

The fascinating etiological clues that pertain to many types of MALT lymphoma have previously been discussed. When appropriate, therapy for an underlying infection is usually the preferred initial treatment approach for MALT lymphomas.

Several distinct cytogenetic abnormalities have been observed in MALT lymphoma. The most common is t(11;18)(q21; q21), which is found in about half of MALT lymphomas.[10] Two genes of interest are involved in t(11;18): *API2*, which is a member of the inhibitor of apoptosis protein (IAP) family; and *MLT*, which plays a role in the activation of NF-kB. A much more infrequent cytogenetic finding in MALT lymphoma is t(1;14),(p22; q32). The *BCL10* gene, which is involved in t(1;14), also probably has an impact on the NF-kB signaling pathway.

Presentation with early stage disease (stage I-II) is a distinctive feature of many MALT lymphomas (Table 1). More often than with any other indolent lymphoma, localized therapy approaches can be appropriate treatment considerations for patients with MALT lymphoma. Radiation therapy and surgery can be effective approaches.

While often localized and responsive to treatment at the time of initial diagnosis, the non-gastric MALT lymphomas are prone to late relapse, even those that are initially detected with localized (stage I-II) disease.[151] Thus, systemic therapy is sometimes also needed. The optimum systemic approach is not clear. Single-agent alkylators, single-agent rituximab, and combination regimens have all been utilized. The disease usually is responsive to systemic therapy approaches.

7.4 Nodal Marginal Zone Lymphoma

Most patients with nodal marginal zone lymphoma present with advanced stage disease (Table 1). In contrast to MALT lymphoma, the outlook with nodal marginal zone lymphoma is no better than with advanced stage follicular lymphoma.[152]

7.5 Splenic Marginal Zone Lymphoma

As with lymphoplasmacytic lymphoma, hepatitis C may play a role in the genesis of some cases of splenic marginal zone lymphoma. Splenomegally is usually the dominant clinical feature in these patients. Bone marrow and peripheral blood involvement are also commonly seen. A serum M-peak is present in about 10-20% of patients. When patients have cytopenias, it is sometimes unclear whether the cytopenias are related to splenic sequestration or to marrow infiltration. Splenectomy is often the most appropriate initial therapeutic intervention. When cytopenias resolve following splenectomy, patients can often remain stable for prolonged periods without further therapy. Eventual progression in the bone marrow, blood, and the lymph nodes can be expected. Systemic therapy approaches that are successful in follicular lymphoma or in CLL are typically also effective in splenic marginal zone lymphoma.

8. PROSPECTS FOR THE FUTURE

Our understanding of the biology of the indolent lymphomas is having an increasing impact on patient management. Etiological clues, such as in gastric MALT lymphoma, can relate directly to therapy decisions. Chemotherapy choices are increasingly likely to be guided by knowledge of the biological pathways that are altered in specific disease entities.   The conventional view that "biological therapy" denotes immunotherapy may need to be re-defined, since many chemotherapeutic agents will be developed with specific biological target pathways in mind.

The horizons of immunotherapy are expanding.   Monoclonal antibody therapy is now standard, either by itself, in conjunction with chemotherapy, or with other biological agents.   Strategies to manipulate the patients' T-cell response are expanding.   Vaccine approaches are improving.   Ex vivo strategies to augment the T-cell response are being explored.   And the risks associated with allogeneic stem cell transplant are decreasing.

The pace of treatment progress seems at times to be as slow as the clinical pace of the indolent lymphoma.   But current biological insights warrant optimism.   Bridging the gap between basic science observations and clinical accomplishments is an increasing challenge.   One key link is patients' willingness to participate in clinical trials.   The medical community needs to advocate participation in clinical trials, so that promising biological observations   can   be   brought   to   clinical   fruition.

Table 1. Clinical Features of Indolent Lymphoma

	FL	SLL	nodal MZL	extra-nodal MZL	Lymph-plasmacytic
frequency	22%	6%	1%	5%	1%
median age (yrs)	59	65	58	60	63
% male	42	53	42	48	53
stage (%)					
I	18	4	13	39	7
II	15	5	13	28	13
III	16	8	34	2	7
IV	51	83	40	31	73
B symptoms (%)	28	33	37	19	
Bulk ≥ 5cm (%)	61	59	36	68	50
Marrow involved (%)	42	72	32	14	73
GI tract involved (%)	4	3	5	50	7

Abbreviations: FL, follicular lymphoma; SLL, small lymphocytic lymphoma; MZL, marginal zone lymphoma.
adapted from Armitage and Weisenburger[3]

Table 2. Molecular Response Correlates with Duration of Clinical Response

Author	Therapy	% Failure-Free if:		P Value
		Molec. Resp	Molec. Non-Resp	
Freedman[47]	BMT	90	29	< 0.01
López-Guillermo[48]	CT ± XT	73	28	< 0.01
Czuczman[49]	Rituximab	76	23	< 0.01

* 5-year FFS data, except Czuczman et al, which is 1 yr

Table 3. Preliminary Results of Randomized Trial Comparing Concurrent R-FND with Sequential FND Followed by RITUXIMAB[90]

	R-FND (N=82)	P Value	FND → R (N=78)
CR%	88	NS	85
CR + PR%	100	NS	96
Surv. (% at 3 yrs)	96	NS	94
FFS (% at 3 yrs):			
all patients	76	0.12	60
Follicular only	84	0.01	59
Molec. Resp %:			
at 6 mo	89	< 0.01	60
at 12 mo	89	0.01	68

Table 4. Stage IV Follicular Lymphoma: 25 Years of Treatment Progress[31]

			% Survival		
Years	Regimen	No. Pts.	5-yr	10-yr	15-yr
1977	CHOP-B	96	64	39	28
1982	CHOP-B → IFN	131	75	52	42
1988	ATT (+ IFN)	136	52	60	-
1992	ATT vs FND (+ IFN)	142	82	-	-
1997	FND vs. R-FND (+IFN)	200	90	-	-

Liu Q, et al: Blood 2003; 102: 398a

9.   REFERENCES

1. Harris NL, Jaffe ES, Diebold J, et al: World Health Organization classification of neoplastic diseases of the hematopoietic and lymphoid tissues: report of the Clinical advisory Committee meeting-Airlie House, Virginia, November 1997. J Clin Oncol 1999; 17: 3853-3849

2. Nathwani BN, Harris NL, Weisenburger D, Isaacson PG, Piris MA, Berger F, Müller-Hermelink HK, Swerdlow SH. Follicular Lymphoma. In: Jaffe ES, Harris NL, Stein H, Vardiman JW, eds. World Health Organization Classification of Tumours: Pathology and Genetics of Tumours of Haematopoietic and Lymphoid Tissues. Lyon, IARC 2001: Pages 162-167

3. Armitage JO, Weisenburger DD: New approach to classifying non-Hodgkin's lymphomas: clinical features of the major histologic subtypes.   Non-Hodgkin's Lymphoma Classification Project. J Clin Oncol 1998; 16: 2780-95

4. Biagi JJ, Seymour JF. Insights into the molecular pathogenesis of follicular lymphoma arising from analysis of geographic variation. Blood 2002; 99: 4265-4275

5. Coiffier B, Thieblemont C, Felman P, et al: Indolent nonfollicular lymphomas: characteristics, treatment, and outcome. Semin Hematol 1999; 36: 198-208

6. Eck M, Schmauβer B, Greiner A, and Müller-Hermelink K: *Helicobacter pylori* in gastric mucosa-associated lymphoid tissue type lymphoma.   In: Fischback W, ed., Gastrointestinal Lymphoma: Future Perspectives. Springer-Verlag Berlin-Heidelberg 2000 (Recent Results in Cancer Research, Vol. 156): pages 9-18

7. Wotherspoon AC, Doglioni C, Diss TC, et al: Regression of primary low-grade B-cell gastric lymphoma of mucosa-associated lymphoid tissue type after eradication of *Helicobacter pylori.* Lancet 1993; 342: 575-577

8. Hofbauer GF, Kessler B, Kempf W, et al: Multilesional primary cutaneous diffuse large B-cell lymphoma responsive to antibiotic treatment. Dermatology 2001; 203: 168-170

9. Ferreri AJM, Guidoboni M, Ponzoni M, et al: Evidence for an association between *Chlamydia psittaci* and ocular adnexal lymphomas. J Natl Cancer Inst 2004; 96: 586-594

10. Auer IA, Gascoyne RD, Connors JM, et al: t(11;18)(q21;q21) is the most common translocation in MALT lymphomas. Ann Oncol 1997; 8: 979-985

11. Willis TG, Jadayel DM, Du MQ, et al: Bcl10 is involved in t(1;14)(p22;q32) of MALT B cell lymphoma and mutated in multiple tumor types. Cell 1999; 96: 35-45

12. Jaffe ES: Follicular lymphoma: Possibility that they are benign tumors of the lymphoid system. JNCI 1983; 70: 401-403

13. Dave S, Wright G, Tan B, et al: Prediction of survival in follicular lymphoma based on molecular features of tumor-Infiltrating immune cells. N Engl J Med 2004; 351: 2159-2169

14. Lossos IS, Alizadeh AA, Diehn M, et al: Transformation of follicular lymphoma to diffuse large-cell lymphoma: Alternative patterns with increased or decreased expression of c-myc and its regulated genes. Proc Natl Acad Sci USA 2002; 99: 8886-8891

15. Elinitoba-Johnson KS, Jenson SD, Abbott RT, et al: Involvement of multiple signaling pathways in follicular lymphoma transformation: p38-mitogenactivated protein kinase as a target for therapy. Proc Natl Acad Sci USA 2003; 100: 7259-7264

16. Glas AM, Kersten, MJ, Delahaye LJMJ, et al: Gene expression profiling in follicular lymphoma to assess clinical aggressiveness and to guide the choice of treatment. Blood 2002; 105: 301-307

17. Rosenwald A, Wright G, Chan WC, et al: The use of molecular profiling to predict survival after chemotherapy for diffuse large-B-cell lymphoma. N Engl J Med 2005; 346: 1937-1947

18. Korsmeyer S. Bcl-2 initiates a new category of oncogenes: Regulators of cell death. Blood 1992;80: 879-886

19. Albinger-Hegyi A, Hochreutener B, Abdou M-T, et al: High frequency of t(14;18)-translocation breakpoints outside of major breakpoint and minor cluster regions in follicular lymphomas. Improved polymerase chain reaction protocols for their detection. Am J Pathol 2002; 160: 823-832

20. Liu NS, Medeiros LJ, Cabanillas F, et al: Prognostic relevance of t(14;18) status in follicular lymphoma. Proc ASCO 2003; 22: 2219 (abstr)

21. Lopez-Guillermo A, Cabanillas F, McDonnell TI, et al: Correlation of bcl-2 rearrangement with clinical characteristics and outcome in indolent follicular lymphoma. Blood 1999; 93: 3081-3087

22. Bosga-Bouwer AG, van Imhoff GW, Boonstra R, et al: Follicular lymphoma grade 3B includes 3 cytogenetically defined subgroups with primary t(14;18), 3q27, or other translocations: t(14;18) and 3q27 are mutually exclusive. Blood 2003; 101: 1145-1154

23. Lee MS, Chang KS, Cabanillas F, et al: Detection of minimal residual cells carrying the t(14;18) by DNA sequence amplification. Science 1987; 237: 175-178

24. Gribben JG, Nuberg D, Barber M, et al: Detection of residual lymphoma cells by polymerase chain reaction in peripheral blood is significantly less predictive for relapse than detection in bone marrow. Blood 1994; 83: 3800-3807

25. Waters JS, Webb A, Cunningham D, et al: Phase I clinical and pharmacokinetic study of bcl-2 antisense oligonucleotide therapy in patients with non-Hodgkin's lymphoma. J Clin Oncol 2000; 18: 1812-1823

26. Horning SJ: Natural history of and therapy for the indolent non-Hodgkin's lymphomas. Semin Oncol 1993; 20: 75-80

27. Brice P, Bastion Y, Lepage E, et al: Comparision in low-tumor-burden follicular lymphomas between an initial no-treatment policy, prednimustine, or interferon alfa: a randomized study from the Groupe d'Etude des Lymphomes Folliculaires. Grope d'Etude des Lymphomes de l'Adulte. J Clin Oncol 1997; 15: 1110-1117

28. Ardeshna KM, Smith P, Norton A, et al: Long-term effect of a watch and wait policy versus immediate systemic treatment for asymptomatic advanced-stage non-Hodgkin lymphoma: a randomized controlled trial. Lancet 2003; 362-: 516-522

29. Young RC, Longo DL, Glatstein E, et al: The treatment of indolent lymphomas: watchful waiting v aggressive combined modality treatment. Semin Hematol 1988; (2 Suppl 2):11-6

30. Horning SJ, Rosenberg SA: The natural history of initially untreated low-grade non-Hodgkin's lymphomas. N Engl J Med 1984; 311: 1471-1475

31. Liu Q, Fayad L, Hagemeister FB, et al: Stage IV indolent lymphoma: 25 years of treatment progress. Blood 2003; 102: 398a (abstr)

32. Van Besien K, Sobocinski KA, Rowlings PA et al: Allogeneic bone marrow transplantation for low-grade lymphoma. Blood 1998; 92: 1832-1836

33. Petersen PM Gospodarowicz M, Tsang R, et al: Long-term outcome in stage I and II follicular lymphoma following treatment with involved field radiation therapy alone. Proc ASCO 2004; 23: 561 (abstr)

34. Hehn ST, Grogan TM, Miller TP: Utility of fine-needle aspiration as a diagnostic technique in lymphoma. J Clin Oncol 2004; 22: 3046-3052

35. Shipp MA, Harrington DP, Anderson JR, et al: The International Non-Hodgkin's Lymphoma Prognostic Factors Project: A predictive model for aggressive non Hodgkin's lymphoma. N Engl J Med 1993; 329 : 987-994

36. Solal-Celigny P, Roy P, Colombat P, et al: Follicular lymphoma international prognostic index. Blood 2004; 104: 1258-1265

37. Lopez-Guillermo A, Montserrat E, Bosch F, et al: Applicability of the International Index for aggressive lymphomas to patients with low-grade lymphoma. J Clin Oncol 1994; 12: 1343-1348

38. Dimoupolous MA, Cabanillas F, Lee JJ, et al: Prognostic role of serum beta 2-microglobulin in Hodgkin's disease. J Clin Oncol 1993; 11: 1108-1111

39. Swan F, Velasquez WS, Tucker S, et al: A new serologic staging system for large-cell lymphomas based on initial ß2-microglobulin and lactate dehydrogenase levels. J Clin Oncol 1989; 7:1518-1527

40. Litam P, Swan F, Cabanillas F, et al: Prognostic value of serum beta-2 microglobulin in low-grade lymphoma. Ann Intern Med 1991; 114: 855-860

41. Johnson PWM, Swinbank K, MacLennan S, et al: Variability of polymerase chain reaction detection of the bcl-2-IgH translocation in an international multicentre study. Ann Oncol 1999; 10: 1349-1354

42. Summers KE, Davies AJ, Matthews J, et al: The relative role of peripheral blood and bone marrow for monitoring molecular evidence of disease in follicular lymphoma by quantitative real-time polymerase chain reaction. Br J Haematol 2002; 118: 563-566

43. Schüler F. Hirt C, Dölken G: Chromosomal translocation t(14;18) in healthy individuals. Semin Cancer Biology 2003; 13: 203-209

44. Price CGA, Meerabux J, Murtagh S, et al: The significance of circulating cells carrying t(14;18) in long remission from follicular lymphoma. J Clin Oncol 1991; 9: 1527-1532

45. Colombat P, Garrigue MA, Lamagnere JP, et al: bcl-2 evaluation in patients in long-term complete remission after bone marrow transplantation. J Clin Oncol 1994; 12: 2516 (letter)

46. Johnson PWM, Price CGA, Smith T, et al: Detection of cells bearing the t(14;18) translocation following myeloablative treatment and autologous bone marrow transplantation for follicular lymphoma. J Clin Oncol 1994; 12: 798-805

47. Freedman AS, Neuberg D, Mauch P, et al: Long-term follow-up of autologous bone marrow transplantation in patients with relapsed follicular lymphoma. Blood 1999; 94: 3325-3333

48. Lopez-Guillermo A, Cabanillas F, McLaughlin P, et al: The clinical significance of molecular response in indolent follicular lymphomas. Blood 1998; 91: 2955-2960

49. Czuczman MS, Grillo-Lopez AJ, McLaughlin P, et al: Clearing of cells bearing the *bcl-2* [t(14;18)] translocation from blood and marrow of patients treated with rituximab alone or in combination with CHOP chemotherapy. Annals of Oncology 2001; 12: 109-114

50. Rambaldi A, Lazzari M, Manzoni C, et al: Monitoring of minimal residual disease after CHOP and rituximab in previously untreated patients with follicular lymphoma. Blood 2002; 99: 856-862

51. Blum R, Seymour JF, Wirth A, et al: Evaluation of 18-FDG-PET in the staging of patients with indolent non-Hodgkin's lymphoma. Ann Oncol 2002; 13 (suppl 2): 45a (abstr)

52. Friedberg JW, Chengazi V: PET scans in the staging of lymphoma: current status. The Oncologist 2003; 8: 438-447

53. Dabaja BS, Ha CS, Wilder RB, Pro B, McLaughlin P, Cabanillas F, Cox JD: Importance of esophagogastroduodenoscopy in the evaluation of non-gastrointestinal mucosa-associated lymphoid tissue lymphoma. Cancer J 2003; 9: 321-324

54. Paryani SB, Hoppe RT, Cox RS, et al: Analysis of non-Hodgkin's lymphomas with nodular and favorable histologies, stages I and II. Cancer 1983; 52: 2300-2307

55. Mac Manus MP and Hoppe RT: Is radiotherapy curative for stage I and II low-grade follicular lymphoma? Results of a long-term follow-up study of patients treated at Stanford University. J Clin Oncol 1996; 14: 1282-1290

56. McLaughlin P, Fuller LM, Velasquez WS, et al: Stage I-II follicular lymphoma: Treatment results for 76 patients. Cancer 1986; 58:1596-1602

57. Seymour JF, Pro B, Fuller LM, et al: Long-term follow-up of a prospective study of combined modality therapy for stage I-II indolent non-Hodgkin's lymphoma. J Clin Oncol 2003; 21: 2115-2122

58. Soybeyran P, Eghbali H, Trojani M, et al: Is there any place for a wait-and-see policy in stage 10 follicular lymphoma? A study of 42 consecutive patients in a single center. Ann Oncol 1996; 7: 713-718

59. Advani R, Rosenberg SA, Horning SJ. Stage I and II follicular non-Hodgkin's lymphoma: long-term follow-up of no initial therapy. J Clin Oncol 2004; 22: 1454-1459

60. Ha CS, Kong JS, McLaughlin P: et al: Stage III follicular lymphoma: long-term follow-up and patterns of failure. Int J Radiat Oncol Biol Phys 2003; 57: 748-754

61. Jacobs JP, Murray KJ, Schultz CJ, et al: Central lymphatic irradiation for stage III nodular malignant lymphoma: Long-term results. J Clin Oncol 1993; 11: 233-238.

62. McLaughlin P., Fuller LM, Velasquez WS, et al: Stage III follicular lymphoma: Durable remissions with a combined chemotherapy-radiotherapy regimen. J Clin Oncol 1987; 5: 867-8741

63. Zelenetz AD, Appelbaum FR, Buadi F, et al: The NCCN non-Hodgkin's lymphoma clinical practice guidelines. Journal of the National Comprehensive Cancer Center Network 2004; 2: 226-336

64. Peterson BA, Petroni GR, Frizzera G, et al: Prolonged single-agent versus combination chemotherapy in indolent follicular lymphomas: A study of the Cancer And Leukemia Group B. J Clin Oncol 2003; 21: 5-15

65. Rigacci L, Federico M, Martelli M, et al: The role of anthracyclines in combination chemotherapy for the treatment of follicular lymphoma: Retrospective study of the Intergruppo Italiano Linfomi on 761 cases. Leuk & Lymphoma 2003; 44: 1911-1917

66. Jones SE, Grozea PN, Metz EN, et al: Improved complete remission rates and survival for patients with large cell lymphoma treated with chemoimmunotherapy. A Southwest Oncology Group Study. Cancer 1983; 51: 1083-1090

67. Rohatiner AZS, Gregory W, Peterson B, et al: A meta-analysis of randomized trials evaluating the role of interferon as treatment for follicular lymphoma. Proc ASCO 1998; 17: 4a (abstr)

68. Allen IE, Ross SD, Borden SP, et al: Meta-analysis to assess the efficacy of interferon-alpha in patients with follicular non-Hodgkin's lymphoma. J Immunother 2001: 58-65

69. Czuczman M, Weaver R, Alkuzweny, et al: Prolonged clinical and molecular remission in patients with low-grade or follicular non-Hodgkin's lymphoma treated with rituximab plus CHOP chemotherapy: 9-year follow-up. J Clin Oncol 2004; 22: 4711-4716

70. Redman J, Cabanillas F, Velasquez W, et al: Phase II trial of fludarabine phosphate in lymphoma: an effective new agent for low-grade lymphoma. J Clin Oncol 1998; 10: 790-794

71. Solal-Celigny P, Brice P, Brousse N, et al: Phase II trial of fludarabine monophosphate as first-line treatment in patients with advanced follicular lymphoma: a multicenter

study by the Groupe d'Etude des Lymphomes de l'Adulte. J Clin Oncol 1996; 14: 514-519

72. McLaughlin P, Hagemeister FB, Romaguera JE, et al: Fludarabine, mitoxantrone, and dexamethasone: an effective new regimen for indolent lymphoma. J Clin Oncol 1996; 14: 1262-1268

73. Zinzani PL, Bendandi M, Magagnoli M, et al: Fludarabine–mitoxantrone combination-containing regimen in recurrent low-grade non-Hodgkin's lymphoma Ann Oncol 1997; 8: 379-383

74. Tsimberidou AM, McLaughlin P, Younes A, et al: Fludarabine, mitoxantrone, dexamethasone (FND) compared with an alternating triple therapy (ATT) regimen in patients with stage IV indolent lymphoma. Blood 2002; 100: 4351-4357

75. Zinzani PL, Pulsoni A, Perrotti A, et al: Fludarabine plus mitoxantrone with and without rituximab versus CHOP with and without rituximab as front-line treatment for patients with follicular lymphoma. J Clin Oncol 2004; 22: 2654-2661

76. Velasquez WS, Lew D, Grogan TM, et al: Combination of fludarabine and mitoxantrone in untreated stages III and IV low-grade lymphoma: S9501. J Clin Oncol 2003; 21: 1996-2003

77. Solal-Celigny P, Lepage E, Brousse N, et al: Doxorubicin-containing regimen with or without interferon alfa-2b for advanced follicular lymphomas: final analysis of survival and toxicity in the Groupe d'Etude des Lymphomes Folliculaires 86 Trial. J Clin Oncol 1998; 16: 2332-2338

78. Verstovsek S, Romaguera JE, Cabanillas F, et al: CHOP-Bleo plus interferon-α for stage IV low grade lymphoma – an update after 13-year follow up: significant improvement in both overall end failure-free survival. Blood 1999; 94 (suppl. 1, part 2): 270b (abstr)

79. Fisher RI, Dana BW, LeBlanc M, et al: Interferon alpha consolidation after intensive chemotherapy does not prolong the progression-free survival of patients with low-grade non-Hodgkin's lymphoma: results of the Southwest Oncology Group randomized phase III study 8809. J Clin Oncol 2000; 18: 2010-2016

80. Cole BF, Solal-Celigny P, Gelber RD, et al: Quality-of-life-adjusted survival analysis of interferon alfa-2b treatment for advanced follicular lymphoma: an aid to clinical decision making. J Clin Oncol 1998; 16: 2339-2344

81. Friedberg JW, Kim H, McCauley M, et al: Combination immunotherapy with a CpG oligonucleotide (1018 ISS) and rituximab in patients with non-Hodgkin lymphoma: increased interferon-α/β- inducible gene expression, without significant toxicity. Blood 2005; 105: 489-495

82. McLaughlin P, Grillo-Lopez AJ, Link BK, et al: Rituximab chimeric antiCD20 monoclonal antibody therapy for relapsed indolent lymphoma: half of patients respond to a four-dose treatment program. J Clin Oncol 1998; 16: 2825-2833

83. Maloney DG, Grillo-Lopez AJ, White CA, et al: IDEC-C2B8 (Rituximab) anti-CD20 monoclonal antibody therapy in patients with relapsed low-grade non-Hodgkin's lymphoma. Blood 1997; 90: 2188-2195

84. Colombat P, Salles G, Brousse N, et al: Rituximab (anti-CD20 monoclonal antibody) as single first-line therapy for patients with follicular lymphoma with a low tumor burden: clinical and molecular evaluation. Blood 2001; 97: 101-106

85. Ghielmini M, Schmitz SF, Cogliatti SB, et al: Prolonged treatment with rituximab in patients with follicular lymphoma significantly increases event-free survival and response duration compared with the standard weekly x 4 schedule. Blood 2004; 103: 4416-4423

86. Hainsworth, JD, Litchy S, Burris HA, et al: rituximab as first-line and maintenance therapy for patients with indolent non-hodgkin's lymphoma. J Clin Oncol 2002; 20: 4261-4267

87. Kimby E, Geisler C, Hagberg H, et al: Rituximab as single agent and in combination with interferon-α-2a as treatment of untreated and first relapse follicular or other low-grade lymphomas. A randomized phase II study. Ann Oncol 2002; 13 (Suppl 2): 85 (abstr)

88. Alas S, Emmanouilides C, Bonavida B: Inhibition of interleukin 10 by rituximab results in down-regulation of bcl-2 and sensitization of B-cell non-Hodgkin's lymphoma to apoptosis. Clin Can Res 2004; 7: 709-723

89. Di Gaetano N, Xiao Y, Erba R, Bassan R, Rambaldi A, Golay J, Introna M: Synergism between fludarabine and rituximab revealed in a follicular lymphoma cell line resistant to the cytotoxic activity of either drug alone. Br J Haematol 2001; 114: 800-809

90. McLaughlin P, Rodriguez MA, Hagemeister FB, et al: Stage IV indolent lymphoma: a randomized study of concurrent vs. sequential use of FND chemotherapy (fludarabine, mitoxantrone, dexamethasone) and rituximab monoclonal antibody therapy, with interferon maintenance. Proc ASCO 2003; 22: 564 (abstr)

91. Marcus R, Imrie K, Belch A, et al: CVP chemotherapy plus rituximab compared with CVP as first-line treatment for advanced follicular lymphoma. Blood online October 2004

92. Hiddemann W, Dreyling MH, Forstpointner R, et al: Combined immuno-chemotherapy (R-CHOP) significantly improves time to treatment failure in first line therapy of follicular lymphoma: Results of a prospective randomized trial of the German Low Grade Lymphoma Study Group (GLSG). Blood 2003; 102: 104a (abstr)

93. Hochster HS, Weller E, Ryan T, et al: Results of E1496: A phase III trial of CVP with or without maintenance rituximab in advanced indolent lymphoma (NHL). Proc ASCO 2004; 23:556 (abstr)

94. Kaminiski MS, Tuck M, Regan, et al: High response rates and durable remissions in patients with previously untreated, advanced-stage, follicular lymphoma treated with tositumomab and iodine I-131 tositumomab (Bexxar®). Blood 2002; 100 (suppl): 356a (abstr) – N Engl J Med 2005, in press

95. Press OW, Unger JM, Braziel RM, et al: A phase 2 trial of CHOP chemotherapy followed by tositumomab/iodine I 131 tositumomab for previously untreated follicular non-Hodgkin lymphoma: Southwest Oncology Group Protocol S9911. Blood 2003; 102: 1606-1612.

96. Leonard JP, Coleman M, Kostakoglu L: Fludarabine monophosphate followed by iodine I 131 tositumomab for untreated low-grade and follicular non-Hodgkin's lymphoma (NHL). Blood 1999; 94: 90a (abstr)

97. Kunkel LA: Idiotype vaccines in the treatment of B-cell non-Hodgkin's lymphoma. Cancer Invest 2004; 22: 97-105

98. Kwak LW, Campbell MJ, Czerwinski DK, et al: Induction of immune responses in patients with B-cell lymphoma against the surface-immunoglobulin idiotype expressed by their tumors. N Engl J Med 1992; 327: 1209-1215

99. Laport GG, Levine BL, Stadtmauer EA, et al: Adoptive transfer of costimulated T cells induces lymphocytosis in patients with relapsed/refractory non-Hodgkin lymphoma following CD34[+]-selected hematopoietic cell transplantation. Blood 2003; 102: 2004-2013

100. Horning SJ, Negrin RS, Hoppe RT, et al: High-dose therapy and autologous bone marrow transplantation for follicular lymphoma in first complete or partial remission: results of a phase II clinical trial. Blood 2001; 97: 404-409

101. Freedman AS, Gribben JG, Neuberg D, et al High-dose therapy and autologous bone marrow transplantation in patients with follicular lymphoma during first remission. Blood 1996; 88: 2780-2786

102. Schouten HC, Qian W, Kvaloy-Schouten S, et al: High-dose therapy improves progression-free survival and survival in relapsed follicular non-Hodgkin's lymphoma: Results from the randomized European CUP Trial. J Clin Oncol 2003; 21: 3918-3927

103. Lenz G, Dreyling M, Schiegnitz E, et al: Myeloablative radiochemotherapy followed by autologous stem cell transplantation in first remission prolongs progression-free survival in follicular lymphoma: results of a prospective, randomized trial of the German Low-Grade Lymphoma Study Group. Blood 2004; 104: 2667-2674

104. Gallagher CJ, Gregory WM, Jones AE, et al: Follicular lymphoma: prognostic factors for response and survival. J Clin Oncol 1986; 4: 1470-1480

105. Khouri IF, Saliba RM, Giralt SA, et al: Nonablative allogeneic hematopoietic transplantation as adoptive immunotherapy for indolent lymphoma: low incidence of toxicity, acute graft-versus-hosts disease, and treatment-related mortality. Blood 2001; 98: 3595-3599

106. Ketterer N, Salles G, Moullet I, et al: Factors associated with successful mobilization of peripheral blood progenitor cells in 200 patients with lymphoid malignancies. Br J Haematol 1998; 103: 235-242

107. Yamauchi T, Nowak BJ, Keating MJ, et al: DNA repair initiated in chronic lymphocytic leukemia lymphocytes by 4-hydroperoxycyclophosphamide is inhibited by fludarabine and clofarabine. Clin Can Res 2001; 7: 580-3589

108. Velasquez WS, McLaughlin P, Tucker S, et al: ESHAP - An effective chemotherapy regimen in refractory and relapsing lymphoma: a 4-year follow-up study. J Clin Oncol 1994; 12: 1169-1176

109. El Gnaoui T, Dupuis J, Joly B, et al: Rituximab, gemcitabine and oxaliplatin (R-GEMOX): A promising regimen for refractory/relapsed B-cell lymphoma. Blood 2004; 104 (Suppl): 681a (abstr)

110. Davis RE, Brown KK, Siebenlist U, et al: Constitutive nuclear factor kappaB activity is required for survival of activated B cell-like diffuse large B cell lymphoma cells. J Exper Med 2001; 194: 1861-1874

111. Goy A, Younes A, McLaughlin P, et al: Phase II study of proteasome inhibitor bortezomib in relapsed or refractory B-cell non-Hodgkin's lymphoma. J Clin Oncol, in press

112. O'Connor O, Wright J, Moskowitz C, et al: A multicenter experience with singe agent bortezomib in non-Hodgkin's lymphoma reveals marked difference in sub-type sensitivity to proteasome inhibition. Blood 2004; 104 (Suppl): 175a (abstr)

113. Link BK, Wang H, Byrd JC: A phase II study of RemitogenT(Hu1D10), a humanized monoclonal antibody in patients with relapsed or refractory follicular, small lymphocytic, or marginal zone/MALT B-cell lymphoma. Blood 2001; 98: 2540a (abstr)

114. Leonard JP, Coleman M, Matthews JC: Phase I/II trial of epratuzumab (humanized anti-CD22 antibody) in non-Hodgkin's lymphoma (NHL). Blood 2002; 100: 358a (abstr)

115. Grossbard ML, Lambert JM, Goldmacher VS, et a: Anti-B4-blocked ricin: a phase I trial of 7-day continuous infusion in patients with B-cell neoplasms. J Clin Oncol 1993; 11: 726-737

116. Vitetta ES, Stone M, Amlot P, et al: Phase I immunotoxin trial in patients with B-cell lymphoma. Cancer Res 1991; 51: 4052-4058

117. Dang NH, Hagemeister FB, Pro B, et al: Phase II study of denileukin diftitox for relapsed/refractory B-cell non-Hodgkin's lymphoma: J Clin Oncol 2004; 22: 4095-4102

118. DeNardo GL, DeNardo SJ, Goldstein DS, et al: Maximum-tolerated dose, toxicity, and efficacy of (131)I-Lym-1 antibody for fractionated radioimmunotherapy of non-Hodgkin's lymphoma. J Clin Oncol 1998; 16: 3246-3256

119. Kaminiski MS, Zelenetz AD, Press OW, et al: Pivotal study of iodine I 121 tositumomab for chemotherapy-refractory low-grade or transformed low-grade B-cell non-Hodgkin's lymphoma. J Clin Oncol 2001; 19: 3918-3928

120. Witzig TE, Gordon LI, Cabanillas F, et al: Randomized controlled trial of yttrium-90-labeled ibritumomab tiuxetan radioimmunotherapy versus rituximab immunotherapy for patients with relapsed or refractory low-grade, follicular, or transformed B-cell non-Hodgkin's lymphoma. J Clin Oncol 2002; 20: 2453-2463

121. Liu SY, Eary JF, Petersondorf SH, et al: Follow-up of relapsed B-cell lymphoma patients treated with iodine-131- labeled anti-CD20 antibody and autologous stem-cell rescue. J Clin Oncol 1998; 16: 3270

122. Leonard JP, Coleman M, Matthews JC, et al: Epratuzumab (anti-CD22) and rituximab (anti-CD20) combination immunotherapy for non-Hodgkin's lymphoma: preliminary response data. Proc ASCO 2002; 21: 266a (abstr)

123. Sacchi S, Federico M, Vitolo U, et al: Clinical activity and safety of combination immunohterapy with IFN-alpha 2a and rituximab in patients with relapsed low grade non-Hodgkin's lymphoma. Haematologica 2001; 86: 951-958

124. Liu NS, Grimm E, Poindexter N: Antibody dependent cellular cytotoxicity and natural killer cell activity in patients with recurrent indolent lymphoma receiving rituximab in combination with GM-CSF. Blood 2003, 102: 411a (abstr)

125. van der Kolk LE, Grillo-López, Baars JW, and van Oers MHJ: Treatment of relapsed B-cell non-Hodgkin's lymphoma with a combination of chimeric anti-CD20 monoclonal antibodies (rituximab) and G-CSF: final report on safety and efficacy. Leukemia 2003; 17: 1658-1664

126. Ansell SM, Witzig TE, Kurtin PJ, et al: Phase I study of interleukin-12 in combination with rituximab in patients with B-cell non-Hodgkin lymphoma. Blood 2002; 99: 67-74

127. Pro B, Smith MR, Younes A, et al: Genasense (Bcl-2 antisense) plus rituximab is active in patients with relapsed or refractory B-cell non-Hodgkin's lymphoma. Blood 2003; 102, (abstr 1491).

128. Rohatiner AZS, Johnson PWM, Price CGA, et al: Myeloablative therapy with autologous bone marrow transplantation as consolidation for recurrent follicular lymphoma. J Clin Oncol 1994; 12: 1177-1184

129. Pedersen-Bjergaard J, Pedersen M, Myhre J, et al: High risk of therapy-related leukemia after BEAM chemotherapy and autologous stem cell transplantation for previously treated lymphomas in mainly related to primary chemotherapy and not to the BEAM-transplantation procedure. Leukemia 1997; 11: 1654-1660

130. Hosing C, Saliba RM, McLaughlin P, et al: Long-term results favor allogeneic over autologous hematopoietic stem cell transplantation in patient with refractory or recurrent indolent non-Hodgkin's lymphoma. Ann Oncol 2003; 14: 737-744

131. Hamblin TJ, Davis Z, Gardiner A, Oscier DG, Stevenson FK: Unmutated IgV (H) genes are associated with a more aggressive form of chronic lymphocytic leukemia. Blood 1999; 94: 1848-1854

132. Staudt LM. Molecular diagnosis of the hematologic cancers. N Engl J Med 2003; 348: 1777-1785

133. Rassenti LZ, Huynh L, Toy TL,et al: ZAP-70 compared with immunoglobulin heavy-chain gene mutation status as a predictor of disease progression in chronic lymphocytic leukemia. N Engl J Med 2004; 351: 893-901

134. Thieblemont C, Nasser V, Felman P, et al: Small lymphocytic lymphoma, marginal zone B-cell lymphoma, and mantle cell lymphoma exhibit distinct gene-expression profiles allowing molecular diagnosis. Blood 2004; 103: 2727-2737

135. Almasri NM, Duque RE, Iturraspe J, et al: Reduced expression of CD20 antigen as a characteristic marker for chronic lymphocytic leukemia. Am J Hematol 1992; 40: 259-263

136. Hainsworth JD, Litchy S, Barton JH, et al: Single-agent rituximab as first-line and maintenance treatment for patients with chronic lymphocytic leukemia or small lymphocytic lymphoma: A phase II trial of the Minnie Pearl Cancer Research Network. J Clin Oncol 2003; 21: 1746-1751

137. Venugopal P, Sivaraman S, Huang XK, et al: Effects of cytokines on CD20 antigen expression on tumor cells from patients with chronic lymphocytic leukemia. Leuk Res 2000; 24: 411-415

138. Keating MJ, Chiorazzi N, Messmer B, et al: Biology and treatment of chronic lymphocytic leukemia. Hematology 2003; 153-175

139. Kay NE, Geyer SM, Lin T, et al: Combination chemotherapy with pentostatin, cyclophosphamide and rituximab induces high rate of remissions including complete responses and achievement of minimal residual disease in previously untreated B-chronic lymphocytic leukemia. Blood 2004; 104 (Suppl): 100a (abstr)

140. Keating MJ, Flinn I, Jain V, et al: Therapeutic role of alemtuzumab (Campth-1H) in patients who have failed fludarabine: results of a large international study. Blood 2002; 99: 3554-3561

141. Owen RG, Treon SP, Al-Katib A, et al: Clinicopathological definition of Waldenstrom's macroglobulinemia: Consensus panel recommendations from the Second International Workshlop on Waldenstrom's Macroglobulinemia. Semin Oncol Oncol 2003; 30: 110-115

142. Offit K, Parsa NZ, Filippa D, et al: (9;14)(p13;q32) denotes a subset of low-grade non-Hodgkin's lymphoma with plasmacytoid differentiation. Blood 1992; 80: 2594-2599

143. Zuckerman E, Zuckerman T: Hepatitis C virus infection in patients with B-cell non-Hodgkin lymphoma. Ann Intern Med 1997; 127: 423-428

144. Pozzato G, Mazzaro C, Crovatto M, et al: Low-grade malignant lymphoma, hepatitis C virus infection, and mixed cryoglobulinemia. Blood 1994; 84: 3047-3053

145. Gertz MA, Anagnostopoulos A, Anderson K, et al: Treatment recommendations in Waldenstrom's macroglobulinemia consensus panel recommendations in Waldenstrom's macroglobulinemia: consensus panel recommendations from the Second International Workshop on Waldenstrom's Macroglobulinemia. Semin Oncol 2003; 30: 121-126

146. Zucca E, Bertoni F, Roggero E, et al: Management of rare forms of lymphoma. Curr Opin Oncol 1998; 10: 377-384

147. Nathwani BN, Anderspm KR, Armitage JO, et al: Marginal zone B-cell lymphoma: A clinical comparison of nodal and mucosa-associated lymphoid tissue types. J Clin Oncol 1999; 17: 2486-2492

148. Arcaini L, Paulli M, Boveri E, et al: Marginal zone-related neoplasms of splenic and nodal origin. Haematologica 2003; 88: 80-93

149. Zucca E, Conconi A, Pedrinis E, et al: Nongastric marginal zone B-cell lymphoma of mucosa-associated lymphoid tissue. Blood 2003; 101: 2489-2495

150. Berger F, Felman P, Sonet A, et al: Nonfollicular small B-cell lymphomas: a heterogeneous group of patients with distinct clinical features and outcome. Blood 1994; 83: 2829-2835

151. Thieblemont C, de la Fouchardiere A, Coiffier B: Nongastric mucosa-associated lymphoid tissue lymphomas. Clin Lymphoma 2003; 3: 212-224

152. Fisher RI, Dahlberg S, Nathwani BN, et al: A clinical analysis of two indolent lymphoma entities: Mantle cell lymphoma and marginal zone lymphoma (including the mucosa-associated lymphoid tissue and monocytoid B-cell subcategories): A Southwest Oncology Group Study. Blood 1995; 85: 1075-1082

Chapter 4

DIFFUSE LARGE B-CELL NHL

Jonathan W. Friedberg, MD and Richard I. Fisher, MD

*University of Rochester Medical Center, James P. Wilmot Cancer Center,
Lymphoma Program 601 Elmwood Avenue, Box 704 Rochester, N.Y. 14642*

1.   INTRODUCTION

Diffuse large B-cell lymphoma (DLBCL) is the most common non-Hodgkin lymphoma in the United States, accounting for 30 to 40 percent of adult NHL.[1] Over the past 10 years, routine incorporation of monoclonal antibody therapy in treatment regimens has favorably impacted overall survival in most subgroups of patients with DLBCL. Additionally, there has been remarkable progress in the understanding of the biological heterogeneity of this disease. Historically, the International Prognostic Factor index (IPI) permitted identification of subsets of patients with large variations in prognosis. There is now accumulating evidence that the clinical behavior of certain DLBCL can be profiled by the expression of molecular markers, which will undoubtedly play a role in the development of new prognostic models that may refine our ability to identify poor-risk patients. With this technology, over the next decade, it is hoped that novel therapeutic targets will be identified, allowing continued improvements in outcome for patients with this disease.

1.1   Clinical features

There has been a striking increase in NHL incidence rates over the last four decades that has been referred to as an epidemic of NHL. The reasons for this are not entirely clear, and can not be explained by the HIV epidemic. Although there have been increases in most histologies, the largest increases have occurred in patients with aggressive lymphomas, including

DLBCL. Although DLBCL can occur at any age, it is, in general, a disease of middle-aged and older adults.[2] Unlike indolent lymphomas that are almost always widely disseminated at diagnosis, diffuse large B cell lymphomas present as early-stage disease in approximately 30% of cases. Patients typically present with a rapidly enlarging symptomatic mass, with B symptoms (fever, unexplained weight loss > 10% over 6 month interval, or night sweats) in one-third of the cases. Up to 40% of diffuse large B-cell lymphomas are extranodal; common sites include the gastrointestinal tract, bone, and CNS.

1.2   Pathology, biology and classification of DLBCL

It is imperative that diagnostic material for DLBCL reviewed by an experienced hematopathologist. Adequate biopsy must include lymph node architecture; fine needle aspiration is insufficient for the diagnosis of DLBCL,[3] and excisional biopsy is preferred over core needle biopsy, whenever possible.

Details of of the pathology of DLBCL are included in Chapter 6. The WHO classification remains in clinical use, and includes DLBCL as a mature B-cell neoplasm.[4] In addition to *de novo* (referred to as primary) disease, DLBCL can also represent progression/transformation (referred to as secondary) of an indolent lymphoma. Immunophenotypically, tumor cells generally express pan B-cell antigens (CD19, CD20, CD22, CD79a), as well as CD45, and monoclonal surface membrane IgM; occasionally other heavy chain isotypes are present. Uncommonly, DLBCL cells are CD10+, CD5+ or surface membrane immunoglobulin (sIg) negative[5,6].

Various morphologic variants and subtypes have been described, including centroblastic, immunoblastic, T-cell/histiocyte rich and anaplastic. However, immunophenotypic and genetic parameters have not helped to delineate distinctive morphologic variants and distinction among these variants has generally met with poor reproducibility.[7] However, the WHO classification also describes three subtypes of DLBCL that can be distinguished by their distinctive clinical features and/or immunophenotypic and genotypic features: mediastinal (thymic) large B-cell lymphoma, intravascular large B-cell lymphoma and primary effusion lymphoma (PEL). The former arises in the mediastinum, presenting as a locally invasive anterior mediastinal mass with frequent airway compromise and superior vena cava syndrome.[8] Primary mediastinal large B cell NHL appears to be linked molecularly to Hodgkin lymphoma.[9] Intravascular large B-cell lymphoma is a rare subtype of extranodal DLBCL characterized by the presence of lymphoma cells only in the lumina of small vessels, particularly capillaries without an extravascular mass.[10]Diagnosis is difficult, and many reported cases have been found at autopsy. PEL is a very rare neoplasm of large B-cells, universally associated with human herpes virus 8 (HHV8), presenting as serous pleural or peritoneal effusions without detectable tumor masses immunocompromised hosts.[11] It has a markedly aberrant phenotype, often with expression of activation and plasma cell-related markers (CD30, CD38 and CD138).

Cytogenetic and molecular analyses are providing additional insights into the pathogenesis of DLBCL. For example, rearrangement of *bcl-2* has been observed to occur in 20% to 30% of patients. A high level of bcl-2 protein occurs in 25 to 80% of DLBCL (depending on the study), and this appears to be associated with a worse prognosis.[12] Similarly the *bcl-6* gene, known to have structural similarities to a class of transcription factors that participate in the control of cell proliferation and differentiation, is rearranged in a subset of DLBCL, and may correlate with a favorable clinical outcome.[13]

A number of recent studies have attempted to define germinal-center and non-germinal center phenotypes in DLBCL, using markers such as bcl-6, CD10 (germinal center) and MUM1/IRF4 and CD138 (post-germinal center). In general, a germinal center immunophenotype, particularly including Bcl-6 expression, has been associated with a better prognosis.

The use of microarray to analyze gene expression has confirmed the long suspected biologic and karyotypic diversity among DLBCL. In 2000, Alizedah et al. first reported on the application of the complementary-DNA(cDNA) microarray techniques to DLBCL, demonstrating that diversity in gene expression among DLBCLs apparently reflected the variation in tumor proliferation rate, host response and differentiation state of the tumor.[14] Subsequently, an international collaboration sought to confirm these findings through examination of gene expression of DLBCL from 240 patients with the use of DNA microarrays.[15] Three subgroups with distinctive gene-expression profiles were identified on the basis of hierarchical clustering: germinal-center B-cell-like, activated B-cell-like, and type 3 diffuse large-B-cell lymphoma. Two common oncogenic events in DLBCL: bcl-2 translocation and c-rel amplification were detected only in the germinal-center B-cell-like subgroup, which had the highest five-year survival rate.

Shipp *et al.* have shown that the outcome of patients with DLBCL treated with standard chemotherapy is influenced by expression of genes that regulate responses to B-receptor signaling, critical serine/threonine phosphorylation pathways and apoptosis.[16] The gene for protein kinase C-beta was identified as highly predictive of poor prognosis, and clinical trials of a PKC-B inhibitor in the treatment of DLBCL have commenced. The same group has identified tumor microenvironment and host inflammatory response as defining features of DLBCL, suggesting rational therapies may target this compartment.[17]

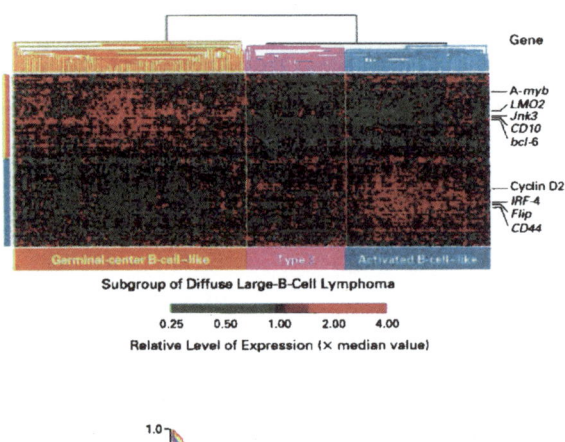

Subgroup of Diffuse Large-B-Cell Lymphoma

0.25   0.50   1.00   2.00   4.00

Relative Level of Expression (× median value)

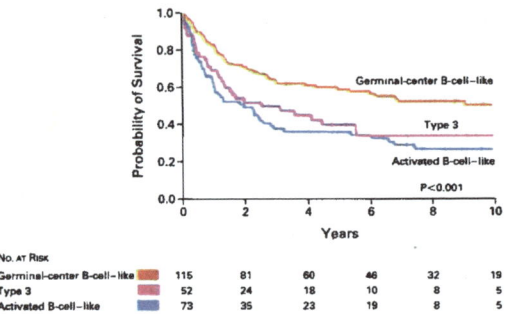

Figure 1. Utilizing microarray technology and hierarchechal clustering algorithm, three subgroups of diffuse large B cell lymphoma can be identified with unique outcomes following standard therapy. The superior outcomes of patients with "Germinal-center B-cell-like" disease is maintained even when controlling for various IPI risk groups. (Reproduced with permission from NEJM, Volume 346, page 1939, 2002)

A recent study from Stanford University attempted to distill the complex gene array signatures into readily adaptable PCR method.[18] They determined that measurement of the expression of six genes: *LMO2, BCL6, FN1, CCND2, SCYA3,* and *BCL2,* by PCR, is sufficient to predict overall survival in diffuse large-B-cell lymphoma, yielding prognostic information similar to that found in the more cumbersome gene array analysis. Ongoing clinical trials should define the optimal clinical role for this technology.

2. STAGING AND PRETREATMENT EVALUATION

Because DLBCL is a potentially curable disease, it is essential that the patient be accurately and completely staged at the time of diagnosis. A careful history and physical examination is critical to determine the potential extent of the disease and subsequent appropriate therapeutic choice. The presence and duration of specific "B" symptoms known to have an adverse prognosis in patients with DLBCL should be ascertained. All patients with DLBCL should have a complete blood count and chemistry survey, including LDH; chest radiograph; computed tomographic (CT) scan of the thorax abdomen and pelvis; and iliac crest bone marrow biopsy (bilateral preferred). Any neurological symptoms should be evaluated with a high volume lumbar puncture for cytologic and chemical analyses of the cerebrospinal fluid, along with MRI evaluation of the brain parenchyma, spine and leptomeninges with gadolinium. Asymptomatic patients with lymphomatous involvement of the testicle, sinus, or with significant numbers of large lymphoma cells in the bone marrow with large cells should also undergo evaluation of the CNS, given the predilection for CNS involvement in these circumstances.

Patients with any history of cardiac disease, symptoms, or above age 40-50, should undergo evaluation of cardiac function with either a radionucleotide ventriculogram or echocardiogram if therapy is to include chest irradiation or an anthracycline.

Positron emission tomography (PET) is a novel functional imaging technique described in detail in Chapter 8. These functional scans are complementary to anatomic imaging, and may improve staging at the time of diagnosis, particularly through the detection of otherwise occult abdominal or splenic disease. Nuclear scintigraphy may also help to characterize a residual mass on anatomic imaging following therapy as either fibrosis or residual active lymphoma.[19] The data supporting widespread use of this modality for clinical decision making in DLBCL remains limited, and largely retrospective. Clearly, positive PET scans at the end of therapy, or in follow-up, warrant confirmatory anatomic imaging and biopsy, since some of these patients may remain in prolonged remission. Ongoing clinical trials incorporating PET in staging and follow-up of patients with DLBCL should better define its role.

The *Ann-Arbor staging system*, designed originally for Hodgkin lymphoma, remains in general use for DLBCL (Table 1).[20] Stage 1 disease is confined to a single lymph node region (I), or is disease involving a single extralymphatic organ or site (IE). Stage II includes involvement of two or more lymph node regions on the same side of the diaphragm, or involvement of an extralymphatic organ or site and its associated regional lymph nodes with or without other lymph node regions on the same side of the diaphragm

(IIE). "Localized disease" commonly refers to stage I or II. Stage III includes patients with involvement of lymph node regions on both sides of the diagphragm, including spleen (IIIS), or localized involvement of an extralymphatic organ (IIIE).   Stage IV includes all patients with disseminated involvement of one or more extralymphatic organs or tissues, with or without associated lymph node involvement. A limitation of the Ann Arbor system in staging patients with DLBCL is that lymph node size, although highly prognostic, is not included. For example, patients with stage II disease that is nonbulky have a better prognosis than do patients with bulky stage II disease (bulk being defined as a tumor mass >10 cm in diameter in one location or a mediastinal mass >1/3 of the thoracic diameter), and probably warrant different therapy.

2.1   International prognostic index

The International Non-Hodgkin's Lymphoma Prognostic Factors Index (IPI) utilized pretreatment prognostic factors in a cohort of over 5000 thousand patients to develop a predictive model of outcome for aggressive NHL.[21]   In an analysis of 2031 aggressive lymphoma patients (majority DLBCL) of all ages, five pretreatment characteristics were found to be independent predictors of death: age ($\leq$60 vs >60), tumor stage I or II (localized) vs III or IV (advanced), the number of extra nodal sites of involvement ($\leq$1 vs >1), patient ECOG performance status 0 or 1 (ambulatory) vs $\geq$2 (not ambulatory) (equivalent Karnofsky scores, greater than or equal to 80 and less than or equal to 70), and serum LDH level (less than or equal to 1 times normal vs. >1 times normal). Each of the individual factors had comparable relative risks and thus could be summed together. The resulting model identified four risk groups with associated five-year survival rates: low risk (0-1, risk factor) 73 %; low intermediate risk (2,risk factors) 51%; high intermediate risk (3 risk factors) 43 %; and high risk (4-5 risk factors) 26 % (Table 2). The increased risk of death was due to both a lower rate of complete responses and a higher rate of relapse from complete response. For example patients in the high risk IPI group had a CR rate of 44% and a five-year survival rate of only 26% as compared to a CR rate of 87% and a five-year survival of 73% in patients in the low risk IPI group. The IPI, summarized in Table 2, should be calculated on all patients at time of diagnosis with DLBCL, prior to beginning therapy.

2.2   Treatment of localized DLBCL

Historically, external beam radiation therapy was employed as a single modality in the therapy of localized DLBCL, with prolonged disease-free survival of approximately 35%.[22] Beginning almost 20 years ago, the results of several large phase II trials suggested that patients who received combined modality programs chemotherapy and involved field radiation had superior outcomes.[23,24] With the success of anthracycline containing combination chemotherapy in treating advanced stage DLBCL (see below), the combination of cyclophosphamide, doxorubicin, vincristine and prednisone (CHOP) chemotherapy with radiation therapy emerged as the strategy of choice for treating localized DLBCL.

More recently, randomized clinical trials have addressed the optimal schedule of chemotherapy in localized DLBCL. The current standard of care for this group of patients was defined by a Southwest Oncology Group (SWOG) study, which randomized 401 patients with non-bulky stage I or II aggressive NHL (mainly DLBCL) to 3 cycles of CHOP followed by involved field radiation (40-50 Gy) or to 8 cycles of CHOP alone.[25] The progression-free survival (PFS) and overall survival (OS) at 5 years were both significantly superior for the combined modality arm (PFS, 77% vs 64%:; OS, 82% vs 72%). Life threatening toxicities were higher in the patients receiving CHOP alone. Interestingly, 10 year follow-up of this trial suggests an increase in late recurrences (> 5 years post therapy) in patients treated with abbreviated chemotherapy and radiation.[26] The OS in both arms showed a continuous rate of death over the first ten years with no evidence of plateau in the survival curve, a finding remarkably different from advanced stage disease treated with CHOP.

When any risk factor (age > 60 years, high LDH, stage II disease and performance status >/= 2) in the stage-modified ("Miller Modification") IPI is present, outcome is inferior to those patients with no risk factors.[27] 5-year overall survival in the SWOG study was 94%,71% and 50% for those with no , 1 or 3 or more of these adverse risk factors respectively. These findings have been confirmed by the Canadian experience utilizing brief chemotherapy and radiation. The overall survival rates at 5 and 10 years were, respectively, 97% and 89% (no factors), 77% and 56% (one or two factors), and 58% and 48% (three factors), and the 5-year and 10-year PFS rates were, respectively, 94% and 89% (no factors), 79% and 73% (one or two factors), and 60% and 50% (three factors).[28]

In another randomized trial, the Eastern Cooperative Oncology Group (ECOG) enrolled 210 patients, and randomized 172 patients who had attained CR after 8 cycles of CHOP to no further therapy or involved field radiation.[29] Disease-free survival (DFS) at 6 years was superior for the combined treatment arm (73% vs 56%), however here was no difference in

OS. Radiation therapy enhanced local control. Patients with 3 or more disease sites or a poor performance status were more likely to fail CHOP with or without radiation therapy.

The GELA group has reported a randomized trial of previously untreated patients less than 61 years old with localized stage I or II aggressive lymphoma and no adverse prognostic factors according to the IPI comparing the standard three cycles of CHOP plus involved-field radiotherapy (329 patients) or chemotherapy alone with dose-intensified doxorubicin, cyclophosphamide, vindesine, bleomycin, and prednisone (ACVBP) plus sequential consolidation (318 patients).[30] Patients with bulk stage II disease, a group known to require more chemotherapy than 3 cycles of CHOP, were included on this trial, unlike the SWOG experience. The five-year estimates of event-free survival were 82 percent for patients receiving ACVBP chemotherapy alone and 74 percent for those receiving standard CHOP + XRT. The respective five-year estimates of overall survival in this trial were 90 percent and 81 percent, respectively.

An early report from the GELA group presented in abstract form, included elderly patients with localized aggressive NHL and an age-adjusted IPI of zero suggests the addition of involved field radiotherapy to 4 courses of CHOP did not improve rates of complete response, 5-year event-free survival, or 5-year overall survival.[31]. Finally, in another preliminary report, SWOG presented a pilot trial adding the monoclonal anti-CD20 antibody rituximab to three cycles of CHOP chemotherapy followed by XRT in patients with at least one adverse risk factor.[32] Progression-free survival (PFS) and overall survival (OS) measured at 2 years was 94% and 95%, respectively, superior to the historical experience without rituximab therapy.

The authors currently recommend 3 cycles of CHOP and rituximab with involved field radiation, for patients with stage I and non-bulky stage II disease, based on survival advantages through the first nine years and less associated toxicity. Patients with bulky disease clearly require more chemotherapy, and highly selected patients with no risk factors may not require radiation. Clinical trials involving new agents such as radioimmunotherapy are currently targeting those patients with more aggressive presentations of early stage DLBCL.

3.   TREATMENT OF ADVANCED STAGE DLBCL

Before the development of multiagent chemotherapy regimens, the median survival of patients with DLBCL was one year. The prototype "first-generation" chemotherapy regimen, CHOP remains the current standard chemotherapy backbone for non-localized DLBCL in the United States. "Second" and Third generation" chemotherapy regimens were designed to deliver six to eight active lymphoma drugs at the highest possible drug dose per unit time. A meta-analysis of five randomized controlled trials, involving over 1,900 patients, failed to show any survival benefit of third generation regimens over standard CHOP.[33] ECOG conducted a randomized trial comparing CHOP to the second generation m-BACOD (low-dose methotrexate with leucovorin rescue, bleomycin, doxorubicin, cyclophosphamide, vincristine, and dexamethasone), and found no difference in response or survival, but increased toxicity with m-BACOD.[34] The definitive evaluation of CHOP chemotherapy was SWOG trial 8516, which compared CHOP, to m-BACOD, ProMACE-CytaBOM (prednisone, doxorubicin, cyclophosphamide, and etoposide, followed by cytarabine, bleomycin, vincristine, and methotrexate with leucovorin rescue), or MACOP-B (methotrexate with leucovorin rescue, doxorubicin, cyclophosphamide, vincristine, prednisone, and bleomycin) in patients with stage II-IV disease.[35] After over six years, there was no difference between CHOP and the newer regimens in progression-free survival, with 5-year estimates of 33-38%, or in overall survival, with 5-year estimates of 45-46%.

The most significant advance in the treatment of advanced stage DLBCL since the publication of the definitive SWOG study involves the addition of rituximab to standard chemotherapy (Table 3). (see chapter 7 for a detailed discussion of monoclonal antibody therapy). Vose et al initially reported a phase II study of rituximab plus CHOP in untreated DLBCL.[36] In the initial report of this study, the overall response rate was 97% (32/33), with 20 CR, and 12 PR. The Groupe d'Etude des Lymphomes de l'Adulte(GELA) published the results of a randomized trial comparing eight courses of standard dose CHOP given every three weeks or to the same regimen plus the monoclonal anti-CD20 antibody rituximab (375 mg/m2) on day 1 of each of the eight cycles of CHOP (CHOP-R).[37] All patients in this trial were over age 60, and had advanced stage DLBCL. Complete response rates of 63 and 76 percent (p = 0.005) and two year overall survivals of 57 and 70 percent were achieved by CHOP and CHOP-R, respectively. The incidence of severe or serious side effects was similar in the two treatment arms. Interestingly, the most profound benefit of rituximab was observed in patients with a low-risk age-adjusted International Prognostic index (0 or 1 adverse prognostic factors, 1-year EFS was 81 and 57 percent for the CHOP-R and CHOP arms, respectively. An unplanned subgroup analysis also suggested particular benefit of rituximab in patients with DLBCL positve for bcl-2, suggesting one mechanism of rituximab in this setting may involve overcoming bcl-2 associated chemotherapy resistance.[38]

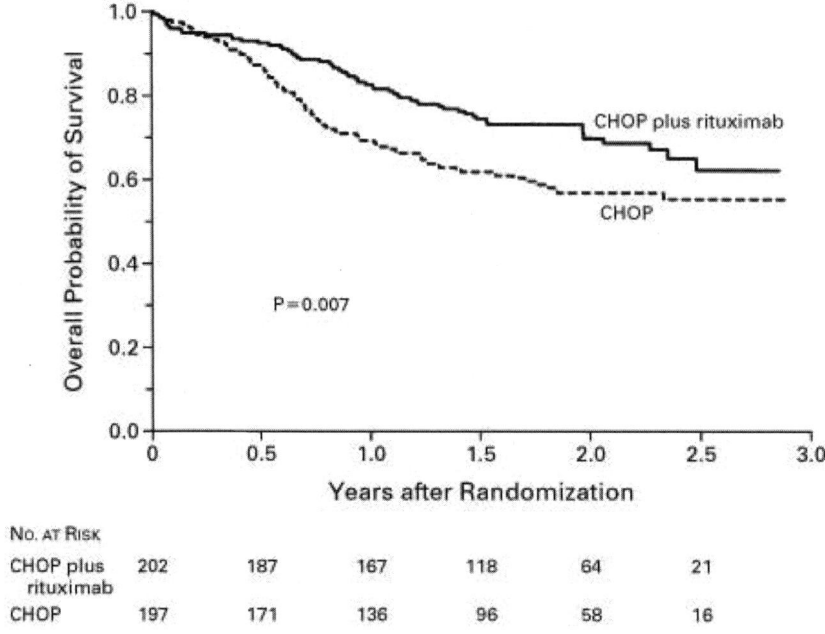

Figure 2. Superior overall survival of patients in the GELA trial treated with CHOP + rituximab (N=202) compared with CHOP (N=197). This survival benefit is maintained through five years of follow up. (Reproduced with permission from NEJM, Volume 346, page 239, 2002.)

A larger (N=632) intergroup United States Study randomized a similar population of elderly patients to CHOP vs. CHOP with rituximab given on an alternating schedule as described in follicular lymphoma.[39] Responding patients then were randomized to receive either rituximab "maintenance" therapy (4 doses q 6 months x 2 years) or no maintenance. The significant interaction between the induction and maintenance therapies makes interpretation of this trial difficult. Preliminary results suggest a progression-free survival benefit to the addition of rituximab; however no overall survival benefit is apparent. Using a weighted analysis to mathematically model two groups being treated with CHOP alone or CHOP plus Rituximab as induction therapy (controlling for maintenance exposure), an overall survival benefit becomes apparent when induction therapy consisted of CHOP combined with rituximab *versus* CHOP alone, of a similar magnitude to that seen in the GELA trial. An important contribution of this trial was lack of benefit to "maintenance" rituximab when rituximab is included as part of the initial chemotherapy regimen.

Preliminary results from the MInT Trial (Mab Thera International Trial), a trial evaluating the combination of CHOP and rituximab in patients younger than age 60, were recently presented.[40] Eligibility criteria included IPI 0,1 only; Stages II – IV or Stage I with bulk; and patients < 60 years of age. Patients received 6 cycles of any one of several CHOP-like regimens followed by radiation therapy (30 – 40 Gray to bulky disease or E lesions). The preliminary report analyzed the first 326 patients. Approximately 30% of the patients had low bulk, early stage disease. Patients receiving rituximab with chemotherapy had a significantly longer 2-year TTF (81% vs. 58 %) compared with those receiving chemotherapy alone. In addition, the 2-year OS significantly favored chemotherapy plus Rituximab (95% vs. 85%, p = 0.0026).

A second treatment modality under evaluation to improve outcomes of DLBCL involves intensifying chemotherapy dose. A major limitation of these efforts is that they did not include rituximab in the treatment regimens. For example, SWOG conducted a pilot study evaluating dose-intensified CHOP, without rituximab, (CHOP-DI: cyclophosphamide 1,600 mg/m^2, doxorubicin 65 mg/m^2, and vincristine 1.4 mg/m^2) with filgrastim support, every 14 days for six planned courses.[41] Treatment with CHOP-DI was safely administered in the cooperative group setting and resulted in survival 14% better compared with historical SWOG controls.

Two large trials from Germany (NHL-B1 and NHL-B2) randomized patients to 6 cycles of CHOP-21 (every three weeks), CHOP-14 (every two weeks), CHOEP-21 (CHOP plus etoposide 100 mg/m(2) d1-d3), or CHOEP-14 in a 2x2 factorial study design. Patients in the 2-weekly regimens received G-CSF starting from day 4. Patients in these trials also received radiotherapy (36 Gy) to sites of initial bulky disease and extranodal disease. One trial (NHL-B2) was limited to patients older than age 60.[42] Five-year event-free and overall survival rates were 32.5% and 40.6%, respectively, for CHOP-21 and 43.8% and 53.3%, respectively, for CHOP-14. Toxicity of CHOP-14 and CHOP-21 was similar, but CHOEP-21 and in particular CHOEP-14 were more toxic.

In the parallel trial (NHL B1) for patients younger than age 61, CHOEP achieved better complete remission (87.6% versus 79.4%; P = .003) and 5-year event-free survival rates (69.2% versus 57.6%; P = .004, primary end point) than CHOP.[43] The benefit of interval reduction was less clear. Although the CHOEP regimens induced more myelosuppression, these regimens were reasonably well tolerated: there were only 3 therapy-associated deaths, one (0.5%) in the CHOEP-21 and 2 (1.1%) in the CHOEP-14 cohort. Additional trials incorporating monoclonal antibody therapy into these intensified programs are ongoing; until these data are available, we do not recommend dose intense regimens outside of a clinical trial setting.

The ultimate dose intensification consists of high dose therapy with autologous stem cell support (ASCT). The PARMA trial in patients with relapsed disease (see below) provides rationale for including this aggressive approach as initial therapy. In the PARMA study, the event-free survival (EFS) and the OS were superior in the high dose therapy group compared with conventional salvage chemotherapy.[44]

ASCT as consolidation after CR, or as induction therapy, has been tested in newly diagnosed untreated DLBCL patients in several phase III trials. In the majority of these trials, poor-risk disease was identified by criteria other than the IPI. A variety of schedules incorporating ASCT have been evaluated: following a CR after a full course of induction therapy;[45] following a full course of induction therapy, regardless of response;[46] or requiring a response [47,48] after abbreviated standard-dose chemotherapy or abbreviated dose-intense chemotherapy;[49,50] and following a "slow" response to induction chemotherapy.[51]

The recently published Groupe Ouest–Est des Leucémies et des Autres Maladies du Sang (GOELAMS) trial randomized 197 consecutive patients to receive either 8 courses of standard CHOP chemotherapy, or a complicated regimen of CEEP (cyclophosphamide, vindesine, epirubicin and prednisone), followed by high doses of methotrexate and cytarabine, BEAM conditioning, and ASCT in responding patients.[52] Overall, 78 percent of the patients completed the assigned treatment; the median follow-up was four years. The estimated event-free survival rate at five years was significantly higher among patients who received ASCT than among patients who received CHOP (55% vs. 37%). A subgroup analysis (retrospectively done) demonstrated a survival benefit in patients with a high intermediate age-adjusted IPI (OS: 74% vs. 44%).

This data is reminiscent of the final report of the LNH87–2 trial of the GELA.[45] In this trial 1,043 patients were initially randomized to treatment with four courses of either of two anthracycline containing regimens (ACVB or NCVB), and then all received the same four additional courses of cyclophosphamide 1,200 mg/m2 given intravenously on day 1, vindesine 2 mg/m2 given intravenously on days 1 and 5, bleomycin 10 mg given intravenously on days 1 and 5, prednisone 60 mg/m2 given orally on days 1 through 5, and intrathecal methotrexate 15 mg on day 2. The study tested ASCT as consolidation, and patients achieving a CR were randomized to additional cycles of sequential chemotherapy or ASCT with CBV (cyclophosphamide, carmustine, and etoposide) conditioning. Similar to the GOELAMS trial, a retrospective analysis determined 451 patients to be of high/intermediate or high-risk utilizing the IPI. The 8-year overall survival (OS) was superior in the ASCT arm at 64%, compared with the sequential chemotherapy arm 49%.

Importantly, in most of the phase III trials reported to date, the high risk patients were not initially identified as the target population for the trial, and subset analysis was performed retrospectively. A major additional concern around ASCT as part of upfront therapy in NHL is the potential risk of long-term fatal toxicities associated with this therapy, particularly MDS and AML, which can exceed 10%.[53,54] With the exception of the aforementioned French studies, the majority of the current mature phase III trials report improved DFS, but not OS with ASCT in patients under age 60, who are in high or high-intermediate IPI risk groups. Moreover, none of the mature trials incorporated rituximab, and it remains unknown if a benefit of transplant is abrogated by the addition of rituximab to the induction or consolidation regimens.

An expert consensus has concluded that the role of ASCT as primary therapy in high-risk NHL patients is not yet defined, and conclusions should await additional randomized phase III trials.[55] Currently, the SWOG and Cancer and Leukemia Group B (CALGB) are enrolling patients to definitively address this question, comparing early versus delayed ASCT for patients with high-intermediate and high risk large cell non-Hodgkin's lymphoma in patients treated with a standard course of CHOP and rituximab therapy. Until this trial is complete, we do not recommend high dose therapy for *de novo* aggressive NHL outside of a clinical trial setting.

3.1   Salvage therapy

The initial step in planning salvage chemotherapy at time of disease progression or recurrence is to determine the goal of treatment. A minority of patients who fail to achieve an initial remission or relapse from complete remission can be cured. This is less likely in elderly patients, those with extensive disease, those with no response to initial therapy, and those with a poor performance status. In such patients less intensive, palliative systemic treatments, with single active chemotherapeutic agents, including vinca alkaloids, alkylating agents, or anthracyclines may be appropriate. Responses to single agent rituximab occur approximately 30% of the time, and are generally of brief duration.[56]   The role of radioimmunotherapy as salvage for DLBCL after a rituximab containing conditioning regimen is limited; in one study responses of brief duration to ibritumomab tiuxetan were observed.[57] External beam radiotherapy may alleviate the symptoms at a particular site of involvement in patients with relapsed diffuse large B-cell lymphoma.

Younger patients should be treated with curative intent, and most commonly receive combination chemotherapy regimens including agents such as cisplatin, ifosfamide, etoposide, and cytarabine, often in combination with rituximab. Memorial-Sloan-Kettering has recently published results of R-ICE chemotherapy (rituximab, ifosfamide, carboplatin, etoposide), in patients with recurrent DLBCL.[58] The CR rate was 53%, significantly better than the 27% CR rate achieved among 147 similar consecutive historical control patients with DLBCL treated with ICE; the PR rate was 25%.

Therefore, this is a very effective cytoreduction and mobilization regimen in patients with NHL, and has become a widely used salvage and stem cell mobilization option for patients eligible for subsequent ASCT.

An international randomized trial referred to as the PARMA study defined the role of ASCT in relapsed DLBCL.[44] Patients on this trial were under age 60 with aggressive NHL who had relapsed after an initial complete remission. Patients were first treated with two courses of conventional DHAP (dexamethasone, cytarabine and cisplatinum) salvage chemotherapy. Those patients responding were then randomized to involved field radiotherapy and high dose chemotherapy with ASCT versus DHAP chemotherapy for 4 cycles followed by involved field radiotherapy. ASCT was associated with a superior failure-free survival (51% vs. 12% at 5 years) and overall survival (53% vs. 32% at 5 years). The number of patients cured of lymphoma with conventional salvage therapy was very low. For eligible patients, therefore, high-dose therapy and ASCT are the treatments of choice in the setting of progressive disease.

The role of allogeneic transplantation in the management of patients with relapsed or primary refractory DLBCL is unclear because of the small number of patients in the literature, the inclusion of patients with various histologies, and the lack of homogeneity with respect to risk factors. Some studies suggest that patients undergoing allogeneic transplantation had lower relapse rates as compared to those undergoing autologous transplantation; others have demonstrated that the type of transplant did not influence either relapse rate or disease-free survival.[59] Significant treatment-related mortality remains the major obstacle of this approach. Ongoing studies in high-risk patients are evaluating nonmyeloablative allogeneic transplantation as an option, particularly for patients with progressive disease following autologous transplantation.[60]

3.2   New Agents and Future Directions

Historically, the development of new agents for the treatment of DLBCL was challenging. The large number of available active agents and the comparatively high complete remissions rate in previously untreated patients meant that a drug required outstanding single agent activity in phase II testing before it was considered for evaluation as a front line agent. In the past 5 years, the paradigm has changed, due in large part to the dramatic success of rituximab, insights of new targets from gene expression profiling, the development of surrogate biological endpoints, and the observation in solid tumors that single agent activity does not predict efficacy in the setting of combination therapy.[61] Chapter 14 focuses on many of these promising novel compounds for DLBCL. As our understanding of the molecular biology of DLBCL continues to evolve, molecular targets will become the focus of many therapeutic trials. Thoughtful clinical investigation remains the key to future progress in DLBCL.

Table 1. Ann Arbor Staging System for Lymphoma

Stage 1	Involvement of a single lymph node region or lymph node structure
Stage 2	Involvement of two or more lymph node regions on the same side of the diaphragm
Stage 3	Involvement of lymph node regions or structures on both sides of the diaphragm
Stage 4	Involvement of extranodal sites beyond 'E' sites

Annotations
   A: no B symptoms.
   B: fever, weight loss >10% over 6 months, or night sweats.
   E: involvement of a single extranodal site contiguous or proximal to known nodal site.

Table 2. International Prognostic Index. Adapted from [21]

Risk Group	Risk Factors	Frequency (%)	CR Rate (%)	2 year Survival (%)	5 year Survival (%)
Low	0,1	35	87	84	73
Low-Intermediate	2	27	67	66	51
High-Intermediate	3	22	55	54	43
High	4,5	16	44	34	26

Score 0 or 1 for each factor. 0= absent, 1= present. Risk factors include: age > 60; LDH > upper limit of normal; stage III or IV disease; performance status >/=2; extranodal sites > 1.

Table 3. Phase III Studies of Chop vs. Chop-R for DLBCL

Study	Population	Therapy	2-Year TTF	2-Year OS
MInT[40]	<60; favorable	CHOP	58%	85%
		CHOP-R	81%	95%
GELA[37]	>60; Advanced Stage	CHOP	40%	60%
		CHOP-R	58%	72%
ECOG-4494[39]	>60; Advanced Stage	CHOP	55%	65%
		CHOP-R	65%	71%

4.   REFERENCES

1. Armitage JO, Weisenburger DD: New approach to classifying non-Hodgkin's lymphomas: clinical features of the major histologic subtypes. Non-Hodgkin's Lymphoma Classification Project. J Clin Oncol 16:2780-95., 1998
2. Greenlee RT, Hill-Harmon MB, Murray T, et al: Cancer statistics, 2001. CA Cancer J Clin 51:15-36, 2001
3. Hehn ST, Grogan TM, Miller TP: Utility of fine-needle aspiration as a diagnostic technique in lymphoma. J Clin Oncol 22:3046-52, 2004
4. Harris NL, Jaffe ES, Diebold J, et al: World Health Organization classification of neoplastic diseases of the hematopoietic and lymphoid tissues: report of the Clinical Advisory Committee meeting-Airlie House, Virginia, November 1997. J Clin Oncol 17:3835-49., 1999
5. Doggett RS, Wood GS, Horning S, et al: The immunologic characterization of 95 nodal and extranodal diffuse large cell lymphomas in 89 patients. Am J Pathol 115:245-52, 1984
6. Stein H, Lennert K, Feller AC, et al: Immunohistological analysis of human lymphoma: correlation of histological and immunological categories. Adv Cancer Res 42:67-147, 1984

7. Harris NL, Jaffe ES, Stein H, et al: Perspective: A Revised European-American Classificiation of Lymphoid Neoplasm: A Proposal from the International Lymphoma Study Group. Blood 84:1361-1392, 1994
8. van Besien K, Kelta M, Bahaguna P: Primary mediastinal B-cell lymphoma: a review of pathology and management. J Clin Oncol 19:1855-64, 2001
9. Savage KJ, Monti S, Kutok JL, et al: The molecular signature of mediastinal large B-cell lymphoma differs from that of other diffuse large B-cell lymphomas and shares features with classical Hodgkin lymphoma. Blood 102:3871-9, 2003
10. Ferreri AJ, Campo E, Seymour JF, et al: Intravascular lymphoma: clinical presentation, natural history, management and prognostic factors in a series of 38 cases, with special emphasis on the 'cutaneous variant'. Br J Haematol 127:173-83, 2004
11. Ascoli V, Lo Coco F, Torelli G, et al: Human herpesvirus 8-associated primary effusion lymphoma in HIV--patients: a clinicopidemiologic variant resembling classic Kaposi's sarcoma. Haematologica 87:339-43, 2002
12. Gascoyne RD, Adomat SA, Krajewski S, et al: Prognostic significance of Bcl-2 protein expression and Bcl-2 gene rearrangement in diffuse aggressive non-Hodgkin's lymphoma. Blood 90:244-51, 1997
13. Offit K, LoCoco F, Louie DC, et al: Rearrangement of the bcl-6 gene as a prognostic marker in diffuse large-cell lymphoma. N.Engl.J.Med. 331:74-80, 1994
14. Alizadeh AA, Eisen MB, Davis RE, et al: Distinct types of diffuse large B-cell lymphoma identified by gene expression profiling. Nature 403:503-11, 2000
15. Rosenwald A, Wright G, Chan WC, et al: The Use of Molecular Profiling to Predict Survival after Chemotherapy for Diffuse Large B-Cell Lymphoma. N.Engl.J.Med. 346:1937-1947, 2002
16. Shipp MA, Ross KN, Tamayo P, et al: Diffuse large B-cell lymphoma outcome prediction by gene-expression profiling and supervised machine learning. Nat Med 8:68-74, 2002
17. Monti S, Savage KJ, Kutok JL, et al: Molecular profiling of diffuse large B-cell lymphoma identifies robust subtypes including one characterized by host inflammatory response. Blood 105:1851-61, 2005
18. Lossos IS, Czerwinski DK, Alizadeh AA, et al: Prediction of survival in diffuse large-B-cell lymphoma based on the expression of six genes. N Engl J Med 350:1828-37, 2004
19. Friedberg JW, Chengazi V: PET Scans in the Staging of Lymphoma: Current Status. Oncologist 8:438-47, 2003
20. Carbone PP, Kaplan HS, Musshoff K, et al: Report of the Committee on Hodgkin's Disease Staging Classification. Cancer Res 31:1860-1, 1971
21. A predictive model for aggressive non-Hodgkin's lymphoma. The International Non-Hodgkin's Lymphoma Prognostic Factors Project. N Engl J Med 329:987-94, 1993.
22. Schein PS, Chabner BA, Canellos GP, et al: Potential for prolonged disease-free survival following combination chemotherapy of non-Hodgkin's lymphoma. Blood 43:181-9, 1974
23. Jones SE, Miller TP, Connors JM: Long-term follow-up and analysis for prognostic factors for patients with limited-stage diffuse large-cell lymphoma treated with initial chemotherapy with or without adjuvant radiotherapy. J Clin Oncol 7:1186-91, 1989
24. Longo DL: Combined modality therapy for localized aggressive lymphoma: enough or too much? J Clin Oncol 7:1179-81, 1989

25. Miller TP, Dahlberg S, Cassady JR, et al: Chemotherapy alone compared with chemotherapy plus radiotherapy for localized intermediate- and high-grade non-Hodgkin's lymphoma. N.Engl.J.Med. 339:21-26, 1998

26. Miller TP, LeBlanc M, Spier C, et al: CHOP alone compared to CHOP plus radiotherapy for early stage aggressive non-Hodgkin's lymphomas: Update of the Southwest Oncology Group (SWOG) randomized trial. Blood 98:724-5a, 2001

27. Miller TP: The limits of limited stage lymphoma. J Clin Oncol 22:2982-4, 2004

28. Shenkier TN, Voss N, Fairey R, et al: Brief chemotherapy and involved-region irradiation for limited-stage diffuse large-cell lymphoma: an 18-year experience from the British Columbia Cancer Agency. J Clin Oncol 20:197-204, 2002

29. Horning SJ, Weller E, Kim K, et al: Chemotherapy with or without radiotherapy in limited-stage diffuse aggressive non-Hodgkin's lymphoma: Eastern Cooperative Oncology Group study 1484. J Clin Oncol 22:3032-8, 2004

30. Reyes F, Lepage E, Ganem G, et al: ACVBP versus CHOP plus radiotherapy for localized aggressive lymphoma. N Engl J Med 352:1197-205, 2005

31. Fillet G, Bonnet C, Mournier N, et al: Radiotherapy is unnecessary in elderly patients with localized aggressive non Hodgkin's lymphoma: Results of the GELA LNH 93-4 study. Blood 100:92a, 2002

32. Miller TP, Unger JM, Spier C, et al: Effect of adding rituximab to three cycles of CHOP plus involved field radiotherapy for limited-stage aggressive diffuse B cell lymphoma, SWOG 0014. Blood 104:48a, 2004

33. Messori A, Vaiani M, Trippoli S, et al: Survival in patients with intermediate or high grade non-Hodgkin's lymphoma: meta-analysis of randomized studies comparing third generation regimens with CHOP. Br J Cancer 84:303-7, 2001

34. Gordon LI, Harrington D, Andersen J, et al: Comparison of a Second-Generation Combination Chemotherapeutic Regimen (m-BACOD) with a Standard Regimen (CHOP) for Advanced Diffuse Non-Hodgkin's Lymphoma. N.Engl.J.Med. 327:1342-1349, 1992

35. Fisher RI, Gaynor ER, Dahlberg S, et al: Comparison of a standard regimen (CHOP) with three intensive chemotherapy regimens for advanced non-Hodgkin's lymphoma. N Engl J Med 328:1002-6, 1993

36. Vose JM, Link BK, Grossbard ML, et al: Phase II study of rituximab in combination with chop chemotherapy in patients with previously untreated, aggressive non-Hodgkin's lymphoma. J Clin Oncol 19:389-97, 2001

37. Coiffier B, Lepage E, Briere J, et al: CHOP chemotherapy plus rituximab compared with CHOP alone in elderly patients with diffuse large-B-cell lymphoma. N Engl J Med 346:235-42, 2002

38. Mounier N, Briere J, Gisselbrecht C, et al: Rituximab plus CHOP (R-CHOP) overcomes bcl-2--associated resistance to chemotherapy in elderly patients with diffuse large B-cell lymphoma (DLBCL). Blood 101:4279-84, 2003

39. Haberman TM, Weller EA, Morrison VA, et al: Phase III trial of rituximab-CHOP vs. CHOP with a second randomization to maintenance rituximab or observation in patients 60 years of age and older with diffuse large B cell lymphoma. Blood 102:6a, 2003

40. Pfreundschuh M, Truemper L, Gill D, et al: First analysis of the completed Mabthera international trial in young patients with low-risk diffuse large B cell lymphoma: addition of rituximab to a CHOP-like regimen significantly improves outcome of all patients with the identification of a very favorable subgroup with IPI=0 and no bulky disease. Blood 104:48a, 2004

41. Blayney DW, LeBlanc ML, Grogan T, et al: Dose-intense chemotherapy every 2 weeks with dose-intense cyclophosphamide, doxorubicin, vincristine, and

prednisone may improve survival in intermediate- and high-grade lymphoma: a phase II study of the Southwest Oncology Group (SWOG 9349). J Clin Oncol 21:2466-73, 2003

42. Pfreundschuh M, Trumper L, Kloess M, et al: Two-weekly or 3-weekly CHOP chemotherapy with or without etoposide for the treatment of elderly patients with aggressive lymphomas: results of the NHL-B2 trial of the DSHNHL. Blood 104:634-41, 2004

43. Pfreundschuh M, Trumper L, Kloess M, et al: Two-weekly or 3-weekly CHOP chemotherapy with or without etoposide for the treatment of young patients with good-prognosis (normal LDH) aggressive lymphomas: results of the NHL-B1 trial of the DSHNHL. Blood 104:626-33, 2004

44. Philip T, Guglielmi C, Hagenbeek A, et al: Autologous bone marrow transplantation as compared with salvage chemotherapy in relapses of chemotherapy-sensitive non-Hodgkin's lymphoma. N Engl J Med 333:1540-5, 1995

45. Haioun C, Lepage E, Gisselbrecht C, et al: Survival benefit of high-dose therapy in poor-risk aggressive non-Hodgkin's lymphoma: Final analysis of the Prospective LNH87-2 Protocol - A Groupe d'Etude des Lymphomes de l'Adulte Study. J.Clin.Oncol. 18:3025-3030, 2000

46. Santini G, Salvagno L, Leoni P, et al: VACOP-B versus VACOP-B plus autologous bone marrow transplantation for advanced diffuse non-Hodgkin's lymphoma: results of a prospective randomized trial by the non-Hodgkin's lymphoma cooperative study group. J.Clin.Oncol. 16:2796-2802, 1998

47. Kluin-Nelemans HC, Zagonel V, Anastasopoulou A, et al: Standard Chemotherapy with or without High-Dose Chemotherapy for Aggressive Non-Hodgkin's Lymphoma: Randomized Phase III EORTC Study. J.Nat.Cancer Inst. 93:22-30, 2000

48. Kaiser U, Uebelacker I, Abel U, et al: A Randomized Study to Evaluate The Use of High-Dose Therapy As Part Of Primary Treatment for 'Aggressive' Lymphoma. J.Clin.Oncol., 2002

49. Gianni AM, Bregni M, Siena S, et al: High dose chemotherapy and autologous bone marrow transplantation compared with MACOP-B in aggressive B-cell lymphoma. N.Engl.J.Med. 336:1290-1297, 1997

50. Gisselbrecht C, Lepage E, Molina T, et al: Shortened First-Line High-Dose Chemotherapy For Patients With Poor-Risk Aggressive Lymphoma. J.Clin.Oncol. 20:2472-2479, 2002

51. Verdonck LF, van Putten WLJ, Hagenbeek A, et al: Comparison of CHOP Chemotherapy with Autologous Bone Marrow Transplantation for Slowly Responding Patients with Aggressive Non-Hodgkin's Lymphoma. N.Engl.J.Med. 332:1045-1051, 1995

52. Milpied N, Deconinck E, Gaillard F, et al: Initial treatment of aggressive lymphoma with high-dose chemotherapy and autologous stem-cell support. N Engl J Med 350:1287-95, 2004

53. Friedberg JW, Neuberg D, Stone RM, et al: Outcome in patients with myelodysplastic syndrome after autologous bone marrow transplantation for non-Hodgkin's lymphoma. J Clin Oncol 17:3128-35, 1999

54. Brown JR, Yeckes H, Friedberg JW, et al: Increasing Incidence of Late Second Malignancies After Conditioning With Cyclophosphamide and Total-Body Irradiation and Autologous Bone Marrow Transplantation for Non-Hodgkin's Lymphoma. J Clin Oncol 23:2208-14, 2005

55. Shipp MA, Abeloff MD, Antman KH, et al: International consensus conference on high-dose therapy with hematopoietic stem cell transplantation in aggressive non-Hodgkin's lymphomas: Report of the jury. J.Clin.Oncol. 17:423-429, 1999

56. Coiffier B, Haioun C, Ketterer N, et al: Rituximab (anti-CD20 monoclonal antibody) for the treatment of patients with relapsing or refractory aggressive lymphoma: a multicenter phase II study. Blood 92:1927-32, 1998

57. Morschhauser F, Huglo D, Martinelli G, et al: Yttrium-90 Ibribumomab tiuxetan for patients with relapsed/refractroy diffuse large B cell lymphoma not appropriate for autologous stem cell transplantation: results of an open-label phase II trial. Blood 104:41a, 2004

58. Kewalramani T, Zelenetz AD, Nimer SD, et al: Rituximab and ICE as second-line therapy before autologous stem cell transplantation for relapsed or primary refractory diffuse large B-cell lymphoma. Blood 103:3684-8, 2004

59. Peggs KS, Mackinnon S, Linch DC: The role of allogeneic transplantation in non-Hodgkin's lymphoma. Br J Haematol 128:153-68, 2005

60. Escalon MP, Champlin RE, Saliba RM, et al: Nonmyeloablative allogeneic hematopoietic transplantation: a promising salvage therapy for patients with non-Hodgkin's lymphoma whose disease has failed a prior autologous transplantation. J Clin Oncol 22:2419-23, 2004

61. Friedberg JW: Developing new monoclonal antibodies for aggressive lymphoma: a challenging road in the rituximab era. Clin Cancer Res 10:5297-8, 2004

Chapter 5

MANTLE CELL LYMPHOMA: CURRENT CONCEPT IN BIOLOGY AND TREATMENT

Jia Ruan, MD, PhD, and John P. Leonard, MD

Center for Lymphoma and Myeloma and Division of Hematology/Oncology, Weill Medical College of Cornell University and New York Presbyterian Hospital, New York, New York, USA

1.   INTRODUCTION

Mantle cell lymphoma (MCL) is a distinct subtype and accounts for approximately 5-10% of non-Hodgkin's lymphomas. The tumor cells are characterized by CD5-positive, CD23-negative follicular mantle B cells with typical t(11; 14)(q13;q32) translocation and cyclin D1 protein over-expression. Four histological subtypes of MCL have been described which include mantle zone, nodular, diffuse, and blastoid forms. MCL commonly occurs in elderly patients with disseminated disease involving lymph nodes, spleen, bone marrow, blood, and the gastrointestinal system. The clinical course is typically more aggressive than indolent lymphomas with median survival of 3-4 years.

Traditional chemotherapy such as CHOP-like regimen produces no cure with usual time to progression of approximately one year. The addition of monoclonal antibody rituximab to the induction chemotherapy, and further consolidation with stem cell transplant in selected patients has yielded more favorable and durable responses. Overall the prognosis for patients with mantle cell lymphoma remains poor and novel strategies are needed. Advancement in molecular biology, DNA microarray technology and proteomics will likely provide important cellular targets for therapeutics development and treatment intervention.

2.   PATHOLOGIC FEATURES OF MANTLE CELL LYMPHOMA

2.1   Definition

The Revised European-American Classification of Lymphoid Neoplasms (REAL) classification incorporated the mantle cell lymphoma (MCL) as a distinct subtype of non-Hodgkin's lymphoma (NHL) in 1994 [1], while earlier systems referred to this entity as centrocytic lymphoma (Kiel classification) or intermediately differentiated lymphocytic lymphoma (Rappaport) [2]. Previously, many cases of mantle cell lymphoma were considered as either small cleaved cell lymphoma or small lymphocytic lymphoma under the Working Formulation [3]. The various names given to this entity complicate analysis of the literature, particularly with regard to historical response to treatment and clinical course. However, it is now appreciated that MCL represents approximately 5-10% of all NHL cases [4, 5] characterized by CD5-positive, CD23-negative follicular mantle B cells with typical t(11; 14)(q13;q32) translocation and cyclin D1 protein overexpression [6].

2.2   Diagnostic Pathology

On histopathology, MCL specimens comprise atypical small to medium-sized follicular mantle B lymphocytes with slightly irregular or "cleaved" nuclei. The tumor cells exhibit either a mantle, nodular or diffuse pattern of growth, or a combination of the three [7]. A large cell or blastic/blastoid variant is also occasionally observed [5]. All histologic patterns are associated with a prominent, irregular meshwork of follicular dendritic cells [8, 9]. Flow cytometric or immunohistochemical analysis typically reveals CD5+ and CD23- malignant B cells with t(11; 14)(q13;q32) translocation and cyclin D1 protein overexpression [7, 10]. The clonal B cells also express pan-B cell antigens CD19, CD20, CD22, and FMC7 in addition to surface IgM and IgD. CD10 and CD23 are usually absent. In some cases it is difficult to distinguish MCL from small lymphocytic lymphoma/chronic lymphocytic leukemia. In general, a greater intensity of surface immunoglobulin and CD20 staining, along with an absence of CD23, favors a diagnosis of MCL.

3.   MOLECULAR PATHOGENESIS OF MANTLE CELL LYMPHOMA

3.1   Genetics

The majority of MCL cases exhibit the t(11;14)(q13;q32) translocation[11, 12] which places the *CCND1* (or *PRAD1*, bcl-1) gene locus on band 11q13 adjacent to the immunoglobulin heavy chain (*IGH*) enhancer region at 14q32, causing cyclin D1 over-expression [13, 14]. In the absence of a secondary genetic mutation, however, the characteristic t(11;14)(q13;q32) and the resultant cyclin D1 overexpression is insufficient for lymphomagenesis [15, 16]. The most common secondary genomic alterations include gains in 3q, 6p, 12q, and losses in 13q, 6q, 9p and 17p [17]. This leads to abnormalities in expression of genes associated with cell cycles including CDK inhibitors p16 [18], p21 [19], and p27 [20], tumor suppressor p53 [21], proto-oncogene myc [22] and genes involved in apoptosis pathways [23]. Array-based comparative genomic hybridization (CGH) analysis on MCL patient samples and cell lines have identified additional novel recurrent genomic alterations including homozygous deletion of proapoptotic BIM at 2q13 [24, 25].

3.2   Cell Cycle Dysregulation

Cyclin D1 in complex with cyclin-dependent kinases 4 (CDK4) phosphorylates and inactivates the retinoblastoma protein and promotes progression through the G1-S phase of the cell cycle [26, 27]. Cyclin D1 overexpression is the hallmark of MCL, but it is not exclusive to this disorder as it can be seen in other hematological malignancies including multiple myeloma [28]. Cyclin D1 mRNA expression has been detected in virtually all MCL specimens by reverse transcription PCR, no expression was observed in reactive lymph nodes or non-mantle cell lymphomas [29, 30]. Similar results have been observed when cyclin D1 protein is assayed by flow cytometry or immunohistochemistry [10, 31]. In a subset of MCL, the half-life of cyclin D1 is prolonged by the deletion of 3' end untranslated regulatory sequences involved in mRNA stability and translational control, which further augments the cyclin D1 overexpression [32].

It is apparent; however, that overexpression of cyclin D1 alone is insufficient for MCL pathogenesis. Cooperation with other proto-oncogenes is necessary for tumor transformation. In pre-clinical studies, concurrent c-myc and cyclin D1 overexpression in transgenic mice results in lymphoma formation [15, 16]. Overexpression of c-myc mRNA has been observed in 38% of MCL patient samples, with a slightly higher frequency in blastoid variants, and is associated with poor prognosis [22, 33]. Mutations in tumor suppressors functioning as inhibitors of cyclin-CDK complexes (such as p15, p16 and p21) is another major mechanism for tumorigenesis in cyclin D1 overexpressing tumors [18, 19, 34]. Mutations and deletions of the tumor suppressor gene p53, which normally increase the expression of CDK inhibitor p21 in the setting of DNA damage, have also been observed in mantle cell lymphoma. These genetic abnormalities likely play a contributing role in etiology, and have been associated with a more aggressive course and poor prognosis [35]. Other associated chromosomal abnormalities include those involving inactivation of the ATM (ataxia telangiectasia mutated) tumor suppressor gene [36-38]. In fact, MCL harbors the highest frequency (43% of MCL case examined) of ATM mutations amongst the different subtypes of lymphomas. The pathogenic and prognostic implications of the ATM mutations in MCL remain to be further defined. Additional candidate genes implicated in MCL pathogenesis include the TCL1 gene located at 14q32 which has been implicated in T-cell prolymphocytic leukemia [39], and BCMSUN gene located on 13q14.3 which is frequently deleted in both mantle cell lymphoma and chronic lymphocytic leukemia tumor samples [40]. Notably, BCL-6 mutations, which are present in the majority of follicular lymphoma cases, are infrequent in MCL, occurring in approximately 10% of cases [41].

3.3   Cellular Proliferation

Mantle cell lymphoma cells express CD40, a tumor necrosis factor receptor family member that regulates B cell proliferation, survival and differentiation [42]. Binding of CD40 with its ligand (CD40L or CD154), may induce cell cycling in some lymphoma cell lines [43]. When primary MCL cells were cultured with a soluble recombinant CD40L trimer, significant proliferation was observed as determined by induction of DNA synthesis (thymidine incorporation assays) and cell cycling [44]. Interleukin-4 as well as IL-10 have been shown to augment these effects [45, 46]. Thus, genetic factors (particularly those related to cyclin D1 overexpression) appear to interact with features of the cellular microenvironment resulting in lymphomagenesis, and elucidation of these processes may ultimately provide novel therapeutic strategies for MCL.

3.4   Gene Expression Profiles

Gene expression profiling using DNA microarrays has made it possible to develop molecular prognostic signatures based on gene expression patterns in order to predict clinical course and treatment response in MCL. It also has the potential to identify novel molecular targets for therapeutics development.   The lymphoma/leukemia molecular profiling project has identified 42 MCL signature genes based upon expression profiling study on a large cohort of newly diagnosed MCL specimens [47].   Collectively, the MCL signature genes are distinct from the genes defining DLBCL and SLL/CLL, but are comparable between the cyclin D1-positive and cycle D1-negative MCL tumors.   20 genes belonging to the proliferation signature have been identified as the sole predictors associated with survival among MCL patients, and can be used to construct a quantitative prognostic model. In cyclin D1-positive tumors, differences in cyclin D1 mRNA level as a result of the 3' UTR genomic alteration in MCL, coupled with deletions of INK4a/ARF locus on 9p21 which encodes two tumor suppressor proteins p16INK4a and p14ARF, appear to be the strongest predictors for tumor proliferation rate and survival, and correlate with the proliferative signature prognostic model.   Deletions of tumor suppressors including the p53 and ATM are not strongly associated with proliferation or survival.   Other investigators have shown in addition to the lymphoproliferative signatures specific for cell cycle control, genes associated with multidrug resistance are up-regulated in MCL [48].   Increased expression of MMP-9, a matrix metalloproteinase involved in metastasis and angiogenesis, in non-B cells and down-regulation of RECK (inhibitor of MMP-9) have also been reported [49].

4.   CLINICAL FEATURES

The development of immunohistochemical and molecular assays for mantle cell lymphoma has allowed for more accurate diagnosis and led to various studies describing the clinical aspects of patients with this disease [5, 50-52].   Patients have a median age of approximately 65 years, and a male predominance is present. Stage III or IV disease is common, in conjunction with disseminated lymphadenopathy and frequent bone marrow involvement.   Most patients have either intermediate-high or high risk characteristics by International Prognostic Index (IPI) criteria. Splenomegaly is observed at diagnosis in approximately half of the patients, while gastrointestinal and Waldeyer's ring sites of disease may also be frequently observed. Lymphoma homing to gastrointestinal track appears to be associated with the expression of integrin $\alpha 4\beta 7$ on the tumor cells [53].

Overall, MCL combines unfavorable features of both indolent and aggressive NHL. As with the indolent lymphomas, the disease is generally incurable, however a more rapid clinical course is observed, with median survival of just 3 to 4 years. Those individuals with the diffuse type of MCL appear to have a shorter median life expectancy (16 months) than individuals with nodular types (50 months) [51]. In contrast, the mantle zone variant exhibits the clinical features of a low-grade lymphoma with 3 year survival rate at 100% [52]. Response to doxorubicine-based regimens correlates with histologic patterns with nodular and diffuse subtypes more resistant to the chemotherapy. Other adverse prognostic indicators include advanced stage disease, B symptoms, poor performance status, and bone marrow involvement. At the molecular level, increased proteosome-mediated degradation of the CDK inhibitor p27 in MCL specimens has been associated with a poor prognosis [54]. The level of Ki-67, a nuclear marker of cell proliferation, is another major prognostic factor (Martinez A Am J Path 2004 164:501-510). An earlier study has reported that the 15% of MCL tumors which do not demonstrate cyclin D1 protein overexpression have a significantly better outcome (86% vs 30% 5 year survival) and may in fact represent a separate entity [12].

5.   TREATMENT

5.1   Results of treatment with conventional chemotherapy

Although most patients present with chemosensitive disease, the typical clinical course for MCL is marked by continuous relapse after the initial therapy. There is no evidence of a cured fraction with conventional chemotherapy. Few prospective therapeutic trials have been reported in mantle cell lymphoma, and results from early studies are difficult to interpret due to variability in diagnostic criteria for study entry and small patient sample sizes. In comparison to other indolent lymphomas such as marginal zone lymphoma, a Southwest Oncology Group (SWOG) study has found lower complete remission rate, and worse failure-free survival and overall survival MCL group treated with CHOP regimen [55]. A randomized multicenter study of cyclophosphamide, vincristine and prednisone (COP) alone or with doxorubicin (CHOP) demonstrated no significant difference in complete (41% vs 58%) or partial (43% vs 31%) remission, relapse-free survival (10 vs 7 months) or overall survival (32 vs 37 months) [56], and therefore both of these regimens are commonly employed in the initial therapy of MCL. The subset of patients with low and low-intermediate risk IPI scores may have a survival benefit when treated with an anthracycline-containing regimen [57]. In a prospective-randomized study from the German Low grade Lymphoma Study Group (GLSG) comparing upfront CHOP vs. MCP (mitoxantrone, chlorambucil and prednisone), 87% overall response rate was detected in the CHOP arm compared to 73% response rate in the MCP arm (p=0.08) [58]. No differences were observed for progression-free survival between the two regimens. The overall survival was slightly higher in the CHOP arm (57% vs. 31% at 5 year, p=0.0578). However, since all patients under the age of 60 recruited after 1998 were assigned to the CHOP arm, the unbalanced patient characteristics between the two arms has made it difficult to interpret the observed differences on the overall survival.

Hyper-CVAD regimen which incorporates hyperfractionated intense-dose cyclophosphamide alternating with high doses of catarabine and methotrexate plus leucovorin rescue was first adapted by the investigators at MD Anderson to treat patients with mantle cell lymphoma. In their series of 45 patients (25 previously untreated and 20 with relapsed disease), CR rate of 38% and PR rate of 55% were achieved after 4 cycles of chemotherapy. 26 responding patients who went on to either autologous or allogeneic transplants all achieved CR. Elderly patients deemed noncandidate for transplant received total of 8 cycles of chemotherapy. For previously untreated patients, the 3 year overall survival was 92% and event-free survival was 72%, significantly improved over previously treated patients and historical controls [59]. The treatment-related mortality was over 10%. Nevertheless, hyper-CVAD remains an effective and intensive therapy for previously untreated younger patients, especially when used in the setting as induction regimen in preparation for ASCT. Recent updates of this study continue to show survival advantage of upfront hyper-CVAD over CHOP.

Purine analogues have also been evaluated in the upfront setting of MCL treatment, although responses in general have been disappointing. The overall response rates with fludarabine or 2-chlorodeoxyadenosine (2-CdA) therapy have been observed in the modest 60% range [60-62]. Time to progression was shorter in MCL compared with other indolent histology subtypes, and treatment-related mortality was 5%, most associated with pancytopenia and infections [61].

Unfortunately, virtually all patients relapse and salvage regimens are generally associated with a lower response rate and shorter time to progression. At the Weill Medical College of Cornell University – New York Presbyterian Hospital, we have commonly utilized the PEP-C regimen in this setting which consists of low-dose prednisone (20 mg), etoposide (50 mg), procarbazine (50 mg) and cyclophosphamide (50 mg) administered orally. Treatment is initiated with daily dosing of all agents until the white blood cell count falls below 3000 (usually occurring within 2-3 weeks). Treatment is held until count recovery from the nadir, and is then reinstituted on a daily, alternate day, or fractionated weekly basis (e.g. 5 of 7 days) titrated to hematologic parameters, i.e. ANC above 1000. The dose per day remains constant, only the number of days per week is altered. Preliminary clinical data have suggested that this regimen is convenient, well tolerated, and is associated with significant clinical activity in mantle cell lymphoma. 19 patients with MCL were evaluated and 16 (84%) demonstrated clinical responses (42% CR, 42% PR). Median duration of MCL patients on this continuous regimen has been 15+ months (range 3 to 42+ months). Toxicities include mild to moderate cytopenias (39% of patients), as well as occasional infections (15%) or gastrointestinal side effects (17%). These findings suggest that the PEP-C regimen can be a useful management option for MCL patients, and a number of them have been maintained on it for several years [63]. The combination of rituximab and thalidomide has also been explored as a salvage regimen for relapsed and refractory disease. A pilot study by Drach et al reported 81% response rate in 16 patients (5 CR and 8 PR) and median PFS of 20.4 months. 1 patient developed grade 4 neutropenia and two thromboembolic events were noted. The authors postulate that the marked clinical activity may relate to both the anti-tumor effect of rituximab and the immune-modulatory function of thalidomide on the tumor micro-environment [64].

5.2   Monoclonal antibody-based therapies

Rituximab, a chimeric antibody directed against the CD20 antigen, has been widely employed as a novel anti-lymphoma therapy. In mantle cell lymphoma, the standard regimen of 4 weekly infusions of 375 mg/m2/week has been demonstrated to have moderate activity, with an overall response rate of 37-38% in the previously untreated or relapsed setting, with a median time to progression of 7 months [65, 66]. While combinations of chemotherapy and rituximab have been explored in order to take advantage of potential synergy between agents, and initial results of a phase II trial of CHOP plus rituximab treatment in newly-diagnosed MCL exhibited a high response rate (48% CR and 48% PR), most patients relapsed with a median progression-free survival of 16.6 months [67]. A fraction (36%) of patients by molecular analysis demonstrated no evidence of bone marrow minimal residual disease after treatment, suggesting that this regimen could be used as an *in vivo* purge for subsequent high dose chemotherapy and autologous stem cell transplantation. However, there was no clear evidence of an advantage measured by PFS for the combination over CHOP alone. Follow-up of this study was too short to assess the efficacy on overall survival. Similar results were reported subsequently by German Low Grade Lymphoma Study Group (GLSG) in a prospective randomized phase III trial comparing CHOP plus rituximab vs. CHOP alone in 122 previously untreated patients [68]. The CHOP-R regimen affords both higher response rate (94% vs. 75%, p=0.005) and longer time to treatment failure (TTF) (median 21 months vs. 14 months, p=0.031) compared to CHOP alone. Interestingly to note, all responders in this trial were randomized again for consolidation treatment using IFN-α vs. myeloablative radio-chemotherapy and autologous stem cell transplant (ASCT) in patients under 60 yrs of age while all older patients received IFN-α. NO differences in PFS or overall survival were observed in the two arms after the second randomization. This clearly indicates that the favorable effect of rituximab, when used in combination with CHOP, has limited impact on response duration and overall survival. Subgroup analysis to compare the survival after autologous transplant following either CHOP-R regimen or CHOP alone was not available to suggest whether improved tumor purging from CHOP-R regimen could translate into improvement on survival. To explore whether addition of rituximab to a more intensive chemotherapy regimen could lead to improved PFS and OS, MD Anderson conducted a phase II trial of R-hyperCVAD alternating with R-M/A (methotrexate and cytarabine) [69]. The observed CR/CRu rate was 87% after 6 cycles of chemotherapy, and the 3-year FFS and OS were 67% and 81%, comparable to those achieved after high-dose consolidation and ASCT. However, the hematologic toxicity was significant during and after therapy including the development of secondary AML. Radio-labeled anti-CD20 antibodies have been studied in the relapsed setting. High overall response rate of 100% (91% CR) and long-lasting remission (estimated 3-year OS of 93%) were reported in 16 heavily pretreated patients when 131-iodine-labeled anti-CD20 antibody tositumomab was use in combination with high-dose chemotherapy followed by ASCT [70].

5.3 Autologous and allogeneic stem cell transplantation

High dose chemotherapy with autologous stem cell transplantation offers clear clinical benefit in relapsed diffuse large B cell NHL. This approach has also been evaluated in attempts to improve upon the limited results of standard dose chemotherapy in MCL. A number of chemotherapy regimens have been employed as induction therapy prior to autologous stem cell transplant (ASCT), including Hyper-CVAD (cyclophosphamide, doxorubicin, vincristine, dexamethasone, with methotrexate and cytarabine) and Dexa-BEAM (dexamethasone, BCNU, etoposide, cytarabine, and melphalan), with resultant high response rates and most patients remaining progression-free 2 to 3 years after therapy [59, 71]. Myeloablative radiochemotherapy combining TBI and cyclophosphamide has also been employed successfully as pre-transplant conditioning regimen [72]. Earlier studies yielded conflicting results. Some series have obtained less promising results with autologous transplantation in MCL, demonstrating that the majority of patients relapse within 2 years [73, 74]. It is possible that failure of purging strategies may contribute to the limited results in autotransplantation [74]. Recently, however, new evidence has indicated that ASCT may have long-term benefit if used earlier during the course of disease. A retrospective analysis from the European Blood and Bone Marrow Transplant Registries showed that subgroup of patients transplanted in first CR had better survival [75]. In the European MCL Network trial, 269 patients in first remission after a CHOP-like regimen were randomized upfront to either myeloablative radiochemotherapy (TBI plus cyclophosphamide) followed by ASCT or conventional α-interferon maintenance [76]. With a median follow-up of 7 years, the PFS at 2 year was 73% for ASCT as compared to 43% for IFN-α. The 3-year survival after ASCT was 83% compared to 77% in the IFN-α arm. Addition of rituximab to pre-transplant conditional regimen and / or post-transplant maintenance therapy has yielded durable remissions in the autologous transplant setting [77, 78]. In a study of 28 patients who were treated with either cisplatin or doxorubicin-based induction chemotherapy followed by high-dose sequential therapy containing rituximab, 21 of 27 patients were in clinical and molecular remission at a median of 21 months. The 54-month estimated OS and event-free survival were 89% and 79% respectively, significantly improved over the historical controls of 42% and 18% respectively. In an updated report from the Nordic MCL project [79], 88 evaluable patients who received induction therapy with maxi-CHOP with high-dose cyclophosphamide (1200 mg/m2), high-dose Ara-C and 2 standard doses of rituximab followed by BEAM/BEAC and ASCT, the 3-

year failure-free survival was 68%, relapse-free survival was 76%, and overall survival was 85%, all favorable compared to historical controls.

Selected patients have been treated with allogeneic stem cell transplantation for mantle cell lymphoma with apparently higher rates of overall and disease-free survival [80, 81]. This strategy has also been utilized in patients with relapsed MCL following autologous stem cell transplant [82]. However, due to the advanced age of this particular patient group, myeloablative allogeneic transplant is prohibitive for most patients. The graft-versus-lymphoma effect which may be present in allogeneic transplantation has now been exploited via "mini-allogeneic transplants" [83]. The combination of fludarabine and total body irradiation has successfully been employed as a reduced intensity pre-transplant conditional regimen in a multi-center study with projected overall and disease-free survivals at 2 years at 65% and 60% respectively [84]. The association between disease response and chronic GVHD was observed, however, non-relapse conditions including GVHD remain the main cause of mortality (24%). Other studies have reported inferior clinical outcomes. Nevertheless, reduced intensity SCT represents a promising salvage strategy that warrants continued and cautious investigation.

5.4 Experiences with Novel Proteasome Inhibitor Bortezomib

Bortezomib, a dipeptidyl boronic acid derivative, selectively inhibits the 26S proteasome which is essential in the degradation of intracellular proteins including p53, nuclear factor kappa B (NF-κB), bcl-2, and cyclin-dependent kinase (cdk) inhibitors such as p21 and p27 . Inhibition of the ubiquitin-proteasome pathway in tumor cells hinders tumor growth by inducing cell cycle arrest, apoptosis and inhibiting tumor metastasis and angiogenesis. Based on its marked efficacy and low toxicity as a single agent in multiple myeloma trials, bortezomib has been approved by the US Food and Drug Administration for the treatment of relapsed or refractory multiple myeloma in 2003. In addition, bortezomib has also shown encouraging clinical activities in NHL including mantle cell lymphoma (MCL) and indolent lymphoma. In a phase I trial using bortezomib in patients with hematologic malignancy refractory to standard therapy [85], 10 patients with NHL were included. 1 patient with mantle cell lymphoma achieved PR after 2 cycles of treatment at dose of 1.38 mg/m^2. In a single-center phase II trial at Memorial Sloan-Kettering Cancer Center using bortezomib at a dose of 1.5 mg/m2 on days 1,4, 8 and 11 per a 3-week-cycle, 1 out of 11 patient with MCL achieved a CRu, 4 patients achieved a PR, and four had stable disease, giving a response rate of 50% [86]. The duration of response appears to be lasting at least 6 months in the responders. The treatment was well-tolerated with electrolyte abnormalities and reversible lymphopenia and thrombocytopenia as the most common toxicities. A lower response rate was observed in the multi-center Canadian trial using bortezomib at 1.3 mg/m2 dose for a maximum of 4 cycles [87]. Overall response of 33% was observed in both previously untreated and treated groups, although CR was rare. Results from these phase II trials demonstrate that bortezomib is an active agent in mantle cell lymphoma. Currently multiple trials are ongoing to further exam its efficacy either as a single agent or in combination with other active regimens including CHOP plus rituximab.

6.   CONCLUSIONS

MCL is recognized as one of the most unfavorable forms of lymphoma, with resistance to chemotherapy and a relatively rapid clinical progression in most cases. Traditional CHOP-like chemotherapy affords moderate response rate but no cure. Addition of monoclonal anti-CD20 antibody rituximab improves response and molecular remission rate, however, the benefit is limited to the duration of the induction chemotherapy and cannot be translated into progression free survival or overall survival advantage. More intensive regimens such as hyper-CVAD are largely prohibitive for most of the patients due to treatment-related toxicities, although the response rate and survival data appears to be superior to CHOP in selected patients, particularly when used in conjunction with autologous stem cell transplant. Emerging transplant data indicates that autologous stem cell transplant, when used early in the course of the disease, may have favorable effect on long term survival in younger patients. Reduced-intensity allogeneic transplant is still early in the experimental stage. For majority of the patients, relapsed and refractory diseases are common. Development of novel therapeutics to improve outcomes in both the upfront and salvage settings is urgently needed.

It is appreciated on the molecular level that cooperating mutations from proto-oncogenes (e.g. c-myc) and tumor suppressor genes such as p53 and cyclin dependent kinase inhibitors, in conjunction with cyclin D1 over-expression and cell cycle dysregulation ultimately leads to mantle cell lymphomagenesis. Acquisition of additional genomic mutations and recruitment of stromal elements including neo-vasculatures within the tumor microenvironment sustain and propagate tumor growth and metastasis. Further delineation of critical gene products regulating lymphoma growth both within the tumor cell and its microenvironment could provide target-specific biologics as a new treatment platform. One such example directly targeting tumor cells is the use of bortezomib (Velcade), a protease inhibitor, in the treatment of mantle cell lymphoma. Trials studying the efficacy of anti-angiogenic reagents such as bevacizumab (Avastin) which targets tumor vascular microenvironment is currently ongoing. Used alone or in combination with chemotherapy, target-specific compound(s) are hoped to bring improved clinical outcome including survival benefit with low toxicities for patients who have this particularly difficult subtype of non-Hodgkin's lymphoma.

7.   REFERENCES

1.   Harris, N.L., Jaffe, E.S., Stein, H., Banks, P.M., Chan, J.K., Cleary, M.L., Delsol, G., De Wolf-Peeters, C., Falini, B. and Gatter, K.C., *A revised european-american classification of lymphoid neoplasms: A proposal from the international lymphoma study group.[see comment]. [review] [296 refs].* Blood., 1994. **84**(5): p. 1361-1392.
2.   Braylan, R.C., Jaffe, E.S. and Berard, C.W., *Malignant lymphomas: Current classification and new observations. [review] [149 refs].* Pathology Annual, 1975. **10**: p. 213-270.
3.   Anonymous, *National cancer institute sponsored study of classifications of non-hodgkin's lymphomas: Summary and description of a working formulation for clinical usage. The non-hodgkin's lymphoma pathologic classification project.* Cancer, 1982. **49**(10): p. 2112-2135.
4.   Anderson, J.R., Armitage, J.O. and Weisenburger, D.D., *Epidemiology of the non-hodgkin's lymphomas: Distributions of the major subtypes differ by geographic locations. Non-hodgkin's lymphoma classification project.* Annals of Oncology, 1998. **9**(7): p. 717-720.
5.   Weisenburger, D.D. and Armitage, J.O., *Mantle cell lymphoma-- an entity comes of age.[see comment]. [review] [119 refs].* Blood, 1996. **87**(11): p. 4483-4494.
6.   Harris, N.L., Jaffe, E.S., Diebold, J., Flandrin, G., Muller-Hermelink, H.K., Vardiman, J., Lister, T.A. and Bloomfield, C.D., *World health organization classification of neoplastic diseases of the hematopoietic and lymphoid tissues: Report of the clinical advisory committee meeting-airlie house, virginia, november 1997.[see comment].* Journal of Clinical Oncology., 1999. **17**(12): p. 3835-3849.
7.   Weisenburger, D.D., *Mantle cell lymphoma*, in *Neoplastic hematopathology*, D. M. Knowles, Editor. 2001, Lippincott Williams & Wilkins: Philadelphia. p. 789-803.
8.   Harris, N.L., Nadler, L.M. and Bhan, A.K., *Immunohistologic characterization of two malignant lymphomas of germinal center type (centroblastic/centrocytic and centrocytic) with monoclonal antibodies. Follicular and diffuse lymphomas of small-cleaved-cell type are related but distinct entities.* American Journal of Pathology, 1984. **117**(2): p. 262-272.
9.   Zukerberg, L.R., Medeiros, L.J., Ferry, J.A. and Harris, N.L., *Diffuse low-grade b-cell lymphomas. Four clinically distinct subtypes defined by a combination of morphologic and immunophenotypic features.[see comment].* American Journal of Clinical Pathology, 1993. **100**(4): p. 373-385.
10.   Zukerberg, L.R., Yang, W.I., Arnold, A. and Harris, N.L., *Cyclin d1 expression in non-hodgkin's lymphomas. Detection by immunohistochemistry.* American Journal of Clinical Pathology, 1995. **103**(6): p. 756-760.

11.   Swerdlow, S.H. and Williams, M.E., *From centrocytic to mantle cell lymphoma: A clinicopathologic and molecular review of 3 decades. [review] [134 refs].* Human Pathology, 2002. **33**(1): p. 7-20.

12.   Yatabe, Y., Suzuki, R., Tobinai, K., Matsuno, Y., Ichinohasama, R., Okamoto, M., Yamaguchi, M., Tamaru, J., Uike, N., Hashimoto, Y., Morishima, Y., Suchi, T., Seto, M. and Nakamura, S., *Significance of cyclin d1 overexpression for the diagnosis of mantle cell lymphoma: A clinicopathologic comparison of cyclin d1-positive mcl and cyclin d1-negative mcl-like b-cell lymphoma.* Blood, 2000. **95**(7): p. 2253-2261.

13.   Rosenberg, C.L., Wong, E., Petty, E.M., Bale, A.E., Tsujimoto, Y., Harris, N.L. and Arnold, A., *Prad1, a candidate bcl1 oncogene: Mapping and expression in centrocytic lymphoma.* Proceedings of the National Academy of Sciences of the United States of America, 1991. **88**(21): p. 9638-9642.

14.   Williams, M.E. and Swerdlow, S.H., *Cyclin d1 overexpression in non-hodgkin's lymphoma with chromosome 11 bcl-1 rearrangement.* Annals of Oncology, 1994. **1**: p. 71-73.

15.   Bodrug, S.E., Warner, B.J., Bath, M.L., Lindeman, G.J., Harris, A.W. and Adams, J.M., *Cyclin d1 transgene impedes lymphocyte maturation and collaborates in lymphomagenesis with the myc gene.* EMBO Journal, 1994. **13**(9): p. 2124-2130.

16.   Lovec, H., Grzeschiczek, A., Kowalski, M.B. and Moroy, T., *Cyclin d1/bcl-1 cooperates with myc genes in the generation of b-cell lymphoma in transgenic mice.* EMBO Journal, 1994. **13**(15): p. 3487-3495.

17.   Au, W.Y., Gascoyne, R.D., Viswanatha, D.S., Connors, J.M., Klasa, R.J. and Horsman, D.E., *Cytogenetic analysis in mantle cell lymphoma: A review of 214 cases.* Leukemia & Lymphoma, 2002. **43**(4): p. 783-791.

18.   Dreyling, M.H., Bullinger, L., Ott, G., Stilgenbauer, S., Muller-Hermelink, H.K., Bentz, M., Hiddemann, W. and Dohner, H., *Alterations of the cyclin d1/p16-prb pathway in mantle cell lymphoma.* Cancer Research, 1997. **57**(20): p. 4608-4614.

19.   Pinyol, M., Hernandez, L., Cazorla, M., Balbin, M., Jares, P., Fernandez, P.L., Montserrat, E., Cardesa, A., Lopez-Otin, C. and Campo, E., *Deletions and loss of expression of p16ink4a and p21waf1 genes are associated with aggressive variants of mantle cell lymphomas.* Blood, 1997. **89**(1): p. 272-280.

20.   Quintanilla-Martinez, L., Davies-Hill, T., Fend, F., Calzada-Wack, J., Sorbara, L., Campo, E., Jaffe, E.S. and Raffeld, M., *Sequestration of p27kip1 protein by cyclin d1 in typical and blastic variants of mantle cell lymphoma (mcl): Implications for pathogenesis.* Blood, 2003. **101**(8): p. 3181-3187.

21.   Greiner, T.C., Moynihan, M.J., Chan, W.C., Lytle, D.M., Pedersen, A., Anderson, J.R. and Weisenburger, D.D., *P53 mutations in mantle cell lymphoma are associated with variant cytology and predict a poor prognosis.* Blood, 1996. **87**(10): p. 4302-4310.

22.   Nagy, B., Lundan, T., Larramendy, M.L., Aalto, Y., Zhu, Y., Niini, T., Edgren, H., Ferrer, A., Vilpo, J., Elonen, E., Vettenranta, K., Franssila, K. and Knuutila, S., *Abnormal expression of apoptosis-related genes in haematological malignancies: Overexpression of myc is poor prognostic sign in mantle cell lymphoma.* British Journal of Haematology, 2003. **120**(3): p. 434-441.

23.   Hofmann, W.K., De Vos, S., Tsukasaki, K., Wachsman, W., Pinkus, G.S., Said, J.W. and Koeffler, H.P., *Altered apoptosis pathways in mantle cell lymphoma detected by oligonucleotide microarray.* Blood, 2001. **98**(3): p. 787-794.

24.   De Leeuw, R.J., Davies, J.J., Rosenwald, A., Bebb, G., Gascoyne, R.D., Dyer, M.J., Staudt, L.M., Martinez-Climent, J.A. and Lam, W.L., *Comprehensive whole genome array cgh profiling of mantle cell lymphoma model genomes.* Human Molecular Genetics, 1827. **13**(17): p. 1827-1837.

25.   Tagawa, H., Karnan, S., Suzuki, R., Matsuo, K., Zhang, X., Ota, A., Morishima, Y., Nakamura, S. and Seto, M., *Genome-wide array-based cgh for mantle cell lymphoma: Identification of homozygous deletions of the proapoptotic gene bim.* Oncogene, 1348. **24**(8): p. 1348-1358.

26. Hunter, T. and Pines, J., *Cyclins and cancer. Ii: Cyclin d and cdk inhibitors come of age.[see comment]. [review] [152 refs]*. Cell, 1994. **79**(4): p. 573-582.

27. Xiao, Z.X., Ginsberg, D., Ewen, M. and Livingston, D.M., *Regulation of the retinoblastoma protein-related protein p107 by g1 cyclin-associated kinases.* Proceedings of the National Academy of Sciences of the United States of America, 1996. **93**(10): p. 4633-4637.

28. Bergsagel, P.L. and Kuehl, W.M., *Critical roles for immunoglobulin translocations and cyclin d dysregulation in multiple myeloma. [review] [30 refs]*. Immunological Reviews, 2003. **194**: p. 96-104.

29. Athanasiou, E., Kotoula, V., Hytiroglou, P., Kouidou, S., Kaloutsi, V. and Papadimitriou, C.S., *In situ hybridization and reverse transcription-polymerase chain reaction for cyclin d1 mrna in the diagnosis of mantle cell lymphoma in paraffin-embedded tissues.* Modern Pathology, 2001. **14**(2): p. 62-71.

30. Bijwaard, K.E., Aguilera, N.S., Monczak, Y., Trudel, M., Taubenberger, J.K. and Lichy, J.H., *Quantitative real-time reverse transcription-pcr assay for cyclin d1 expression: Utility in the diagnosis of mantle cell lymphoma.* Clinical Chemistry, 2001. **47**(2): p. 195-201.

31. Elnenaei, M.O., Jadayel, D.M., Matutes, E., Morilla, R., Owusu-Ankomah, K., Atkinson, S., Titley, I., Mandala, E.M. and Catovsky, D., *Cyclin d1 by flow cytometry as a useful tool in the diagnosis of b-cell malignancies.* Leukemia Research, 2001. **25**(2): p. 115-123.

32. Rimokh, R., Berger, F., Bastard, C., Klein, B., French, M., Archimbaud, E., Rouault, J.P., Santa Lucia, B., Duret, L., Vuillaume, M. and Et Al., *Rearrangement of ccnd1 (bcl1/prad1) 3' untranslated region in mantle-cell lymphomas and t(11q13)-associated leukemias.* Blood, 1994. **83**(12): p. 3689-3696.

33. Hernandez, L., Hernandez, S., Bea, S., Pinyol, M., Ferrer, A., Bosch, F., Nadal, A., Fernandez, P.L., Palacin, A., Montserrat, E. and Campo, E., *C-myc mrna expression and genomic alterations in mantle cell lymphomas and other nodal non-hodgkin's lymphomas.* Leukemia, 1999. **13**(12): p. 2087-2093.

34. Koduru, P.R., Zariwala, M., Soni, M., Gong, J.Z., Xiong, Y. and Broome, J.D., *Deletion of cyclin-dependent kinase 4 inhibitor genes p15 and p16 in non-hodgkin's lymphoma.* Blood, 1995. **86**(8): p. 2900-2905.

35. Louie, D.C., Offit, K., Jaslow, R., Parsa, N.Z., Murty, V.V., Schluger, A. and Chaganti, R.S., *P53 overexpression as a marker of poor prognosis in mantle cell lymphomas with t(11;14)(q13;q32).* Blood, 1995. **86**(8): p. 2892-2899.

36. Stilgenbauer, S., Schaffner, C., Winkler, D., Ott, G., Leupolt, E., Bentz, M., Moller, P., Muller-Hermelink, H.K., James, M.R., Lichter, P. and Dohner, H., *The atm gene in the pathogenesis of mantle-cell lymphoma.* Annals of Oncology, 2000. **1**: p. 127-130.

37. Schaffner, C., Idler, I., Stilgenbauer, S., Dohner, H. and Lichter, P., *Mantle cell lymphoma is characterized by inactivation of the atm gene.* Proceedings of the National Academy of Sciences of the United States of America, 2000. **97**(6): p. 2773-2778.

38. Fang, N.Y., Greiner, T.C., Weisenburger, D.D., Chan, W.C., Vose, J.M., Smith, L.M., Armitage, J.O., Mayer, R.A., Pike, B.L., Collins, F.S. and Hacia, J.G., *Oligonucleotide microarrays demonstrate the highest frequency of atm mutations in the mantle cell subtype of lymphoma.* Proceedings of the National Academy of Sciences of the United States of America, 2003. **100**(9): p. 5372-5377.

39. Narducci, M.G., Pescarmona, E., Lazzeri, C., Signoretti, S., Lavinia, A.M., Remotti, D., Scala, E., Baroni, C.D., Stoppacciaro, A., Croce, C.M. and Russo, G., *Regulation of tcl1 expression in b- and t-cell lymphomas and reactive lymphoid tissues.* Cancer Research, 2000. **60**(8): p. 2095-2100.

40. Mertens, D., Wolf, S., Bullinger, L., Ohl, S., Schaffner, C., Dohner, H., Stilgenbauer, S. and Lichter, P., *Bcmsun, a candidate gene for b-cell chronic lymphocytic leukemia and mantle-cell lymphoma, has an independently expressed homolog on 1p22-p31, bcmsun-like.* International Journal of Cancer, 2000. **88**(5): p. 692-697.

41.   Capello, D., Vitolo, U., Pasqualucci, L., Quattrone, S., Migliaretti, G., Fassone, L., Ariatti, C., Vivenza, D., Gloghini, A., Pastore, C., Lanza, C., Nomdedeu, J., Botto, B., Freilone, R., Buonaiuto, D., Zagonel, V., Gallo, E., Palestro, G., Saglio, G., Dalla-Favera, R., Carbone, A. and Gaidano, G., *Distribution and pattern of bcl-6 mutations throughout the spectrum of b-cell neoplasia.* Blood, 2000. **95**(2): p. 651-659.

42.   Gordon, J., *Cd40 and its ligand: Central players in b lymphocyte survival, growth, and differentiation. [review] [35 refs].* Blood Reviews, 1995. **9**(1): p. 53-56.

43.   Wang, H., Grand, R.J., Milner, A.E., Armitage, R.J., Gordon, J. and Gregory, C.D., *Repression of apoptosis in human b-lymphoma cells by cd40-ligand and bcl-2: Relationship to the cell-cycle and role of the retinoblastoma protein.* Oncogene, 1996. **13**(2): p. 373-379.

44.   Andersen, N.S., Larsen, J.K., Christiansen, J., Pedersen, L.B., Christophersen, N.S., Geisler, C.H. and Jurlander, J., *Soluble cd40 ligand induces selective proliferation of lymphoma cells in primary mantle cell lymphoma cell cultures.* Blood, 2000. **96**(6): p. 2219-2225.

45.   Castillo, R., Mascarenhas, J., Telford, W., Chadburn, A., Friedman, S.M. and Schattner, E.J., *Proliferative response of mantle cell lymphoma cells stimulated by cd40 ligation and il-4.* Leukemia, 2000. **14**(2): p. 292-298.

46.   Visser, H.P., Tewis, M., Willemze, R. and Kluin-Nelemans, J.C., *Mantle cell lymphoma proliferates upon il-10 in the cd40 system.* Leukemia, 1483. **14**(8): p. 1483-1489.

47.   Rosenwald, A., Wright, G., Wiestner, A., Chan, W.C., Connors, J.M., Campo, E., Gascoyne, R.D., Grogan, T.M., Muller-Hermelink, H.K., Smeland, E.B., Chiorazzi, M., Giltnane, J.M., Hurt, E.M., Zhao, H., Averett, L., Henrickson, S., Yang, L., Powell, J., Wilson, W.H., Jaffe, E.S., Simon, R., Klausner, R.D., Montserrat, E., Bosch, F., Greiner, T.C., Weisenburger, D.D., Sanger, W.G., Dave, B.J., Lynch, J.C., Vose, J., Armitage, J.O., Fisher, R.I., Miller, T.P., Leblanc, M., Ott, G., Kvaloy, S., Holte, H., Delabie, J. and Staudt, L.M., *The proliferation gene expression signature is a quantitative integrator of oncogenic events that predicts survival in mantle cell lymphoma.[see comment].* Cancer Cell, 2003. **3**(2): p. 185-197.

48.   Thieblemont, C., Nasser, V., Felman, P., Leroy, K., Gazzo, S., Callet-Bauchu, E., Loriod, B., Granjeaud, S., Gaulard, P., Haioun, C., Traverse-Glehen, A., Baseggio, L., Bertucci, F., Birnbaum, D., Magrangeas, F., Minvielle, S., Avet-Loiseau, H., Salles, G., Coiffier, B., Berger, F. and Houlgatte, R., *Small lymphocytic lymphoma, marginal zone b-cell lymphoma, and mantle cell lymphoma exhibit distinct gene-expression profiles allowing molecular diagnosis.* Blood, 2004. **103**(7): p. 2727-2737.

49.   Ek, S., Hogerkorp, C.M., Dictor, M., Ehinger, M. and Borrebaeck, C.A., *Mantle cell lymphomas express a distinct genetic signature affecting lymphocyte trafficking and growth regulation as compared with subpopulations of normal human b cells.* Cancer Research, 2002. **62**(15): p. 4398-4405.

50.   Samaha, H., Dumontet, C., Ketterer, N., Moullet, I., Thieblemont, C., Bouafia, F., Callet-Bauchu, E., Felman, P., Berger, F., Salles, G. and Coiffier, B., *Mantle cell lymphoma: A retrospective study of 121 cases. [review] [44 refs].* Leukemia., 1998. **12**(8): p. 1281-1287.

51.   Weisenburger, D.D., Vose, J.M., Greiner, T.C., Lynch, J.C., Chan, W.C., Bierman, P.J., Dave, B.J., Sanger, W.G. and Armitage, J.O., *Mantle cell lymphoma. A clinicopathologic study of 68 cases from the nebraska lymphoma study group. [review] [54 refs].* American Journal of Hematology., 2000. **64**(3): p. 190-196.

52.   Majlis, A., Pugh, W.C., Rodriguez, M.A., Benedict, W.F. and Cabanillas, F., *Mantle cell lymphoma: Correlation of clinical outcome and biologic features with three histologic variants.* Journal of Clinical Oncology, 1664. **15**(4): p. 1664-1671.

53.   Geissmann, F., Ruskone-Fourmestraux, A., Hermine, O., Bourquelot, P., Belanger, C., Audouin, J., Delmer, A., Macintyre, E.A., Varet, B. and Brousse, N., *Homing receptor alpha4beta7 integrin expression predicts digestive tract involvement in mantle cell lymphoma.* American Journal of Pathology, 1701. **153**(6): p. 1701-1705.

54. Chiarle, R., Budel, L.M., Skolnik, J., Frizzera, G., Chilosi, M., Corato, A., Pizzolo, G., Magidson, J., Montagnoli, A., Pagano, M., Maes, B., De Wolf-Peeters, C. and Inghirami, G., *Increased proteasome degradation of cyclin-dependent kinase inhibitor p27 is associated with a decreased overall survival in mantle cell lymphoma.* Blood, 2000. **95**(2): p. 619-626.

55. Fisher, R.I., Dahlberg, S., Nathwani, B.N., Banks, P.M., Miller, T.P. and Grogan, T.M., *A clinical analysis of two indolent lymphoma entities: Mantle cell lymphoma and marginal zone lymphoma (including the mucosa-associated lymphoid tissue and monocytoid b-cell subcategories): A southwest oncology group study.* Blood, 1075. **85**(4): p. 1075-1082.

56. Meusers, P., Engelhard, M., Bartels, H., Binder, T., Fulle, H.H., Gorg, K., Gunzer, U., Havemann, K., Kayser, W., Konig, E. and Et Al., *Multicentre randomized therapeutic trial for advanced centrocytic lymphoma: Anthracycline does not improve the prognosis.* Hematological Oncology, 1989. **7**(5): p. 365-380.

57. Zucca, E., Roggero, E., Pinotti, G., Pedrinis, E., Cappella, C., Venco, A. and Cavalli, F., *Patterns of survival in mantle cell lymphoma.* Annals of Oncology, 1995. **6**(3): p. 257-262.

58. Nickenig, C., Dreyling, M., Schiegnitz, E., Pfreundschuh, M., Truemper, L.H., Reiser, M., Wandt, H., Lengfelder, E., Ludwig, W., Berdel, W.E., Metzner, B., Hess, G., Forstpointner, R., Parwaresch, R., Hasford, J., Unterhalt, M. and Hiddemann, W., *Chop improves response rates but not overall survival in follicular and mantle cell lymphoma (mcl) - results of a randomized trial of the german low grade lymphoma study group (glsg) [abstract].* Blood, 2004. **104**: p. 611a.

59. Khouri, I.F., Romaguera, J., Kantarjian, H., Palmer, J.L., Pugh, W.C., Korbling, M., Hagemeister, F., Samuels, B., Rodriguez, A., Giralt, S., Younes, A., Przepiorka, D., Claxton, D., Cabanillas, F. and Champlin, R., *Hyper-cvad and high-dose methotrexate/cytarabine followed by stem-cell transplantation: An active regimen for aggressive mantle-cell lymphoma.* Journal of Clinical Oncology., 1998. **16**(12): p. 3803-3809.

60. Meusers, P. and Hense, J., *Management of mantle cell lymphoma. [review] [91 refs].* Annals of Hematology, 1999. **78**(11): p. 485-494.

61. Foran, J.M., Rohatiner, A.Z., Coiffier, B., Barbui, T., Johnson, S.A., Hiddemann, W., Radford, J.A., Norton, A.J., Tollerfield, S.M., Wilson, M.P. and Lister, T.A., *Multicenter phase ii study of fludarabine phosphate for patients with newly diagnosed lymphoplasmacytoid lymphoma, waldenstrom's macroglobulinemia, and mantle-cell lymphoma.* Journal of Clinical Oncology, 1999. **17**(2): p. 546-553.

62. Zinzani, P.L., Magagnoli, M., Moretti, L., De Renzo, A., Battista, R., Zaccaria, A., Guardigni, L., Mazza, P., Marra, R., Ronconi, F., Lauta, V.M., Bendandi, M., Gherlinzoni, F., Gentilini, P., Ciccone, F., Cellini, C., Stefoni, V., Ricciuti, F., Gobbi, M. and Tura, S., *Randomized trial of fludarabine versus fludarabine and idarubicin as frontline treatment in patients with indolent or mantle-cell lymphoma.* Journal of Clinical Oncology, 2000. **18**(4): p. 773-779.

63. Coleman, M., Leonard, J.P., Lee, C. and Al., E., *The pep-c (c3) oral combination chemotherapy regimen for refractory / relapsed lymphoma:Daily prednisone, etoposide, procarbazine and cyclophosphamide.* Blood., 1999. **94**: p. 94a.

64. Kaufmann, H., Raderer, M., Wohrer, S., Puspok, A., Bankier, A., Zielinski, C., Chott, A. and Drach, J., *Antitumor activity of rituximab plus thalidomide in patients with relapsed/refractory mantle cell lymphoma.* Blood, 2004. **104**(8): p. 2269-2271.

65. Foran, J.M., Rohatiner, A.Z., Cunningham, D., Popescu, R.A., Solal-Celigny, P., Ghielmini, M., Coiffier, B., Johnson, P.W., Gisselbrecht, C., Reyes, F., Radford, J.A., Bessell, E.M., Souleau, B., Benzohra, A. and Lister, T.A., *European phase ii study of rituximab (chimeric anti-cd20 monoclonal antibody) for patients with newly diagnosed mantle-cell lymphoma and previously treated mantle-cell lymphoma, immunocytoma, and small b-cell lymphocytic lymphoma.[erratum appears in j clin oncol 2000 may;18(9):2006].* Journal of Clinical Oncology, 2000. **18**(2): p. 317-324.

66.   Foran, J.M., Cunningham, D., Coiffier, B., Solal-Celigny, P., Reyes, F., Ghielmini, M., Johnson, P.W., Gisselbrecht, C., Bradburn, M., Matthews, J. and Lister, T.A., *Treatment of mantle-cell lymphoma with rituximab (chimeric monoclonal anti-cd20 antibody): Analysis of factors associated with response.* Annals of Oncology, 2000. **1**: p. 117-121.

67.   Howard, O.M., Gribben, J.G., Neuberg, D.S., Grossbard, M., Poor, C., Janicek, M.J. and Shipp, M.A., *Rituximab and chop induction therapy for newly diagnosed mantle-cell lymphoma: Molecular complete responses are not predictive of progression-free survival.* Journal of Clinical Oncology., 2002. **20**(5): p. 1288-1294.

68.   Lenz, G., Dreyling, M., Hoster, E., Wormann, B., Duhrsen, U., Metzner, B., Eimermacher, H., Neubauer, A., Wandt, H., Steinhauer, H., Martin, S., Heidemann, E., Aldaoud, A., Parwaresch, R., Hasford, J., Unterhalt, M. and Hiddemann, W., *Immunochemotherapy with rituximab and cyclophosphamide, doxorubicin, vincristine, and prednisone significantly improves response and time to treatment failure, but not long-term outcome in patients with previously untreated mantle cell lymphoma: Results of a prospective randomized trial of the german low grade lymphoma study group (glsg).* Journal of Clinical Oncology, 2005. **23**(9): p. 1984-1992.

69.   Romaguera, J., Fayad, L., Rodriguez, M.A., Hagemeister, F., Pro, B., Mclaughlin, P., Younes, A., Samaniego, F., Goy, A., Sarris, A.H., Dang, N.H., Medeiros, L.J., Katz, R., Gagneja, H., Samuels, B. and Cabanillas, F., *Rituximab plus hypercvad (r-hcvad) alternating with rituximab plus high-dose methotrexate-cytarabine (r-m/a) in untreated mantle cell lymphoma (mcl): Prolonged follow-up confirms high rates of failure-free survival (ffs) and overall survival (os) [abstract].* Blood, 2004. **104**: p. 128a.

70.   Gopal, A.K., Rajendran, J.G., Petersdorf, S.H., Maloney, D.G., Eary, J.F., Wood, B.L., Gooley, T.A., Bush, S.A., Durack, L.D., Martin, P.J., Matthews, D.C., Appelbaum, F.R., Bernstein, I.D. and Press, O.W., *High-dose chemo-radioimmunotherapy with autologous stem cell support for relapsed mantle cell lymphoma.* Blood, 2002. **99**(9): p. 3158-3162.

71.   Josting, A., Reiser, M., Wickramanayake, P.D., Rueffer, U., Draube, A., Sohngen, D., Tesch, H., Wolf, J., Diehl, V. and Engert, A., *Dexa-beam: An effective regimen for cytoreduction prior to high-dose chemotherapy with autologous stem cell support for patients with relapsed/refractory mantle-cell lymphoma.* Leukemia & Lymphoma, 2000. **37**(1-2): p. 185-187.

72.   Haas, R., Brittinger, G., Meusers, P., Murea, S., Goldschmidt, H., Wannenmacher, M. and Hunstein, W., *Myeloablative therapy with blood stem cell transplantation is effective in mantle cell lymphoma.* Leukemia, 1975. **10**(12): p. 1975-1979.

73.   Freedman, A.S., Neuberg, D., Gribben, J.G., Mauch, P., Soiffer, R.J., Fisher, D.C., Anderson, K.C., Andersen, N., Schlossman, R., Kroon, M., Ritz, J., Aster, J. and Nadler, L.M., *High-dose chemoradiotherapy and anti-b-cell monoclonal antibody-purged autologous bone marrow transplantation in mantle-cell lymphoma: No evidence for long-term remission.[see comment].* Journal of Clinical Oncology., 1998. **16**(1): p. 13-18.

74.   Vose, J.M., Bierman, P.J., Weisenburger, D.D., Lynch, J.C., Bociek, Y., Chan, W.C., Greiner, T.C. and Armitage, J.O., *Autologous hematopoietic stem cell transplantation for mantle cell lymphoma.* Biology of Blood & Marrow Transplantation, 2000. **6**(6): p. 640-645.

75.   Vandenberghe, E., Ruiz De Elvira, C., Loberiza, F.R., Conde, E., Lopez-Guillermo, A., Gisselbrecht, C., Guilhot, F., Vose, J.M., Van Biesen, K., Rizzo, J.D., Weisenburger, D.D., Isaacson, P., Horowitz, M.M., Goldstone, A.H., Lazarus, H.M. and Schmitz, N., *Outcome of autologous transplantation for mantle cell lymphoma: A study by the european blood and bone marrow transplant and autologous blood and marrow transplant registries.* British Journal of Haematology, 2003. **120**(5): p. 793-800.

76.   Dreyling, M., Lenz, G., Schiegnitz, E., Van Hoof, A., Gisselbrecht, C. and Al., E., *Early consolidation with myeloablative radiochemotherapy followed by autologous stem cell transplantation in first remission significantly prolongs progression-free survival in mantle*

cell lymphoma - long term follow up of a prospective randomized trial of the european mcl network [abstract]. Blood, 2004. **104**: p. 7a.

77.   Magni, M., Di Nicola, M., Devizzi, L., Matteucci, P., Lombardi, F., Gandola, L., Ravagnani, F., Giardini, R., Dastoli, G., Tarella, C., Pileri, A., Bonadonna, G. and Gianni, A.M., *Successful in vivo purging of cd34-containing peripheral blood harvests in mantle cell and indolent lymphoma: Evidence for a role of both chemotherapy and rituximab infusion.* Blood, 2000. **96**(3): p. 864-869.

78.   Gianni, A.M., Magni, M., Martelli, M., Di Nicola, M., Carlo-Stella, C., Pilotti, S., Rambaldi, A., Cortelazzo, S., Patti, C., Parvis, G., Benedetti, F., Capria, S., Corradini, P., Tarella, C. and Barbui, T., *Long-term remission in mantle cell lymphoma following high-dose sequential chemotherapy and in vivo rituximab-purged stem cell autografting (r-hds regimen).* Blood, 2003. **102**(2): p. 749-755.

79.   Geisler, C.H., Elonen, E., Kolstad, A., Laurell, A. and Al., E., *Nordic mantle cell lymphoma (mcl) project: Prolonged follow-up of 86 patients treated with beam/beac + pbsct confirms that addition of high-dose ara-c and rituximab to chop induction + in-vivo purging with rituximab increases clinical and molecular response rates, pcr-neg. Grafts, failure-free, relapse-free and overall survival [abstract].* Blood, 2004. **104**: p. 8a.

80.   Khouri, I.F., Lee, M.S., Romaguera, J., Mirza, N., Kantarjian, H., Korbling, M., Albitar, M., Giralt, S., Samuels, B., Anderlini, P., Rodriguez, J., Von Wolff, B., Gajewski, J., Cabanillas, F. and Champlin, R., *Allogeneic hematopoietic transplantation for mantle-cell lymphoma: Molecular remissions and evidence of graft-versus-malignancy.* Annals of Oncology, 1293. **10**(11): p. 1293-1299.

81.   Kroger, N., Hoffknecht, M., Kruger, W., Zeller, W., Renges, H., Stute, N., Zschaber, R. and Zander, A.R., *Allogeneic bone marrow transplantation for refractory mantle cell lymphoma.* Annals of Hematology, 2000. **79**(10): p. 578-580.

82.   Martinez, C., Carreras, E., Rovira, M., Urbano-Ispizua, A., Esteve, J., Perales, M., Fernandez, F. and Montserrat, E., *Patients with mantle-cell lymphoma relapsing after autologous stem cell transplantation may be rescued by allogeneic transplantation.* Bone Marrow Transplantation, 2000. **26**(6): p. 677-679.

83.   Khouri, I.F., Lee, M.S., Saliba, R.M., Jun, G., Fayad, L., Younes, A., Pro, B., Acholonu, S., Mclaughlin, P., Katz, R.L. and Champlin, R.E:, *Nonablative allogeneic stem-cell transplantation for advanced/recurrent mantle-cell lymphoma.* Journal of Clinical Oncology, 2003. **21**(23): p. 4407-4412.

84.   Maris, M.B., Sandmaier, B.M., Storer, B.E., Chauncey, T., Stuart, M.J., Maziarz, R.T., Agura, E., Langston, A.A., Pulsipher, M., Storb, R. and Maloney, D.G., *Allogeneic hematopoietic cell transplantation after fludarabine and 2 gy total body irradiation for relapsed and refractory mantle cell lymphoma [abstract].* Blood, 2004. **104**: p. 809a.

85.   Orlowski, R.Z., Stinchcombe, T.E., Mitchell, B.S., Shea, T.C., Baldwin, A.S., Stahl, S., Adams, J., Esseltine, D.L., Elliott, P.J., Pien, C.S., Guerciolini, R., Anderson, J.K., Depcik-Smith, N.D., Bhagat, R., Lehman, M.J., Novick, S.C., O'connor, O.A. and Soignet, S.L., *Phase i trial of the proteasome inhibitor ps-341 in patients with refractory hematologic malignancies.* Journal of Clinical Oncology, 2002. **20**(22): p. 4420-4427.

86.   O'connor, O.A., Wright, J., Moskowitz, C., Muzzy, J., Macgregor-Cortelli, B., Stubblefield, M., Straus, D., Portlock, C., Hamlin, P., Choi, E., Dumetrescu, O., Esseltine, D., Trehu, E., Adams, J., Schenkein, D. and Zelenetz, A.D., *Phase ii clinical experience with the novel proteasome inhibitor bortezomib in patients with indolent non-hodgkin's lymphoma and mantle cell lymphoma. [see comment].* Journal of Clinical Oncology, 2005. **23**(4): p. 676-684.

87.   Belch, A., Kouroukis, C.T., Crump, M., Sehn, L., Gascoyne, R.D., Klasa, R.J., Jean, P. and Eisenhauer, E., *Phase ii trial of bortezomib in mantle cell lymphoma [abstract].* Blood, 2004. **104**: p. 608a.

Chapter 6

T-CELL NON-HOGDKIN'S LYMPHOMA

Andrew M. Evens, DO, MS,[1] Christiane Querfeld, MD,[2] and
Steven T. Rosen, MD[1]

[1]Department of Medicine and [2]Dermatology, Division of Hematology/Oncology Northwestern University Feinberg School of Medicine and the Robert H. Lurie Comprehensive Cancer Center of Northwestern University 676 N. St. Clair, Suite 850 Chicago, IL 60611

1. INTRODUCTION

T-cell non-Hodgkin's lymphoma (NHL) represents approximately 10% to 15% of all lymphomas diagnosed in Western countries.[1-4] Varied geographic frequency of T-cell NHL has been documented ranging from 18.3% of NHL diagnosed in Hong Kong to 1.5% in Vancouver, British Columbia. This may in part be a reflection of increased exposure to pathogenic factors such as human T-cell leukemia virus-1 (HTLV-1) and Epstein Barr virus (EBV) in Asian nations.[1] T-cell NHL commonly presents with extranodal disease and often contain varying amounts of necrosis/apoptosis on biopsy specimens making differentiation between a reactive process and diagnosis on neoplasm challenging. Immunophenotypic, cytogenetic, and molecular analyses have enhanced diagnostic capabilities as well as improved classification and prognostication for T-cell NHL. The current World Health Organization (WHO) classification recognizes 11 distinct clinicopathologic disorders encompassing the spectrum of T-cell malignancies (See Table 1).[5] The broad spectrum of pathologic subtypes with varied clinical behavior poses a challenge to the systematic study of these diseases. Furthermore, these distinct T-cell NHL subtypes have unique characteristics and often warrant individualized diagnostic and therapeutic treatment strategies. Some agents that play a special role in the therapy of T-cell NHL include nucleoside analogues, denileukin diftitox (Ontak), retinoids, rexinoids and alpha-interferon. The precise role of transplantation for T-cell lymphoma patients has not been fully defined, but several case series have documented the feasibility of autologous and allogeneic transplant with reported long-term survival rates similar to transplanted B-cell NHL.   We review herein the etiology, pathology, diagnosis and treatment strategies for patients with T-cell NHL described according to specific clinicopathologic disease subtype.

2.   CLASSIFICATION

T-cell lymphomas commonly present with extranodal disease and often contain varying amounts of necrosis/apoptosis on biopsy specimens making differentiation between a reactive process and diagnosis of neoplasm challenging.[6] Moreover, the confirmation of a diagnosis of T-cell lymphoma may be difficult based on clinical, morphologic and immunophenotypic grounds as this data are often identifiable for a malignant process, but not specific for a particular NHL or for an exact subtype of T-cell lymphoma.[7] Over the last few decades, significant advances have been made in the field of molecular biology.   Cytogenetic and molecular analyses have not only enhanced diagnostic capabilities (NHL vs. reactive process), but have also allowed for the differentiation and prognostication of particular subgroups within the T-cell NHL category.[8]   The REAL and subsequent WHO classification have combined the morphologic, genetic, immunophenotypic, and clinical T-cell NHL characteristics to define distinct subtypes not completely described in the earlier Working Formulation and Kiel classifications (See Table 1).[4,5]   The NHL Classification Project validated the varied T-cell NHL clinicopathologic subtypes.[1]

3.   ETIOLOGY

Genetic alterations involved in lymphoma oncogenesis include chromosome rearrangements, disruption of tumor suppressor genes and an increase in the number of copies of genes (gene amplification). Moreover, infection of cells by viruses and bacteria such as HTLV-I,[9] EBV,[10] human herpes virus-8 (HHV-8),[11] hepatitis C[12] and helicobacter pylori[13] may also contribute to lymphogenesis.

Chromosome rearrangements contribute to altered gene function through varied mechanisms such as protooncogene activation and deregulation of gene expression.   The primary mechanism of protooncogene activation in lymphoma is reciprocal and balanced chromosomal translocations. These translocations are mostly recurrent and non-random in NHL.   The majority of chromosome translocations in NHL involve the juxtaposition of a protooncogene from one chromosome next to regulatory sequences of a partner chromosome. This contributes to control of the protooncogene by a promoter associated with an immunoglobulin (Ig) or T-cell receptor (TCR) gene. The two subtypes of TCR's that T-cell lymphocytes express are gamma-delta (γδ) or alpha-beta (αβ).[14] Approximately 95% of normal T lymphocytes express the αβ heterodimer, while the minority of T lymphocytes express the γδ heterodimer.[15] Alpha-beta T-cells develop predominantly in the thymus, while γδ T-cells may develop in extra-thymic locations such as the skin, intestinal epithelium and spleen.[16,17] The four TCR genes are arranged in germline configuration in non-continuous segments of variable (V), diversity (D), joining (J) and constant (C) regions. The precise mechanism by which translocation of TCR and Ig genes occur is not known, but it appears to in part involve dysfunctional gene remodeling including V-D-J recombination, isotype switching and somatic hypermutation.[18] T-cell neoplasms may have rearrangements involving the site of TCR α and δ genes on chromosome 14,[19] or more rarely, chromosome 7 (7q34-36 and 7p15), the site of TCR β and γ genes.[20] Many of the genes located at the breakpoints of recurring chromosome translocations have been identified.[21] The majority of translocated genes encode transcription factors.[21,22] Transcription factors are involved in the initiation of gene transcription and cell differentiation. The most common result of chromosome translocations in lymphomas that involve TCR and/or Ig genes is deregulation of gene expression with irregular or over-expression in cells that normally do not express this gene. Few lymphomas have been recognized to contain translocations that produce a fusion protein, such as the t(2;5)(p23;q35) translocation in anaplastic large cell lymphoma (ALCL) that results in expression of the nucleophosim (NPM)-anaplastic lymphoma kinase (ALK) protein.

Inactivation of tumor suppressor genes may also play a role in lymphogenesis. The most common mechanism of tumor suppressor inactivation occurs through the Knudson two-hit model where a reduction of homozygosity leads to tumor formation, for example, following germline deletion of one allele and somatic mutation of the other.[23] Tumor suppressor genes identified with NHL include p53, p15 and p16.[24] Moreover, specific chromosomal deletions that have been detected in NHL (including some T-cell lymphomas), such as 3p, 6q, 13q and 17p, may represent sites of yet to be identified tumor suppressor loci.[25-27] Other mediators that may be involved in lymphogenesis include the cyclin-dependent kinase (cdk) inhibitors, such as p21[(Waf1)].[28] A function of the p21[(Waf1)] protein includes the arrest of cells in G_1-phase checkpoint by associating with cyclin-cdk complexes, but the exact factors critical for apoptosis have not been clearly defined.[29]   The gene for the p21$^{(Waf1)}$ protein has been identified as a downstream target of p53 in regulating cell cycle progression through G_1.[30] Induction of p21$^{(Waf1)}$ has also been demonstrated to occur through a p53-independent pathway.[31]

Gene amplification leads to an increase in the number of copies of a gene in the genome of a cell, which may contribute to lymphogenesis.[32]   Gene amplification has been identified mostly in B-cell lymphomas (e.g., REL gene), although amplification of TCR genes in varied T-cell lymphomas has been described.[33] Random genomic instability, as seen in many epithelial cancers, is not a characteristic of the more stable lymphoma genome. Defects in DNA mismatch repair that manifest as genomic microsatellite instability are also less recognized in lymphoma, as compared to various hereditary solid tumor syndromes and rare sporadic cancers.[34,35]

4.   PROGNOSIS

The optimal therapeutic strategy for T-cell NHL is in evolution. The T-cell disorders have been a challenge to evaluate. Few randomized or multi-institution clinical trials comparing chemotherapeutic or other treatment modalities for T-cell NHL have been reported. This is in part due to not only the overall lower incidence and prevalence compared to other malignancies, but also the heterogeneity of disease and the infrequent documentation of a clonal immunophenotypic marker for T-cells make a timely and definite diagnosis difficult. Although, approximately 5,000 patients will be diagnosed in the United States in 2003, which is more than the 3,600 and 4,300 cases of acute lymphoblastic leukemia and chronic myelogenous leukemia, that will be diagnosed, respectively.[36]

Several studies have documented that T-cell phenotype is an independent poor prognostic factor among all NHL diagnoses on multivariate analysis.[3,4] When analyzing T-cell NHL populations, 5-year overall survival (OS) rates have ranged from to 26% to 41%.[3,4,37] Moreover, contemporary studies have demonstrated significantly worse survival when T-cell NHL (all histologies) has been directly compared to aggressive B-cell NHL with 5-year OS rates ranging from 39% to 41% versus 52% to 63%, respectively.[3,37] Gallamini and colleagues recently analyzed PTCL-noc patients and showed in multivariate analysis that the number of factors: age > 60, Eastern Cooperative Oncology Group (ECOG) performance status 2 to 4, LDH above normal, and bone marrow involvement independently predicted for survival (no adverse factors = 5-year and 10-year OS of 62.3% and 54.9%, respectively; 1 factor = 5-year and 10-year OS of 52.9% and 38.8%, respectively; 2 factors = 5-year and 10-year OS of 32.9% and 18.0%, respectively; 3 or 4 factors = 5-year and 10-year OS of 18.3 and 12.6%, respectively; p= 0.0000, log rank 66.79).[38]

When large populations of T-cell NHL have been analyzed, some have documented variable survival rates among different T-cell histologies (anaplastic large cell lymphoma [ALK-positive] > peripheral T-cell lymphoma, not otherwise specified > extranodal NK/T-cell lymphoma-nasal type > angioimmunoblastic lymphoma > subcutaneous panniculitis-like T-cell lymphoma > hepatosplenic T-cell lymphoma > enteropathy-type intestinal T-cell lymphoma),[4,37,39] while others have not.[1,40] The majority of T-cell NHL studies have established that the International Prognostic Index (IPI) significantly predicts outcome in patients.[3,4,41] However, it is important to recognize that few reports have included sufficient numbers of less common T-cell NHL diagnoses such as subcutaneous panniculitis-like T-cell lymphoma, hepatosplenic T-cell lymphoma and enteropathy-type intestinal T-cell lymphoma to allow sufficient prognostic and survival comparisons. One report showed that within the entire subset of T-cell lymphoma that EBV-positivity was associated with significantly inferior survival rates compared to EBV-negative T-cell lymphoma.[42]

5. SPECIFIC DISEASE TYPES

5.1 Peripheral T-cell lymphoma, not otherwise characterized (PTCL-noc)

PTCL-noc is predominantly a nodal lymphoma that represents the most common T-cell lymphoma subtype in Western countries comprising approximately 50-60% of T-cell lymphomas and 5% to 7% of all NHL.[1] PTCL-noc usually affects male adults (1.5 male-to-female ratio) with a median age of 61 years (range 17-90) in a large study with 25% of patients presenting in stage I or IIE, 12% stage III and 63% stage IV.[1] PTCL-noc patients from this study commonly presented with unfavorable characteristics including B symptoms (40%), elevated LDH (66%), bulky tumor ≥ 10 cm (11%), non-ambulatory performance status (29%) and extranodal disease (56%) leading to the majority of patients (53%) falling into the unfavorable IPI category (score of 3 to 5). Other smaller studies of PTCL-noc patients have corroborated male preponderance, B symptoms and extranodal disease (bone marrow > liver > skin > lung and bone).[37,43]

T-cell NHL is also associated with hemophagocytic syndrome, preceding, during or while disease is in remission.[44-46] Hemophagocytic syndrome is characterized by high fever, skin lesions, lung infiltrates, jaundice, hepatosplenomegaly, liver dysfunction, coagulation abnormalities, pancytopenia, and a benign prominent histiocytic proliferation with hemophagocytosis in addition to the proliferation of atypical T-lymphocytes or immunoblasts in the bone marrow, lymph node, spleen, and liver. Cytokines released from EBV-infected T-lymphocytes, such as tumor necrosis factor-alpha, lead to the histiocytic activation and the subsequent hemophagocytosis.[47]

5.1.1 Pathology

Earlier studies of peripheral T-cell NHL recognized a variety of morphologic subtypes based on cell size by diffuse small cleaved, mixed cell, large cell and immunoblastic. In addition, the term lymphoepitheliod (Lennert's) lymphoma is considered a cytopathologic variant for cases rich in epitheliod cells. However, reliable histological definitions based on these morphologic subtypes have not been defined. Moreover, no clinical differences have been demonstrated based on these varied histologic subgroups. Most PTCL-noc cases contain a combination of small and large atypical T-cells with frequently admixed eosinophils and/or epitheliod histiocytes. T-cell associated antigens such as CD2, CD3, CD5 and CD7 are variably expressed on immunophenotypic analysis, although one of the mature T-cell antigens (CD5 or CD7) is usually lost. Furthermore, CD4 is more commonly expressed than CD8, although some PTCL-noc tumors may be double negative (CD4-CD8-). Genetic analysis is often useful in establishing a T-cell neoplastic diagnosis.

5.1.2 Molecular

Some studies have suggested that TCR gene rearrangements are rare in PTCL-noc, although these findings may be dependent on the laboratory techniques employed to determine TCR clonality.[48] Studies in PTCL-noc that incorporated more sensitive clonality techniques such as PCR documented rearranged TCR genes in many cases.[49] Moreover, analysis of γ TCR loci may provide a higher diagnostic yield than β TCR loci for the study of PTCL-noc clonality.[50] Lepretre et al analyzed 49 consecutive cases of PTCL-noc and demonstrated that only 3 cases involved chromosome 7q35 rearrangement (none for 7p15) and 2 cases were associated with 14q11.[48] Importantly, chromosome analysis in this study was performed using metaphase cytogenetics, thereby likely decreasing the sensitivity for detecting TCR rearrangements. Overall, cytogenetic aberrations in PTCL-noc are common with approximately 70-90% of abnormal metaphases documented in most series (See Table 2).[8,48] Schlegelberger et al reported that chromosome analysis in PTCL allowed for separation of PTCL into low and high-grade categories, but the prognostic significance of this distinction has not been established.[3,8] Moreover, many studies reporting on PTCL-noc cytogenetics have included very small patient numbers and used older lymphoma disease classifications.

Lepretre et al recently described their results in 71 untreated patients with PTCL, of which included 49 patients with PTCL-noc diagnosis (2 patients with hepatosplenic and 20 patients with AIL).[48] Good-quality metaphases were obtained in 90% of PTCL-noc patients and 78% of these patients had documented chromosome abnormalities. Moreover, 25 of 38 (90%) of cases with chromosome abnormalities contained complex karyotypes ($\geq$ 3 changes). Of all 71 cases in their series (including 20 cases of AIL), 40 patients demonstrated numerical abnormalities with the most common changes being trisomies 3 (15.7%), 5 (14%), 7 (14%), 21 (14%), 8 (12.2%) and 19 (12.2%) and losses of chromosomes 13 (14%), 10 (10.5%) and Y (10.5%). Trisomies 3, 5 and 7 have been reported commonly to be associated with the broad category of T-cell lymphoma.[8] Although these trisomies are not unique to specific T-cell lymphoma subtypes.[51] The most common chromosomal structural abnormalities identified in Lepretre et al series were chromosome 6 (31.5%; mainly due to 6q deletions, 19.2%), 1q (22.8%), 7q (22.8%), 9p (19.4%), 9q (19.2%), 4q (19.2%), 3q (19.2%), 2p (17.5%), 1p (17.5%) and 14q (17.5%).[48] Chromosome 1 changes and 6q deletions have been commonly associated with both B and T-cell NHL.[51] Age greater than 60, stage III/IV and elevated lactate dehydrogenase (LDH) were associated with significantly shorter survival in the 71 patients from the Lepretre et al study. No significant statistical difference was found with overall survival and chromosomal abnormalities with regards to the entire population in their series or for independent histologic subtypes.

It has been suggested that a tumor suppressor gene(s) on 6q may be involved in this and other T-cell lymphomas, although this putative tumor suppressor gene has not been identified.[52,53] A Japanese study documented p53 gene mutations in 5 of 5 peripheral T-cell lymphoma cases (post-renal transplant).[54] Their study also demonstrated that 25% of cases had k-ras mutations and one-third of cases showed mutations of c-kit and beta-catenin genes. Other studies have established that a significant minority of PTCL-noc overexpress p53 protein (contributing to functional inactivation of p53), while p53 mutations have been documented less commonly.[55,56] Furthermore, as compared to p53-negative cases, p53-positive cases have been shown to contain significantly higher proliferative activity, less frequent expression of the downstream p21$^{(Wafl)}$ protein and frequent expression of Bcl-2.[55,57] Prognostic studies in PTCL-noc have demonstrated that p53 protein overexpression and mutation of p53 correlate significantly with increased treatment failure and worse overall and disease-free survival in multivariate analysis (with 1-year survival rates in one study of 0% versus 64% with mutated and normal p53, respectively).[55-57] Some studies in PTCL-noc have documented abnormalities of retinoblastoma gene expression at the transcriptional and/or post-transcriptional level.[55] Further study is needed into the molecular pathogenesis of PTCL-noc specifically regarding abnormalities in the p53 and Rb gene pathways.

5.1.3   Treatment

In many of the prognostic studies discussed above, most T-cell NHL patients were treated in the same manner as intermediate-grade B-cell patients with anthracycline-based combination chemotherapy including regimens such as CHOP alone or CHOP alternating with DHAP (dexamethasone, cisplatin and cytarabine), mBACOD (adriamycin, cyclophosphamide, vincristine, bleomycin, methotrexate and decadron) or ACVB (adriamycin, cyclophosphamide, vindesine, bleomycin and prednisone) or VIM-3 (mitoxantrone, ifosfamide, methyl-GAG, Vehem, prednisone and methotrexate) or CVP (cyclophosphamide, vincristine and prednisone), CHOP or CHOP with etoposide or COPBLAM (cyclophosphamide, vincristine, prednisone, bleomycin, adriamycin and procarbazine).[3,4,39] Randomized trials comparing CHOP (cyclophosphamide, adriamycin, vincristine and prednisone) to other combination regimens confirmed CHOP as a standard regimen for intermediate-grade B-cell NHL,[58,59] unfortunately these trials do not allow for subset analysis of T-cell patients. Rituximab should not be included in the treatment for PTCL-noc (unless other conditions exist such as immune thrombocytopenic purpura) as CD20 is not expressed. Moreover, combined T-cell (from disease) and B-cell (from rituximab) suppression may result in prohibitive morbidity and mortality.

Other therapeutic agents tested in T-cell NHL include purine and pyrimidine analogues, denileukin ditox, and retinoic acid/interferon-alfa (IFN-α) combination. Nucleoside analogues, such as 2'-deoxycoformin (dCF; pentostatin), fludarabine and 2-chlorodeoxyadenosine (2-CdA) have been tested mostly in patients with cutaneous NHL, although several anecdotal reports have reported activity in other T-cell NHL subtypes.[60,61] Administered as intravenous bolus daily over 3 days (at an initial dose of 5 mg/m^2/day, repeated every 3 to 4 weeks) response rates to the adenosine deaminase (ADA) inhibitor, pentostatin, are 50% (7% complete remission) in single institution phase II studies with median duration of responses of 4 to 6 months.[61,62] Other trials have reported lower response rates (15 to 20%) for pentostatin in PTCL-noc.[63,64] One trial analyzed response according to CD26 status since CD26 is a surface glycoprotein with an important role in T-cell function as the ADA binding protein.[62,65] However, 5 of 9 CD26-negative patients responding to pentostatin.[61] The pyrimidine antimetabolite, gemcitabine, has activity in relapsed/refractory T-cell NHL as a single agent with reported response rates of 60% in small single-institution studies.[66,67] Gemcitabine has also been studied in combination with cisplatin and methylprednisone with encouraging early results in relapsed Hodgkin's disease and NHL.[68]

Denileukin diftitox (DAB$_{389}$IL-2, Ontak), is a novel recombinant fusion protein consisting of peptide sequences for the enzymatically active and membrane active and membrane translocation domains of diptheria toxin with recombinant interleukin-2 (CD25 receptor) that has been studied mostly in cutaneous T-cell NHL although clinical benefit has been reported in other T-cell NHL patients.[69,70] Huang and colleagues studied 17 patients with relapsed T-cell NHL using 13-cis-retinoic acid with IFN-α.[71] A response rate of 31% was documented in 4 of 6 ALCL patients and 1 of 7 PTCL-noc, although median survival for the entire group of patients was 3.6 months. The MD Anderson group also documented similar response rates to IFN-α therapy (combined with isotretinoin) in patients with relapsed T-cell NHL and Hodgkin's disease.[72] Treatment for hemophagocytic syndrome associated with T-cell NHL is difficult as most chemotherapy and antiviral agents are typically ineffective, although etoposide has proven some benefit.[73]

5.2   Angioimmunoblastic T-cell lymphoma (AITL)

AITL, also known as angioimmunoblastic lymphadenopathy with dysproteinemia, is one of the more common T-cell lymphomas accounting for 15-20% of cases and 4-6% of all lymphoma.[1] Mean age of presentation is 57 to 65 with a slight male predominance and the majority of patients present with stage III or IV disease.[1,37,43,74] AITL is commonly a systemic disease with nodal involvement with various associated disease features such as organomegaly, B symptoms (50-70%), skin rash, pruritis, pleural effusions, arthritis, eosinophilia and varied immunologic abnormalities (positive Coombs' test, cold agglutins, hemolytic anemia, antinuclear antibodies, rheumatoid factors, cryoglobulins and polyclonal hypergammaglobulinemia).[43,74]

5.2.1   Pathology

AITL is characterized by a polymorphous infiltrate of lymph nodes with nodal architecture commonly effaced with opened and dilated peripheral sinuses. There is often significant proliferation of high endothelial venules and follicular dendritic cells. The lymphoid cells commonly consist of a mixture of small and medium sized lymphocytes with plasma cells and B-immunoblasts, while clusters of epitheliod histiocytes and many eosinophils may be present. T-cell associated antigens are usually expressed and CD4 expression is more common than CD8. Clusters of follicular dendritic cells (CD21+) are often present around proliferated venules.

5.2.2   Molecular

Histologic diagnosis of AITL may be difficult, therefore demonstration of TCR clonality is often important for diagnosis of malignancy. The TCR genes (usually β) are rearranged in approximately 70-100% of patients with AITL when performing Southern blot analyses for rearranged alleles or detection of clonal products after PCR.[75,76] Furthermore, these series documented Ig genes (heavy chain) to be rearranged in 0-15% of cases. Feller et al documented that specific patterns of clonal gene rearrangement correlate with prognosis in AITL.[77] They showed that patients with concomitant TCR β-chain gene and Ig gene rearrangements often presented with hemolytic anemia, experienced spontaneous transient remissions (and remissions following steroids), but did not respond as well to chemotherapy and had worse overall survival compared to patients with "TCR-only" clonality (no Ig gene rearrangements). Some histologic cases of AIL may demonstrate oligo-clonality, while other cases may show regression or appearance of clonality.[33,78] One detailed retrospective pathologic study of 22 AITL biopsy cases, documented γ-TCR clonality in 16 of 22 patients, β-TCR clonality in 16 of 22, Ig clonality in 6/22, PCR oligoclonal products in 3/22.[78] Moreover, 'functional' γ-TCR, β-TCR and Ig clonality was demonstrated by sequence analyses of PCR products in 6 of 12, 9 of 11 and 8 of 8 cases respectively.   'Functional' TCR and/or Ig oligo-clones were detected in 6 of 20 cases with 11 cases showing 'nonfunctional' TCR and Ig sequences.[78] Further study is warranted to determine the importance of the heterogeneous forms of clonality and the significance of functional versus non-functional sequences in AITL.

Conventional cytogenetics (metaphase analysis) will detect chromosomal abnormalities in approximately 70-80% of patients with AITL (See Table 2).[8,48,79,80] One study incorporating interphase FISH analysis increased the number of aberrant chromosomes identified to 90% of patients and more than 40% of patients were noted to have oligo-clonal clones.[81] Trisomies 3 and 5 and an additional X chromosome are the most frequent cytogenetic abnormalities detected in AITL patients and complex karyotypes are common.[48,80,81] Fifty to seventy-five percent of patients with AITL will have trisomy 3 and/or trisomy 5 clones.[48,82] In a retrospective cytogenetic analysis of 50 patients with AITL, the presence of complex karyotype was associated with inferior survival in multivariate analysis.[79] Other potential mechanisms of lymphogenesis such as downstream $p21^{(Waf1)}$ abnormalities, dependent or independent of p53 protein overexpression,[55] and N-ras[83] have rarely been documented to be associated with AITL. Prospective studies are needed to confirm these results and to further explore potential proto-oncogenes involved in AITL.

B-cell EBV genomes are detected by PCR (for presence of EBV-DNA) and/or FISH analysis (for EBV-encoded small nuclear RNA's, or EBER-1) in approximately 80-100% of AITL-involved lymph nodes.[10,84,85] The exact role of EBV in the pathogenesis of AITL is not known, although recent research has demonstrated significant interplay between AITL and the survival and clonal expansion of EBV.[85,86]

5.2.3 Treatment

Spontaneous disease regression is seen on rare occasions, although AITL typically follows an aggressive clinical course. Treatment with anthracycline-based combination chemotherapy results in complete remission (CR) rates of 50% to 70% of AITL patients, although only 10-30% of patients are long-term survivors.[1,3,4,37,39,87] One prospective, non-randomized multicenter study treated newly diagnosed 'stable' AITL patients with single-agent prednisone and combination chemotherapy for relapsing/refractory patients or initially if 'life-threatening' disease was present at diagnosis.[88] Complete remission was 29% with single-agent prednisone while CR for relapsed/refractory or patients treated initially with combination chemotherapy was 56% and 64%, respectively. With a median follow-up of 28 months (range, 7 to 53), the overall survival (OS) and disease-free survival (DFS) was 40.5% (CI, 24% to 56%) and 32.3% (CI, 17% to 47%), respectively, although median OS was 15 months. There are anecdotal reports of relapsed AITL patients who have responded to immunosuppressive therapy, such as low-dose methotrexate/prednisone[89,90] as well as reported responses to purine analogue treatment.[91-93] Furthermore, cyclosporine has demonstrated activity in relapsed AITL patients in case reports and Eastern Cooperative Oncology Group is studying this in a prospective study.[94,95]

5.3   Anaplastic large-cell lymphoma (ALCL), T/null cell, primary systemic type

ALCL, primary systemic type, accounts for approximately 2% to 3% of all NHL.[4,37] This disease mainly involves lymph nodes, although extranodal sites may be involved (not exclusively the skin; see cutaneous CD30+ ALCL section below). As will be discussed below in the molecular section, this disease may be divided in part based on the expression of the tyrosine kinase anaplastic lymphoma kinase (ALK), created from a balanced chromosome translocation. When heterogeneous patient populations are analyzed, the prevalence of ALK-positivity in primary systemic ALCL cases is 50-60%.[96,97] ALK-positive ALCL is typically diagnosed in men prior to age 35 (male to female ratio: 3.0) with frequent systemic symptoms, extranodal and advanced stage disease.[43,98] ALK-negative patients are usually older (median age, 61 years) with a male to female ratio of 0.9 with similar high incidence of extranodal disease.[96,98] In addition to the prognostic importance of ALK-positivity, the IPI has been identified as an independent prognostic factor within the group of ALK-positive ALCL patients with reported 5-year OS of 94% versus 41% for IPI 0 or 1 and 2 to 4, respectively.[98] This better prognosis is apparent despite ALK-positive patients more commonly presenting with poorer performance status and more advanced stage disease compared to ALK-negative disease.

5.3.1   Pathology

The morphology of ALCL, systemic type, consists of large lymphoid cells with pleomorphic or multiple prominent nuclei and abundant cytoplasm. The tumor cells grow in a cohesive pattern and sinusoidal spread in the lymph nodes. The tumor cells express CD30 and either T-cell or no specific lineage antigens (null cell). The T-cell antigens CD3, CD43, and/or CD45 and epithelial membrane antigen are commonly expressed, while CD15 is negative. Furthermore, ALCL tumor cells often express a mature activated T-cell phenotype (HLA-DR, CD25+) and cytotoxic granules are usually present.

5.3.2   Molecular

Studies applying Southern blot techniques to detect TCR gene rearrangements in ALCL have shown inconsistencies between TCR rearrangements and immunophenotype.[99,100] More updated studies using PCR analysis for TCR rearrangements have demonstrated clonal rearrangements in most cases of T-cell and null-type ALCL (70-90%) with clonal β genes being more commonly detected than γ gene rearrangements.[101,102] Furthermore, genotypic studies have improved the classification of the varied ALCL disease subtypes. Clonal rearrangements of the TCR in histologic designated "B-cell ALCL" has rarely been documented confirming that "B-cell ALCL" is genetically different than T-cell ALCL and likely represent a variant of diffuse large, B-cell lymphoma.[101,103,104]

Beginning in 1988, it was demonstrated that ALCL is associated with the chromosome translocation t(2;5).[105,106] This nonrandom t(2;5) chromosome translocation has been cloned and is known to cause the fusion of the nucleophosim (NPM) gene located at 5q35 to the gene at 2p23 encoding the receptor tyrosine kinase, ALK, resulting in the fusion protein NPM-ALK (See Table 2).[107-111] The transcription of the 80-kd chimeric fusion protein NPM-ALK (also known as p80) results as a consequence of the ALK gene coming under the control of the NPM promoter.[112] Further characterization of the properties of NPM, ALK and NPM-ALK has been described in detail elsewhere.[113] The presence of NPM-ALK may be detected by RT-PCR[109] and FISH techniques.[114] Polyclonal (ALK11) and monoclonal (ALK1 and ALKc) antibodies specific for the ALK portion of the molecule have been established that stain both the cytoplasm and nucleus in tissues containing the NPM-ALK translocation, which is documented in approximately 50-90% of primary systemic ALCL cases.[108] When heterogeneous patient populations are analyzed, the prevalence of ALK-positivity in primary systemic ALCL cases is 50-60%.[96] Several series have documented that up to 30% of ALK-positive ALCL cases are found to be negative for the t(2;5) translocation, suggesting that other fusion proteins and chromosome translocations are involved with the 2q23 ALK gene other than NPM.[108,115,116] Other fusion partners to the ALK gene include non-muscle tropomyosin (TPM3) forming t(1;2)(q21;23) creating the chimeric protein TPM3-ALK,[117-120] tropomyosin receptor kinase-fused gene (TFG) forming t(2;3)(p23;q21) resulting in the TFG-ALK protein,[118,119,121] clathrin heavy polypeptide-like gene (CLTCL) forming t(2;22) resulting in the CLTCL-ALK protein[122] and 5-aminoimidazole-4-carboxamide-1-beta-D-ribonucleotide-transformylase/inosine-monophosphate- cyclohydrolase enzymatic activities (ATIC) caused by the inversion(2) (p23;q35) resulting in ATIC-ALK[123-125] (See Table 3). ALK-positive diffuse large B-cell lymphoma has been recently reported is characterized by a simple or complex t(2;17)(p23;q23) that involves the CLTC gene at chromosome band 17q23 and the ALK gene at chromosome band 2p23.[126]

The determination of ALK-positivity is important as it denotes a significant favorable prognosis with reported 5-year overall survival rates of 71% to 80% versus 15% to 46% for ALK-negative ALCL cases when treated with anthracycline-based therapy.[96,116,127] Moreover, the prognosis for ALK-positive and ALK-negative ALCL groups may be further divided based on CD56 positivity (neural cell-adhesion molecule), which portends a significantly worse outcome when it is expressed in either ALCL subgroup.[97] The expression of the ALK gene is not confined to ALCL thus decreasing the positive predictive value of this testing. Other disease entities that rarely express the ALK gene include neuroblastoma, rhabdomyosarcoma and inflammatory myofibroblastic tumors.[110,128-130] There are also reports of the detection of ALK genes in non-neoplastic and "normal" peripheral blood cells.[108,131] This data confirms that indiscriminate molecular testing should be avoided, but rather should be a compliment to a detailed clinical and histologic workup.

Other mechanisms of oncogenesis in ALCL include anti-apoptosis (increased bcl-2),[132] hypermethylation,[133] c-myc expression,[134] and EBV infection.[135] Furthermore, the NPM/ALK fusion protein has been demonstrated to constitutively activate the downstream phosphatidylinositol 3-kinase (PI3K)-Akt pathway suggesting that this pathway may be involved in the molecular pathogenesis of ALCL.[136,137] DNA gene array technology is also being applied to continue to enhance our understanding of the oncogenic pathways involved in ALCL.[138]

5.3.3   Treatment

Therapy for pediatric ALCL is often based on prognostic risk factors with treatment regimens modeled after high-grade B-cell NHL protocols. Following a brief cytoreductive prephase, short, intensified poly-agent chemotherapy is administered with the number of cycles dependent on stage of disease.[139] Therapy for adult ALCL, systemic type, has commonly included anthracycline-based regimens such as CHOP chemotherapy.[98,103] Autologous hematopoietic stem cell transplantation (HSCT) in first complete remission has been advocated by some groups, although this approach warrants prospective validation (see HSCT section below).

5.4   Cutaneous T-cell Lymphomas

Cutaneous T-cell lymphomas (CTCL) constitute a group of cutaneous non-Hodgkin lymphomas with clonal expansions of T-lymphocytes into the skin. Several entities are recognized by classification systems such as the European Organization for Research and Treatment of Cancer (EORTC) and WHO classification that are based on morphological, histopathological, and molecular features (See Table 4).[140-143] The etiology of CTCL remains largely unknown. Microbiologic theories suggesting a contributory role in the pathogenetic events leading to monoclonal T-cell proliferation have not been verified. However, chronic antigen stimulation mediated via Toll-like receptors (TLRs), antigen-specific T-cell receptors (TCR), and/or immunmodulatory receptors such as CD40 remain theoretical considerations. CTCL originate from T-lymphocytes with preference for the skin microenvironment without extracutaneous manifestations after presentation and at 6 months thereafter.[144] Adhesion molecules and chemokines have been associated with T-cell trafficking into the skin.[145] Cutaneous lymphocyte antigen (CLA) initiates skin homing by mediating E-selectin-dependent trafficking of T cells to skin.[146]

5.5 Mycosis fungoides/Sézary syndrome

Mycosis fungoides (MF) represents the most common type of CTCL comprising 50% of CTCL with a male predominance of approximately 2:1 and a predominance of African-American patients of 1.6:1. It has a yearly incidence of 0.36 cases per 100,000 population that has remained constant over the last decade.[147] Clinical and histologic diagnosis of MF has proved to be difficult, since in early stages it may resemble other dermatoses such as eczematous dermatitis, psoriasis, and parapsoriasis.[148] More recently, observations about invisible MF cases with recalcitrant pruritus were reported.[149] MF with follicular mucinosis and pagetoid reticulosis are distinct variants of MF.[150,151]

5.5.1 Pathology

Characteristic histologic features of classical MF/SS are a papillary dermal band-like infiltrate with atypical lymphocytes with hyperchromatic, hyperconvoluted nuclei, variable findings of inflammatory cells, and epidermotropism with infrequently seen Pautrier's microabscesses.[152] Most MF/SS cases bear the phenotype of the CD4+ T-helper/inducer lymphocyte. Only a minute number of cases are of the cytotoxic/suppressor T-cell subset expressing the CD4−/CD8+ phenotype.[153] A clonal gene rearrangement of the T-cell receptor can be detected in many cases.[154] In advanced stages, an aberrant phenotype with loss of T-cell markers is a common finding.

The clinical course of MF is characterized by a chronic indolent progression. A limited number of patients progress into more aggressive and advanced disease with either cutaneous or extracutaneous tumor manifestations. The reason for the slow progression of most patient's CTCL is not known. Control of tumor growth by an effective antitumor immune response is suspected. Dendritic cells are found to induce and maintain antitumor immunity.[155] In addition, activated dendritic cells stimulate T cells towards an IL-12-dependent T-helper cell type 1 (T_h1) response with secretion of interferon-gamma.[156] Patients with advanced MF and SS have been shown to display a T_h1/ T-helper cell type2 (T_h2) imbalance with a predominant type 2 immune response followed by an impaired cell-mediated immunity.[157]

5.5.2   Molecular

Several genes have been suspected to be involved in the pathogenesis of MF/SS. Acquired defects in apoptosis through inactivation of the *p16* gene and silencing of p*15* have been reported.[158,159] In addition, activation of signal transducer and transcription activator 1 (STAT1), STAT3, IL-15, IL-16, decreased expression or infrequent mutations of FAS, overexpression of bcl-2, and increased activity of telomerase with shortened telomeres have been found to be associated in the tumorgenesis.[160-163] Allelic losses at 1p, 9p, 10q, and 17p with gains in chromosome 4q, 18, and 17q, microsatellite instability, and rarely mutations of *p53* in primary CTCL have also been reported.[164]

The most important predictive factor for survival remains the T classification, extracutaneous manifestation, and patient age.[165] In addition, several independent adverse prognostic factors have been identified including large cell transformation, follicular mucinosis, thickness of tumor infiltrate, and increased lactic dehydrogenase (LDH).[166,167] Patients with large Sézary-cells were also found to have a worse prognosis. A high Sézary cell count, loss of T-cell markers such as CD5 and CD7, existence of a T-cell clone in the blood and chromosomal abnormalities in T-cells are also independently associated with a poor outcome.[165] The presence of cytotoxic $CD8^+$ T-lymphocytes in the dermal infiltrate, as well as the density of epidermal Langerhans cells greater than 90 cells/mm^2 is associated with a better prognosis.[168] Gamma-delta phenotype has recently been shown to correlate with a poor prognosis compared to alpha-beta.[169]

5.5.3   Treatment

Clinically, MF is characterized by erythematous patches, evolving into plaques or tumors; however, the progress is variable.[170] It is classified as an indolent lymphoma by the EORTC. Sézary syndrome is the aggressive, leukemic, and erythrodermic variant of CTCL, which is characterized by circulating, atypical, malignant T-lymphocytes with cerebriform nuclei (Sézary cells), and lymphadenopathy.[171] MF/SS are commonly referred to as CTCL. For staging purposes the tumor node metastasis (TNM) system is most commonly used (See Table 5 and Table 6).[172]

5.5.4 Treatment of early stage disease

At present, CTCL are regarded to as incurable. In early CTCL the cell-mediated immune response is usually normal. Therefore, the majority of these cases can be treated successfully with topical modalities. Early aggressive therapy does not improve the prognosis of patients with CTCL.[173] The skin-targeted modalities include psoralens with ultraviolet light A (PUVA), narrowband-ultraviolet light B (NB-UVB), skin electron beam radiation, as well as topical preparations of steroids, retinoids, carmustine, and nitrogen mustard. PUVA is probably the preferred treatment option. Several studies confirmed high remission rates in early stages of MF. Herrmann et al. reported complete remissions in 65% of patients.[174] However, long-term PUVA therapy is associated with an increased risk of squamous cell carcinoma and malignant melanoma.[175] Narrowband-UVB phototherapy (NB-UVB) is considered to be less carcinogenic and may be an alternative treatment option in early stage MF.[176] However, the remission time is short. A few cases have been reported showing that UVA_1 phototherapy is also effective.[177] CTCL are radiosensitive and radiation therapy is effective in controlling localized tumors. –Total skin electron radiation has proven efficacy in treating early stage MF with 95% CR and 50% long-term-remission rate.[178] However, this complex technique should be reserved for centers with extensive experience, because of its potential toxicity.

In clinical trials, the RXR specific retinoid bexarotene demonstrated efficacy in a topical gel formulation for cutaneous lesions in patients with early stage CTCL.[179] Treatment-limiting toxic effects were associated with mild to moderate skin irritation. A long-term follow-up study of patients with CTCL stage IA and IB treated with topical nitrogen mustard demonstrated its efficacy with an overall response rate of 83%, and complete response rate of 50%.[180] No secondary malignancies related to therapy were reported. Less than 10% of patients experienced contact hypersensitivity reactions. Topical Carmustine (BCNU) shows similar results, however patients may develop progressing teleangiectasias from treatment.[181]

5.5.5 Treatment of advanced stage MF/SS

A limited number of patients progress into more aggressive and advanced disease with either cutaneous or extracutaneous tumor manifestations. Treatment goals in advanced stages should be to reduce tumor burden, to relieve symptoms, and to decrease the risk of transformation into aggressive lymphoma. Established treatment options include mono- or polychemotherapy including COP or CHOP regimens, extracorporeal photopheresis, interferons, retinoids, monoclonal antibodies and recombinant toxins. Combinations are frequently used.

In advanced stages there is a dominant T_h2 cytokine response leading to an impaired immune response. Treatments such as biologic response modifiers target the reconstitution of immune function and are probably superior to standard chemotherapies in this regard.[182] Interferon-alpha is probably the most effective treatment in advanced MF with overall response rates ranging from 50% to 80%.[183] Side effects are dose related and most common are flu-like symptoms. Interferon-alpha is often used in combination with retinoids, PUVA, electron beam radiation, and extracorporeal photopheresis.[184] The combination therapy of IFN-α and PUVA resulted in high response rates in more than 90% of patients and shows superiority to other combinations.[185]

The therapeutic efficacy of some retinoids in CTCL has been confirmed in several, small, monotherapy studies.[185] Response rates range from 44% to 67%. Combinations with PUVA and retinoids achieved clinical response with less exposure to UVA.[186] Bexarotene, a new US Food and Drug Administration (FDA) approved synthetic retinoid for refractory CTCL that selectively binds to retinoid X receptors has been studied in two multicenter phase II-III clinical trials for refractory early and advanced stage patients.[187,188] An overall response rate of 54% of patients with refractory early stage and 45% of patients with refractory advanced stage has been reported. The most common adverse effects are hyperlipidemia and hypothyroidism. Retrospective comparison data suggest that there is little difference in efficacy between bexarotene and agents such as all-trans retinoic acid (retinoic acid receptor-specific retinoid), but clear differences in toxicity exists.[189]

Chemotherapy is not curative and can palliate patients who relapse or do not respond to biologic response modifiers/retinoids. A recent published multicenter study demonstrated high efficacy of pegylated liposomal doxorubicin monotherapy with an overall response rate of 88% and a low rate of adverse effects compared with other chemotherapy protocols in patients with CTCL.[190] Temozolomide, a new oral alkylating agent, is being evaluated in a phase II trial for patients with relapsed MF and SS. Patients with MF/SS have been shown to have low levels of DNA repair enzyme O^6 alkylguanine DNA alkyltransferase (AGT) and may be particularly sensitive to this alkylator.[191]

New treatments include recombinant toxins such as denileukin diftitox (interleukin-2 receptor specific fusion protein combined with diphtheria toxin). A phase III study initiated for patients with refractory or advanced CTCL showed results with a 30% response rate. Reported adverse effects are similar to interferon-alpha however, a significant number of patients developed vascular leak syndrome.[192] Investigational approaches include monoclonal antibodies such as alemtuzumab. Alemtuzumab is a humanized monoclonal antibody directed against the lymphocyte surface antigen CD52, which is abundantly expressed on normal and most malignant T-lymphocytes.[193] A recently published study of alemtuzumab in 22 patients with advanced MF/SS recorded a clinical response in 55% of cases with 32% complete remission.[194] In selected instances young patients with advanced or biologically aggressive CTCL may benefit from allogeneic stem cell transplantation regimen to induce a graft-versus-lymphoma response.[195] Other investigational approaches are immunomodulatory cytokines such as recombinant interleukin (rIL)-12 and unmethylated cytosine-phosphorothiolated guanine-containing (CpG) DNA to enhance innate antitumor immune mechanisms via activation of dendritic cells and cytotoxic T-cell responses.[196,197] The therapeutic benefit of CpG DNA in addition to peptide-based vaccines is also being evaluated.[198]

5.6 Lymphomatoid papulosis

5.6.1 Pathology

Lymphomatoid papulosis (LyP) is most commonly associated with MF, CD30[+] large T-cell lymphoma, and Hodgkin's disease.[199] Three histologic types have been identified, characterized as type A, B, and C. Type A and C consist of large lymphocytes resembling Reed-Sternberg cells. Type A cells are embedded in a dense inflammatory background, whereas type C cells form large sheets imitating CD30[+] large T-cell lymphoma. Type B simulates classical MF features with epidermotropism and a dermal band-like infiltrate composed of small to medium-sized cells.[200] LyP lesions occasionally exhibit clonal gene rearrangements. Identical clones have been found in associated CTCL.[201] Recently published immunohistochemical data suggest that fascin expression in LyP may become a predictive marker for development of second lymphoid malignancy.[202] Low or loss of CD134 expression may also predict disease progression.[203]

5.6.2 Treatment

LyP represents a benign, chronic recurrent, self-healing, papulonodular and papulonecrotic CD30[+] skin eruption.[204] However, 10 to 20% of patients may develop a lymphoid malignancy, but the prognosis for patients with LyP is otherwise excellent, showing a 100% 5-year survival. There is no curative treatment available. LyP is managed by observation, intralesional steroid injection, ultraviolet light therapy, or low-dose methotrexate.

5.7   Anaplastic large-cell lymphoma, CD30+ cutaneous type

Primary systemic CD30+ ALCL and primary cutaneous CD30+ ALCL represent identical morphologic entities, but they are clinically distinct diseases.[113,205]

5.7.1   Pathology

The neoplastic cells of primary cutaneous CD30[+] large T-cell lymphoma (CD30[+] LTCL) are of the CD4[+] helper T-cell phenotype with CD30 expression. This tumor has an excellent prognosis as confirmed in several studies, in contrast to the transformation of MF to a CD30[-] large cell variant. It shows histological and immunophenotypic overlap with LyP. Therefore, clinical features are important in distinguishing CD30[+] LTCL from LyP. Cytomorphology shows a diffuse, non-epidermotropic infiltrate with cohesive sheets of large CD30[+] lymphocytes. In most cases tumor cells show anaplastic features, less commonly a pleomorphic or immunoblastic appearance. However, there is no difference in the prognosis and survival rate. Primary cutaneous CD30[+] LTCL rarely carry the t(2;5) translocation and are usually ALK negative. These lesions may undergo spontaneous regression, as does the lesions of LyP. The mechanism of tumor regression remains unknown. CD30 ligand-mediated cytotoxicity may participate in the pathophysiology of clinical regression.[206]   A few cases have been reported showing that CD30/CD56 coexpression is associated with a disease progression, as well as increased Fascin level.[202,207]   In cases with progression, point mutations and deletions on TGF-β receptor genes I, and II have been found leading to the loss of its tumor suppressive properties.[207,208]

5.7.2   Treatment

CD30[+] LTCL presenting *de novo*, typically arises in solitary or localized nodules. It comprises approximately 9% of CTCL and typically affects older patients.[113]   Regional lymph node involvement is seen in 25% of patients at presentation. According to the WHO classification, this entity is also known as anaplastic large T-cell lymphoma.   Spot radiation or surgical excision is the preferred treatment with systemic chemotherapy reserved for cases with large tumor burden and extracutaneous involvement. More recently there has been reported efficacy of recombinant interferon-γ and combined treatment with bexarotene and interferon-alpha 2a.[209,210]

5.8   CD30-negative cutaneous large T-cell lymphoma

5.8.1   Pathology

Primary cutaneous CD30⁻ large T-cell lymphomas (CD30⁻LTCL) do not produce T_h2 cytokines and do not express CD30.[211] Microscopically, a dense nodular or diffuse infiltrate characterized by pleomorphic medium or large-sized cells and immunoblastic lymphocytes is present. Large cells comprise over 30% and might resemble classical MF undergoing large cell transformation.

5.8.2   Treatment

These lymphomas are aggressive neoplasms with an estimated 15% 5-year survival rate.[212] Patients present with solitary, localized or generalized plaques, nodules, or tumors without spontaneous regression. Multi-agent systemic chemotherapy is recommended in most cases, with radiotherapy limited to localized disease.

5.9   Pleomorphic T-cell lymphomas with small/medium cells

5.9.1   Pathology

Small/medium-sized pleomorphic CTCL type appears clinically with single erythematous to violaceous nodules or tumors and accounts for less than 3% of CTCL cases.[140] Most cases have an unfavorable prognosis with a median survival of $\leq$ 24 months, however, the CD3⁺, CD4⁺, CD8⁻ subtype with limited lesions might be associated with a better prognosis with a reported 45% 5-year survival rate.[213] Other risk factors predicting tumor progression or dissemination have not been identified. Histopathology shows a dermal dense, diffuse, or nodular infiltrate comprising small and medium sized pleomorphic cells with variable epidermotropism.[214] Most cases express a classic T-helper cell phenotype and do not express CD30.

5.9.2   Treatment

The optimal therapy of pleomorphic T-cell lymphomas with small/medium cells has not been defined. Localized lesions have been treated with radiation or surgical excision. Only short-term outcome have been reported. Patients with generalized skin disease or progression have been treated effectively with systemic treatments including multi-agent chemotherapy, retinoids, interferons and monoclonal antibodies.

5.10   Subcutaneous panniculitis-like T-cell lymphoma (SCPTCL)

SCPTCL is a rare T-cell lymphoma that infiltrates the subcutaneous fat without dermal and epidermal involvement causing erythematous to violaceous nodules and/or plaques and is often associated with a systemic hemophagocytic syndrome.[215-217] Moreover, a controversial entity known as cytophagic histiocytic panniculitis (CHP) has been described as an inflammatory disease (also often associated with hemophagocytic syndrome) with possible connection to SCPTCL.[218,219] CHP is a disease that has been recognized to have diverse outcomes ranging from indolent to aggressive/fatal clinical courses.[218,219] It may overlap clinically and histologically with angiocentric lymphoma.

5.10.1   Pathology

SCPTCL is a rare T-cell lymphoma localized to subcutaneous tissue consisting of a mixture of small, medium and large atypical cells with prominent tumor necrosis and karyorrhexis. The neoplastic lymphocytes often rim individual adipocytes. Benign/reactive histiocytes may be present with associated phagocytosis of red cells or nuclear debris. Necrosis of fat and connective tissue is always seen, but not with angiodestruction. The phenotype consists of pan-T-cell antigens that are more commonly CD8+ > CD4-CD8- > CD4+, while CD56 is usually negative. Histologic diagnosis is not precise for SCPTCL and may be associated with a broad morphologic differential diagnosis including erythema nodosum, lupus profundus, erythema induratum and benign lobular panniculitis.[220] Genotypic studies are often critical in confirming a neoplastic diagnosis.[216,217]

5.10.2   Molecular

PCR gene rearrangement studies have recently demonstrated that CHP is likely part of the same clinicopathologic spectrum of SCPTCL, with SCPTCL representing a neoplastic clonal process, while CHP represents pre-malignant lymphoid disease.[217,219,221] Gonzalez et al first documented in 1991 a subcutaneous T-cell lymphoma associated with hemophagocytic syndrome and β-TCR chain clonality.[222] Since then, numerous small case reports have documented the entity of SCPTCL and it has been recognized as a separate T-cell lymphoma in the REAL and current WHO classification.[223,224] Most reports demonstrated a monoclonal TCR (commonly γ-gene rearrangement) and many cases were EBV positive (See Table 2). Retrospective case series with somewhat larger patient numbers have corroborated the clonality of TCR in the majority of cases of SCPTCL, but have not validated an association with EBV.[215-217,225,226] Kumar et al study of 16 cases of SCPTCL showed 8 of 9 cases had clonal TCR-γ gene rearrangements while 10 cases were negative for Epstein-Barr viral sequences.[215] Moreover, molecular usage studies of TCR γ-gene segments in SCPTCL have demonstrated that the Vγ2 gene is primarily expressed.[216,225,227] This is in contrast to other T-cell lymphomas such as hepatosplenic lymphoma where the Vγ1 gene is preferentially expressed.[225,227] The TCR-γ gene consists of 6 varied Vγ gene segments, although $\gamma\delta$ T-cells express the Vγ1 or Vγ2 genes in approximately 95% of cases.[15,227,228] It has been shown that normal $\gamma\delta$ T-lymphocytes that reside in the intestine, spleen and thymus mainly express the Vγ1 gene, while normal $\gamma\delta$ T-lymphocytes in the skin, tonsils and peripheral blood primarily express Vγ2 genes.[15,227] This indicates that $\gamma\delta$ T-cell lymphomas such as hepatosplenic and SCPTCL are derived from local lymphoid tissue. This may be potentially helpful not only for accurate diagnosis, classification and monitoring of minimal residual disease (MRD) with $\gamma\delta$ T-cell lymphomas, but also may contribute to discovery of molecular directed therapies for these often difficult-to-treat diseases.[216] Chromosome abnormalities and proto-oncogenes associated with SCPTCL have been rarely reported in the literature. Mizutani and colleagues documented t(1;6)(11q;21p) in one patient with SCPTCL.[229]

5.10.3   Treatment

Clinical course of SCPTCL is variable ranging from indolent disease to rapidly fatal fulminant hemophagocytosis.[216,217] When treatment is warranted, most patients respond to systemic combination chemotherapy or local radiation therapy, although median survival is typically less than 2 years.[216] One case report described a SCPTCL patient with durable response following fludarabine, mitoxantrone and dexamethasone (FND) therapy.[230]

5.11   Hepatosplenic T-cell lymphoma (HSTCL)

HSTCL is an uncommon T-cell lymphoma that is seen mainly in young males (median age 35) presenting with B symptoms, prominent hepatosplenomegaly, mild anemia, neutropenia, thrombocytopenia (commonly severe), significant peripheral blood lymphocytosis, rare lymphadenopathy and is often associated with an aggressive clinical course (median survival 12 to 14 months).[231-233]

5.11.1   Pathology

This neoplasm infiltrates the sinuses of the liver, bone marrow (2/3 of patients) and splenic red pulp. HSTCL tumor cells are usually homogenous, medium-sized lymphoid cells with round nuclei, moderately condensed chromatin and moderate pale cytoplasm. Erythrophagocytosis may be present in the spleen and bone marrow and circulating peripheral blood tumor cells are seen in approximately 25% to 50% of patients. The tumor cells are usually CD4-CD8- (85%), positive for CD2, CD3 and CD7 (negative for CD5) and express CD56 in 70% to 80% of cases.[233] TIA-1 is present in almost all cases, but commonly granzyme B and perforin are not present indication a non-activated cytotoxic T-cell phenotype. Cells usually express the gamma/delta T-cell receptor (Vd1+/Vd2-/Vd3-), but are negative for EBV.[233]

5.11.2   Molecular

Similar to other T-cell lymphomas already discussed, detection of clonal TCR gene rearrangements may prove essential in establishing a diagnosis of HSTCL especially with complex histologic cases.[234] HSTCL likely arises from $\gamma\delta$ T-cells of the hepatic sinusoids and splenic red pulp and most cases of HSTCL are demonstrated to have clonal TCR γ-gene or δ-gene rearrangements with a cytotoxic T-cell phenotype (See Table 2).[15,225,235] Moreover, the Vγ1 or Vδ1 genes are preferentially expressed in this disease reflecting in part the normal localization of $\gamma\delta$ T-lymphocytes that reside in the spleen, intestinal tissue and thymus.[216,225,227,233] An $\alpha\beta$ T-cell phenotype has been described with HSTCL.[54,236] These infrequent $\alpha\beta$ HSTCL cases interestingly occurred more commonly in women, but otherwise were characterized by similar clinicopathologic and cytogenetic features similar to γδ HSTCL. The primary recurrent chromosome abnormality in HSTCL demonstrated in many of cases is isochrome (i) 7(10q),[48,231,233,237] although not all series have documented i(7q) abnormalities in HSTCL.[216,238] Furthermore, i(7q) is not specific for HSTCL as this karyotype has been reported in acute leukemia, prolymphocytic leukemia and Wilms' tumor.[216,239] Trisomy 8 has been frequently observed in HSTCL.[48] Other chromosome aberrations less frequently detected in HSTCL include deletion 11q, t(1;14)(q21;q13), der(21)t(7;21) and complex karyotype.[216,237,240]

Abnormal expression of p21, p53 or other oncogenic gene pathways have not been identified in HSTCL.[55,241] Reports of associated EBV have been conflicting, but some reports have documented strong EBER-1 expression in cases of HSTCL.[226,231,242] As previously discussed, a significant minority of HSTCL is recognized in post-transplant patients.[216,243] Again conflicting results regarding EBV positivity in this post-transplant T-cell lymphoma population have been reported, but the majority of cases have not documented associated EBV or other viruses.[243,244]

5.11.3 Treatment

The clinical course of HSTCL is commonly aggressive despite multiagent chemotherapy,[233] although rare patients may exhibit indolent disease [personal communication, Dr. Jane Winter]. Anecdotal reports have described activity with the purine analogue, pentostatin, in relapsed HSTCL patients.[245] Approximately 10% to 20% of HSTCL cases arise in immunocompromised patients, predominantly in the solid organ transplant setting.[246] Furthermore, post-transplant T-cell lymphoproliferative disorders typically do not respond to reduction in immunosuppression alone and often have a very aggressive clinical course with median survival commonly measured in weeks to months.[216,246,247]

5.12 Extranodal NK/T-cell lymphoma, nasal and nasal-type

Extranodal NK/T-cell lymphoma, nasal and nasal-type, formerly known as angiocentric lymphoma, is rare in Western countries being more prevalent in Asia and populations of Peru.[248-250] The disease commonly presents in men at the median age of 50. This entity is associated with EBV and is typically characterized by extranodal presentation and localized stage I/II disease, but with angiodestructive proliferation and an aggressive clinical course.[251-253] These tumors have a predilection for the nasal cavity and paranasal sinuses ("nasal"), although the "nasal-type" designation encompasses other extranodal sites of NK/T-cell lymphomatous disease (skin, gastrointestinal, testis, kidney, upper respiratory tract and rarely orbit/eye). Cases resembling hydroa vacciniforme-like eruptions have been reported sharing common cytologic and cytogenetic abnormalities.[254]

5.12.1   Pathology

Extranodal NK/T-cell lymphoma is designated "NK/T" secondary to the uncertainty of its cellular origin. The characteristic histologic feature is an angiodestructive pattern with frequent necrosis. This lymphoma was also formerly known as "lethal midline granuloma". The tumor cells consist of a mixture of small, medium and large cells, but most are large dysplastic cells. The immunophenotype expresses NK antigens (CD16, CD56, CD57) with surface and cytoplasmic CD3 and cytotoxic granules (granzyme B and TIA-1). CD8-positivity is more common than CD4-CD8-, while CD4+ is rare.

5.12.2   Molecular

Most molecular studies of this disease have included small patient numbers, but many studies have been reported. The rearrangement of TCR genes has been inconsistently identified in this disease, being described anywhere from 0 to 60% in various studies.[28,255-257] When present, γδ rearrangements are more common, while Ig rearrangements are germline (See Table 2). Studies have suggested that separation into distinct NK-cell and T-cell categories is feasible based on lineage-specific TCR rearrangements and immunophenotype.[257] Cytogenetic abnormalities are common in extranodal NK/T-cell lymphoma, nasal type. Most reports have identified deletions of chromosome 6 (q21~25) to be the most frequent recurrent cytogenetic abnormality.[258] Siu and colleagues demonstrated consistent patterns of allelic abnormalities with loss of heterozygosity (LOH) at chromosome 6q in 91% of nasal lymphoma cases versus 50% of non-nasal NK lymphoma cases.[259] Furthermore, they observed LOH at 13q in 33% of cases at presentation of disease, but in 100% of cases at relapse. A recent study by Ko et al documented frequent losses at 1p, 17p and 12q and gains at 2q, 13q and 10q with infrequent chromosome 6q aberration.[256] Other reported non-random chromosome abnormalities include isochromes 6p, 1q, 17q and 7q, 11q aberrations, +X and +8 (See Table 2).[260]

Identification of oncogenes related to extranodal NK/T-cell lymphoma has been difficult, in part related to sufficient recovery of viable, non-necrotic tissue for appropriate analyses.   p53 has been shown to be overexpressed in many cases of extranodal NK/T-cell lymphomas, nasal type.[241,250]   However, p53 mutations are much more infrequently identified.[250,261] Mutations of k-ras have been described in this lymphoma.[54]

Overexpression p21 and p16 has been documented in NK/T-cell lymphoma, but the patterns of expression have been variable.[241,262] It is not clear whether p21 overexpression is directly involved in the pathogenic process. EBV may play a role in the oncogenesis of extranodal NK/T-cell lymphoma, nasal type. EBER-1 RNA transcripts are detectable in the majority of cells in nearly all cases.[28,250,256,263] Moreover, EBV-latent membrane protein (LMP-1) is expressed in most cases.[28]

5.12.3 Treatment

Combined modality therapy incorporating adriamycin-based chemotherapy (minimum 6 cycles for patients with stage III or IV disease), involved-field (IF) radiation (median dose 50 Gy, range 30 to 67 Gy)[251] and intrathecal prophylaxis is recommended for extranodal NK/T-cell lymphoma-nasal patients, although the benefit of the addition of chemotherapy to radiation has not been confirmed for limited stage disease.[252,253] Response rates for NK/T-cell lymphoma, nasal, have been reported to be near 85% (two-thirds CR) following radiation alone, although 50% of patients will experience local relapse and 25% systemic relapse with a predilection to extranodal sites such as testis, orbit, skin, gastrointestinal tract and central nervous system.[264,265] Li and colleagues recently reported on 77 patients with NK/T-cell sinonasal lymphoma (56 locoregional, 21 systemic disease) with 5-year OS rate of 36% (median follow-up, 89 months).[265]

Kim and colleagues showed 5-year DFS for patients with stage I/II disease 34% to 38% and OS 57% to 65%, although systemic disease progression was often fatal.[252,264] Li and colleagues showed in Taiwan that combined chemotherapy/radiation or radiation alone resulted in better survival compared to chemotherapy alone (5-year survival rates, 59%, 50%, and 15%, respectively; P = 0.01) in patients with NK/T-cell sinonasal locoregional disease.[265] Li and colleagues in China retrospectively compared stage IE patients who received IF radiation alone versus combined chemotherapy with radiotherapy.[253] Of note, this group divided IE patients into limited (confined to nasal cavity) and extensive (presenting with extension beyond the nasal cavity) stage IE disease. Limited stage IE patients survived longer than extensive IE patients overall (5-year OS 90% versus 57%, respectively, P <0.001). Moreover, comparing radiation alone to combined modality therapy, the 5-year OS was not significantly different for both limited stage IE, 89% and 92%, respectively, as well as extensive IE disease at 54% of 58%, respectively.

Patients with systemic disease have poor long-term survival (5-year overall survival 20% to 25%) with high locoregional (over 50%) and systemic failure rates (over 70%).[253,265]   The traditional approach for stage III and IV extranodal NK/T-cell lymphoma-nasal is combined modality therapy with adriamycin-based chemotherapy and radiation therapy.[251,253]

6.   ENTEROPATHY-TYPE INTESTINAL T-CELL LYMPHOMA (EITCL)

EITCL (also known as intestinal T-cell lymphoma) is a rare T-cell lymphoma of intraepithelial lymphocytes that commonly presents with multiple circumferential jejunal ulcers in adults with a prior brief history of gluten-sensitive enteropathy.[266] EITCL accounts for less than 1% of NHL's according to the International Lymphoma Study Group and has been recognized to have a poor prognosis with reported 5-year overall survival and disease-free survival rates of 20% and 3%, respectively.[266] This is in part related to many patients presenting with poor performance status and varied complications of locally advanced disease by the time a diagnosis of EITCL has been confirmed.

EITCL may present without antecedent celiac history, but most patients have abdominal pain and weight loss. Evidence of celiac serologic markers such as positive anti-gliadin antibodies and/or HLA types such as DQA1*0501/DQB1*0201/DRB1*0304 may be present at diagnosis of EITCL.[267,268] Moreover, these genotypes may represent celiac patients at higher risk for development of EITCL.[268,269] Small-bowel perforation or obstruction, gastrointestinal bleeding and enterocolic fistulae are recognized complications of this disease.[266]

6.1.1   Pathology

EITCL may be a difficult diagnosis to establish on histologic grounds alone. The tumor cells contain a combination of small, medium and large (anaplastic) cells, and reactive histiocytes are often seen. The immunophenotype consists of pan-T-cell antigens, usually CD8+ and the mucosal lymphoid antigen, CD103, is often expressed.

6.1.2   Molecular

Earlier diagnosis is warranted and molecular and genetic techniques may expedite the diagnosis of this disease when applied in the appropriate clinical circumstance, which would hopefully translate into improved long-term outcomes.[270] The TCR genes are rearranged in nearly all cases of

EITCL (more commonly γ than β).[271-273] Moreover, TCR gene rearrangements are often present in patients with EITCL who have evolved from sprue.[272-275] Daum and colleagues compared 8 patients with overt EITCL to 13 patients of celiac disease caused by a defined disorder, 3 patients with refractory sprue evolving into overt EITCL and to 2 patients with ulcerative jejunitis.[271] They demonstrated clonal TCR-γ gene rearrangement with PCR in all resected jejunal specimens of the EITCL patients. Furthermore, 4 of 8 duodenal biopsy specimens from overt EITCL patients demonstrated positive clonality compared to 2 of 3 with refractory sprue evolving into overt EITCL, 2 of 2 with ulcerative jejunitis (a disease associated with increased risk for development of EITCL),[276] 1 of 6 with refractory sprue and no patients with sprue caused by a defined disorder.

Chromosomal aberrations have rarely been reported with EITCL (See Table 2). Obermann and colleagues recently found loss of heterozygosity at chromosome 9p21 associated with EITCL.[277] One report documented that 22 of 23 EITCL tumors stained for p53 with 9 of 19 cases studied having collections of small lymphocytes in the affected bowel expressing p53.[273] The role of p53 in the oncogenesis of EITCL is not known. Varied reports have documented EBV positivity (by PCR and FISH with EBER-1 analysis) in association with EITCL including cases of EBV-related EITCL PTLD suggesting a possible etiologic role of EBV in the pathogenesis of EITCL.[278-281] Furthermore, analysis comparing the prevalence of EBV in Mexican versus European EITCL cases demonstrated that there are significant epidemiologic differences in EBV association (100% versus 10%, respectively).[280]

6.1.3   Treatment

Following diagnosis of EITCL, adriamycin-based combination chemotherapy should be considered for each patient and aggressive nutritional support with parenteral or enteral feeding is critical in the care of these patients.[266] Patients with known celiac disease should adhere to a gluten-free diet. 18F-fluoro-deoxy-glucose positron emission tomography (FDG-PET) may be a useful imaging tool for clinical evaluation of EITCL patients.[282]

7.   ADULT T-CELL LEUKEMIA/LYMPHOMA (ATL)

ATL was first described in 1977 by Uchiyama and colleagues.[283] They detailed 16 patients with morphologically heterogenous leukemic cells with indented/lobulated nuclei. Thirteen of the 16 patients had originated from the same area of southern Japan. The retrovirus, HTLV-1, has been documented to be critical to the development of ATL.[284] HTLV-1 is known to cause diseases other than ATL, including tropical spastic paraparesis/HTLV-1-associated myelopathy, infective dermatitis and uveitis. In endemic areas in Japan, approximately 10% to 35% of the population is infected with HTLV-1.[285] Among these carriers, the overall risk of ATL is approximately 2.5% in patients who live to age 70.[286] Two to 6% of the Caribbean population are HTLV-1 carriers, while less than 1% of the population in lower risk areas such as the United States and Europe are seropositive.[287,288] HTLV-1 is transmitted through sexual intercourse, transfused blood products (products containing white blood cells; not fresh frozen plasma), shared needles, breast milk and vertical transmission.[283,284,289,290] Transfusion of HTLV-1-contaminated blood products results in seroconversion in approximately 30% to 50% of patients at a median of 51 days.[290]

The clinical features of 187 ATL patients included median age onset 55 years, lymphadenopathy (72%), skin lesions (53%), hepatomegaly (47%), splenomegaly (25%) and hypercalcemia (28%) present at diagnosis.[285] The differential diagnosis between cutaneous ATL and MF is often difficult. Cellular immune suppression is often seen in HTLV-1 and ATL leading to strongyloides infection in a significant minority of patients.[291] ATL is separated into 4 subtypes divided on clinicopathologic features and prognosis: actue, lymphoma, chronic and smoldering.[292] Shimoyama and colleagues reported on the characteristics of 818 ATL patients in 1991.[292] Patients with acute type present with hypercalcemia, leukemic manifestations and tumor lesions and have the worst prognosis with median survival of approximately 6 months. Lymphoma type patients present with low circulating abnormal lymphocytes (<1%) and nodal, liver, splenic, central nervous system, bone, gastrointestinal disease and have median survival of 10 months. Chronic type patients present with > 5% abnormal circulating lymphocytes and had a median survival of 24 months, while smoldering type patients median survival had not yet been reached.

7.1.1   Pathology

Abnormal T-lymphocytes are often seen in patients peripheral blood smear with cells having indented or lobulated nuclei (leading to the term "flower cells"). HTLV-1 is a single-stranded, diploid RNA virus that enters T-cells and integrates into the host DNA as a provirus.[293-295] HTLV-1 encodes three structural genes (*pol, gag* and *tax*) and two regulatory genes (*tax* and *rex*). Tax, a potent HTLV-1 transcription activator, plays an important role in HTLV-1-induced transformation and resistance to apoptosis in part through the induction of IKB-alpha degradation, resulting in the activation of the NF-KB pathway.[296] HTLV-1 promotes other genetic events including deletion of the tumor suppressor genes, p15INK4B and p16INK4A.[297] It is not known if HTLV-1 has direct carcinogenetic activity or is a virus that is involved in a multi-step process of evolution of genetic instability.[9,298,299] Adult T-cell leukemia cells often express CD2, CD3, CD4, CD25, CD52 and CD122 antigens.[300]

7.1.2   Molecular

Itoyama and colleagues examined the cytogenetic abnormalities in 50 newly diagnosed ATL patients.[9] Immunophenotypic analysis was divided into 2 categories: 1) the more usual/common CD4+CD8- or 2) the unusual CD4-CD8+, CD4+CD8+ or CD4-CD8- phenotypes. The unusual phenotypes were found in 19% and 17% of patients with acute ATL and lymphomatous ATL, respectively, compared to 0% of chronic ATL patients. All 50 patients had abnormal karyotypes with most patients having simple numerical and clonal structural abnormalities with almost all chromosomes being affected. Multiple chromosome breaks (> six) aneuploidy were significantly more frequent in the combined acute and lymphoma subtypes compared to chronic ATL. Moreover, multiple chromosomal breaks (> six) and abnormalities of 1p, 1p22, 1q, 1q10-22, 3q, 3q10-12, 3q21 and 17q were associated with significantly overall shorter survival. Using comparative genomic hybridization in 64 ATL patients, Tsukasaki and colleagues documented that chromosome imbalances, losses and gains were more frequently observed in aggressive ATL as compared to indolent disease.[299] Gains in 1q and 4q were significantly more common with aggressive ATL, whereas gain of 7q was associated with good prognosis within the group of aggressive disease patients.

7.1.3   Treatment

ATL is an aggressive neoplasm with resistance to conventional chemotherapy, in part due to resistance of tax-induced apoptosis and overexpression of P-glycoprotein (the product of multidrug resistance-1 gene).[9,301,302] Patients may initially respond to combination chemotherapy, but unfortunately response durations are brief (5 to 7 months).[285,303-305] El-Sabban and colleagues combined arsenic trioxide (As_2O_3) with IFN-α, which induced cell cycle arrest and apoptosis.[301] This combination induced the degradation of tax, which was associated with an upregulation of IKB-alpha with a subsequent major decrease in RelA DNA binding NF-KB complexes. Bazarbachi and colleagues have corroborated this data as they demonstrated high synergy between IFN-α and As_2O_3 with respect to cellular proliferation, cell cycle arrest and induction of apoptosis both in HTLV-1 transformed cell lines and primary ATL cells in culture.[306,307] Furthermore, all-trans retinoic acid (ATRA) has been demonstrated to have an effect on ATL cell cycle progression, which may have implications for the clinical application of ATRA in ATL.[308]

Response rates of 70 to 90% to combination IFN-α and zidovudine therapy have been demonstrated in ATL with associated increased median survival rates compared to historical control (11 to 18 months versus 4 to 8 months, respectively).[309,310] A recent clinical trial that investigated initial cytoreductive therapy with CHOP followed by antinucleoside, IFN-α and oral etoposide therapy demonstrated encouraging results.[311] Other agents with anecdotal activity in ATL include irinotecan and the purine analogues (2-deoxycoformcin and 2-chlorodeoxyadenosine),[312-314] although 2-deoxycoformcin did not appear to improve outcomes when added to combination chemotherapy.[315] Future research should include the investigation of antibodies such as denileukin deftitox and CAMPATH.[300,316,317]

8.   HEMATOPOIETIC STEM CELL
TRANSPLANTATION (HSCT)

The exact role of autologous or allogeneic HSCT in T-cell NHL has not been defined. An accepted standard of care for patients with relapsed, chemotherapy-sensitive DLBCL is high-dose chemotherapy followed by autologous peripheral stem cell rescue (in other words, autologous HSCT).[318] Randomized trials comparing salvage chemotherapy alone to chemotherapy with autologous HSCT for relapsed T-cell NHL have not been completed, although results of retrospective analyses appear promising. Several case series have reported the outcome of patients with relapsed T-cell NHL following autologous and allogeneic HSCT.[319-324] PTCL-noc and ALCL were the predominant subtypes in these trials and 3-year OS and DFS rates ranged from 39% to 58% and 37% to 48%, respectively, following autologous HSCT (median follow-up of 36 to 43 months).[319,321] Furthermore, high IPI (≥ 2) significantly predicted a worse outcome in 2 of the above-described trials,[320,321] while one did not.[319] Furthermore, ALCL (versus non-ALCL) predicted an improved outcome in the largest trial (3-year OS 79% versus 44%, respectively, P=0.08).[319]

Song et al recently compared relapsed/refractory T-cell NHL to DLBCL patients who received autologous HSCT over the same time period with outcome analysis according to T-cell pathologic subtype.[322] Over a 12-year period, 29 T-cell NHL patients with relapsed and 7 patients with primary refractory disease were compared to 97 patients with relapsed DLBCL. With a median follow-up of 42 months, T-cell NHL patients had a 17% treatment related mortality (TRM) with 3-year OS and DFS of 48% and 37%, respectively, compared to 53% and 42%, respectively, for DLBCL patients (non-significant). They documented no significant outcome differences according to T-cell subtype, although PTCL-noc patients had a trend for inferior 3-year DFS of 28% compared to 67% for ALCL. Several other case series and case reports have confirmed the feasibility of autologous HSCT with reported long-term survival for other rarer relapsed T-cell NHL subtypes, including EITCL,[325] extranodal NK/T-cell lymphoma-nasal,[326] SCPTCL,[327] HSTCL,[233] ATL[328] and AIL.[329] Rodriguez and colleagues recently showed that patients with primary refractory T-cell NHL may experience long-term survival similar to primary refractory B-cell NHL when salvaged with autologous HSCT.[330] It appears from the non-randomized studies described above that patients with relapsed or refractory T-cell NHL may gain similar benefit to autologous HSCT as DLBCL patients. Prospective randomized studies are warranted.

HSCT in first remission remains controversial. Some groups advocate autologous HSCT for ALCL patients in first CR in part due to the presumption that IPI does not correlate with prognosis in ALCL. French and Italian investigators have documented long-term survival rates of approximately 90% for ALCL patients in first CR for who actually received an autologous HSCT.[331,332] These results are encouraging, but systemic ALCL (especially ALK-positive) have the best prognosis among T-cell NHL subtypes and recent studies have confirmed a significant correlation of IPI to OS and DFS.[98] Prospective, randomized trials need to be performed to confirm these observations, especially in higher risk patients, such as ALCL patients with high IPI and/or CD56-positive and/or ALK-negative disease.[96-98,205]

Small case series and anecdotal reports have described the feasibility and long-term survival for patients with relapsed T-cell NHL following matched-sibling and unrelated allogeneic HSCT (including reduced-intensity conditioning), including patients with chemotherapy-resistant T-cell NHL and patients with hemophagocytic syndrome.[320,321,333-335]

9.   RADIATION THERAPY

Due to the paucity of clinical trials, the integration of radiation therapy into the treatment plan of most T-cell NHL patients often models that of B-cell NHL. Compared to DLBCL, T-cell NHL more commonly presents with stage III/IV disease (48% and 74% respectively)[4] and T-cell patients frequently present with combined nodal and extranodal disease at diagnosis (especially PTCL-noc, ALCL and AIL),[1,3,37,43] thereby often obviating the need for the addition of radiation to chemotherapy. Studies specifically addressing the benefits of radiation therapy to bulky sites for T-cell NHL patients with advanced disease have not been done.

Extranodal NK/T-cell lymphoma, nasal and nasal-type, is one T-cell lymphoma subtype where radiation plays a major role in the therapeutic plan (see above).[251-253,264] This is due in part to that extranodal NK/T-cell lymphoma-nasal patients commonly present with stage I/II disease (80%).[251]

10.   EMERGING THERAPIES

Identification of relevant protooncogenes and tumor suppressor genes involved in the pathogenesis of T-cell NHL such as the NPM/ALK fusion protein, p53 and retinoblastoma (RB) gene, cyclin dependent kinase (such as p15INK4b, p16INK4a, p21WAF1), histone deacetylation inhibitors and infectious etiologies (EBV and Helicobacter pylori) as well as their interplay with the various regulatory pathways of cell cycle progression and apoptosis represent potential candidates for molecular-based therapy. Identification of specific fusion products such as NPM-ALK will facilitate the production of targeted treatments such as anti-sense oligodeoxynucleotides and monoclonal antibody therapies directed towards specific fusion proteins. Gene therapy using adenoviral vector-mediated wild-type p53 gene transfer is being evaluated and may have application in certain T-cell lymphomas.[336] In addition to denileukin ditox, several other recombinant chimeric immunotoxins have been successfully produced, such as anti-CD30 (member of tumor necrosis factor receptor), in order to target CD30-positive NHL (expressed in: ALCL and Reed Sternberg cells of Hodgkin's disease >> PTCL-noc = EITCL = nasal-type > HSTCL = SCPTCL).[337] Tumor suppressor genes, such as p53 and RB are commonly altered in diseases such as ATL.[338] A monoclonal antibody directed against the human transferrin receptor (TfR) HTLV-1-infected cells (mAb A24) is under development, as HTLV-1 cells constitutively express high levels of surface TfR.[339] Cell cycle regulatory genes, such as cyclin dependent kinase inhibitors, are often inactivated by hypermethylation, which contributes to increased cell cycle progression.[297] Cyclin dependent kinase modulators such as Flavopiridol, broadly inhibit cyclin dependent kinase and promote cell cycle block. Importantly, these agents can induce apoptosis and modulate transcriptional events regardless of bcl-2 or p53 status.[340,341] Other intracellular signaling pathways such as the protein kinase C modulating agents, UCN-01 and Bryostatin, are also being examined alone or in combination with cytotoxic chemotherapy in NHL.[342,343] Future molecular studies in T-cell NHL are likely to provide additional disease-specific molecular perturbations and chromosomal translocations with important diagnostic and therapeutic implications. Furthermore, histone deacetylase (HDAC) inhibitors (such as depsipeptide) increase histone acetylation leading to cellular differentiation, decreased cell proliferation and induction of cell death, and are being examined in patients with T-cell NHL.[344] The role of viral pathogenesis in T-cell NHL tumor development continues to be studied as a potential target of drug therapy.[345]

The expanding knowledge into the cellular and molecular mechanisms of T-cell NHL oncogenesis needs to be validated in excised lymphomatous tissue. Prior limitations in tissue-based research may be averted through use of technology such as cDNA microarray. The identification and description of specific gene and protein expression with T-cell NHL through gene expression profiling is warranted.[346] Identification of T-cell tumor-specific epitopes are being identified and studied in an attempt to develop rationale vaccine strategies for patients with T-cell NHL.[347,348] This research may not only lead to more advanced T-cell NHL tumor classification to allow accurate prediction of patients course of disease, but may also further elucidate the molecular oncogenesis of T-cell NHL in order to develop patient-tailored therapy including discovery of molecular targeted therapy.

11. CONCLUSIONS

A significant amount of data has accumulated over the last few decades regarding the molecular and clinical characteristics of T-cell lymphoma NHL. Characterization of clonal TCR gene rearrangements has often allowed earlier detection of T-cell lymphoma and specific gene patterns may correlate with prognosis. Gamma-delta TCR clonality now represents the more common TCR rearrangement in SCPTCL, HSTCL, extranodal NK/T-cell lymphoma, and EITCL, and when present often represent cases with more aggressive clinical courses. Improved molecular techniques such as RT-PCR and FISH have allowed documentation of recurring, non-random chromosome abnormalities such as deletion 6q in extranodal NK/T-cell lymphoma, nasal type, i7(10q) in HSTCL, complex karyotypes in PTCL-NOC, trisomies 3 and 5 in AIL and t(2;5)(p23;35) with systemic anaplastic T-cell lymphoma. Moreover, the distinct T-cell NHL subtypes often warrant individualized diagnostic and therapeutic strategies, such as the associated CHP and hemophagocytic syndrome with SCPTCL, the chromosomal translocation, t(2;5), leading to NPM-ALK fusion protein, viral pathogenesis EBV and HTLV-I associated with extranodal NK/T-cell lymphoma--nasal type and ATL, respectively, and the role of radiation therapy in extranodal NK/T-cell lymphoma-nasal type. In addition to CHOP chemotherapy, other active therapeutic agents in T-cell NHL have been identified that include purine and pyrimidine analogues, denileukin ditox, retinoids and IFN-α. Furthermore, identification of the relevant genes involved in the pathogenesis of T-cell lymphoma such as the NPM/ALK fusion protein, p53, cyclin dependent kinase inhibitors (including p15, p16 and p21), and EBV as well as their interplay with the various regulatory pathways of cell cycle progression and apoptosis represent potential candidates for molecular-based therapy. Prospective, multi-institution clinical trials remain critically important in order to determine the most effective treatment regimens that will continue to improve cure rates in these aggressive, yet treatable and often curable diseases.

Table 1. T-cell lymphomas according to WHO classification

Mature (peripheral) T-cell lymphoma/neoplasms[1]
Peripheral T-cell lymphoma, not otherwise characterized
Angioimmunoblastic T-cell lymphoma
Anaplastic large-cell lymphoma, T/null cell, primary systemic type
Anaplastic large-cell lymphoma, T/null cell, primary cutaneous type
Subcutaneous panniculitis-like T-cell lymphoma
Hepatosplenic gamma-delta T-cell lymphoma
Extranodal NK/T-cell lymphoma, nasal type
Enteropathy-type T-cell lymphoma
Adult T-cell lymphoma/leukemia (HTLV1+)
Mycoses Fungoides/Sezary Syndrome
Precursor T-cell lymphoma/neoplasms
Precursor T-lymphoblastic lymphoma/leukemia (precursor T-cell acute lymphoblastic leukemia)

[1]T-cell prolymphocytic leukemia, T-cell granular lymphocytic leukemia and Aggressive NK-cell leukemia are also included in this category.

Table 2. Characteristic genetic and molecular features of T-cell lymphomas

Lymphoma Histologic subtype	Chromosome Translocations	TCR gene rearrangement	Protooncogene involved	Protooncogene mechanism and function
Peripheral T-cell (not otherwise characterized)	Often complex Numerical: +3, +5, +21, -13, +8, +19, -10, -Y Structural: del(6q), 1q, 7q, 9p, 9q, 4q,2p, 1p, Inv(14)(q11); t(7)(q35):	$\alpha\beta > \gamma\delta$	?p53 ?Rb gene TCRA/D TCRB/G ?c-kit ?k-ras ?beta-catenin	Functional inactivation and/or mutation TF—deregulation
Angioimmunoblastic	+3 and +5 >> +X	$\alpha\beta = \gamma\delta$	EBV (in many cases) ?p53 ?n-ras	?viral oncogenesis ?p21
Anaplastic T-cell (systemic)	t(2;5)(p23;q35); less common t(1;2), t(2;3), t(2;22) or inv(2)	$\alpha\beta >> \gamma\delta$	NPM/ALK* ?c-myc ?hypermethylation ?EBV	Fusion protein—ALK is a TK; ?PI3K activation

Lymphoma Histologic subtype	Chromosome Translocations	TCR gene rearrangement	Protooncogene involved	Protooncogene mechanism and function
Subcutaneous panniculitis-like	t(1;6)(11q;21p) rarely	γδ > αβ	--	--
Hepatosplenic	i(7)(10q) and +8	γδ >> αβ	?EBV	--
Extranodal T-cell (nasal)	del 6 (q21~25) most frequent; Numerical: +13q, -1p, -17p, -12q, +2q, +10q, ,+X, and -11q, Structural: isochromes 6p, 1q, 17q; del(11q)	γδ >> αβ	EBV (in nearly all cases) ?p53	?viral oncogenesis overexpression, ?p21, p16
Enteropathy-type intestinal	LOH 9p21	γδ > αβ > NK	EBV (geographic variation) ?p53	--

*See Table 3 for complete characteristics.

Abbreviations: ND, None described; TCR, T-cell receptor; TF, transcription factor; TK, tyrosine kinase; PI3K, phosphatidylinositol 3-kinase-Akt pathway; LOH, loss of heterozygosity.

Table 3. Characteristics of fusion proteins associated with ALK-positive ALCL

Genetic aberration	Frequency	Fusion protein connected with TK domain of ALK 2p23	Size of fusion protein	Staining pattern
t(2;5)	73%	NPM	80kd	Cytoplasmic and nuclear
t(1;2)	17%	TPM3	104kd	Cytoplasmic and nuclear
t(2;3)	2.5%	TFG	97kd	Cytoplasmic
t(2;22)	2.5%	CLTCL	96kd	Granular cytoplasmic
inv(2)	2.5%	ATIC	250kd	Cytoplasmic

Abbreviations: TK, tyrosine kinase; ALK, anaplastic lymphoma kinase; ALCL, anaplastic large cell lymphoma; NPM, nucleophosim gene; TPM3, nonmuscle tropomyosin; TFG, tropomyosin receptor kinase-fused gene; CLTCL, clathrin heavy polypeptide-like gene; ATIC, 5-aminoimidazole-4-carboxamide-1-beta-D-ribonucleotide transformylase/inosine monophosphate cyclohydrolase; inv, inversion.

Table 4. EORTC classification for primary cutaneous T-cell lymphomas and corresponding categories in the WHO classification

EORTC	WHO
Cutaneous T-cell lymphoma	
Indolent	
Mycosis fungoides	Mycosis fungoides
Mycosis fungoides variants	Mycosis fungoides variants
Follicular MF	Follicular MF
Pagetoid reticulosis	Pagetoid reticulosis
CD30$^+$ large T-cell lymphoma	Primary cutaneous CD30$^+$ ALCL (CD30$^+$ lymphoproliferative diseases including lymphomatoid papulosis)
Lymphomatoid Papulosis	
Aggressive	
Sézary syndrome	Sézary syndrome
CD30$^-$ large T-cell lymphoma	Peripheral T-cell lymphoma, unspecified
Provisional entities	
CTCL, pleomorphic, small/medium-sized	Peripheral T-cell lymphoma, unspecified
Subcutaneous panniculitis-like T-cell lymphoma	Subcutaneous panniculitis-like T-cell lymphoma
Granulomatous slack skin	Granulomatous slack skin

Table 5. TNMB classification for MF/SS

T (skin)	
T1	limited patch/plaque (<10% of BSA)
T2	generalized patch/plaque(>10% of BSA)
T3	tumors
T4	generalized erythroderma
N (nodes)	
N0	no clinically abnormal peripheral lymphnodes
N1	clinically abnormal peripheral lymphnodes
NP0	biopsy performed, not CTCL
NP1	biopsy performed, CTCL
LNO	uninvolved
LN1	reactive lymph node
LN2	dermatopathic node, small clusters of convoluted cells (< 6 cells per cluster)
LN3*	dermatopathic node, small clusters of convoluted cells (> 6 cells per cluster)
LN4*	lymph node effacement
M (viscera)	
M0	no visceral metastasis
M1	visceral metastasis
B (blood)	
B0	atypical circulating cells not present (<5%)
B1	atypical circulating cells present (>5%)

Abbreviation: TNMB, tumor, node, metastasis, blood
*Pathologically involved lymph nodes

Table 6. Stage Classification for MS/SS

Stage	T	N	NP	M
IA	1	0	0	0
IB	2	0	0	0
IIA	1/2	1	0	0
IIB	3	0/1	0	0
III	4	0/1	0	0
IVA	1-4	0/1	1	0
IVB	1-4	0/1	0/1	1

12.   REFERENCES

1.   Rudiger T, Weisenburger DD, Anderson JR, et al. Peripheral T-cell lymphoma (excluding anaplastic large-cell lymphoma): results from the Non-Hodgkin's Lymphoma Classification Project. Ann Oncol. 2002;13:140-149.

2.   Armitage JO, Weisenburger DD. New approach to classifying non-Hodgkin's lymphomas: clinical features of the major histologic subtypes. Non-Hodgkin's Lymphoma Classification Project. J Clin Oncol. 1998;16:2780-2795.

3.   Gisselbrecht C, Gaulard P, Lepage E, et al. Prognostic significance of T-cell phenotype in aggressive non-Hodgkin's lymphomas. Groupe d'Etudes des Lymphomes de l'Adulte (GELA). Blood. 1998;92:76-82.

4.   Melnyk A, Rodriguez A, Pugh WC, Cabannillas F. Evaluation of the Revised European-American Lymphoma classification confirms the clinical relevance of immunophenotype in 560 cases of aggressive non-Hodgkin's lymphoma. Blood. 1997;89:4514-4520.

5.   Harris NL, Jaffe ES, Diebold J, et al. World Health Organization classification of neoplastic diseases of the hematopoietic and lymphoid tissues: report of the Clinical Advisory Committee meeting-Airlie House, Virginia, November 1997. J Clin Oncol. 1999;17:3835-3849.

6.   Rosenberg SA. Classification of lymphoid neoplasms. Blood. 1994;84:1359-1360.

7.   Borowitz MJ, Reichert TA, Brynes RK, et al. The phenotypic diversity of peripheral T-cell lymphomas: the Southeastern Cancer Study Group experience. Hum Pathol. 1986;17:567-574.

8.   Schlegelberger B, Feller AC. Classification of peripheral T-cell lymphomas: cytogenetic findings support the updated Kiel classification. Leuk Lymphoma. 1996;20:411-416.

9.   Itoyama T, Chaganti RS, Yamada Y, et al. Cytogenetic analysis and clinical significance in adult T-cell leukemia/lymphoma: a study of 50 cases from the human T-cell leukemia virus type-1 endemic area, Nagasaki. Blood. 2001;97:3612-3620.

10.   Weiss LM, Jaffe ES, Liu XF, Chen YY, Shibata D, Medeiros LJ. Detection and localization of Epstein-Barr viral genomes in angioimmunoblastic lymphadenopathy and angioimmunoblastic lymphadenopathy-like lymphoma. Blood. 1992;79:1789-1795.

11.   Luppi M, Barozzi P, Maiorana A, et al. Human herpesvirus-8 DNA sequences in human immunodeficiency virus-negative angioimmunoblastic lymphadenopathy and benign lymphadenopathy with giant germinal center hyperplasia and increased vascularity. Blood. 1996;87:3903-3909.

12.   Bianco E, Marcucci F, Mele A, et al. Prevalence of hepatitis C virus infection in lymphoproliferative diseases other than B-cell non-Hodgkin's lymphoma, and in myeloproliferative diseases: an Italian Multi-Center case-control study. Haematologica. 2004;89:70-76.

13.   Ohnita K, Isomoto H, Mizuta Y, et al. Helicobacter pylori infection in patients with gastric involvement by adult T-cell leukemia/lymphoma. Cancer. 2002;94:1507-1516.

14.   Hayday AC, Barber DF, Douglas N, Hoffman ES. Signals involved in gamma/delta T cell versus alpha/beta T cell lineage commitment. Semin Immunol. 1999;11:239-249.

15.   Falini B, Flenghi L, Pileri S, et al. Distribution of T cells bearing different forms of the T cell receptor gamma/delta in normal and pathological human tissues. J Immunol. 1989;143:2480-2488.

16.   Ota Y, Kobata T, Seki M, et al. Extrathymic origin of V gamma 1/V delta 6 T cells in the skin. Eur J Immunol. 1992;22:595-598.

17.   Bandeira A, Itohara S, Bonneville M, et al. Extrathymic origin of intestinal intraepithelial lymphocytes bearing T-cell antigen receptor gamma delta. Proc Natl Acad Sci U S A. 1991;88:43-47.

18. Kuppers R, Dalla-Favera R. Mechanisms of chromosomal translocations in B cell lymphomas. Oncogene. 2001;20:5580-5594.

19. Croce CM, Isobe M, Palumbo A, et al. Gene for alpha-chain of human T-cell receptor: location on chromosome 14 region involved in T-cell neoplasms. Science. 1985;227:1044-1047.

20. Foroni L, Foldi J, Matutes E, et al. Alpha, beta and gamma T-cell receptor genes: rearrangements correlate with haematological phenotype in T cell leukaemias. Br J Haematol. 1987;67:307-318.

21. Drexler HG, MacLeod RA, Borkhardt A, Janssen JW. Recurrent chromosomal translocations and fusion genes in leukemia-lymphoma cell lines. Leukemia. 1995;9:480-500.

22. Rabbitts TH. Chromosomal translocation master genes, mouse models and experimental therapeutics. Oncogene. 2001;20:5763-5777.

23. Knudson AG. Antioncogenes and human cancer. Proc Natl Acad Sci U S A. 1993;90:10914-10921.

24. Liggett WH, Jr., Sidransky D. Role of the p16 tumor suppressor gene in cancer. J Clin Oncol. 1998;16:1197-1206.

25. Johansson B, Billstrom R, Kristoffersson U, et al. Deletion of chromosome arm 3p in hematologic malignancies. Leukemia. 1997;11:1207-1213.

26. Hauptschein RS, Gamberi B, Rao PH, et al. Cloning and mapping of human chromosome 6q26-q27 deleted in B-cell non-Hodgkin lymphoma and multiple tumor types. Genomics. 1998;50:170-186.

27. Migliazza A, Bosch F, Komatsu H, et al. Nucleotide sequence, transcription map, and mutation analysis of the 13q14 chromosomal region deleted in B-cell chronic lymphocytic leukemia. Blood. 2001;97:2098-2104.

28. Kanavaros P, Lescs MC, Briere J, et al. Nasal T-cell lymphoma: a clinicopathologic entity associated with peculiar phenotype and with Epstein-Barr virus. Blood. 1993;81:2688-2695.

29. Harper JW, Adami GR, Wei N, Keyomarsi K, Elledge SJ. The p21 Cdk-interacting protein Cip1 is a potent inhibitor of G1 cyclin-dependent kinases. Cell. 1993;75:805-816.

30. el-Deiry WS, Tokino T, Velculescu VE, et al. WAF1, a potential mediator of p53 tumor suppression. Cell. 1993;75:817-825.

31. Gartenhaus RB. Microsatellite instability in hematologic malignancies. Leuk Lymphoma. 1997;25:455-461.

32. Rao PH, Houldsworth J, Dyomina K, et al. Chromosomal and gene amplification in diffuse large B-cell lymphoma. Blood. 1998;92:234-240.

33. Willenbrock K, Roers A, Seidl C, Wacker HH, Kuppers R, Hansmann ML. Analysis of T-cell subpopulations in T-cell non-Hodgkin's lymphoma of angioimmunoblastic lymphadenopathy with dysproteinemia type by single target gene amplification of T cell receptor- beta gene rearrangements. Am J Pathol. 2001;158:1851-1857.

34. Gamberi B, Gaidano G, Parsa N, et al. Microsatellite instability is rare in B-cell non-Hodgkin's lymphomas. Blood. 1997;89:975-979.

35. Prolla TA. DNA mismatch repair and cancer. Curr Opin Cell Biol. 1998;10:311-316.

36. Jemal A, Murray T, Samuels A, Ghafoor A, Ward E, Thun MJ. Cancer statistics, 2003. CA Cancer J Clin. 2003;53:5-26.

37. Pellatt J, Sweetenham J, Pickering RM, Brown L, Wilkins B. A single-centre study of treatment outcomes and survival in 120 patients with peripheral T-cell non-Hodgkin's lymphoma. Ann Hematol. 2002;81:267-272.

38. Gallamini A, Stelitano C, Calvi R, et al. Peripheral T-cell lymphoma unspecified (PTCL-U): a new prognostic model from a retrospective multicentric clinical study. Blood. 2003.

39.   Reiser M, Josting A, Soltani M, et al. T-cell non-Hodgkin's lymphoma in adults: clinicopathological characteristics, response to treatment and prognostic factors. Leuk Lymphoma. 2002;43:805-811.

40.   Karakas T, Bergmann L, Stutte HJ, et al. Peripheral T-cell lymphomas respond well to vincristine, adriamycin, cyclophosphamide, prednisone and etoposide (VACPE) and have a similar outcome as high-grade B-cell lymphomas. Leuk Lymphoma. 1996;24:121-129.

41.   Ansell SM, Habermann TM, Kurtin PJ, et al. Predictive capacity of the International Prognostic Factor Index in patients with peripheral T-cell lymphoma. J Clin Oncol. 1997;15:2296-2301.

42.   Cheng AL, Su IJ, Chen YC, Uen WC, Wang CH. Characteristic clinicopathologic features of Epstein-Barr virus-associated peripheral T-cell lymphoma. Cancer. 1993;72:909-916.

43.   Arrowsmith ER, Macon WR, Kinney MC, et al. Peripheral T-cell lymphomas: clinical features and prognostic factors of 92 cases defined by the revised European American lymphoma classification. Leuk Lymphoma. 2003;44:241-249.

44.   Takahashi N, Chubachi A, Kume M, et al. A clinical analysis of 52 adult patients with hemophagocytic syndrome: the prognostic significance of the underlying diseases. Int J Hematol. 2001;74:209-213.

45.   Goldschmidt N, Amir G, Krieger M, Gilead L, Paltiel O. Fatal hemophagocytic syndrome in a patient with panniculitis-like T-cell lymphoma and no clinical evidence of disease. Leuk Lymphoma. 2003;44:1803-1806.

46.   Su IJ, Wang CH, Cheng AL, Chen RL. Hemophagocytic syndrome in Epstein-Barr virus-associated T-lymphoproliferative disorders: disease spectrum, pathogenesis, and management. Leuk Lymphoma. 1995;19:401-406.

47.   Lay JD, Chuang SE, Rowe M, Su IJ. Epstein-barr virus latent membrane protein-1 mediates upregulation of tumor necrosis factor-alpha in EBV-infected T cells: implications for the pathogenesis of hemophagocytic syndrome. J Biomed Sci. 2003;10:146-155.

48.   Lepretre S, Buchonnet G, Stamatoullas A, et al. Chromosome abnormalities in peripheral T-cell lymphoma. Cancer Genet Cytogenet. 2000;117:71-79.

49.   Theodorou I, Bigorgne C, Delfau MH, et al. VJ rearrangements of the TCR gamma locus in peripheral T-cell lymphomas: analysis by polymerase chain reaction and denaturing gradient gel electrophoresis. J Pathol. 1996;178:303-310.

50.   Theodorou I, Raphael M, Bigorgne C, et al. Recombination pattern of the TCR gamma locus in human peripheral T-cell lymphomas. J Pathol. 1994;174:233-242.

51.   Schouten HC, Sanger WG, Weisenburger DD, Armitage JO. Chromosomal abnormalities in patients with non-cutaneous T-cell non-Hodgkin's lymphoma. The Nebraska Lymphoma Study Group. Eur J Cancer. 1990;26:618-622.

52.   Hatta Y, Yamada Y, Tomonaga M, Miyoshi I, Said JW, Koeffler HP. Detailed deletion mapping of the long arm of chromosome 6 in adult T-cell leukemia. Blood. 1999;93:613-616.

53.   Tagawa H, Miura I, Suzuki R, Suzuki H, Hosokawa Y, Seto M. Molecular cytogenetic analysis of the breakpoint region at 6q21-22 in T-cell lymphoma/leukemia cell lines. Genes Chromosomes Cancer. 2002;34:175-185.

54.   Hoshida Y, Hongyo T, Nakatsuka S, et al. Gene mutations in lymphoproliferative disorders of T and NK/T cell phenotypes developing in renal transplant patients. Lab Invest. 2002;82:257-264.

55.   Kanavaros P, Bai M, Stefanaki K, et al. Immunohistochemical expression of the p53, mdm2, p21/Waf-1, Rb, p16, Ki67, cyclin D1, cyclin A and cyclin B1 proteins and apoptotic index in T-cell lymphomas. Histol Histopathol. 2001;16:377-386.

56.   Moller MB, Gerdes AM, Skjodt K, Mortensen LS, Pedersen NT. Disrupted p53 function as predictor of treatment failure and poor prognosis in B- and T-cell non-Hodgkin's lymphoma. Clin Cancer Res. 1999;5:1085-1091.

57. Pescarmona E, Pignoloni P, Puopolo M, et al. p53 over-expression identifies a subset of nodal peripheral T-cell lymphomas with a distinctive biological profile and poor clinical outcome. J Pathol. 2001;195:361-366.

58. Gordon LI, Harrington D, Andersen J, et al. Comparison of a second-generation combination chemotherapeutic regimen (m-BACOD) with a standard regimen (CHOP) for advanced diffuse non-Hodgkin's lymphoma. N Engl J Med. 1992;327:1342-1349.

59. Fisher RI, Gaynor ER, Dahlberg S, et al. Comparison of a standard regimen (CHOP) with three intensive chemotherapy regimens for advanced non-Hodgkin's lymphoma. N Engl J Med. 1993;328:1002-1006.

60. Kurzrock R. Therapy of T cell lymphomas with pentostatin. Ann N Y Acad Sci. 2001;941:200-205.

61. Tsimberidou AM, Giles F, Duvic M, Fayad L, Kurzrock R. Phase II study of pentostatin in advanced T-cell lymphoid malignancies: update of an M.D. Anderson Cancer Center series. Cancer. 2004;100:342-349.

62. Dang NH, Hagemeister FB, Duvic M, et al. Pentostatin in T-non-Hodgkin's lymphomas: efficacy and effect on CD26+ T lymphocytes. Oncol Rep. 2003;10:1513-1518.

63. Mercieca J, Matutes E, Dearden C, MacLennan K, Catovsky D. The role of pentostatin in the treatment of T-cell malignancies: analysis of response rate in 145 patients according to disease subtype. J Clin Oncol. 1994;12:2588-2593.

64. Monfardini S, Sorio R, Cavalli F, et al. Pentostatin (2'-deoxycoformycin, dCF) in patients with low-grade (B-T-cell) and intermediate- and high-grade (T-cell) malignant lymphomas: phase II study of the EORTC Early Clinical Trials Group. Oncology. 1996;53:163-168.

65. Aldinucci D, Poletto D, Lorenzon D, et al. CD26 expression correlates with a reduced sensitivity to 2'-deoxycoformycin-induced growth inhibition and apoptosis in T-cell leukemia/lymphomas. Clin Cancer Res. 2004;10:508-520.

66. Sallah S, Wan JY, Nguyen NP. Treatment of refractory T-cell malignancies using gemcitabine. Br J Haematol. 2001;113:185-187.

67. Zinzani PL, Magagnoli M, Bendandi M, et al. Therapy with gemcitabine in pretreated peripheral T-cell lymphoma patients. Ann Oncol. 1998;9:1351-1353.

68. Chau I, Harries M, Cunningham D, et al. Gemcitabine, cisplatin and methylprednisolone chemotherapy (GEM-P) is an effective regimen in patients with poor prognostic primary progressive or multiply relapsed Hodgkin's and non-Hodgkin's lymphoma. Br J Haematol. 2003;120:970-977.

69. LeMaistre CF, Saleh MN, Kuzel TM, et al. Phase I trial of a ligand fusion-protein (DAB389IL-2) in lymphomas expressing the receptor for interleukin-2. Blood. 1998;91:399-405.

70. Talpur R, Apisarnthanarax N, Ward S, Duvic M. Treatment of refractory peripheral T-cell lymphoma with denileukin diftitox (ONTAK). Leuk Lymphoma. 2002;43:121-126.

71. Huang CL, Lin ZZ, Su IJ, et al. Combination of 13-cis retinoic acid and interferon-alpha in the treatment of recurrent or refractory peripheral T-cell lymphoma. Leuk Lymphoma. 2002;43:1415-1420.

72. Tsimberidou AM, Giles F, Romaguera J, Duvic M, Kurzrock R. Activity of interferon-alpha and isotretinoin in patients with advanced, refractory lymphoid malignancies. Cancer. 2004;100:574-580.

73. Imashuku S, Kuriyama K, Sakai R, et al. Treatment of Epstein-Barr virus-associated hemophagocytic lymphohistiocytosis (EBV-HLH) in young adults: a report from the HLH study center. Med Pediatr Oncol. 2003;41:103-109.

74. Siegert W, Nerl C, Agthe A, et al. Angioimmunoblastic lymphadenopathy (AILD)-type T-cell lymphoma: prognostic impact of clinical observations and laboratory findings at presentation. The Kiel Lymphoma Study Group. Ann Oncol. 1995;6:659-664.

75.   Weiss LM, Strickler JG, Dorfman RF, Horning SJ, Warnke RA, Sklar J. Clonal T-cell populations in angioimmunoblastic lymphadenopathy and angioimmunoblastic lymphadenopathy-like lymphoma. Am J Pathol. 1986;122:392-397.

76.   Suzuki H, Namikawa R, Ueda R, et al. Clonal T cell population in angioimmunoblastic lymphadenopathy and related lesions. Jpn J Cancer Res. 1987;78:712-720.

77.   Feller AC, Griesser H, Schilling CV, et al. Clonal gene rearrangement patterns correlate with immunophenotype and clinical parameters in patients with angioimmunoblastic lymphadenopathy. Am J Pathol. 1988;133:549-556.

78.   Lipford EH, Smith HR, Pittaluga S, Jaffe ES, Steinberg AD, Cossman J. Clonality of angioimmunoblastic lymphadenopathy and implications for its evolution to malignant lymphoma. J Clin Invest. 1987;79:637-642.

79.   Schlegelberger B, Zwingers T, Hohenadel K, et al. Significance of cytogenetic findings for the clinical outcome in patients with T-cell lymphoma of angioimmunoblastic lymphadenopathy type. J Clin Oncol. 1996;14:593-599.

80.   Kaneko Y, Maseki N, Sakurai M, et al. Characteristic karyotypic pattern in T-cell lymphoproliferative disorders with reactive "angioimmunoblastic lymphadenopathy with dysproteinemia-type" features. Blood. 1988;72:413-421.

81.   Schlegelberger B, Zhang Y, Weber-Matthiesen K, Grote W. Detection of aberrant clones in nearly all cases of angioimmunoblastic lymphadenopathy with dysproteinemia-type T-cell lymphoma by combined interphase and metaphase cytogenetics. Blood. 1994;84:2640-2648.

82.   Schlegelberger B, Nolle I, Feller AC, Bauer E, Grote W. Angioimmunoblastic lymphadenopathy with trisomy 3: the cells of the malignant clone are T cells. Hematol Pathol. 1990;4:179-183.

83.   Klinman DM, Steinberg AD, Mushinski JF. Effect of cyclophosphamide therapy on oncogene expression in angioimmunoblastic lymphadenopathy. Lancet. 1986;2:1055-1058.

84.   Smith JL, Hodges E, Quin CT, McCarthy KP, Wright DH. Frequent T and B cell oligoclones in histologically and immunophenotypically characterized angioimmunoblastic lymphadenopathy. Am J Pathol. 2000;156:661-669.

85.   Anagnostopoulos I, Hummel M, Finn T, et al. Heterogeneous Epstein-Barr virus infection patterns in peripheral T-cell lymphoma of angioimmunoblastic lymphadenopathy type. Blood. 1992;80:1804-1812.

86.   Brauninger A, Spieker T, Willenbrock K, et al. Survival and clonal expansion of mutating "forbidden" (immunoglobulin receptor-deficient) epstein-barr virus-infected b cells in angioimmunoblastic t cell lymphoma. J Exp Med. 2001;194:927-940.

87.   Sallah S, Gagnon GA. Angioimmunoblastic lymphadenopathy with dysproteinemia: emphasis on pathogenesis and treatment. Acta Haematol. 1998;99:57-64.

88.   Siegert W, Agthe A, Griesser H, et al. Treatment of angioimmunoblastic lymphadenopathy (AILD)-type T-cell lymphoma using prednisone with or without the COPBLAM/IMVP-16 regimen. A multicenter study. Kiel Lymphoma Study Group. Ann Intern Med. 1992;117:364-370.

89.   Quintini G, Iannitto E, Barbera V, et al. Response to low-dose oral methotrexate and prednisone in two patients with angio-immunoblastic lymphadenopathy-type T-cell lymphoma. Hematol J. 2001;2:393-395.

90.   Gerlando Q, Barbera V, Ammatuna E, Franco V, Florena AM, Mariani G. Successful treatment of angioimmunoblastic lymphadenopathy with dysproteinemia-type T-cell lymphoma by combined methotrexate and prednisone. Haematologica. 2000;85:880-881.

91.   Tsatalas C, Margaritis D, Kaloutsi V, Martinis G, Kotsianidis I, Bourikas G. Successful treatment of angioimmunoblastic lymphadenopathy with dysproteinemia-type T-cell lymphoma with fludarabine. Acta Haematol. 2001;105:106-108.

92. Hast R, Jacobsson B, Petrescu A, Hjalmar V. Successful treatment with fludarabine in two cases of angioimmunoblastic lymphadenopathy with dysproteinemia. Leuk Lymphoma. 1999;34:597-601.

93. Sallah S, Wehbie R, Lepera P, Sallah W, Bobzien W. The role of 2-chlorodeoxyadenosine in the treatment of patients with refractory angioimmunoblastic lymphadenopathy with dysproteinemia. Br J Haematol. 1999;104:163-165.

94. Murayama T, Imoto S, Takahashi T, Ito M, Matozaki S, Nakagawa T. Successful treatment of angioimmunoblastic lymphadenopathy with dysproteinemia with cyclosporin A. Cancer. 1992;69:2567-2570.

95. Takemori N, Kodaira J, Toyoshima N, et al. Successful treatment of immunoblastic lymphadenopathy-like T-cell lymphoma with cyclosporin A. Leuk Lymphoma. 1999;35:389-395.

96. Gascoyne RD, Aoun P, Wu D, et al. Prognostic significance of anaplastic lymphoma kinase (ALK) protein expression in adults with anaplastic large cell lymphoma. Blood. 1999;93:3913-3921.

97. Suzuki R, Kagami Y, Takeuchi K, et al. Prognostic significance of CD56 expression for ALK-positive and ALK-negative anaplastic large-cell lymphoma of T/null cell phenotype. Blood. 2000;96:2993-3000.

98. Falini B, Pileri S, Zinzani PL, et al. ALK+ lymphoma: clinico-pathological findings and outcome. Blood. 1999;93:2697-2706.

99. Simonitsch I, Panzer-Gruemayer ER, Ghali DW, et al. NPM/ALK gene fusion transcripts identify a distinct subgroup of null type Ki-1 positive anaplastic large cell lymphomas. Br J Haematol. 1996;92:866-871.

100. Tkachuk DC, Griesser H, Takihara Y, et al. Rearrangement of T-cell delta locus in lymphoproliferative disorders. Blood. 1988;72:353-357.

101. Foss HD, Anagnostopoulos I, Araujo I, et al. Anaplastic large-cell lymphomas of T-cell and null-cell phenotype express cytotoxic molecules. Blood. 1996;88:4005-4011.

102. Chhanabhai M, Adomat SA, Gascoyne RD, Horsman DE. Clinical utility of heteroduplex analysis of TCR gamma gene rearrangements in the diagnosis of T-cell lymphoproliferative disorders. Am J Clin Pathol. 1997;108:295-301.

103. Weisenburger DD, Anderson JR, Diebold J, et al. Systemic anaplastic large-cell lymphoma: results from the non-Hodgkin's lymphoma classification project. Am J Hematol. 2001;67:172-178.

104. Haralambieva E, Pulford KA, Lamant L, et al. Anaplastic large-cell lymphomas of B-cell phenotype are anaplastic lymphoma kinase (ALK) negative and belong to the spectrum of diffuse large B-cell lymphomas. Br J Haematol. 2000;109:584-591.

105. Kaneko Y, Frizzera G, Edamura S, et al. A novel translocation, t(2;5)(p23;q35), in childhood phagocytic large T-cell lymphoma mimicking malignant histiocytosis. Blood. 1989;73:806-813.

106. Fischer P, Nacheva E, Mason DY, et al. A Ki-1 (CD30)-positive human cell line (Karpas 299) established from a high-grade non-Hodgkin's lymphoma, showing a 2;5 translocation and rearrangement of the T-cell receptor beta-chain gene. Blood. 1988;72:234-240.

107. Weisenburger DD, Gordon BG, Vose JM, et al. Occurrence of the t(2;5)(p23;q35) in non-Hodgkin's lymphoma. Blood. 1996;87:3860-3868.

108. Pulford K, Lamant L, Morris SW, et al. Detection of anaplastic lymphoma kinase (ALK) and nucleolar protein nucleophosmin (NPM)-ALK proteins in normal and neoplastic cells with the monoclonal antibody ALK1. Blood. 1997;89:1394-1404.

109. Lamant L, Meggetto F, al Saati T, et al. High incidence of the t(2;5)(p23;q35) translocation in anaplastic large cell lymphoma and its lack of detection in Hodgkin's disease. Comparison of cytogenetic analysis, reverse transcriptase-polymerase chain reaction, and P-80 immunostaining. Blood. 1996;87:284-291.

110. Morris SW, Kirstein MN, Valentine MB, et al. Fusion of a kinase gene, ALK, to a nucleolar protein gene, NPM, in non-Hodgkin's lymphoma. Science. 1994;263:1281-1284.

111. Yee HT, Ponzoni M, Merson A, et al. Molecular characterization of the t(2;5) (p23; q35) translocation in anaplastic large cell lymphoma (Ki-1) and Hodgkin's disease. Blood. 1996;87:1081-1088.

112. Fujimoto J, Shiota M, Iwahara T, et al. Characterization of the transforming activity of p80, a hyperphosphorylated protein in a Ki-1 lymphoma cell line with chromosomal translocation t(2;5). Proc Natl Acad Sci U S A. 1996;93:4181-4186.

113. Stein H, Foss HD, Durkop H, et al. CD30(+) anaplastic large cell lymphoma: a review of its histopathologic, genetic, and clinical features. Blood. 2000;96:3681-3695.

114. Mathew P, Sanger WG, Weisenburger DD, et al. Detection of the t(2;5)(p23;q35) and NPM-ALK fusion in non-Hodgkin's lymphoma by two-color fluorescence in situ hybridization. Blood. 1997;89:1678-1685.

115. Benharroch D, Meguerian-Bedoyan Z, Lamant L, et al. ALK-positive lymphoma: a single disease with a broad spectrum of morphology. Blood. 1998;91:2076-2084.

116. Falini B, Pulford K, Pucciarini A, et al. Lymphomas expressing ALK fusion protein(s) other than NPM-ALK. Blood. 1999;94:3509-3515.

117. Lamant L, Dastugue N, Pulford K, Delsol G, Mariame B. A new fusion gene TPM3-ALK in anaplastic large cell lymphoma created by a (1;2)(q25;p23) translocation. Blood. 1999;93:3088-3095.

118. Pulford K, Falini B, Cordell J, et al. Biochemical detection of novel anaplastic lymphoma kinase proteins in tissue sections of anaplastic large cell lymphoma. Am J Pathol. 1999;154:1657-1663.

119. Rosenwald A, Ott G, Pulford K, et al. t(1;2)(q21;p23) and t(2;3)(p23;q21): two novel variant translocations of the t(2;5)(p23;q35) in anaplastic large cell lymphoma. Blood. 1999;94:362-364.

120. Siebert R, Gesk S, Harder L, et al. Complex variant translocation t(1;2) with TPM3-ALK fusion due to cryptic ALK gene rearrangement in anaplastic large-cell lymphoma. Blood. 1999;94:3614-3617.

121. Hernandez L, Pinyol M, Hernandez S, et al. TRK-fused gene (TFG) is a new partner of ALK in anaplastic large cell lymphoma producing two structurally different TFG-ALK translocations. Blood. 1999;94:3265-3268.

122. Touriol C, Greenland C, Lamant L, et al. Further demonstration of the diversity of chromosomal changes involving 2p23 in ALK-positive lymphoma: 2 cases expressing ALK kinase fused to CLTCL (clathrin chain polypeptide-like). Blood. 2000;95:3204-3207.

123. Trinei M, Lanfrancone L, Campo E, et al. A new variant anaplastic lymphoma kinase (ALK)-fusion protein (ATIC-ALK) in a case of ALK-positive anaplastic large cell lymphoma. Cancer Res. 2000;60:793-798.

124. Wlodarska I, De Wolf-Peeters C, Falini B, et al. The cryptic inv(2)(p23q35) defines a new molecular genetic subtype of ALK-positive anaplastic large-cell lymphoma. Blood. 1998;92:2688-2695.

125. Ma Z, Cools J, Marynen P, et al. Inv(2)(p23q35) in anaplastic large-cell lymphoma induces constitutive anaplastic lymphoma kinase (ALK) tyrosine kinase activation by fusion to ATIC, an enzyme involved in purine nucleotide biosynthesis. Blood. 2000;95:2144-2149.

126. Gascoyne RD, Lamant L, Martin-Subero JI, et al. ALK-positive diffuse large B-cell lymphoma is associated with Clathrin-ALK rearrangements: report of 6 cases. Blood. 2003;102:2568-2573.

127. Shiota M, Fujimoto J, Semba T, Satoh H, Yamamoto T, Mori S. Hyperphosphorylation of a novel 80 kDa protein-tyrosine kinase similar to Ltk in a human Ki-1 lymphoma cell line, AMS3. Oncogene. 1994;9:1567-1574.

128. Lamant L, Pulford K, Bischof D, et al. Expression of the ALK tyrosine kinase gene in neuroblastoma. Am J Pathol. 2000;156:1711-1721.

129. Falini B, Bigerna B, Fizzotti M, et al. ALK expression defines a distinct group of T/null lymphomas ("ALK lymphomas") with a wide morphological spectrum. Am J Pathol. 1998;153:875-886.
130. Griffin CA, Hawkins AL, Dvorak C, Henkle C, Ellingham T, Perlman EJ. Recurrent involvement of 2p23 in inflammatory myofibroblastic tumors. Cancer Res. 1999;59:2776-2780.
131. Trumper L, Pfreundschuh M, Bonin FV, Daus H. Detection of the t(2;5)-associated NPM/ALK fusion cDNA in peripheral blood cells of healthy individuals. Br J Haematol. 1998;103:1138-1144.
132. ten Berge RL, Meijer CJ, Dukers DF, et al. Expression levels of apoptosis-related proteins predict clinical outcome in anaplastic large cell lymphoma. Blood. 2002;99:4540-4546.
133. Pinyol M, Cobo F, Bea S, et al. p16(INK4a) gene inactivation by deletions, mutations, and hypermethylation is associated with transformed and aggressive variants of non-Hodgkin's lymphomas. Blood. 1998;91:2977-2984.
134. Inghirami G, Macri L, Cesarman E, Chadburn A, Zhong J, Knowles DM. Molecular characterization of CD30+ anaplastic large-cell lymphoma: high frequency of c-myc proto-oncogene activation. Blood. 1994;83:3581-3590.
135. Herbst H, Dallenbach F, Hummel M, et al. Epstein-Barr virus DNA and latent gene products in Ki-1 (CD30)-positive anaplastic large cell lymphomas. Blood. 1991;78:2666-2673.
136. Bai RY, Ouyang T, Miething C, Morris SW, Peschel C, Duyster J. Nucleophosmin-anaplastic lymphoma kinase associated with anaplastic large-cell lymphoma activates the phosphatidylinositol 3-kinase/Akt antiapoptotic signaling pathway. Blood. 2000;96:4319-4327.
137. Slupianek A, Nieborowska-Skorska M, Hoser G, et al. Role of phosphatidylinositol 3-kinase-Akt pathway in nucleophosmin/anaplastic lymphoma kinase-mediated lymphomagenesis. Cancer Res. 2001;61:2194-2199.
138. Gaiser T, Thorns C, Merz H, Noack F, Feller AC, Lange K. Gene profiling in anaplastic large-cell lymphoma-derived cell lines with cDNA expression arrays. J Hematother Stem Cell Res. 2002;11:423-428.
139. Seidemann K, Tiemann M, Schrappe M, et al. Short-pulse B-non-Hodgkin lymphoma-type chemotherapy is efficacious treatment for pediatric anaplastic large cell lymphoma: a report of the Berlin-Frankfurt-Munster Group Trial NHL-BFM 90. Blood. 2001;97:3699-3706.
140. Willemze R, Kerl H, Sterry W, et al. EORTC classification for primary cutaneous lymphomas: a proposal from the Cutaneous Lymphoma Study Group of the European Organization for Research and Treatment of Cancer. Blood. 1997;90:354-371.
141. Russell-Jones R. World Health Organization classification of hematopoietic and lymphoid tissues: implications for dermatology. J Am Acad Dermatol. 2003;48:93-102.
142. Sander CA, Flaig MJ, Jaffe ES. Cutaneous manifestations of lymphoma: a clinical guide based on the WHO classification. World Health Organization. Clin Lymphoma. 2001;2:86-100; discussion 101-102.
143. Chan JK, Banks PM, Cleary ML, et al. A revised European-American classification of lymphoid neoplasms proposed by the International Lymphoma Study Group. A summary version. Am J Clin Pathol. 1995;103:543-560.
144. Fink-Puches R, Zenahlik P, Back B, Smolle J, Kerl H, Cerroni L. Primary cutaneous lymphomas: applicability of current classification schemes (European Organization for Research and Treatment of Cancer, World Health Organization) based on clinicopathologic features observed in a large group of patients. Blood. 2002;99:800-805.
145. Drillenburg P, Pals ST. Cell adhesion receptors in lymphoma dissemination. Blood. 2000;95:1900-1910.

146. Kansas GS. Selectins and their ligands: current concepts and controversies. Blood. 1996;88:3259-3287.

147. Weinstock MA, Gardstein B. Twenty-year trends in the reported incidence of mycosis fungoides and associated mortality. Am J Public Health. 1999;89:1240-1244.

148. Zackheim HS, McCalmont TH. Mycosis fungoides: the great imitator. J Am Acad Dermatol. 2002;47:914-918.

149. Pujol RM, Gallardo F, Llistosella E, et al. Invisible mycosis fungoides: a diagnostic challenge. J Am Acad Dermatol. 2002;47:S168-171.

150. van Doorn R, Scheffer E, Willemze R. Follicular mycosis fungoides, a distinct disease entity with or without associated follicular mucinosis: a clinicopathologic and follow-up study of 51 patients. Arch Dermatol. 2002;138:191-198.

151. Haghighi B, Smoller BR, LeBoit PE, Warnke RA, Sander CA, Kohler S. Pagetoid reticulosis (Woringer-Kolopp disease): an immunophenotypic, molecular, and clinicopathologic study. Mod Pathol. 2000;13:502-510.

152. Fung MA, Murphy MJ, Hoss DM, Grant-Kels JM. Practical evaluation and management of cutaneous lymphoma. J Am Acad Dermatol. 2002;46:325-357; quiz, 358-360.

153. Lu D, Patel KA, Duvic M, Jones D. Clinical and pathological spectrum of CD8-positive cutaneous T-cell lymphomas. J Cutan Pathol. 2002;29:465-472.

154. Delfau-Larue MH, Laroche L, Wechsler J, et al. Diagnostic value of dominant T-cell clones in peripheral blood in 363 patients presenting consecutively with a clinical suspicion of cutaneous lymphoma. Blood. 2000;96:2987-2992.

155. Luftl M, Feng A, Licha E, Schuler G. Dendritic cells and apoptosis in mycosis fungoides. Br J Dermatol. 2002;147:1171-1179.

156. Lee BN, Duvic M, Tang CK, Bueso-Ramos C, Estrov Z, Reuben JM. Dysregulated synthesis of intracellular type 1 and type 2 cytokines by T cells of patients with cutaneous T-cell lymphoma. Clin Diagn Lab Immunol. 1999;6:79-84.

157. Rook AH, Vowels BR, Jaworsky C, Singh A, Lessin SR. The immunopathogenesis of cutaneous T-cell lymphoma. Abnormal cytokine production by Sezary T cells. Arch Dermatol. 1993;129:486-489.

158. Navas IC, Algara P, Mateo M, et al. p16(INK4a) is selectively silenced in the tumoral progression of mycosis fungoides. Lab Invest. 2002;82:123-132.

159. Scarisbrick JJ, Woolford AJ, Calonje E, et al. Frequent abnormalities of the p15 and p16 genes in mycosis fungoides and sezary syndrome. J Invest Dermatol. 2002;118:493-499.

160. Qin JZ, Kamarashev J, Zhang CL, Dummer R, Burg G, Dobbeling U. Constitutive and interleukin-7- and interleukin-15-stimulated DNA binding of STAT and novel factors in cutaneous T cell lymphoma cells. J Invest Dermatol. 2001;117:583-589.

161. Dereure O, Levi E, Vonderheid EC, Kadin ME. Infrequent Fas mutations but no Bax or p53 mutations in early mycosis fungoides: a possible mechanism for the accumulation of malignant T lymphocytes in the skin. J Invest Dermatol. 2002;118:949-956.

162. Nielsen M, Kaltoft K, Nordahl M, et al. Constitutive activation of a slowly migrating isoform of Stat3 in mycosis fungoides: tyrphostin AG490 inhibits Stat3 activation and growth of mycosis fungoides tumor cell lines. Proc Natl Acad Sci U S A. 1997;94:6764-6769.

163. Garatti SA, Roscetti E, Trecca D, Fracchiolla NS, Neri A, Berti E. bcl-1, bcl-2, p53, c-myc, and lyt-10 analysis in cutaneous lymphomas. Recent Results Cancer Res. 1995;139:249-261.

164. Mao X, Lillington D, Scarisbrick JJ, et al. Molecular cytogenetic analysis of cutaneous T-cell lymphomas: identification of common genetic alterations in Sezary syndrome and mycosis fungoides. Br J Dermatol. 2002;147:464-475.

165. Kim YH, Liu HL, Mraz-Gernhard S, Varghese A, Hoppe RT. Long-term outcome of 525 patients with mycosis fungoides and Sezary syndrome: clinical prognostic factors and risk for disease progression. Arch Dermatol. 2003;139:857-866.

166. Grange F, Bagot M. [Prognosis of primary cutaneous lymphomas]. Ann Dermatol Venereol. 2002;129:30-40.

167. Vergier B, de Muret A, Beylot-Barry M, et al. Transformation of mycosis fungoides: clinicopathological and prognostic features of 45 cases. French Study Group of Cutaneious Lymphomas. Blood. 2000;95:2212-2218.

168. Hoppe RT, Medeiros LJ, Warnke RA, Wood GS. CD8-positive tumor-infiltrating lymphocytes influence the long-term survival of patients with mycosis fungoides. J Am Acad Dermatol. 1995;32:448-453.

169. Toro JR, Liewehr DJ, Pabby N, et al. Gamma-delta T-cell phenotype is associated with significantly decreased survival in cutaneous T-cell lymphoma. Blood. 2003;101:3407-3412.

170. Querfeld C, Guitart J, Kuzel TM, Rosen ST. Primary cutaneous lymphomas: a review with current treatment options. Blood Rev. 2003;17:131-142.

171. Vonderheid EC, Bernengo MG, Burg G, et al. Update on erythrodermic cutaneous T-cell lymphoma: report of the International Society for Cutaneous Lymphomas. J Am Acad Dermatol. 2002;46:95-106.

172. Bunn PA, Jr., Lamberg SI. Report of the Committee on Staging and Classification of Cutaneous T-Cell Lymphomas. Cancer Treat Rep. 1979;63:725-728.

173. Rosen ST, Foss FM. Chemotherapy for mycosis fungoides and the Sezary syndrome. Hematol Oncol Clin North Am. 1995;9:1109-1116.

174. Herrmann JJ, Roenigk HH, Jr., Hurria A, et al. Treatment of mycosis fungoides with photochemotherapy (PUVA): long-term follow-up. J Am Acad Dermatol. 1995;33:234-242.

175. Stern RS, Bolshakov S, Nataraj AJ, Ananthaswamy HN. p53 mutation in nonmelanoma skin cancers occurring in psoralen ultraviolet a-treated patients: evidence for heterogeneity and field cancerization. J Invest Dermatol. 2002;119:522-526.

176. Gathers RC, Scherschun L, Malick F, Fivenson DP, Lim HW. Narrowband UVB phototherapy for early-stage mycosis fungoides. J Am Acad Dermatol. 2002;47:191-197.

177. Plettenberg H, Stege H, Megahed M, et al. Ultraviolet A1 (340-400 nm) phototherapy for cutaneous T-cell lymphoma. J Am Acad Dermatol. 1999;41:47-50.

178. Jones GW, Kacinski BM, Wilson LD, et al. Total skin electron radiation in the management of mycosis fungoides: Consensus of the European Organization for Research and Treatment of Cancer (EORTC) Cutaneous Lymphoma Project Group. J Am Acad Dermatol. 2002;47:364-370.

179. Breneman D, Duvic M, Kuzel T, Yocum R, Truglia J, Stevens VJ. Phase 1 and 2 trial of bexarotene gel for skin-directed treatment of patients with cutaneous T-cell lymphoma. Arch Dermatol. 2002;138:325-332.

180. Kim YH, Martinez G, Varghese A, Hoppe RT. Topical nitrogen mustard in the management of mycosis fungoides: update of the Stanford experience. Arch Dermatol. 2003;139:165-173.

181. Zackheim HS. Topical carmustine (BCNU) in the treatment of mycosis fungoides. Dermatol Ther. 2003;16:299-302.

182. Siegel RS, Pandolfino T, Guitart J, Rosen S, Kuzel TM. Primary cutaneous T-cell lymphoma: review and current concepts. J Clin Oncol. 2000;18:2908-2925.

183. Rupoli S, Barulli S, Guiducci B, et al. Low dose interferon-alpha2b combined with PUVA is an effective treatment of early stage mycosis fungoides: results of a multicenter study. Cutaneous-T Cell Lymphoma Multicenter Study Group. Haematologica. 1999;84:809-813.

184. Chiarion-Sileni V, Bononi A, Fornasa CV, et al. Phase II trial of interferon-alpha-2a plus psolaren with ultraviolet light A in patients with cutaneous T-cell lymphoma. Cancer. 2002;95:569-575.

185. Molin L, Thomsen K, Volden G, et al. Oral retinoids in mycosis fungoides and Sezary syndrome: a comparison of isotretinoin and etretinate. A study from the Scandinavian Mycosis Fungoides Group. Acta Derm Venereol. 1987;67:232-236.

186. Suchin KR, Cucchiara AJ, Gottleib SL, et al. Treatment of cutaneous T-cell lymphoma with combined immunomodulatory therapy: a 14-year experience at a single institution. Arch Dermatol. 2002;138:1054-1060.

187. Duvic M, Hymes K, Heald P, et al. Bexarotene is effective and safe for treatment of refractory advanced-stage cutaneous T-cell lymphoma: multinational phase II-III trial results. J Clin Oncol. 2001;19:2456-2471.

188. Heald P, Mehlmauer M, Martin AG, Crowley CA, Yocum RC, Reich SD. Topical bexarotene therapy for patients with refractory or persistent early-stage cutaneous T-cell lymphoma: results of the phase III clinical trial. J Am Acad Dermatol. 2003;49:801-815.

189. Querfeld C, Guitart J, Rademaker A, Fung SB, Kuzel TM. Comparison of selective RAR and RXR retinoid mediated efficacy, tolerance, and survival in refractory cutaneous T-cell lymphoma. J Am Acad Dermatol. 2004; in press.

190. Wollina U, Dummer R, Brockmeyer NH, et al. Multicenter study of pegylated liposomal doxorubicin in patients with cutaneous T-cell lymphoma. Cancer. 2003;98:993-1001.

191. Dolan ME, McRae BL, Ferries-Rowe E, et al. O6-alkylguanine-DNA alkyltransferase in cutaneous T-cell lymphoma: implications for treatment with alkylating agents. Clin Cancer Res. 1999;5:2059-2064.

192. Foss FM. DAB(389)IL-2 (ONTAK): a novel fusion toxin therapy for lymphoma. Clin Lymphoma. 2000;1:110-116; discussion 117.

193. Dearden CE, Matutes E, Catovsky D. Alemtuzumab in T-cell malignancies. Med Oncol. 2002;19 Suppl:S27-32.

194. Lundin J, Hagberg H, Repp R, et al. Phase 2 study of alemtuzumab (anti-CD52 monoclonal antibody) in patients with advanced mycosis fungoides/Sezary syndrome. Blood. 2003;101:4267-4272.

195. Guitart J, Wickless SC, Oyama Y, et al. Long-term remission after allogeneic hematopoietic stem cell transplantation for refractory cutaneous T-cell lymphoma. Arch Dermatol. 2002;138:1359-1365.

196. Zaki MH, Wysocka M, Everetts SE, et al. Synergistic enhancement of cell-mediated immunity by interleukin-12 plus interleukin-2: basis for therapy of cutaneous T cell lymphoma. J Invest Dermatol. 2002;118:366-371.

197. Jakob T, Walker PS, Krieg AM, Udey MC, Vogel JC. Activation of cutaneous dendritic cells by CpG-containing oligodeoxynucleotides: a role for dendritic cells in the augmentation of Th1 responses by immunostimulatory DNA. J Immunol. 1998;161:3042-3049.

198. Davila E, Celis E. Repeated administration of cytosine-phosphorothiolated guanine-containing oligonucleotides together with peptide/protein immunization results in enhanced CTL responses with anti-tumor activity. J Immunol. 2000;165:539-547.

199. Wang HH, Myers T, Lach LJ, Hsieh CC, Kadin ME. Increased risk of lymphoid and nonlymphoid malignancies in patients with lymphomatoid papulosis. Cancer. 1999;86:1240-1245.

200. LeBoit PE. Lymphomatoid papulosis and cutaneous CD30+ lymphoma. Am J Dermatopathol. 1996;18:221-235.

201. Steinhoff M, Hummel M, Anagnostopoulos I, et al. Single-cell analysis of CD30+ cells in lymphomatoid papulosis demonstrates a common clonal T-cell origin. Blood. 2002;100:578-584.

202. Kempf W, Levi E, Kamarashev J, et al. Fascin expression in CD30-positive cutaneous lymphoproliferative disorders. J Cutan Pathol. 2002;29:295-300.

203. Gniadecki R, Rossen K. Expression of T-cell activation marker CD134 (OX40) in lymphomatoid papulosis. Br J Dermatol. 2003;148:885-891.

204. Bekkenk MW, Geelen FA, van Voorst Vader PC, et al. Primary and secondary cutaneous CD30(+) lymphoproliferative disorders: a report from the Dutch Cutaneous Lymphoma Group on the long-term follow-up data of 219 patients and guidelines for diagnosis and treatment. Blood. 2000;95:3653-3661.

205. Tilly H, Gaulard P, Lepage E, et al. Primary anaplastic large-cell lymphoma in adults: clinical presentation, immunophenotype, and outcome. Blood. 1997;90:3727-3734.

206. Mori M, Manuelli C, Pimpinelli N, et al. CD30-CD30 ligand interaction in primary cutaneous CD30(+) T-cell lymphomas: A clue to the pathophysiology of clinical regression. Blood. 1999;94:3077-3083.

207. Natkunam Y, Warnke RA, Haghighi B, et al. Co-expression of CD56 and CD30 in lymphomas with primary presentation in the skin: clinicopathologic, immunohistochemical and molecular analyses of seven cases. J Cutan Pathol. 2000;27:392-399.

208. Schiemann WP, Pfeifer WM, Levi E, Kadin ME, Lodish HF. A deletion in the gene for transforming growth factor beta type I receptor abolishes growth regulation by transforming growth factor beta in a cutaneous T-cell lymphoma. Blood. 1999;94:2854-2861.

209. Yagi H, Tokura Y, Furukawa F, Takigawa M. Th2 cytokine mRNA expression in primary cutaneous CD30-positive lymphoproliferative disorders: successful treatment with recombinant interferon-gamma. J Invest Dermatol. 1996;107:827-832.

210. French LE, Shapiro M, Junkins-Hopkins JM, Vittorio CC, Rook AH. Regression of multifocal, skin-restricted, CD30-positive large T-cell lymphoma with interferon alfa and bexarotene therapy. J Am Acad Dermatol. 2001;45:914-918.

211. Vermeer MH, Tensen CP, van der Stoop PM, et al. Absence of T(H)2 cytokine messenger RNA expression in CD30-negative primary cutaneous large T-cell lymphomas. Arch Dermatol. 2001;137:901-905.

212. Beljaards RC, Meijer CJ, Van der Putte SC, et al. Primary cutaneous T-cell lymphoma: clinicopathological features and prognostic parameters of 35 cases other than mycosis fungoides and CD30-positive large cell lymphoma. J Pathol. 1994;172:53-60.

213. Bekkenk MW, Vermeer MH, Jansen PM, et al. Peripheral T-cell lymphomas unspecified presenting in the skin: analysis of prognostic factors in a group of 82 patients. Blood. 2003;102:2213-2219.

214. Friedmann D, Wechsler J, Delfau MH, et al. Primary cutaneous pleomorphic small T-cell lymphoma. A review of 11 cases. The French Study Group on Cutaneous Lymphomas. Arch Dermatol. 1995;131:1009-1015.

215. Kumar S, Krenacs L, Medeiros J, et al. Subcutaneous panniculitic T-cell lymphoma is a tumor of cytotoxic T lymphocytes. Hum Pathol. 1998;29:397-403.

216. Salhany KE, Macon WR, Choi JK, et al. Subcutaneous panniculitis-like T-cell lymphoma: clinicopathologic, immunophenotypic, and genotypic analysis of alpha/beta and gamma/delta subtypes. Am J Surg Pathol. 1998;22:881-893.

217. Marzano AV, Berti E, Paulli M, Caputo R. Cytophagic histiocytic panniculitis and subcutaneous panniculitis-like T-cell lymphoma: report of 7 cases. Arch Dermatol. 2000;136:889-896.

218. Barron DR, Davis BR, Pomeranz JR, Hines JD, Park CH. Cytophagic histiocytic panniculitis. A variant of malignant histiocytosis. Cancer. 1985;55:2538-2542.

219. Craig AJ, Cualing H, Thomas G, Lamerson C, Smith R. Cytophagic histiocytic panniculitis--a syndrome associated with benign and malignant panniculitis: case comparison and review of the literature. J Am Acad Dermatol. 1998;39:721-736.

220. Requena L, Sanchez Yus E. Panniculitis. Part II. Mostly lobular panniculitis. J Am Acad Dermatol. 2001;45:325-361; quiz 362-324.

221. Wick MR, Patterson JW. Cytophagic histiocytic panniculitis--a critical reappraisal. Arch Dermatol. 2000;136:922-924.

222. Gonzalez CL, Medeiros LJ, Braziel RM, Jaffe ES. T-cell lymphoma involving subcutaneous tissue. A clinicopathologic entity commonly associated with hemophagocytic syndrome. Am J Surg Pathol. 1991;15:17-27.

223. Romero LS, Goltz RW, Nagi C, Shin SS, Ho AD. Subcutaneous T-cell lymphoma with associated hemophagocytic syndrome and terminal leukemic transformation. J Am Acad Dermatol. 1996;34:904-910.

224. Sajben FP, Schmidt C. Subcutaneous T-cell lymphoma: a case report and additional observations. Cutis. 1996;58:297-302.

225. Przybylski GK, Wu H, Macon WR, et al. Hepatosplenic and subcutaneous panniculitis-like gamma/delta T cell lymphomas are derived from different Vdelta subsets of gamma/delta T lymphocytes. J Mol Diagn. 2000;2:11-19.

226. Macon WR, Levy NB, Kurtin PJ, et al. Hepatosplenic alphabeta T-cell lymphomas: a report of 14 cases and comparison with hepatosplenic gammadelta T-cell lymphomas. Am J Surg Pathol. 2001;25:285-296.

227. Kadin ME. Cutaneous gamma delta T-cell lymphomas--how and why should they be recognized? Arch Dermatol. 2000;136:1052-1054.

228. Takihara Y, Tkachuk D, Michalopoulos E, et al. Sequence and organization of the diversity, joining, and constant region genes of the human T-cell delta-chain locus. Proc Natl Acad Sci U S A. 1988;85:6097-6101.

229. Mizutani Y, Iwamasa K, Arai J, Sakai I, Yasukawa M, Fujita S. [Subcutaneous panniculitic T-cell lymphoma with chromosomal abnormalities and large granular lymphocytes morphology]. Rinsho Ketsueki. 2000;41:519-523.

230. Au WY, Ng WM, Choy C, Kwong YL. Aggressive subcutaneous panniculitis-like T-cell lymphoma: complete remission with fludarabine, mitoxantrone and dexamethasone. Br J Dermatol. 2000;143:408-410.

231. Cooke CB, Krenacs L, Stetler-Stevenson M, et al. Hepatosplenic T-cell lymphoma: a distinct clinicopathologic entity of cytotoxic gamma delta T-cell origin. Blood. 1996;88:4265-4274.

232. Weidmann E. Hepatosplenic T cell lymphoma. A review on 45 cases since the first report describing the disease as a distinct lymphoma entity in 1990. Leukemia. 2000;14:991-997.

233. Belhadj K, Reyes F, Farcet JP, et al. Hepatosplenic gammadelta T-cell lymphoma is a rare clinicopathologic entity with poor outcome: report on a series of 21 patients. Blood. 2003;102:4261-4269.

234. Weirich G, Sandherr M, Fellbaum C, et al. Molecular evidence of bone marrow involvement in advanced case ot Tgammadelta lymphoma with secondary myelofibrosis. Hum Pathol. 1998;29:761-765.

235. Farcet JP, Gaulard P, Marolleau JP, et al. Hepatosplenic T-cell lymphoma: sinusal/sinusoidal localization of malignant cells expressing the T-cell receptor gamma delta. Blood. 1990;75:2213-2219.

236. Suarez F, Wlodarska I, Rigal-Huguet F, et al. Hepatosplenic alphabeta T-cell lymphoma: an unusual case with clinical, histologic, and cytogenetic features of gammadelta hepatosplenic T-cell lymphoma. Am J Surg Pathol. 2000;24:1027-1032.

237. Alonsozana EL, Stamberg J, Kumar D, et al. Isochromosome 7q: the primary cytogenetic abnormality in hepatosplenic gammadelta T cell lymphoma. Leukemia. 1997;11:1367-1372.

238. Wong KF, Zhang YM, Chan JK. Cytogenetic abnormalities in natural killer cell lymphoma/leukaemia--is there a consistent pattern? Leuk Lymphoma. 1999;34:241-250.

239. Labal de Vinuesa M, Slavutsky I, Larripa I. Presence of isochromosomes in hematologic diseases. Cancer Genet Cytogenet. 1987;25:47-54.

240. Rossbach HC, Chamizo W, Dumont DP, Barbosa JL, Sutcliffe MJ. Hepatosplenic gamma/delta T-cell lymphoma with isochromosome 7q, translocation t(7;21), and tetrasomy 8 in a 9-year-old girl. J Pediatr Hematol Oncol. 2002;24:154-157.

241. Petit B, Leroy K, Kanavaros P, et al. Expression of p53 protein in T- and natural killer-cell lymphomas is associated with some clinicopathologic entities but rarely related to p53 mutations. Hum Pathol. 2001;32:196-204.

242. Ohshima K, Haraoka S, Harada N, et al. Hepatosplenic gammadelta T-cell lymphoma: relation to Epstein-Barr virus and activated cytotoxic molecules. Histopathology. 2000;36:127-135.

243. Francois A, Lesesve JF, Stamatoullas A, et al. Hepatosplenic gamma/delta T-cell lymphoma: a report of two cases in immunocompromised patients, associated with isochromosome 7q. Am J Surg Pathol. 1997;21:781-790.

244. Labouyrie E, Morel D, Boiron JM, et al. Peripheral T-cell lymphoma in a chronically immunosuppressed renal transplant patient. Mod Pathol. 1995;8:355-359.

245. Iannitto E, Barbera V, Quintini G, Cirrincione S, Leone M. Hepatosplenic gammadelta T-cell lymphoma: complete response induced by treatment with pentostatin. Br J Haematol. 2002;117:995-996.

246. Hanson MN, Morrison VA, Peterson BA, et al. Posttransplant T-cell lymphoproliferative disorders--an aggressive, late complication of solid-organ transplantation. Blood. 1996;88:3626-3633.

247. Leblond V, Dhedin N, Mamzer Bruneel MF, et al. Identification of prognostic factors in 61 patients with posttransplantation lymphoproliferative disorders. J Clin Oncol. 2001;19:772-778.

248. Arber DA, Weiss LM, Albujar PF, Chen YY, Jaffe ES. Nasal lymphomas in Peru. High incidence of T-cell immunophenotype and Epstein-Barr virus infection. Am J Surg Pathol. 1993;17:392-399.

249. Jaffe ES, Chan JK, Su IJ, et al. Report of the Workshop on Nasal and Related Extranodal Angiocentric T/Natural Killer Cell Lymphomas. Definitions, differential diagnosis, and epidemiology. Am J Surg Pathol. 1996;20:103-111.

250. Quintanilla-Martinez L, Franklin JL, Guerrero I, et al. Histological and immunophenotypic profile of nasal NK/T cell lymphomas from Peru: high prevalence of p53 overexpression. Hum Pathol. 1999;30:849-855.

251. Cheung MM, Chan JK, Lau WH, et al. Primary non-Hodgkin's lymphoma of the nose and nasopharynx: clinical features, tumor immunophenotype, and treatment outcome in 113 patients. J Clin Oncol. 1998;16:70-77.

252. Kim GE, Lee SW, Chang SK, et al. Combined chemotherapy and radiation versus radiation alone in the management of localized angiocentric lymphoma of the head and neck. Radiother Oncol. 2001;61:261-269.

253. Li YX, Coucke PA, Li JY, et al. Primary non-Hodgkin's lymphoma of the nasal cavity: prognostic significance of paranasal extension and the role of radiotherapy and chemotherapy. Cancer. 1998;83:449-456.

254. Zhang Y, Nagata H, Ikeuchi T, et al. Common cytological and cytogenetic features of Epstein-Barr virus (EBV)-positive natural killer (NK) cells and cell lines derived from patients with nasal T/NK-cell lymphomas, chronic active EBV infection and hydroa vacciniforme-like eruptions. Br J Haematol. 2003;121:805-814.

255. Yoon TY, Lee HT, Chang SH. Nasal-type T/natural killer cell angiocentric lymphoma, Epstein-Barr virus-associated, and showing clonal T-cell receptor gamma gene rearrangement. Br J Dermatol. 1999;140:505-508.

256. Ko YH, Ree HJ, Kim WS, Choi WH, Moon WS, Kim SW. Clinicopathologic and genotypic study of extranodal nasal-type natural killer/T-cell lymphoma and natural killer precursor lymphoma among Koreans. Cancer. 2000;89:2106-2116.

257. Chiang AK, Chan AC, Srivastava G, Ho FC. Nasal T/natural killer (NK)-cell lymphomas are derived from Epstein-Barr virus-infected cytotoxic lymphocytes of both NK- and T-cell lineage. Int J Cancer. 1997;73:332-338.

258. Siu LL, Wong KF, Chan JK, Kwong YL. Comparative genomic hybridization analysis of natural killer cell lymphoma/leukemia. Recognition of consistent patterns of genetic alterations. Am J Pathol. 1999;155:1419-1425.

259. Siu LL, Chan V, Chan JK, Wong KF, Liang R, Kwong YL. Consistent patterns of allelic loss in natural killer cell lymphoma. Am J Pathol. 2000;157:1803-1809.

260. Tien HF, Su IJ, Tang JL, et al. Clonal chromosomal abnormalities as direct evidence for clonality in nasal T/natural killer cell lymphomas. Br J Haematol. 1997;97:621-625.

261. Sakajiri S, Kawamata N, Egashira M, Mori K, Oshimi K. Molecular analysis of tumor suppressor genes, Rb, p53, p16INK4A, p15INK4B and p14ARF in natural killer cell neoplasms. Jpn J Cancer Res. 2001;92:1048-1056.

262. Quintanilla-Martinez L, Kremer M, Keller G, et al. p53 Mutations in nasal natural killer/T-cell lymphoma from Mexico: association with large cell morphology and advanced disease. Am J Pathol. 2001;159:2095-2105.

263. Chiang AK, Wong KY, Liang AC, Srivastava G. Comparative analysis of Epstein-Barr virus gene polymorphisms in nasal T/NK-cell lymphomas and normal nasal tissues: implications on virus strain selection in malignancy. Int J Cancer. 1999;80:356-364.

264. Kim GE, Cho JH, Yang WI, et al. Angiocentric lymphoma of the head and neck: patterns of systemic failure after radiation treatment. J Clin Oncol. 2000;18:54-63.

265. Li CC, Tien HF, Tang JL, et al. Treatment outcome and pattern of failure in 77 patients with sinonasal natural killer/T-cell or T-cell lymphoma. Cancer. 2004;100:366-375.

266. Gale J, Simmonds PD, Mead GM, Sweetenham JW, Wright DH. Enteropathy-type intestinal T-cell lymphoma: clinical features and treatment of 31 patients in a single center. J Clin Oncol. 2000;18:795-803.

267. Lin HJ, Rotter JI, Conte WJ. Use of HLA marker associations and HLA haplotype linkage to estimate disease risks in families with gluten-sensitive enteropathy. Clin Genet. 1985;28:185-198.

268. Howell WM, Leung ST, Jones DB, et al. HLA-DRB, -DQA, and -DQB polymorphism in celiac disease and enteropathy-associated T-cell lymphoma. Common features and additional risk factors for malignancy. Hum Immunol. 1995;43:29-37.

269. Clerget-Darpoux F, Bouguerra F, Kastally R, et al. High risk genotypes for celiac disease. C R Acad Sci III. 1994;317:931-936.

270. Schmitt-Graff A, Daum S, Hummel M, Zemlin M, Stein H, Riecken EO. Presence of clonal T-cell receptor gene rearrangements provides evidence of widespread intramucosal intestinal T-cell lymphoma. Z Gastroenterol. 1996;34:680-685.

271. Daum S, Weiss D, Hummel M, et al. Frequency of clonal intraepithelial T lymphocyte proliferations in enteropathy-type intestinal T cell lymphoma, coeliac disease, and refractory sprue. Gut. 2001;49:804-812.

272. Cellier C, Delabesse E, Helmer C, et al. Refractory sprue, coeliac disease, and enteropathy-associated T-cell lymphoma. French Coeliac Disease Study Group. Lancet. 2000;356:203-208.

273. Murray A, Cuevas EC, Jones DB, Wright DH. Study of the immunohistochemistry and T cell clonality of enteropathy-associated T cell lymphoma. Am J Pathol. 1995;146:509-519.

274. Bagdi E, Diss TC, Munson P, Isaacson PG. Mucosal intra-epithelial lymphocytes in enteropathy-associated T-cell lymphoma, ulcerative jejunitis, and refractory celiac disease constitute a neoplastic population. Blood. 1999;94:260-264.

275. Carbonnel F, Grollet-Bioul L, Brouet JC, et al. Are complicated forms of celiac disease cryptic T-cell lymphomas? Blood. 1998;92:3879-3886.

276. Ashton-Key M, Diss TC, Pan L, Du MQ, Isaacson PG. Molecular analysis of T-cell clonality in ulcerative jejunitis and enteropathy-associated T-cell lymphoma. Am J Pathol. 1997;151:493-498.

277. Obermann E, Diss T, Hamoudi R, et al. Loss of heterozygosity at chromosome 9p21 is a frequent finding in enteropathy-type T-cell lymphoma. J Pathol. 2004;202:252-262.

278. Lavergne A, Brocheriou I, Delfau MH, Copie-Bergman C, Houdart R, Gaulard PH. Primary intestinal gamma-delta T-cell lymphoma with evidence of Epstein-Barr virus. Histopathology. 1998;32:271-276.

279. Kim YS, Kim JB, Kang YK, Nam ES, Park SH, Kim I. Viral genotypes and p53 expression in Epstein-Barr virus-associated primary malignant lymphomas of the intestines. Hum Pathol. 1999;30:1146-1152.

280. Quintanilla-Martinez L, Lome-Maldonado C, Ott G, et al. Primary non-Hodgkin's lymphoma of the intestine: high prevalence of Epstein-Barr virus in Mexican lymphomas as compared with European cases. Blood. 1997;89:644-651.

281. Abe Y, Muta K, Ohshima K, et al. Cytotoxic T-cell lymphoma diffusely involving the entire gastrointestinal tract associated with Epstein-Barr virus and tubercle bacilli infection. Int J Hematol. 2000;71:379-384.

282. Hoffmann M, Vogelsang H, Kletter K, Zettinig G, Chott A, Raderer M. 18F-fluoro-deoxy-glucose positron emission tomography (18F-FDG-PET) for assessment of enteropathy-type T cell lymphoma. Gut. 2003;52:347-351.

283. Uchiyama T, Yodoi J, Sagawa K, Takatsuki K, Uchino H. Adult T-cell leukemia: clinical and hematologic features of 16 cases. Blood. 1977;50:481-492.

284. Poiesz BJ, Ruscetti FW, Gazdar AF, Bunn PA, Minna JD, Gallo RC. Detection and isolation of type C retrovirus particles from fresh and cultured lymphocytes of a patient with cutaneous T-cell lymphoma. Proc Natl Acad Sci U S A. 1980;77:7415-7419.

285. Takatsuki K, Matsuoka M, Yamaguchi K. Adult T-cell leukemia in Japan. J Acquir Immune Defic Syndr Hum Retrovirol. 1996;13 Suppl 1:S15-19.

286. Mueller N, Okayama A, Stuver S, Tachibana N. Findings from the Miyazaki Cohort Study. J Acquir Immune Defic Syndr Hum Retrovirol. 1996;13 Suppl 1:S2-7.

287. Hanchard B. Adult T-cell leukemia/lymphoma in Jamaica: 1986-1995. J Acquir Immune Defic Syndr Hum Retrovirol. 1996;13 Suppl 1:S20-25.

288. Taylor GP. The epidemiology of HTLV-I in Europe. J Acquir Immune Defic Syndr Hum Retrovirol. 1996;13 Suppl 1:S8-14.

289. Nyambi PN, Ville Y, Louwagie J, et al. Mother-to-child transmission of human T-cell lymphotropic virus types I and II (HTLV-I/II) in Gabon: a prospective follow-up of 4 years. J Acquir Immune Defic Syndr Hum Retrovirol. 1996;12:187-192.

290. Chen YC, Wang CH, Su IJ, et al. Infection of human T-cell leukemia virus type I and development of human T-cell leukemia lymphoma in patients with hematologic neoplasms: a possible linkage to blood transfusion. Blood. 1989;74:388-394.

291. Pagliuca A. Strongyloides hyperinfection in adult T-cell leukaemia/lymphoma. Br J Haematol. 1999;105:1.

292. Shimoyama M. Diagnostic criteria and classification of clinical subtypes of adult T-cell leukaemia-lymphoma. A report from the Lymphoma Study Group (1984-87). Br J Haematol. 1991;79:428-437.

293. Yoshida M. Molecular biology of HTLV-I: recent progress. J Acquir Immune Defic Syndr Hum Retrovirol. 1996;13 Suppl 1:S63-68.

294. Franchini G. Molecular mechanisms of human T-cell leukemia/lymphotropic virus type I infection. Blood. 1995;86:3619-3639.

295. Nagafuji K, Harada M, Teshima T, et al. Hematopoietic progenitor cells from patients with adult T-cell leukemia-lymphoma are not infected with human T-cell leukemia virus type 1. Blood. 1993;82:2823-2828.

296. Evens AM, Gartenhaus RB. Molecular etiology of mature T-cell non-Hodgkin's lymphomas. Front Biosci. 2003;8:d156-175.

297. Hofmann WK, Tsukasaki K, Takeuchi N, Takeuchi S, Koeffler HP. Methylation analysis of cell cycle control genes in adult T-cell leukemia/lymphoma. Leuk Lymphoma. 2001;42:1107-1109.

298. Tsukasaki K, Tsushima H, Yamamura M, et al. Integration patterns of HTLV-I provirus in relation to the clinical course of ATL: frequent clonal change at crisis from indolent disease. Blood. 1997;89:948-956.

299. Tsukasaki K, Krebs J, Nagai K, et al. Comparative genomic hybridization analysis in adult T-cell leukemia/lymphoma: correlation with clinical course. Blood. 2001;97:3875-3881.

300. Zhang Z, Zhang M, Goldman CK, Ravetch JV, Waldmann TA. Effective therapy for a murine model of adult T-cell leukemia with the humanized anti-CD52 monoclonal antibody, Campath-1H. Cancer Res. 2003;63:6453-6457.

301. El-Sabban ME, Nasr R, Dbaibo G, et al. Arsenic-interferon-alpha-triggered apoptosis in HTLV-I transformed cells is associated with tax down-regulation and reversal of NF-kappa B activation. Blood. 2000;96:2849-2855.

302. Kuwazuru Y, Hanada S, Furukawa T, et al. Expression of P-glycoprotein in adult T-cell leukemia cells. Blood. 1990;76:2065-2071.

303. Shimoyama M, Ota K, Kikuchi M, et al. Major prognostic factors of adult patients with advanced T-cell lymphoma/leukemia. J Clin Oncol. 1988;6:1088-1097.

304. Taguchi H, Kinoshita KI, Takatsuki K, et al. An intensive chemotherapy of adult T-cell leukemia/lymphoma: CHOP followed by etoposide, vindesine, ranimustine, and mitoxantrone with granulocyte colony-stimulating factor support. J Acquir Immune Defic Syndr Hum Retrovirol. 1996;12:182-186.

305. Sparano JA, Wiernik PH, Strack M, Leaf A, Becker N, Valentine ES. Infusional cyclophosphamide, doxorubicin, and etoposide in human immunodeficiency virus- and human T-cell leukemia virus type I-related non-Hodgkin's lymphoma: a highly active regimen. Blood. 1993;81:2810-2815.

306. Bazarbachi A, El-Sabban ME, Nasr R, et al. Arsenic trioxide and interferon-alpha synergize to induce cell cycle arrest and apoptosis in human T-cell lymphotropic virus type I-transformed cells. Blood. 1999;93:278-283.

307. Nasr R, Rosenwald A, El-Sabban ME, et al. Arsenic/interferon specifically reverses 2 distinct gene networks critical for the survival of HTLV-1-infected leukemic cells. Blood. 2003;101:4576-4582.

308. Dierov J, Sawaya BE, Prosniak M, Gartenhaus RB. Retinoic acid modulates a bimodal effect on cell cycle progression in human adult T-cell leukemia cells. Clin Cancer Res. 1999;5:2540-2547.

309. Matutes E, Taylor GP, Cavenagh J, et al. Interferon alpha and zidovudine therapy in adult T-cell leukaemia lymphoma: response and outcome in 15 patients. Br J Haematol. 2001;113:779-784.

310. Hermine O, Allard I, Levy V, Arnulf B, Gessain A, Bazarbachi A. A prospective phase II clinical trial with the use of zidovudine and interferon-alpha in the acute and lymphoma forms of adult T-cell leukemia/lymphoma. Hematol J. 2002;3:276-282.

311. Besson C, Panelatti G, Delaunay C, et al. Treatment of adult T-cell leukemia-lymphoma by CHOP followed by therapy with antinucleosides, alpha interferon and oral etoposide. Leuk Lymphoma. 2002;43:2275-2279.

312. Tsuda H, Takatsuki K, Ohno R, et al. Treatment of adult T-cell leukaemia-lymphoma with irinotecan hydrochloride (CPT-11). CPT-11 Study Group on Hematological Malignancy. Br J Cancer. 1994;70:771-774.

313. Yamaguchi K, Yul LS, Oda T, et al. Clinical consequences of 2'-deoxycoformycin treatment in patients with refractory adult T-cell leukaemia. Leuk Res. 1986;10:989-993.

314. Tobinai K, Uike N, Saburi Y, et al. Phase II study of cladribine (2-chlorodeoxyadenosine) in relapsed or refractory adult T-cell leukemia-lymphoma. Int J Hematol. 2003;77:512-517.

315. Tsukasaki K, Tobinai K, Shimoyama M, et al. Deoxycoformycin-containing combination chemotherapy for adult T-cell leukemia-lymphoma: Japan Clinical Oncology Group Study (JCOG9109). Int J Hematol. 2003;77:164-170.

316. Waldmann TA, White JD, Goldman CK, et al. The interleukin-2 receptor: a target for monoclonal antibody treatment of human T-cell lymphotrophic virus I-induced adult T-cell leukemia. Blood. 1993;82:1701-1712.

317. Di Venuti G, Nawgiri R, Foss F. Denileukin Diftitox and Hyper-CVAD in the Treatment of Human T-Cell Lymphotropic Virus 1-Associated Acute T-Cell Leukemia/Lymphoma. Clin Lymphoma. 2003;4:176-178.

318. Philip T, Guglielmi C, Hagenbeek A, et al. Autologous bone marrow transplantation as compared with salvage chemotherapy in relapses of chemotherapy-sensitive non-Hodgkin's lymphoma. N Engl J Med. 1995;333:1540-1545.

319. Blystad AK, Enblad G, Kvaloy S, et al. High-dose therapy with autologous stem cell transplantation in patients with peripheral T cell lymphomas. Bone Marrow Transplant. 2001;27:711-716.

320. Kahl C, Leithauser M, Wolff D, et al. Treatment of peripheral T-cell lymphomas (PTCL) with high-dose chemotherapy and autologous or allogeneic hematopoietic transplantation. Ann Hematol. 2002;81:646-650.

321. Rodriguez J, Munsell M, Yazji S, et al. Impact of high-dose chemotherapy on peripheral T-cell lymphomas. J Clin Oncol. 2001;19:3766-3770.

322. Song KW, Mollee P, Keating A, Crump M. Autologous stem cell transplant for relapsed and refractory peripheral T-cell lymphoma: variable outcome according to pathological subtype. Br J Haematol. 2003;120:978-985.

323. Rodriguez J, Caballero MD, Gutierrez A, et al. High-dose chemotherapy and autologous stem cell transplantation in peripheral T-cell lymphoma: the GEL-TAMO experience. Ann Oncol. 2003;14:1768-1775.

324. Jantunen E, Wiklund T, Juvonen E, et al. Autologous stem cell transplantation in adult patients with peripheral T-cell lymphoma: a nation-wide survey. Bone Marrow Transplant. 2004;33:405-410.

325. Jantunen E, Juvonen E, Wiklund T, Putkonen M, Nousiainen T. High-dose therapy supported by autologous stem cell transplantation in patients with enteropathy-associated T-cell lymphoma. Leuk Lymphoma. 2003;44:2163-2164.

326. Au WY, Lie AK, Liang R, et al. Autologous stem cell transplantation for nasal NK/T-cell lymphoma: a progress report on its value. Ann Oncol. 2003;14:1673-1676.

327. Mukai HY, Okoshi Y, Shimizu S, et al. Successful treatment of a patient with subcutaneous panniculitis-like T-cell lymphoma with high-dose chemotherapy and total body irradiation. Eur J Haematol. 2003;70:413-416.

328. Watanabe J, Kondo H, Hatake K. Autologous stem cell transplantations for recurrent adult T cell leukaemia/lymphoma using highly purified CD34+ cells derived from cryopreserved peripheral blood stem cells. Leuk Lymphoma. 2001;42:1115-1117.

329. Schetelig J, Fetscher S, Reichle A, et al. Long-term disease-free survival in patients with angioimmunoblastic T-cell lymphoma after high-dose chemotherapy and autologous stem cell transplantation. Haematologica. 2003;88:1272-1278.

330. Rodriguez J, Caballero MD, Gutierrez A, et al. High dose chemotherapy and autologous stem cell transplantation in patients with peripheral T-cell lymphoma not achieving complete response after induction chemotherapy. The GEL-TAMO experience. Haematologica. 2003;88:1372-1377.

331. Deconinck E, Lamy T, Foussard C, et al. Autologous stem cell transplantation for anaplastic large-cell lymphomas: results of a prospective trial. Br J Haematol. 2000;109:736-742.

332. Fanin R, Sperotto A, Silvestri F, et al. The therapy of primary adult systemic CD30-positive anaplastic large cell lymphoma: results of 40 cases treated in a single center. Leuk Lymphoma. 1999;35:159-169.

333. Okamura T, Kishimoto T, Inoue M, et al. Unrelated bone marrow transplantation for Epstein-Barr virus-associated T/NK-cell lymphoproliferative disease. Bone Marrow Transplant. 2003;31:105-111.

334. Harashima N, Kurihara K, Utsunomiya A, et al. Graft-versus-Tax response in adult T-cell leukemia patients after hematopoietic stem cell transplantation. Cancer Res. 2004;64:391-399.

335. Imashuku S, Hibi S, Todo S, et al. Allogeneic hematopoietic stem cell transplantation for patients with hemophagocytic syndrome (HPS) in Japan. Bone Marrow Transplant. 1999;23:569-572.

336. Buttgereit P, Schakowski F, Marten A, et al. Effects of adenoviral wild-type p53 gene transfer in p53-mutated lymphoma cells. Cancer Gene Ther. 2001;8:430-439.

337. Nagata S, Onda M, Numata Y, et al. Novel anti-CD30 recombinant immunotoxins containing disulfide-stabilized Fv fragments. Clin Cancer Res. 2002;8:2345-2355.

338. Hatta Y, Koeffler HP. Role of tumor suppressor genes in the development of adult T cell leukemia/lymphoma (ATLL). Leukemia. 2002;16:1069-1085.

339. Moura IC, Lepelletier Y, Arnulf B, et al. A neutralizing monoclonal antibody (mAb A24) directed against the transferrin receptor induces apoptosis of tumor T lymphocytes from ATL patients. Blood. 2004;103:1838-1845.

340. Senderowicz AM. Development of cyclin-dependent kinase modulators as novel therapeutic approaches for hematological malignancies. Leukemia. 2001;15:1-9.

341. Byrd JC, Shinn C, Waselenko JK, et al. Flavopiridol induces apoptosis in chronic lymphocytic leukemia cells via activation of caspase-3 without evidence of bcl-2 modulation or dependence on functional p53. Blood. 1998;92:3804-3816.

342. Blackhall FH, Ranson M, Radford JA, et al. A phase II trial of bryostatin 1 in patients with non-Hodgkin's lymphoma. Br J Cancer. 2001;84:465-469.

343. Harvey S, Decker R, Dai Y, et al. Interactions between 2-fluoroadenine 9-beta-D-arabinofuranoside and the kinase inhibitor UCN-01 in human leukemia and lymphoma cells. Clin Cancer Res. 2001;7:320-330.

344. Piekarz RL, Robey R, Sandor V, et al. Inhibitor of histone deacetylation, depsipeptide (FR901228), in the treatment of peripheral and cutaneous T-cell lymphoma: a case report. Blood. 2001;98:2865-2868.

345. Bariol C, Field A, Vickers CR, Ward R. Regression of gastric T cell lymphoma with eradication of Helicobacter pylori. Gut. 2001;48:269-271.

346. Fillmore GC, Lin Z, Bohling SD, et al. Gene expression profiling of cell lines derived from T-cell malignancies. FEBS Lett. 2002;522:183-188.

347. Passoni L, Gambacorti-Passerini C. ALK a novel lymphoma-associated tumor antigen for vaccination strategies. Leuk Lymphoma. 2003;44:1675-1681.

348. Thirdborough SM, Radcliffe JN, Friedmann PS, Stevenson FK. Vaccination with DNA encoding a single-chain TCR fusion protein induces anticlonotypic immunity and protects against T-cell lymphoma. Cancer Res. 2002;62:1757-1760.

Chapter 7

MONOCLONAL ANTIBODIES IN THE TREATMENT OF NON-HODGKIN'S LYMPHOMA

Richard R. Furman MD, Morton Coleman MD, Daniel Muss and John P. Leonard, MD

Center for Lymphoma and Myeloma, Division of Hematology and Medical Oncology and Weill Medical College of Cornell University and New York Presbyterian Hospital New York, NY

1.   INTRODUCTION

Non-Hodgkin's lymphomas are a heterogeneous group of malignancies that result from the clonal expansion of mature lymphocytes that are unable to terminally differentiate. Each lymphoma is derived from a lymphocyte that is frozen at a particular stage of development and often retains many of the immunophenotypic, morphologic, and molecular markers of the corresponding lymphocyte stage. Thus, lymphocyte development is well marked by the expression of a series of differentiation antigens, termed "cluster of differentiation" (CD) antigens. These characteristics serve as the basis for the World Health Organization (WHO) Classification of Lymphoid Neoplasms [1]. These proteins are also valuable markers for diagnosing and classifying lymphomas, as well as reliable targets for therapy.

The goal of cancer therapy is to eliminate the cancer cells without harming the patient. For lymphomas, chemotherapy and radiation therapy have been the mainstay of treatment. Both of these modalities are quite effective at killing malignant cells, but suffer from a lack of specificity. Many chemotherapeutic agents target rapidly proliferating cells. These cells are most often the malignant cells, but also include hair follicles, bone marrow, and gastrointestinal mucosa, resulting in alopecia, myelosuppression, and mucositis. These and other toxicities that develop limit the doses of chemotherapy that can be utilized in treatment. If the cancer treatment could be delivered specifically to the cancer cells, there would be the expectation of less associated toxicity. The therapy could then be delivered safer and possibly in higher doses, with possible greater effectiveness. Antibodies offer a means to target specific cells in the body, limiting toxicity of non-target lesions.

The specificity of antibody targeted therapy result from features of both the antibody and the antigen. Through the processes of VDJ recombination, somatic hypermutation, and base addition, the immune system is able to generate antibodies that possess extraordinary specificity. One antibody will bind to one antigen without any cross reactivity to other antigens. The second level of specificity is derived from the selection an antigen whose expression is restricted to the targeted cells. The ideal antigen would be one only expressed on malignant cells. Given the ontogenic relationship between lymphomas and normal lymphocytes, the antigens expressed on lymphomas are almost always expressed by their non-malignant counterparts. The damage that might result due to the expression of an antigen on both normal and malignant lymphocytes is minimized by the ability to regenerate normal lymphocytes after therapy, limiting the duration and severity of immunosuppression.

Targeted antigens are cell surface based or soluble molecules. For cell surface based targets, an ideal antigen would fulfill several criteria, including: 1) restricted expression of the antigen so as to spare non-targeted tissues; 2) the antigen should be intensely expressed in order to bind adequate numbers of antibodies; 3) the antigen's cell surface expression should not be modulated so the antibody will remain on the surface once bound to the antigen; and 4) the antigen should not be present in a soluble or secreted form so as to not block the antibody from reaching the targeted cell or generating soluble immune complexes. Soluble molecules are typically cytokines or survival factors whose absence will impair the survival of the malignant cell.

Antibodies eliminate cancer cells through several potential mechanisms: 1) complement dependent cytotoxicity; 2) antibody dependent cellular cytotoxicity; 3) delivery of a toxin or radiation to the target cell; and 4) signaling through the target antigen. Mechanisms 1-3 are mediated by the Fc portion of the antibody. The fourth mechanism of action is mediated by the antigen binding domain of the antibody. Antibodies directed against surface based antigens that are currently being investigated for possible therapeutic use include those against CD3, CD20, CD22, CD23, CD25, CD30, CD40, CD74, and CD80. Antibodies targeting soluble molecules include: vascular endothelial derived growth factor (VEGF), IL-1, IL-6, and tumor necrosis factor-alpha (TNF-α).

There are several different processes used to generate monoclonal antibodies which result in structures with varying degrees of similarity to human immunoglobulins. The first monoclonal antibodies generated were produce by hybridoma technology. Animals, typically mice, were vaccinated with the target antigen. Since technologies to purify the antigen were relatively primitive and there was a need for the antigen to maintain its native conformation in order for the generated antibody to have relevance, whole cells bearing the antigen were used. The B lymphocytes from the spleen of the vaccinated mouse were then purified and fused with a murine myeloma cell line. The cells that were successfully fused were then screened for production of the desired antibody. The antibody-producing hybridomas were then cultured and the monoclonal antibodies collected from the culture supernatant. Antibodies generated in this manner were termed fully murine as they appeared as completely murine in their sequence.

The next technique to be utilized generated "chimeric" monoclonal antibodies. In this process, murine monoclonal antibodies were cleaved into their F(ab')2 and Fc portions. The F(ab')$_2$ fragments were isolated and then fused to Fc fragments that were derived from human cell lines. Subsequently, the antibodies are produced by cloning the cDNA for the chimeric antibody into mammalian cells adapted for high-volume production of antibodies. These antibodies therefore are one part murine and one part human. Since the antigen binding part is derived from the murine antibody, the original specificity for the target antigen is maintained. Since the Fc portion of the molecule is human, this antibody possesses the ability to activate all of the effector functions expected from the class of antibody.

A newer technique involves generating murine antibodies as previously described, but then sequencing the complimentary determining region (CDR). The antigen binding properties of an antibody are determined by the three dimensional structure of the antigen binding pocket or CDR. This structure is defined by the amino acid sequence, and ultimately, the DNA sequence. Once the DNA sequence is determined, it can be cloned into a human immunoglobulin gene of an antibody producing cell line. This "humanized" antibody is fully human in its structure except for the few amino acids that comprise the CDR region. Further advances include the use of transgenic mice that are genetically engineered to generate fully human antibodies.

Human or humanized antibodies offer several possible advantages over murine and chimeric monoclonal antibodies. First, murine and chimeric antibodies have foreign sequences present that might cause the recipient to develop a humoral immune response against the antibody. These human anti-murine antibodies (HAMA) or human anti-chimeric antibodies (HACA) might preclude subsequent clinical use of the therapeutic antibody or lead to severe infusion related toxicities. These HAMA or HACA could bind to the therapeutic antibodies and either neutralize them, by binding in a manner that prevents the therapeutic antibody from binding its target, or result in a more rapid clearance of the therapeutic antibody by the formation of immune complexes. Humanized antibodies, by their nature of possessing fewer foreign sequences would be less likely to generate a host immune response or human anti-human antibodies (HAHA). A second advantage afforded by humanized antibodies is the presence of a functioning Fc domain. The effector functions of antibodies, namely complement activation and antibody dependent cellular cytotoxicity, are mediated by the Fc portion of the antibody. Antibodies that possess functioning Fc domains are able to activate the host's immune response to destroy targeted cells. Chimeric antibodies, since they possess human Fc domains, do activate the immune system, while murine antibodies do so usually to a lesser extent. Thus, murine antibodies are more dependent upon other mechanisms for causing destruction of their target cell, such as radiation or toxin. Third, antibodies bearing human Fc domains generally have a longer half-life than their murine counterparts. In the remaining parts of this review, we will present data related to specific antibodies.

2.   RITUXIMAB

Rituximab (IDEC-C2B8), the first monoclonal antibody to be approved for a cancer indication in the US, received approval from the Food and Drug Administration (FDA) in November 1997. Rituximab is approved as treatment for patients with relapsed or refractory, low-grade or follicular, CD20-positive, B-cell non-Hodgkin's lymphoma. Rituximab is an IgG1 kappa chimeric monoclonal antibody directed against the CD20 molecule whose expression is restricted to only B lymphocytes [2]. Rituximab's murine variable regions are derived from the murine anti-CD20 antibody, 2B8 [3]. Rituximab is composed of two heavy chains of 451 amino acids and two light chains of 213 amino acids, with an approximate molecular weight of 145 kD. Rituximab is produced by Chinese Hamster Ovary (CHO) cells that contain the human/murine cDNA sequences for rituximab and secrete the antibody in large quantities into culture, where it is purified by affinity and ion exchange chromatography. Rituximab binds to the CD20 antigen with a high affinity, 5 x 10-9 mol/L, through its murine variable regions located on both the light and heavy immunoglobulin chains [3].

CD20 is solely expressed on normal and malignant B cells [4, 5]. Its expression is first detectable at the pre-B cell stage of lymphocyte development, when cytoplasmic μH chains are first produced and its expression remains present at high levels until the lymphoplasmactyoid lymphocyte stage when it begins to become down regulated. CD20 is not expressed on plasma cells, the most terminally differentiated B cell. This is of significance since rituximab will not target all the earliest B lymphocyte progenitors or plasma cells, allowing continuation of some antibody production and replenishment of normal B lymphocytes. The CD20 molecule is expressed on over 90% of B-cell lymphomas [2, 4].

CD20 is believed to play a role in regulating the activation, proliferation, and differentiation of B cells through its regulation of transmembrane calcium conductance that is responsive to signaling through the B-cell receptor [6-8]. CD20 possess four transmembrane domains with its C- and N-termini both located within the cytoplasm. Initial experiments supported the idea that CD20 does not internalize [9], is tightly bound in the membrane and not present in the plasma [4]. Subsequent work demonstrated the presence of low amounts of circulating CD20 in the plasma in healthy controls, and significantly elevated levels in patients with CLL [10, 11]. In the CLL patients, the level of circulating CD20 was identified as an independent prognostic indicator [11]. In addition to its spectrum of expression profile, CD20 serves as a good therapeutic target because it is a transmembrane protein whose presence is most likely required for B lymphocyte survival. Thus, it is well anchored to the cell and there is very low potential for the development of CD20 negative B cells through selection.

The exact mechanism of action for rituximab remains debated, but most likely depends upon a combination of: 1) complement activation [3, 12-14]; 2) antibody dependent cellular cytoxicity (ADCC) [12, 15, 16]; and 3) antibody mediated apoptosis involving signaling through the CD20 protein [17-22]. In support of complement dependent cytotoxicity are several observations. The Fc portion of rituximab binds human C1q effectively, initiating the complement cascade [3]. Blocking CD55 and CD59, cellular based inhibitors of complement, increased lymphoma cells' sensitivity to rituximab and levels of CD55 correlated with resistance to rituximab in vitro [12, 14]. And cells cultured in complement depleted media appeared to be less sensitive to the effects of rituximab [13]. Other investigators have not found a correlation between inhibitors of complement and sensitivity to rituximab [23]. It is interesting to note that rituximab has anecdotally demonstrated some activity when used for intrathecal treatment, given that cerebrospinal fluid is not expected to have complement or cells to mediate ADCC [24, 25].

The importance of ADCC has been demonstrated in a series of experiments by Clynes, et al [15]. They demonstrated that mice deficient in the activating FcγRIIIA receptor were unable to arrest transplanted tumors in vivo with rituximab. Whereas, mice deficient in the inhibitory FcγRIIB receptor demonstrate more ADCC. In humans, the best evidence in support of a role for ADDC comes from studies of gene polymorphisms for two activating Fc receptors, FcγRIIIa and FcγRIIa [16, 26]. For FcγRIIIa, the polymorphism results in either a phenylalanine (F) or a valine (V) at amino acid position 158. Human IgG1 binds more strongly to V/V phenotype compared to the F/F or F/V phenotypes. Since FcγRIIIa is mediates ADCC involving NK cells and macrophages, it was hypothesized that the Fc receptors with higher binding avidity would result in a better response to rituximab. The overall response rates at two and twelve months after rituximab therapy in one lymphoma subtype were 100% and 90% of the patients with V/V phenotype, compared to 67% and 51% for patients with either F/V or F/F phenotypes. An additional study by Weng and Levy supported the finding by Cartron, and also identified a polymorphism of amino acid 131 of the FcγRIIa receptor that correlated with outcome.

Although rituximab is not the physiologic ligand for CD20, its binding initiates a series of signaling cascades. These signaling pathways impact upon the cell, often leading to apoptosis. Alas demonstrated that rituximab leads to a decrease in STAT3 activity, resulting in decreased Bcl-2 expression and apoptosis [22]. Others have shown similar effects on signaling pathways between anti-CD20 and anti-B-cell receptor mediated apoptosis [18]. Jazirehi and colleagues demonstrated a decrease in Bcl-XL levels in response to rituximab and that this was mediated through inhibition of NF-κB [19, 20].

The phase I study of rituximab investigated the administration of single doses of the antibody at doses from 10 to 500 mg/m^2. No dose-limiting toxicities (DLTs) were noted in this study [27]. Given the pharmacokinetics observed for rituximab, a second phase I study was performed using a repetitive dosing scheme [28]. In this study, doses of 125, 250, and 375 mg/m^2 were administered weekly for four doses. Once again, no DLTs were observed, with the only adverse events observed being infusional related (fever, chills, rigor, rash, respiratory symptoms, or hypotension) and mild (grades 1 and 2). 375 mg/m^2 was selected as the dose for subsequent phase II development.

The initial phase II study of rituximab demonstrated rituximab treatment to be feasible and effective, with a response rate of 46%, with 8% CRs and

38% PRs, in patients with relapsed low-grade lymphoma [29]. The pivotal study utilized this same dosing scheme of 375 mg/m^2 weekly x four in a multicenter, open-label, single-arm study involving 166 patients with relapsed or refractory low-grade or follicular B-cell lymphoma [30]. Patients with tumor masses >10 cm or with a circulating lymphocyte count of >5000/μl were excluded from the study. The overall response rate was 48% with 6% complete response (CR) and 42% partial responses (PR) rates. The median duration of response was 11.2 months, with a range of 1.9 to 42.1+). Multivariate analysis of the data demonstrated a higher response rate in patients with IWF histologic subtypes B, C, and D compared to IWF subtype A (58% vs. 12%), higher in patients whose largest lesion was <5 cm vs. >5 cm in greatest diameter (53% vs. 38%), and higher in patients with chemosensitive relapse as compared to chemoresistant relapse (53% vs. 36%).

Most patients demonstrated a rapid decrease in the number of peripheral blood B cells by day four, which remained nearly undetectable until approximately six months post-treatment, followed by a slow gradual recovery. Mean serum immunoglobulin levels remained stable over the course of the study, with IgG and IgA levels remaining within the normal range, but IgM levels falling slightly below the lower limits of normal. One out of 166 patients developed a HACA response at day 50, which was not associated with any clinical or laboratory abnormalities. Tumor response correlated with serum rituximab concentrations, with responding patients having a higher median serum concentration at all time points during treatment, but with the difference being statistically significant pre-dose for infusions 2 and 4 as well as post-treatment infusion #4.

Given the tolerability and effectiveness of rituximab in the relapsed setting, Witzig and colleagues from the North Central Cancer Treatment Group studied rituximab in patients with untreated patients with follicular grade I, NHL. As might be expected with untreated patients, they demonstrated an overall response rate of 72%, with a 36% CR rate. The median time to progression was 2.2 years with only 56% of the patients progressing with a median follow-up of only 2.6 years [31]. Rituximab thus may serve as a potential means to delay the exposure of patients to chemotherapy and its resulting toxicities. It will be even more important to determine the numbers of these patients who respond to retreatment with rituximab. When rituximab retreatment was investigated in patients with relapsed, low-grade NHL who had previously demonstrated a response of at least six months, Davis, et al. reported an overall response rate (ORR) of 40%, with 11% complete responses (CR) and 30% partial responses (PR) [32].

While rituximab does demonstrate substantial activity with acceptable toxicity, the benefits of the standard dosing schedule are transient, with relapse expected. A number of investigators have attempted to improve outcomes through modifications of the dose and schedule. Pharmacokinetic analysis from the pivotal trial indicated that 4 doses of rituximab at 375 mg/m2 do not achieve steady state serum concentrations [30]. Piro conducted a phase II study of eight weekly doses of rituximab (375 mg/m2/dose) [33]. This dosing schedule led to higher serum concentrations of rituximab than the four weekly doses (464.7 vs. approximately 538.1 μg/ml), an ORR of 57%, with 14% CRs and 43% PRs and a median time to progression of 19.4+ months, with serum concentrations of rituximab strongly correlating with response. The median rituximab serum concentration was higher for responders compared to non-responders at all time points. Additionally, IWF type A patients (CLL/SLL) had significantly lower serum antibody levels than the other types of low-grade lymphoma. This correlation of serum rituximab levels and response was also seen in the pivotal study [30]. It is worth noting that post-infusion serum levels plateaued after the sixth infusion.

Another modification of the standard dosing scheme for rituximab involves "maintenance" dosing. Since disease progression tends to occur after six months in responders, Hainsworth, et al. studied a regimen involving re-administration of four doses of rituximab to responding patients with low-grade lymphomas every six months for two years [34]. The ORR to the initial four-dose course of rituximab was 47% (7% CR, 40% PR), with 45% of patients demonstrating stable disease. With maintenance therapy, the response rates improved dramatically, achieving an ORR of 73% with a CR rate of 37%. 59% of the patients who initially had stable disease achieved an objective response with continued therapy. In these 16 late responders, responses were achieved after the second course of rituximab in eight, after the third course for six, and after the fourth course for two. The progression-free survival for the entire group was 34 months.

Two studies attempted to further investigate the importance of maintenance rituximab treatment. In the first study, conducted by the Swiss Group for Clinical Cancer Research (SAKK), newly diagnosed or relapsed follicular lymphoma patients received induction therapy with rituximab 375 mg/m^2/week for four weeks [35]. Patients with a response or stable disease were then randomized to either observation or treatment with a single infusion of rituximab 375 mg/m^2 every two months for four infusions starting at week 12. With median follow-up of 35 months, median event-free survival was 12 months in the observation arm versus 23 months in the prolonged treatment arm.

The second study, conducted by the Minnie Pearl Cancer Research Network, involved patients with previously treated low-grade lymphoma. Patients received the standard four week course of rituximab at 375 mg/m2/day as initial therapy [36]. Patients with objective response or stable disease were randomized to receive either maintenance rituximab therapy consisting of a standard four week course administered at six month intervals for up to two years or retreatment with rituximab at the time of lymphoma progression. Final overall and complete response rates were higher in the maintenance group compared to the retreatment group (52% vs. 35% and 27% vs. 4% respectively). Progression-free survival was prolonged in the maintenance group compared to the retreatment group (31.3 vs. 7.4 months; p=0.007). Importantly, there was no difference in the duration of rituximab benefit between the maintenance and retreatment arms (31.3 vs. 27.4 months). There are several important differences between the SAKK and Minnie Pearl Cancer Research Network studies. First, the dose and schedule utilized as maintenance for the studies differed. Whether repeated single infusions at two month intervals (SAKK) or four infusions repeated at six month intervals (Minnie Pearl) would be more effective would depend upon the whether constant low-level exposure or achieving higher peak serum concentrations were more important. Second, and more importantly, the Minnie Pearl group included retreatment at relapse in their analysis. This is very important given the response rate of 40% and a response duration of 18 months seen with rituximab retreatment [32].

Another interesting approach to optimize rituximab effectiveness involved monitoring serum levels of rituximab [37]. Patients with any CD20 positive lymphoma other than CLL/SLL received four weekly infusions of rituximab 375 mg/m2. Serum rituximab levels were monitored for one year in patients without progressive disease. Patients received a single infusion of rituximab when the serum level decreased below 25 μg/ml. The ORR was 59%, with 27% CRs, and median progression-free survival for all patients of 19 months. In patients with low-grade lymphomas, the ORR was 63%, with 36% CRs and a median progression free survival that has not been reached with 25 months of follow-up. The frequency of re-dosing required in this trial supports the concept of a three month re-administration schedule to support serum levels.

Overall, these studies suggest that "maintenance" immunotherapy with rituximab in indolent lymphoma may enhance RR, CR and PFS, however retreating patients with rituximab at the time of disease progression results in a similar overall duration of benefit and may require less utilization of resources. At this point, it appears that either maintenance rituximab or rituximab retreatment at progression are reasonable strategies in patients with indolent lymphoma with an initial response to rituximab treatment.

Long term effects of either strategy with respect to overall survival remain to be determined.

3. CHEMOIMMUNOTHERAPY COMBINATIONS FOR INDOLENT NHL

Another means for utilizing rituximab is in combination with chemotherapy. These chemoimmunotherapy regimens attempt to take advantage of an additive or even synergistic effect of combining chemotherapy with rituximab through concurrent or sequential administration. The strategy for combination chemotherapy is based upon several hypothesized mechanisms. In the first theory, rituximab increases the sensitivity of the lymphoma cells to chemotherapy. This occurs by rituximab altering intracellular signaling pathways or by causing a "double hit" resulting in the cells being more sensitive to chemotherapy. The second hypothesis is that the rituximab will eliminate those cancer cells that are not eliminated by the chemotherapy because of resistance to the chemotherapy.

The first clinical trial to evaluate the safety and efficacy of combination chemoimmunotherapy was done by Czuczman, et al. and involved 40 patients with low-grade and follicular NHL, 38 of who had received prior therapy, enrolled between April 1994 and March 1996 [38]. Patients received six cycles of CHOP chemotherapy at standard doses with two infusions of rituximab administered before the first cycle, single infusions before the third and fifth cycles, and two infusions after the sixth cycle. This study demonstrated an ORR of 100% (87% CR) with a median time to progression of 82.3 months. Ten years after the study's inception, 42% of patients remained in remission.

Czuczman and colleagues have also studied concurrent fludarabine and rituximab in patients with low-grade and follicular NHL [39]. Forty patients were treated with six cycles of fludarabine (25 mg/m^2/d for 5 days every 28 days) plus two infusions of rituximab prior to the first cycle, single infusions with the second, fourth and sixth cycles, and two final infusions four weeks after the final fludarabine treatment. The ORR was 90%, with 80% CRs, and median duration of response that had not been reached at months. Molecular remissions were achieved in 88% of the patient who were positive for the 14;18 translocation at enrollment.

The first randomized study comparing concurrent chemoimmunotherapy to chemotherapy alone in follicular lymphoma was reported by Marcus and colleagues [40]. 321 patients with previously untreated, stage III and IV follicular lymphoma (and generally adverse prognostic features) were randomized to treatment with eight cycles of CVP chemotherapy every 21 days (notably at a perhaps attenuated cyclophosphamide dose of 750 mg/m²/cycle) with or without concurrent rituximab administered on day 1 of each cycle. Overall and complete response rates were 81% and 41% in the R-CVP arm and were 57% and 10% in the CVP arm, respectively (p<0.0001). Median time to progression was 32 months vs. 15 months (p<0.0001). One important feature was that there was no evidence of increased toxicity when rituximab was added to CVP with the exception of infusion related toxicities. Although these data are compelling, the reported follow-up was short and not reported for overall survival.

The German Low-grade Lymphoma Study Group compared treatment with fludarabine, cyclophosphamide, and mitoxantrone with and without rituximab as treatment for relapsed and refractory follicular and mantle cell lymphoma [41]. The addition of rituximab increased the ORR to 79% (33% CRs, 45% PRs) from 58% (13% CRs, 45% PRs), and was associated with a significantly longer progression-free survival (16 versus 10 months) and overall survival (not reached versus 24 months).

Another approach investigated has been the use of rituximab followed by short duration chemotherapy (CVP or CHOP for 3 cycles) [42]. The intention of this combination is to minimize chemotherapy-related toxicities by limiting the amount of chemotherapy necessary to achieve the necessary response. This type of approach is of particular importance when treating elderly patients or patients who might be expected to receive many repetitive cycles of chemotherapy, as seen with follicular lymphomas. A trial of 86 patients showed an overall response rate of 93% (55% CR) with 4 year progression-free survival of 62%. The promising results in these initial studies are limited by the small sample size (and potential patient selection issues) and lack of a chemotherapy-only control group, though they have served as the basis for larger follow-up studies in broader settings.

Zinzani and co-investigators investigated the use of sequential chemotherapy followed by rituximab. They compared a regimen of fludarabine plus mitoxantrone (+/- rituximab) to CHOP (+/- rituximab) in 140 patients with previously untreated follicular lymphoma [43]. This study added rituximab treatment after chemotherapy only in those patients with persistent clinical or molecular evidence of lymphoma. The FM arm demonstrated higher CR rates than the CHOP arm (68% vs. 42%), with 39% of the FM and 19% of the CHOP treated patients achieving molecular remissions after chemotherapy alone. Overall, rituximab improved the rate of molecular CR from 29% to 61% (71% in FM and 51% in CHOP treated patients). However, with a median follow-up of 19 months, there was no difference observed in progression-free or overall survival amongst any of the different treatment groups. When these data mature, an important analysis will be to determine whether there is a benefit to be gained by using rituximab to convert a clinical CR to a molecular CR in patients with a follicular lymphoma.

Patients treated on study by Zanzani, et al. received four doses of rituximab after completing their chemotherapy. The next step in the use of rituximab was to investigate utilizing "maintenance" rituximab after chemotherapy. This is based upon the data emerging regarding the benefits or maintenance therapy with single agent rituximab. Two randomized, controlled studies investigating the use of rituximab maintenance after chemotherapy were undertaken by McLaughlin (from the M.D. Anderson Cancer Center) and the Eastern Cooperative Oncology Group (ECOG). McLaughlin compared treatment with fludarabine, mitoxantrone, and dexamethasone (FND) plus concurrent rituximab followed by α-interferon (α-IFN) to FND followed by α-IFN plus rituximab in patients with follicular NHL. After 30 months of follow-up, no significant differences in response rates or survival have been identified between the treatment groups [44].

In the study conducted by ECOG (E1496), untreated patients with indolent NHL were initially treated with CVP chemotherapy followed by randomization to either observation or maintenance rituximab administered as 4 weekly doses every six months for two years [45]. Patients who received rituximab after CVP had significantly higher PFS at two and four years post-randomization (74% and 58%, respectively) compared with those who only received CVP (42% and 34%, respectively). This improvement in PFS with rituximab maintenance was seen in all tumor histologies, in patients with bulky disease, and in patients with evidence of minimal residual disease following induction therapy. Although a difference in survival has not been observed after a median follow-up of 1.2 years, this trial provides the first randomized evidence that adding rituximab maintenance to chemotherapy in untreated patients who achieve a response or stable disease can prolong response duration.

The European Organization for Research and Treatment of Cancer (EORTC) is currently conducting a randomized study of CHOP vs. concurrent CHOP-R followed by a secondary randomization to either observation or maintenance rituximab (375 mg/m^2 for one dose every three months) in patients with recurrent follicular lymphoma [46]. The trial was stopped at the second planned interim analysis because of a significant difference in CR rate for CHOP-R versus CHOP (30.4% vs. 18.1%). Additionally, rituximab maintenance has also demonstrated a longer PFS at 1 year and 3 years compared to observation (80.2% and 67.7%, respectively, vs. 54.9% and 31.2% respectively).

4.   CHEMOIMMUNOTHERAPY IN AGGRESSIVE LYMPHOMA

Coiffier and colleagues demonstrated in a phase II study of single agent rituximab in aggressive lymphomas an ORR of 31% (9% CRs, 22% PRs) [47]. Even with single agent rituximab being less effective in aggressive lymphomas than in indolent lymphomas, there still remains the potential benefit of combination chemotherapy and immunotherapy. A phase II study of rituximab given on day 1 combined with standard dose CHOP given on day 3 demonstrated an ORR of 94% (61% CRs, 33% PRs). With a minimum follow-up of 24 months, 88% of patients remained alive and free of disease.

The Groupe d'Etude des Lymphomes de l'Adulte (GELA) conducted the first phase III, randomized study comparing eight cycles of CHOP to rituximab plus CHOP (R-CHOP) as treatment for DLBCL in previously untreated patients over the age of 60 years [48, 49]. In this study, patients randomized to receive R-CHOP received both the rituximab and CHOP chemotherapy on day 1 of the cycle. With a median follow-up of five years, R-CHOP produced statistically significant improvements over CHOP in terms of CR rate (76% vs. 63%), 5-year PFS (54% vs. 30%), and 5-yr OS (58% vs. 45%).

More recently, the Mabthera International Trial (MinT) evaluated the addition of concurrent rituximab to a CHOP-like regimen in younger, good-prognosis patients younger than 60 years of age [50]. With median follow-up of two years, the addition of rituximab to chemotherapy resulted in higher CR rates (81 vs. 67%), longer 2-year TTF rates (76% vs. 60%), and better 2 year OS (94% vs. 87%). Follow-up continues, and data on potential benefits of rituximab in patient subgroups (chemotherapy type, bulk of disease, use of radiation treatment, prognosis) are anticipated.

The ECOG 4494 trial investigated the use of CHOP plus rituximab in elderly patients with diffuse large B-cell lymphoma utilizing a 2 x 2 factorial design [51, 52]. Patients were first randomized to treatment with either CHOP chemotherapy with rituximab administered prior to cycle 1 and concurrently with cycles 3, 5, and 7 or CHOP alone. Responding patients were then randomized to either observation or maintenance rituximab administered as a 4-week course every six months for two years. The ORR was not different between the induction regimens, 79% for R-CHOP and 76% for CHOP alone. Weighted analysis was performed to enable each randomization to be examined individually. The data demonstrated an improvement in time-to-treatment failure (TTF) for R-CHOP compared to CHOP induction at three years (52% vs. 39%), and in overall survival at three years (67% vs. 58%). Likewise, maintenance rituximab prolonged

TTF compared to observation, but with no difference in overall survival. Overall, in the patients reaching the second randomization, the 2-year TTF was 77%, 79%, 74%, and 45% for R-CHOP, R-CHOP + MR, CHOP + MR, and CHOP, respectively.   These findings indicate that maintenance rituximab improved TTF in patients treated with CHOP alone (HR .45, *P* =.004), but did not provide any additional benefit to patients treated with R-CHOP (HR = .93, *P* = .81). The primary findings of the study confirm the benefits of CHOP-R induction therapy over CHOP alone, and also suggest that with R-CHOP induction regimen, maintenance rituximab therapy is unnecessary in DLBCL. It could thus be said that it does not matter when rituximab is administered as part of a CHOP induction regimen for DLBCL, so long as it is administered at some point.

Current studies are evaluating the effects of rituximab in combination with other regimens (such as dose-adjusted EPOCH) in DLBCL and other lymphoma histologies with varying results [41, 53, 54].

5.   CHEMOIMMUNOTHERAPY IN HIV-ASSOCIATED LYMPHOMAS

The addition of rituximab to standard CHOP chemotherapy improves the outcome for non-HIV infected patients with diffuse large B-cell lymphoma and has rapidly become the standard of care [48, 50]. In HIV-associated diffuse large B-cell lymphomas the addition of rituximab to standard cytotoxic chemotherapy remains quite controversial. There have been three reports of patients treated with rituximab in combination with chemotherapy, only one of which was a phase III study. The AIDS Malignancies Consortium (AMC) recently updated their AMC010 study which compared standard CHOP chemotherapy to R-CHOP, with responders to R-CHOP receiving three single monthly doses of rituximab as maintenance [55]. The overall CR rate for R-CHOP was 58% compared to 47% for CHOP. This represented a 22% increase in the CR rate, but did not reach statistical significance. Likewise, for time to progression, progression-free survival, and overall survival there was a trend in favor of R-CHOP compared to CHOP (125 vs. 85, 45 vs. 38, and 139 vs. 110 weeks respectively), but none of the data reached statistical significance. It is worth noting that the study was statistically designed to detect an increase in CR rate (the primary endpoint of the study) of 50% from the addition of rituximab to CHOP. Even in view of the lack of statistical significance, the improvements seen with rituximab added to CHOP are suggestive of a potential benefit.

However, these data must be interpreted with caution. There was a marked increase in death due to treatment related infection with the addition of rituximab (14% vs. 2%). There are several hypotheses as to why there was the increase in infection-related mortality with rituximab treatment, including hypogammaglobulinemia [56], prolongation of the neutropenia through cytokines [57], and autoantibody production [58]. This prolonged neutropenia and infection-related deaths were not seen in the studies investigating the combination of rituximab and chemotherapy in non-HIV associated lymphomas, suggesting that the deaths may have been the result of the combination of hypogammaglobulinemia and the CD4 cell lymphopenia seen in HIV patients. To support this belief, the risk of death due to infection were greatest in those patients with a T-cell count of less than 50 cells/mm^3.

In contrast to the AMC study, three other groups published results of their respective phase II studies investigating rituximab in combination with chemotherapy for aggressive lymphomas in HIV positive patients documenting high CR rates without an increase in infectious mortality. The Agence Nationale Recherche SIDA (ANRS) in France treated sixty-one patients as part of their ANRS 085 study [59, 60]. They demonstrated a CR rate of 77%, with a two-year OS of 64% and a two-year DFS of 83%. Although bacterial infections were observed in 34% of patients, only two toxic deaths were seen. Only seven of the 40 patients who achieved a CR have relapsed after 18 months of follow-up. It should be noted that 28% of these patients had aggressive lymphomas other than diffuse, large B-cell lymphoma (i.e. Burkitt's) that would portend a worse prognosis.

Spina, et al. reported on a pooled analysis of three phase II studies investigating rituximab in combination with infusional cyclophosphamide, doxorubicin, and etoposide (R-CDE) in HIV positive patients with aggressive lymphomas [61]. In this series of 74 patients, 72% of patients had diffuse, large cell histology. They report a 70% CR rate, with an estimated two-year failure-free survival and overall survival rates of 59% and 64% respectively. Twenty-three percent of patients developed non-opportunistic infections, with six patients (8%) dying secondary to infection (two bacterial, four opportunistic infections). For comparison, response rates for CDE in HIV lymphomas reported in a separate study included a CR rate of 44%, two-year failure-free survival and overall survival rates of 36% and 43% respectively, with 20% developing grades 3 or 4 infection and no deaths in the post-HAART cohort of patients [62].

As can be seen from the three studies, response rates are increased, but at the risk of serious infections. These studies were not standardized with regard to infectious prophylaxis or the use of granulocyte colony stimulating factors. Therefore, in the right patients with the correct precautions, there may be potential gain from the use of rituximab in combination with chemotherapy for aggressive lymphomas in HIV positive patients.

6.   ALEMTUZUMAB

Alemtuzumab (Campath-1H) is a genetically engineered humanized IgG1 monoclonal antibody directed against CD52. Alemtuzumab, named Campath after *Cam*bridge *Path*ology, was first developed in 1983 as a rat monoclonal antibody that was very effective in reducing graft-versus-host disease following allogeneic bone marrow transplantation. The antigen binding determinants of the Alemtuzumab antibody were eventually cloned into human immunoglobulin producing cells generating a humanized monoclonal antibody. As a humanized antibody, it was believed that alemtuzumab would be more effective at mediating Fc-mediated activities with decreased immunogenicity. Alemtuzumab was first used clinically in 1988 in a patient with refractory lymphoma [63]. But it was not until 1991 that the CD52 antigen was cloned and recognized as the target for alemtuzumab.

CD52 is a glycosylphosphatidylinositol-anchored glycoprotein which is non-modulating antigen and expressed at high density on all lymphocytes and monocytes, but not on granulocytes, erythrocytes, platelets, and hematopoietic stem cells [64, 65]. CD52 is one of the most abundantly expressed membrane glycoproteins, with lymphocytes possessing almost 450,000 molecules per cell. CD52 is almost universally expressed on lymphomas, with more intense expression seen on normal and malignant T cells compared to normal and malignant B cells, as well as on low-grade compared to aggressive lymphomas [66]. Alemtuzumab was demonstrated to be more effective against blood and bone marrow disease compared to lymph node disease, as well as against indolent disease compared to aggressive disease [67]. These data lead to the initial development of alemtuzumab for use in the treatment of patients with CLL. Alemtuzumab is able to fill a niche where rituximab is less effective because of the low-intensity of CD20 expression present on CLL cells. Based upon data generated from the pivotal study, Campath was approved by the FDA in 2000 for treatment of patients with CLL who have relapsed after fludarabine therapy [68].

Since T-cell lymphomas do not express CD20, they represent another area where rituximab is not of value. Peripheral T-cell lymphomas represent 5-10% of NHLs and typically have a poorer prognosis than B-cell lymphomas [1]. Anthracycline-containing chemotherapy regimens are expected to result in long term survival in only approximately 30-40% of patients [69, 70]. Early studies suggested that responses to alemtuzumab correlated with levels of CD52 expression, further supporting a role for alemtuzumab in T-cell lymphomas [71]. Investigators began to utilize Campath in T-cell lymphomas in an analogous manner to rituximab in B-cell lymphomas. Several phase II studies have been performed utilizing alemtuzumab as single agent treatment delivered either by intravenous or subcutaneous injection for either B or T-cell lymphomas.

Three studies investigating alemtuzumab in patients with NHL demonstrated response rates of 16%, 20%, and 44% [72-74]. When Lundin and colleagues analyzed eight patients with mycosis fungoides separately, they identified an ORR of 50%, with 2 CRs. Enblad conducted a trial involving patients with chemotherapy refractory peripheral T-cell lymphomas [75] and demonstrated an ORR of 36% (5 of 14), including 3 CRs. In this trial, hematologic and infectious complications were considerable, and resulted in the study closing prematurely with five deaths attributed in part to alemtuzumab. Given the refractory nature of these patients' disease, the authors concluded that alemtuzumab has considerable activity, and may be sufficiently safe in less heavily treated patients. The same group tested alemtuzumab in twenty-two patients with advanced mycosis fungoides [76], and achieved an ORR was 55%, with 32% of patients achieving a CR. In this study, ten patients developed infections, resulting in one death due to pulmonary aspergillosis. Four patients developed CMV reactivation, with all four responding to IV ganciclovir. The infectious complications in this study appeared more manageable, supporting a role for the further development of alemtuzumab as a treatment for lymphomas. Another approach to reduce the infectious complications was studied by Zinzani, et al [77]. This involved a dosing regimen of 10 mg (instead of 30 mg) administered intravenously three times a week for four weeks. In the ten patients treated, there were six responses, with four PRs and two CRs. Only one infection was noted, which was CMV reactivation adequately treated with ganciclovir. As supportive therapies improve (such as through the use of valganciclovir) and more clinical experience is obtained with alemtuzumab, higher response rates with safer outcomes could be expected.

7.   OTHER IMMUNOTHERAPIES UNDER EXPLORATION IN NHL

The use of other biologic agents either alone or in combination with rituximab is an appealing strategy to avoid the toxicity of chemotherapy or to enhance its efficacy.   Immunostimulatory agents are under active investigation for this purpose.   Interleukin-2 (IL-2) administration expands and activates circulating natural killer (NK) cell populations, which potentially improves antibody-dependent cellular cytotoxicity (ADCC). Since ADCC is an important mechanism of rituximab activity, IL-2 in combination with rituximab might have synergistic effects. Additionally, as previously discussed, less benefit is derived from rituximab use in patients with certain Fc receptor polymorphisms.   In an attempt to investigate this combination, IL-2 was administered at escalating doses from 4.5 to 14 million units subcutaneously three times per week in conjunction with four weekly standard rituximab doses [78]. In this phase I study, most patients responded.   Higher circulating NK cell numbers and increased ADCC activity were seen with IL-2 therapy and correlated with clinical response. Eisenbeis and colleagues have evaluated the combination of IL-2 plus rituximab in patients with rituximab-refractory indolent lymphoma[79]. Since this patient population was resistant to rituximab, the observation of any tumor shrinkage would be significant.   Clinical responses were identified in five of 23 patients.   When the Fc receptor polymorphisms of these patients were examined, it was noted that all of the responding patients analyzed had the phenylalanine polymorphism at position 158.   This polymorphism is associated generally less affective ADCC and less favorable outcome with rituximab. These findings are consistent with the hypothesis that IL-2 may be able to overcome rituximab-resistance when it is related to relatively less effective ADCC due to Fc receptor polymorphism.

Immunostimulatory sequences of DNA in the form of CpG oligonucleotides have a wide range of immune effects including enhancement of antigen presentation and cytokine induction (supporting ADCC). Friedberg and colleagues conducted a phase I trial with 4 doses of a CpG oligodeoxynucleotide (1018 ISS) with rituximab and noted clinical responses with minimal toxicity.[35] Interestingly, correlative studies demonstrated that CpG administration was associated with a dose-related increase in expression of several interferon-inducible genes, a reassuring sign of biological effects. CpG administration is under active exploration both as a single agent and in combination with other therapies in lymphoma as well as other malignancies.

Other investigators have attempted to improve upon rituximab therapy by creating new variations of CD20-directed antibodies. Preclinical studies have been conducted with a number of these agents which have been designed to either have human or humanized structure (other than murine or chimeric) to improve pharmacokinetics and reduce immunogenicity, or to have enhanced complement-mediated cytotoxicity or ADCC.[36,37] Such agents have moved into phase I clinical trials in some cases, and clinical responses have been observed. Whether the theoretical advantages to these antibody modifications translate to clinical benefit for patients remains to be determined.

Alternative targets for monoclonal antibodies (particularly in B cell malignancies) are also under evaluation. The CD22 antigen is widely expressed in normal and malignant B cells and plays a role in B cell activation and trafficking.[38] We conducted phase I trials of epratuzumab, a humanized anti-CD22 antibody, and demonstrated a favorable toxicity profile at doses of up to 1000 mg/m2/week administered for 4 weeks.[39, 40] Clinical responses were noted in follicular NHL and in diffuse large B cell lymphoma. In some cases these have lasted for greater than one year, and second responses (upon retreatment at progression) have been noted. Epratuzumab is currently under active investigation in combination with rituximab, with CHOP-R chemotherapy, as well as in other B cell malignancies and in autoimmune disease.

8. RADIOIMMUNOTHERAPY

Given the exquisite radiosensitivity of low-grade NHL, the attachment of a radioisotope to a monoclonal antibody can enhance the activity of the antibody through the addition of targeted radiation [80]. The monoclonal antibody serves as the means to deliver the radiation directly to the intended target. When conventional radiation is delivered by external beam radiation, normal and malignant tissues are irradiated. For tumors that are not localized, avoiding the normal tissues becomes impossible with this modality. The antibody delivers the radioisotope into proximity of the intended target. When the radioisotope decays, the radiation is released to damage the target cell, typically by inducing DNA strand breaks, leading to apoptosis of the cell. The radiation is delivered not only to the antibody bound targeted cell, but also to neighboring cells that are located within the path length of the radiation. This "cross-fire" effect results in therapeutic benefit if the neighboring cells are tumor cells not bound by antibody, or toxicity if the neighboring cell is a non-malignant cell. This is of particular concern with low-grade lymphomas as they frequently involve the bone marrow and hematopoietic stem cells are very radiosensitive. Thus, myelosuppression is one of the dose limiting toxicities for RIT.

Two such agents have been FDA approved, Yttrium-90 ibritumomab tiuxetan (Zevalin, Biogen Idec) and Iodine-131 tositumomab (Bexxar, Corixa and GlaxoSmithKline), for use in patients with CD20+ transformed or non-transformed follicular lymphoma whose disease is refractory to rituximab and has relapsed following chemotherapy. Both radioimmunoconjugates chelate their radioisotope to a murine antibody against the CD20 antigen. Since the therapeutic modality is radiation, there is less need for a human Fc portion of the immunoglobulin to be present to elicit ADCC or CDC. Utilization of the murine antibody allowed for quicker and simpler therapeutic development of RIT, and is associated with a shorter antibody half-life (potentially resulting in less circulation of unbound radiolabled antibody which can result in non-specific radiation-related toxicity).

One possible problem with a murine antibody is the potential development by the patient of an antibody against mouse antibodies, or HAMA (human anti-murine antibody) antibodies. This HAMA antibody may impair the effectiveness of RIT, or subsequent immunotherapy utilizing murine antibodies, or result in the development of infusion related toxicities. Patients who initially received RIT were at low-risk for developing HAMA as a result of their immune dysfunction secondary to numbers of prior chemotherapies they received. In the pivotal trial of I-131 tositumomab in low-grade NHL, a HAMA rate of only 8% was seen [81]. Patients enrolled on this study had a median of four prior chemotherapy regimens. In the phase I/II study of Y-90 ibritumomab tiuxetan 2% of patients developed HAMA or HACA antibodies [82, 83]. These data compare to a HAMA rate of 63% seen when Kaminski studied I-131 tositumomab as initial therapy in patients with follicular lymphoma [84]. Once again, it is unclear what the clinical implications are of the development of a HAMA, but Kaminski reported that among the 23 patients in whom HAMA levels were more than five times the lowest level of detection, the five-year rate of PFS was 35%, compared with 70% for the remaining 53 patients. Additionally, more patients in the subgroup with high HAMA titers experienced grade 2 or higher fever, myalgias, arthralgias, or rash [84].

I-131 tositumomab and Y-90 ibritumomab tiuxetan utilize different radioisotopes. The I-131 beta emissions travel on average 0.4 mm, or several cell diameters. The beta emissions from Y-90 are of higher energy, resulting in a longer path length compared with I-131 (5 mm). This translates into an optimal target diameter for Y-90 of 3.4 cm compared with 0.34 cm for I-131 [85]. This higher beta energy may be an advantage where deeper penetration is desired, but a disadvantage where it will result in greater toxicity. Additionally, I-131 emits gamma radiation which allows for imaging to be performed using external gamma cameras, in order to determine dosimetry. Since Y-90 does not emit gamma radiation, any dosimetry performed needs to employ a surrogate isotope, in this case indium-111 labeled ibritumomab tiuxetan.

I-131 tositumomab is individually dosed for each patient based on dosimetry calculations, while Y-90 ibritumomab tiuxetan is dosed based on weight. For I-131 tositumomab the dose is calculated to deliver a dose of total-body radiation of 75 cGy, while for Y-90 ibritumomab tiuxetan is typically given at 0.4 mCi/kg, with maximum 32 mCi [82, 86]. Both RITs were found to require dose reductions in patients who had platelet counts between 100-149,000 /μL, as well as recommendations for not treating patients with greater than 25% bone marrow involvement.

In its pivotal study, responses to I-131 tositumomab treatment were compared to the efficacy seen with the patient's last qualifying chemotherapy (LQC) regimen [81]. This enabled refractory patients to be studied without needing to utilize a comparator arm, since these patients had already demonstrated refractoriness to chemotherapy and if subsequent chemotherapy were to be given responses were expected to be less frequent and shorter in duration. All patients treated on protocol had either not responded or had a response of less than six months to their LQC. An ORR of 65%, with 20% CRs, was seen for I-131 tositumomab compared to 28%, with 3% CRs) after the LQC. The median response duration for those patients achieving a CR after I-131 tositumomab had not been reached after 47 months of follow-up, compared to 6.1 months after LQC. Given the refractory nature of these patients' disease, these responses are of particular significance.

In the pivotal study for Y-90 ibritumomab tiuxetan, patients with low-grade, follicular, or transformed B-cell NHL were randomized by Witzig and colleagues to treatment with Y-90 ibritumomab tiuxetan or rituximab [87]. The ORR and CR rate for the two groups were 80% and 30% for Y-90 ibritumomab tiuxetan and 56% and 16% for rituximab. Additionally, more durable responses (greater than six months in length) were seen with Y-90 ibritumomab tiuxetan than rituximab.

In Witzig study, the labeled and unlabeled antibodies differed not just in regard to the presence of the radioisotope, but also since Y-90 ibritumomab tiuxetan is a murine antibody, while rituximab is a chimeric antibody. Two studies were conducted utilizing the same antibody with and without an attached radioisotope that confirmed the importance of the radioisotope to the anti-CD20 therapy. In a trial that compared I-131 labeled tositumomab to unlabeled tositumomab, Davis and colleagues demonstrated ORRs of

55% versus 19%, with 33% CRs versus 8% CRs, for I-131 labeled
tositumomab versus unlabeled tositumomab [80].   In a second study,
Horning evaulated I-131 tositumomab in patients who had previously
received rituximab [88]. The prior responses to rituximab demonstrated by
the 40 patients in this study included 24 patients without any response, 11
patients with responses of less than six months, and five patients with
responses greater than six months. The ORR was 65%, with a CR rate of
38%, for all the patients in the study, and a progression free survival for
responders of 24.5 months. There was no correlation between the response
to I-131 tositumomab to that of the rituximab, indicating that refractoriness
to rituximab does not predict for a poor response to I-131 tositumomab.

In an attempt to maximize the benefits of RIT for patients, I-131
tositumomab was evaluated in indolent or transformed B-cell NHL at first or
second relapse showed a response rate of 76%, with a CR rate of 49% [89].
Median overall duration of remission was 1.3 years, and approximately one-
fourth of the patients remained in a continuous remission ranging from 2.6+
to 5.2+ years after treatment. Kaminski and colleagues assessed the utility
of radioimmunotherapy as initial therapy for follicular lymphoma [84].
Seventy-six patients with untreated, advanced stage follicular lymphoma
were treated with a single course of I-131 tositumomab. The overall
response rate was 95%, including 75% complete responses. Eighty percent
of the assessable patients achieved a molecular remissions based on
polymerase chain reaction assessment for BCL2 gene rearrangements. After
a median follow-up of greater than five years, estimated progression-free
survival was 6.1 years. Treatment was well tolerated. As previously
discussed, HAMA formation occurred in 63% of these patients, far greater
than the eight percent reported in the earlier studies of heavily pretreated
patients.

These findings have led to further studies which will ultimately help to
determine the utility of RIT as a component for initial therapy for indolent
lymphoma. A phase II study conducted by the Southwest Oncology Group
investigated CHOP followed by I-131 tositumomab as initial therapy in
patients with follicular lymphoma [90]. Preliminary results appear quite
favorable, with an ORR 90%, a CR rate of 67%, and a two-year progression
free survival of 81%. As a follow-up, the Southwest Oncology Group and
Cancer and Leukemia Group B are currently conducting a randomized trial
of CHOP plus concurrent rituximab versus CHOP followed by I-131
tositumomab as first therapy for follicular NHL.

Another approach has been to evaluate the use of radioimmunotherapy in
conjunction with autologous stem cell transplantation. Early studies
investigated I-131 tositumomab as a single agent at myeloablative doses of
approximately 25 Gy in place of chemotherapy as part of an autologous stem

cell transplant for patients with relapsed lymphoma [91, 92]. The dose limiting toxicity for RIT is myelosuppression. By utilizing stem cell rescue to overcome this toxicity, the dose of radiation can be increased to the tolerance of the next most sensitive organ. This allows the radiation to be increased form 75 cGy to 25 Gy, an increase in radiation dose of more than 30 fold. This study consisted primarily of patients with low-grade lymphoma. The strategy was to utilize radiation to overcome the presence of any resistance to chemotherapy in previously treated patients. Eighteen of 21 patients (86%) responded, with a 76% CR rate, and a 62% two-year progression free survival.

RIT is also under evaluation in an autologous stem cell transplant approach in combination with chemotherapy. In a phase I study of RIT in combination with BEAM (carmustine, etoposide, cytarabine, and melphalan) chemotherapy for patients refractory to chemotherapy a dose of 75 cGy was found to be tolerable [93]. The three-year overall survival and event free survival for this study after a median follow-up of 38 months were 55% and 39% respectively. These patients would not have been considered eligible for standard autologous stem cell transplants given the chemorefractory nature of their disease, making any responses noteworthy.

One concern related to RIT is the potential exposure of myelopoietic stem cells in the bone marrow to be exposed to radiation. Since most lymphomas invade the bone marrow, there is significant opportunity for toxicity due to "cross-fire". In the short term, this results in pancytopenia. In most cases, this will resolve without complications. Long term, there has been some concern that the use of RIT will lead to myelodysplastic syndromes (MDS) and secondary acute myeloid leukemia (AML), both of which carry poor prognoses. Patients with lymphomas that have been heavily pretreated with chemotherapy are at a significant risk for developing MDS or AML. When the data for I-131 tositumomab are analyzed in aggregate, the annualized incidence for the development of either AML or MDS is 1.6% per year [94]. This rate is consistent with what would be expected for this group of patients treated only with chemotherapy, suggesting no increase risk of AML or MDS from the addition of RIT. To further support this, when the patients who underwent RIT as initial therapy are examined, and thus had no chemotherapy exposure, no cases of AML or MDS were identified.

9.   CONCLUSIONS

The addition of monoclonal antibodies to the armamentarium of treatment options has dramatically altered the care of patients with lymphoma. In addition to representing effective therapies that are often not cross-resistant with standard cytotoxic agents, antibodies offer treatment without many of the toxicities associated with chemotherapy. This has provide a new option for many patients who otherwise were unable to receive treatment because of co-morbid illnesses or cytopenias. Additionally, there is the potential for treating patients early in their diseases with the intent of delaying the exposure to the toxicities of chemotherapy, possibly allowing patients to enjoy better quality of lives. When patients do require chemotherapy, monoclonal antibodies appear to make the chemotherapy more effective. Future research includes efforts to further improve the utility of our current antibodies as well as the identification of novel targets. Currently, a considerable challenge exists in defining the optimal dose, schedule and sequence of antibody therapies among the range of active treatment options. Nonetheless, it is evident that these approaches have improved outcomes for patients with lymphoma, and that additional efforts to further develop antibody-based treatment strategies are clearly warranted.

10.   REFERENCES

1   Harris NL, Jaffe ES, Stein H, Vardiman JW, eds. World Health Organization Classification of Tumours. Pathology and Genetics of Tumours of Haematopoietic and Lymphoid Tissues. 2001, IARC Press: Lyon.

2   Nadler LM, Ritz J, Hardy R, *et al.* A unique cell surface antigen identifying lymphoid malignancies of B cell origin. *J Clin Invest* 1981, 67:134-140.

3   Reff ME, Carner K, Chambers KS, *et al.* Depletion of B cells in vivo by a chimeric mouse human monoclonal antibody to CD20. *Blood* 1994, 83:435-445.

4   Anderson KC, Bates MP, Slaughenhoupt BL, *et al.* Expression of human B cell-associated antigens on leukemias and lymphomas: a model of human B cell differentiation. *Blood* 1984, 63:1424-1433.

5   Tedder TF, Streuli M, Schlossman SF, Saito H. Isolation and structure of a cDNA encoding the B1 (CD20) cell-surface antigen of human B lymphocytes. *Proc Natl Acad Sci U S A* 1988, 85:208-212.

6   Tedder TF, Boyd AW, Freedman AS, *et al.* The B cell surface molecule B1 is functionally linked with B cell activation and differentiation. *J Immunol* 1985, 135:973-979.

7   Tedder TF, Engel P. CD20: a regulator of cell-cycle progression of B lymphocytes. *Immunol Today* 1994, 15:450-454.

8   Riley JK, Sliwkowski MX. CD20: a gene in search of a function. *Semin Oncol* 2000, 27:17-24.

9   Press OW, Appelbaum F, Ledbetter JA, *et al.* Monoclonal antibody 1F5 (anti-CD20) serotherapy of human B cell lymphomas. *Blood* 1987, 69:584-591.

10   Giles FJ, Vose JM, Do KA, *et al.* Circulating CD20 and CD52 in patients with non-Hodgkin's lymphoma or Hodgkin's disease. *Br J Haematol* 2003, 123:850-857.

11   Manshouri T, Do KA, Wang X, *et al.* Circulating CD20 is detectable in the plasma of patients with chronic lymphocytic leukemia and is of prognostic significance. *Blood* 2003, 101:2507-2513.

12   Golay J, Zaffaroni L, Vaccari T, *et al.* Biologic response of B lymphoma cells to anti-CD20 monoclonal antibody rituximab in vitro: CD55 and CD59 regulate complement-mediated cell lysis. *Blood* 2000, 95:3900-3908.

13   Manches O, Lui G, Chaperot L, *et al.* In vitro mechanisms of action of rituximab on primary non-Hodgkin lymphomas. *Blood* 2003, 101:949-954.

14   Bellosillo B, Villamor N, Lopez-Guillermo A, *et al.* Complement-mediated cell death induced by rituximab in B-cell lymphoproliferative disorders is mediated in vitro by a caspase-independent mechanism involving the generation of reactive oxygen species. *Blood* 2001, 98:2771-2777.

15   Clynes RA, Towers TL, Presta LG, Ravetch JV. Inhibitory Fc receptors modulate in vivo cytoxicity against tumor targets. *Nat Med* 2000, 6:443-446.

16   Weng WK, Levy R. Two immunoglobulin G fragment C receptor polymorphisms independently predict response to rituximab in patients with follicular lymphoma. *J Clin Oncol* 2003, 21:3940-3947.

17   Shan D, Ledbetter JA, Press OW. Signaling events involved in anti-CD20-induced apoptosis of malignant human B cells. *Cancer Immunol Immunother* 2000, 48:673-683.

18   Mathas S, Rickers A, Bommert K, *et al.* Anti-CD20- and B-cell receptor-mediated apoptosis: evidence for shared intracellular signaling pathways. *Cancer Res* 2000, 60:7170-7176.

19   Jazirehi AR, Huerta-Yepez S, Cheng G, Bonavida B. Rituximab (chimeric anti-CD20 monoclonal antibody) inhibits the constitutive nuclear factor-{kappa}B signaling pathway in non-Hodgkin's lymphoma B-cell lines: role in sensitization to chemotherapeutic drug-induced apoptosis. *Cancer Res* 2005, 65:264-276.

20   Jazirehi AR, Vega MI, Chatterjee D, *et al.* Inhibition of the Raf-MEK1/2-ERK1/2 signaling pathway, Bcl-xL down-regulation, and chemosensitization of non-Hodgkin's lymphoma B cells by Rituximab. *Cancer Res* 2004, 64:7117-7126.

21   Byrd JC, Kitada S, Flinn IW, *et al.* The mechanism of tumor cell clearance by rituximab in vivo in patients with B-cell chronic lymphocytic leukemia: evidence of caspase activation and apoptosis induction. *Blood* 2002, 99:1038-1043.

22   Alas S, Bonavida B. Rituximab Inactivates Signal Transducer and Activation of Transcription 3 (STAT3) Activity in B-Non-Hodgkin's Lymphoma through Inhibition of the Interleukin 10 Autocrine/Paracrine Loop and Results in Down-Regulation of Bcl-2 and Sensitization to Cytotoxic Drugs. *Cancer Res* 2001, 61:5137-5144.

23   Weng WK, Levy R. Expression of complement inhibitors CD46, CD55, and CD59 on tumor cells does not predict clinical outcome after rituximab treatment in follicular non-Hodgkin lymphoma. *Blood* 2001, 98:1352-1357.

24   Pels H, Schulz H, Manzke O, *et al.* Intraventricular and intravenous treatment of a patient with refractory primary CNS lymphoma using rituximab. *J Neurooncol* 2002, 59:213-216.

25   Rubenstein JL, Combs D, Rosenberg J, *et al.* Rituximab therapy for CNS lymphomas: targeting the leptomeningeal compartment. *Blood* 2003, 101:466-468.

26   Cartron G, Dacheux L, Salles G, *et al.* Therapeutic activity of humanized anti-CD20 monoclonal antibody and polymorphism in IgG Fc receptor FcgammaRIIIa gene. *Blood* 2002, 99:754-758.

27   Maloney DG, Liles TM, Czerwinski DK, *et al.* Phase I clinical trial using escalating single-dose infusion of chimeric anti-CD20 monoclonal antibody (IDEC-C2B8) in patients with recurrent B-cell lymphoma. *Blood* 1994, 84:2457-2466.

28   Maloney DG, Grillo-Lopez AJ, Bodkin DJ, *et al.* IDEC-C2B8: results of a phase I multiple-dose trial in patients with relapsed non-Hodgkin's lymphoma. *J Clin Oncol* 1997, 15:3266-3274.

29   Maloney DG, Grillo-Lopez AJ, White CA, *et al.* IDEC-C2B8 (Rituximab) anti-CD20 monoclonal antibody therapy in patients with relapsed low-grade non-Hodgkin's lymphoma. *Blood* 1997, 90:2188-2195.

30   McLaughlin P, Grillo-Lopez AJ, Link BK, *et al.* Rituximab chimeric anti-CD20 monoclonal antibody therapy for relapsed indolent lymphoma: half of patients respond to a four-dose treatment program. *J Clin Oncol* 1998, 16:2825-2833.

31   Witzig TE, Vukov AM, Habermann TM, *et al.* Rituximab therapy for patients with newly diagnosed, advanced-stage, follicular grade I non-Hodgkin's lymphoma: a phase II trial in the North Central Cancer Treatment Group. *J Clin Oncol* 2005, 23:1103-1108.

32   Davis TA, Grillo-Lopez AJ, White CA, *et al.* Rituximab anti-CD20 monoclonal antibody therapy in non-Hodgkin's lymphoma: safety and efficacy of re-treatment. *J Clin Oncol* 2000, 18:3135-3143.

33   Piro LD, White CA, Grillo-Lopez AJ, *et al.* Extended Rituximab (anti-CD20 monoclonal antibody) therapy for relapsed or refractory low-grade or follicular non-Hodgkin's lymphoma. *Ann Oncol* 1999, 10:655-661.

34   Hainsworth JD, Litchy S, Burris HA, III, *et al.* Rituximab as First-Line and Maintenance Therapy for Patients With Indolent Non-Hodgkin's Lymphoma. *J Clin Oncol* 2002, 20:4261-4267.

35   Ghielmini M, Schmitz SF, Cogliatti SB, *et al.* Prolonged treatment with rituximab in patients with follicular lymphoma significantly increases event-free survival and response duration compared with the standard weekly x 4 schedule. *Blood* 2004, 103:4416-4423.

36   Hainsworth JD, Litchy S, Shaffer DW, *et al.* Maximizing therapeutic benefit of rituximab: maintenance therapy versus re-treatment at progression in patients with indolent non-Hodgkin's lymphoma--a randomized phase II trial of the Minnie Pearl Cancer Research Network. *J Clin Oncol* 2005, 23:1088-1095.

37   Gordan LN, Grow WB, Pusateri A, *et al.* Phase II Trial of Individualized Rituximab Dosing for Patients With CD20-Positive Lymphoproliferative Disorders. *J Clin Oncol* 2005, 23:1096-1102.

38   Czuczman MS, Weaver R, Alkuzweny B, *et al.* Prolonged clinical and molecular remission in patients with low-grade or follicular non-Hodgkin's lymphoma treated with rituximab plus CHOP chemotherapy: 9-year follow-up. *J Clin Oncol* 2004, 22:4711-4716.

39   Czuczman MS, Koryzna A, Mohr A, *et al.* Rituximab in combination with fludarabine chemotherapy in low-grade or follicular lymphoma. *J Clin Oncol* 2005, 23:694-704.

40   Marcus R, Imrie K, Belch A, *et al.* CVP chemotherapy plus rituximab compared with CVP as first-line treatment for advanced follicular lymphoma. *Blood* 2005, 105:1417-1423.

41   Forstpointner R, Dreyling M, Repp R, *et al.* The addition of rituximab to a combination of fludarabine, cyclophosphamide, mitoxantrone (FCM) significantly increases the response rate and prolongs survival as compared with FCM alone in patients with relapsed and refractory follicular and mantle cell lymphomas: results of a prospective randomized study of the German Low-Grade Lymphoma Study Group. *Blood* 2004, 104:3064-3071.

42   Hainsworth JD, Litchy S, Morrissey LH, *et al.* Rituximab plus short-duration chemotherapy as first-line treatment for follicular non-Hodgkin's lymphoma: a phase II trial of the minnie pearl cancer research network. *J Clin Oncol* 2005, 23:1500-1506.

43   Zinzani PL, Pulsoni A, Perrotti A, *et al.* Fludarabine plus mitoxantrone with and without rituximab versus CHOP with and without rituximab as front-line treatment for patients with follicular lymphoma. *J Clin Oncol* 2004, 22:2654-2661.

44   McLaughlin P, Rodriguez MA, Hagemeister FB, *et al.* Stage IV indolent lymphoma: A randomized study of concurrent vs. sequential use of FND chemotherapy (fludarabine, mitoxantrone, dexamethasone) and rituximab (R) monoclonal antibody therapy, with interferon maintenance. *Proc Am Soc Clin Oncol* 2003, 22:564 (abstract 2269).

45   Hochster HS, Weller E, Ryan T, *et al.* Results of E1496: A phase III trial of CVP with or without maintenance rituximab in advanced indolent lymphoma (NHL). *Proc Am Soc Clin Oncol* 2004, 23:556 (abstract 6502).

46   Van Oers MHJ, Van Glabbeke M, Teodorovic I, *et al.* Chimeric Anti-CD20 Monoclonal Antibody (Rituximab; Mabtheraa) in Remission Induction and Maintenance Treatment of Relapsed /Resistant Follicular Non-Hodgkin's Lymphoma : A Phase III Randomized Intergroup Clinical Trial. *Blood* 2004, 104:169a (abstract 586).

47   Coiffier B, Haioun C, Ketterer N, *et al.* Rituximab (anti-CD20 monoclonal antibody) for the treatment of patients with relapsing or refractory aggressive lymphoma: a multicenter phase II study. *Blood* 1998, 92:1927-1932.

48   Coiffier B, Lepage E, Briere J, *et al.* CHOP Chemotherapy plus Rituximab Compared with CHOP Alone in Elderly Patients with Diffuse Large-B-Cell Lymphoma. *N Engl J Med* 2002, 346:235-242.

49   Feugier P, Van Hoof A, Sebban C, *et al.* Long-Term Results of the R-CHOP Study in the Treatment of Elderly Patients With Diffuse Large B-Cell Lymphoma: A Study by the Groupe d'Etude des Lymphomes de l'Adulte. *J Clin Oncol* 2005, 23:4117-4126.

50   Pfreundschuh M, Truemper L, Gill D, *et al.* First analysis of the completed Mabthera international (Mint) trial in young patients with low-risk diffuse large B-cell lymphoma (DLBCL): Addition of rituximab to a CHOP-like regimen significantly improves outcome of all patients with the identification of a very favorable subgroup with IPI=O and no bulky disease. *Blood* 2004, 104:48a (abstract 157).

51   Habermann TM, Weller EA, Morrison VA, *et al.* Phase III trial of rituximab-CHOP (R-CHOP) vs. CHOP with a second randomization to maintenance rituximab (MR) or observation in patients 60 years of age and older with diffuse large B-cell lymphoma (DLBCL). *Blood* 2003, 102:(abstract 8).

52   Habermann TM, Weller E, Morrison VA, *et al.* Rituximab-CHOP versus CHOP with or without maintenance rituximab in patients 60 years of age or older with diffuse large B-cell lymphoma (DLBCL). *Blood* 2004, 104:(abstract 127).

53   Ghielmini M, Schmitz SF, Cogliatti S, *et al.* Effect of single-agent rituximab given at the standard schedule or as prolonged treatment in patients with mantle cell lymphoma: a study of the Swiss Group for Clinical Cancer Research (SAKK). *J Clin Oncol* 2005, 23:705-711.

54   Lenz G, Dreyling M, Hoster E, *et al.* Immunochemotherapy with rituximab and cyclophosphamide, doxorubicin, vincristine, and prednisone significantly improves response and time to treatment failure, but not long-term outcome in patients with previously untreated mantle cell lymphoma: results of a prospective randomized trial of the German Low Grade Lymphoma Study Group (GLSG). *J Clin Oncol* 2005, 23:1984-1992.

55   Kaplan LD, Lee JY, Ambinder RF, *et al.* Rituximab does not improve clinical outcome in a randomized phase III trial of CHOP with or without rituximab in patients with HIV-associated non-Hodgkin's lymphoma: AIDS-malignancies consortium trial 010. *Blood* 2005,

56   Miles SA, McGratten M. Persistent panhypogammaglobulinemia after CHOP-rituximab for HIV-related lymphoma. *J Clin Oncol* 2005, 23:247-248.

57   Dunleavy K, Hakim F, Kim HK, *et al.* B-cell recovery following rituximab-based therapy is associated with perturbations in stromal derived factor-1 and granulocyte homeostasis. *Blood* 2005, 106:795-802.

58   Voog E, Morschhauser F, Solal-Celigny P. Neutropenia in patients treated with rituximab. *N Engl J Med* 2003, 348:2691-2694; discussion 2691-2694.

59   Boue F, Gabarre J, Gisselbrecht C, *et al.* CHOP chemotherapy plus rituximab in HIV patients with high grade lymphoma-Results of an ANRS trial. *Blood* 2002, 100:470a (abstract 1824).

60   Spina M, Tirelli U. HIV-related non-Hodgkin's lymphoma (HIV-NHL) in the era of highly active antiretroviral therapy (HAART): some still unanswered questions for clinical management. *Ann Oncol* 2004, 15:993-995.

61   Spina M, Jaeger U, Sparano JA, *et al.* Rituximab plus infusional cyclophosphamide, doxorubicin, and etoposide in HIV-associated non-Hodgkin lymphoma: pooled results from 3 phase 2 trials. *Blood* 2005, 105:1891-1897.

62   Sparano JA, Lee S, Chen MG, *et al.* Phase II trial of infusional cyclophosphamide, doxorubicin, and etoposide in patients with HIV-associated non-Hodgkin's lymphoma: an Eastern Cooperative Oncology Group Trial (E1494). *J Clin Oncol* 2004, 22:1491-1500.

63   Hale G, Dyer MJ, Clark MR, *et al.* Remission induction in non-Hodgkin lymphoma with reshaped human monoclonal antibody CAMPATH-1H. *Lancet* 1988, 2:1394-1399.

64   Xia MQ, Hale G, Lifely MR, *et al.* Structure of the CAMPATH-1 antigen, a glycosylphosphatidylinositol-anchored glycoprotein which is an exceptionally good target for complement lysis. *Biochem J* 1993, 293 (Pt 3):633-640.

65   Hale G, Xia MQ, Tighe HP, *et al.* The CAMPATH-1 antigen (CDw52). *Tissue Antigens* 1990, 35:118-127.

66   Salisbury JR, Rapson NT, Codd JD, *et al.* Immunohistochemical analysis of CDw52 antigen expression in non-Hodgkin's lymphomas. *J Clin Pathol* 1994, 47:313-317.

67   Dyer MJ, Hale G, Hayhoe FG, Waldmann H. Effects of CAMPATH-1 antibodies in vivo in patients with lymphoid malignancies: influence of antibody isotype. *Blood* 1989, 73:1431-1439.

68   Keating MJ, Flinn I, Jain V, *et al.* Therapeutic role of alemtuzumab (Campath-1H) in patients who have failed fludarabine: results of a large international study. *Blood* 2002, 99:3554-3561.

69   Gisselbrecht C, Gaulard P, Lepage E, *et al.* Prognostic significance of T-cell phenotype in aggressive non-Hodgkin's lymphomas. Groupe d'Etudes des Lymphomes de l'Adulte (GELA). *Blood* 1998, 92:76-82.

70   Melnyk A, Rodriguez A, Pugh WC, Cabannillas F. Evaluation of the Revised European-American Lymphoma classification confirms the clinical relevance of immunophenotype in 560 cases of aggressive non-Hodgkin's lymphoma. *Blood* 1997, 89:4514-4520.

71   Ginaldi L, De Martinis M, Matutes E, *et al.* Levels of expression of CD52 in normal and leukemic B and T cells: correlation with in vivo therapeutic responses to Campath-1H. *Leuk Res* 1998, 22:185-191.

72   Khorana A, Bunn P, McLaughlin P, *et al.* A phase II multicenter study of CAMPATH-1H antibody in previously treated patients with nonbulky non-Hodgkin's lymphoma. *Leuk Lymphoma* 2001, 41:77-87.

73   Uppenkamp M, Engert A, Diehl V, *et al.* Monoclonal antibody therapy with CAMPATH-1H in patients with relapsed high- and low-grade non-Hodgkin's lymphomas: a multicenter phase I/II study. *Ann Hematol* 2002, 81:26-32.

74   Lundin J, Osterborg A, Brittinger G, *et al.* CAMPATH-1H monoclonal antibody in therapy for previously treated low-grade non-Hodgkin's lymphomas: a phase II multicenter study. European Study Group of CAMPATH-1H Treatment in Low-Grade Non-Hodgkin's Lymphoma. *J Clin Oncol* 1998, 16:3257-3263.

75   Enblad G, Hagberg H, Erlanson M, *et al.* A pilot study of alemtuzumab (anti-CD52 monoclonal antibody) therapy for patients with relapsed or chemotherapy-refractory peripheral T-cell lymphomas. *Blood* 2004, 103:2920-2924.

76   Lundin J, Hagberg H, Repp R, *et al.* Phase 2 study of alemtuzumab (anti-CD52 monoclonal antibody) in patients with advanced mycosis fungoides/Sezary syndrome. *Blood* 2003, 101:4267-4272.

77   Zinzani PL, Alinari L, Tani M, *et al.* Preliminary observations of a phase II study of reduced-dose alemtuzumab treatment in patients with pretreated T-cell lymphoma. *Haematologica* 2005, 90:702-703.

78   Gluck WL, Hurst D, Yuen A, *et al.* Phase I studies of interleukin (IL)-2 and rituximab in B-cell non-hodgkin's lymphoma: IL-2 mediated natural killer cell expansion correlations with clinical response. *Clin Cancer Res* 2004, 10:2253-2264.

79   Eisenbeis CF, Leonard J, Rosenblatt J, *et al.* Conversion of antibody-resistant cancer patients to antibody-sensitive: Investigation of Fc receptor polymorphisms and response to IL-2 and rituximab treatment in rituximab-refractory NHL patients. *Proc Am Soc Clin Oncol* 2004, 22:(abstract 2534).

80   Davis TA, Kaminski MS, Leonard JP, *et al.* The radioisotope contributes significantly to the activity of radioimmunotherapy. *Clin Cancer Res* 2004, 10:7792-7798.

81   Kaminski MS, Zelenetz AD, Press OW, *et al.* Pivotal study of iodine I 131 tositumomab for chemotherapy-refractory low-grade or transformed low-grade B-cell non-Hodgkin's lymphomas. *J Clin Oncol* 2001, 19:3918-3928.

82   Witzig TE, White CA, Wiseman GA, *et al.* Phase I/II trial of IDEC-Y2B8 radioimmunotherapy for treatment of relapsed or refractory CD20(+) B-cell non-Hodgkin's lymphoma. *J Clin Oncol* 1999, 17:3793-3803.

83   Gordon LI, Molina A, Witzig T, *et al.* Durable responses after ibritumomab tiuxetan radioimmunotherapy for CD20+ B-cell lymphoma: long-term follow-up of a phase 1/2 study. *Blood* 2004, 103:4429-4431.

84   Kaminski MS, Tuck M, Estes J, *et al.* 131I-tositumomab therapy as initial treatment for follicular lymphoma. *N Engl J Med* 2005, 352:441-449.

85   Gordon LI, Witzig TE, Wiseman GA, *et al.* Yttrium 90 ibritumomab tiuxetan radioimmunotherapy for relapsed or refractory low-grade non-Hodgkin's lymphoma. *Semin Oncol* 2002, 29:87-92.

86   Knox SJ, Goris ML, Trisler K, *et al.* Yttrium-90-labeled anti-CD20 monoclonal antibody therapy of recurrent B-cell lymphoma. *Clin Cancer Res* 1996, 2:457-470.

87   Witzig TE, Gordon LI, Cabanillas F, *et al.* Randomized controlled trial of yttrium-90-labeled ibritumomab tiuxetan radioimmunotherapy versus rituximab immunotherapy for patients with relapsed or refractory low-grade, follicular, or transformed B-cell non-Hodgkin's lymphoma. *J Clin Oncol* 2002, 20:2453-2463.

88   Horning SJ, Younes A, Jain V, *et al.* Efficacy and safety of tositumomab and iodine-131 tositumomab (Bexxar) in B-cell lymphoma, progressive after rituximab. *J Clin Oncol* 2005, 23:712-719.

89   Davies AJ, Rohatiner AZ, Howell S, *et al.* Tositumomab and iodine I 131 tositumomab for recurrent indolent and transformed B-cell non-Hodgkin's lymphoma. *J Clin Oncol* 2004, 22:1469-1479.

90   Press OW, Unger JM, Braziel RM, *et al.* A phase 2 trial of CHOP chemotherapy followed by tositumomab/iodine I 131 tositumomab for previously untreated follicular non-Hodgkin lymphoma: Southwest Oncology Group Protocol S9911. *Blood* 2003, 102:1606-1612.

91   Press OW, Eary JF, Appelbaum FR, *et al.* Phase II trial of 131I-B1 (anti-CD20) antibody therapy with autologous stem cell transplantation for relapsed B cell lymphomas. *Lancet* 1995, 346:336-340.

92   Liu SY, Eary JF, Petersdorf SH, *et al.* Follow-up of relapsed B-cell lymphoma patients treated with iodine-131-labeled anti-CD20 antibody and autologous stem-cell rescue. *J Clin Oncol* 1998, 16:3270-3278.

93   Vose JM, Bierman PJ, Enke C, *et al.* Phase I trial of iodine-131 tositumomab with high-dose chemotherapy and autologous stem-cell transplantation for relapsed non-Hodgkin's lymphoma. *J Clin Oncol* 2005, 23:461-467.

94   Bennett JM, Kaminski MS, Leonard JP, *et al.* Assessment of treatment-related myelodysplastic syndromes and acute myeloid leukemia in patients with non-Hodgkin lymphoma treated with tositumomab and iodine I131 tositumomab. *Blood* 2005, 105:4576-4582.

Chapter 8

BLOOD AND BONE MARROW TRANSPLANTATION FOR PATIENTS WITH HODGKIN'S AND NON-HODGKIN'S LYMPHOMA

Ian W. Flinn, M.D., Ph.D. and Jesus G. Berdeja

The Sidney Kimmel Comprehensive Cancer Center at Johns Hopkins Bunting-Blaustein Cancer Research Building, 1650 Orleans Street/Room 388, Baltimore, MD 21231-1000

1.   INTRODUCTION

Most lymphomas are initially sensitive to chemotherapy and radiation. Unfortunately, many patients will relapse with their disease. Dose escalation of chemotherapy is often limited by hematopoetic toxicity. The realization that a significantly higher dose of chemotherapy or chemoradiotherapy could be delivered to a patient by reconstituting their marrow with hematopoetic stem cells paved the way to autologous blood or marrow transplantation (ABMT) for patients with lymphoma. Initial studies were performed in refractory patients. These studies demonstrated the feasibility of this approach and ushered in more definitive trials in patients with homogenous histologies.

1.1   ABMT for Aggressive NHL

Numerous studies have demonstrated that patients could be salvaged with ABMT after failing conventional therapy[1-11]. The different endpoints and retrospective nature of most of these studies hinders direct comparisons.

Differences in outcomes most likely reflect differences in patient prognostic factors rather than true differences in the therapy delivered. Outcomes were noted to be better in patients who were sensitive to conventional salvage dose therapy. Forty percent of these patients experienced long-term disease-free survival (DFS).[4]. Patients who were resistant to salvage therapy faired less well with the expectation of cure between 10 and 30%. Patients who never entered remission generally had less than a 10% chance of long-term survival. To further evaluate the utility of ABMT in patient with sensitive relapsed disease, the Parma Group conducted a randomized trial comparing ABMT with conventional salvage therapy in patients with intermediate or high grade lymphoma[12]. After two cycles of DHAP chemotherapy, patients with sensitive disease were randomly assigned to complete a total of six cycles of DHAP or to proceed with ABMT. One hundred and nine patients were randomized. Overall survival was 53% at five years in the ABMT group and 32% in the conventional-treatment group (p=.038) (see figure 1). Event-free survival (EFS) was 46% in the ABMT group and 12% in the conventional treatment group (p = .001). The study firmly established ABMT as the standard of care for patients with relapsed, chemotherapy-sensitive aggressive lymphomas.

1.2   ABMT for Low- Grade Lymphoma

The efficacy of ABMT for patients with low-grade lymphoma is less well established.   The indolent lymphomas are generally regarded as incurable with conventional therapies except when localized. However, they are responsive to cytotoxic chemotherapy and radiotherapy and complete remissions are frequently achieved. As is the case with more aggressive lymphomas, durable remissions can be achieved with ABMT. However, unlike ABMT for aggressive lymphomas, plateaus in the survival cures are not seen in patients with low-grade lymphoma, suggesting that ABMT is not curative for most patients with these histologies.

Although most patients with low-grade lymphoma will ultimately relapse with their disease, large registry studies from the United States and Europe have demonstrated that durable remissions can be achieved with this approach[13]. Furthermore, the recent publication of the CUP trial indicates that there is a survival advantage in favor of ABMT for patients who have chemotherapy-sensitive disease after relapsing from initial therapy. In this study, patients with relapsed follicular lymphoma received 3 cycles of salvage chemotherapy. Patients who achieved at least a partial remission were randomized to further chemotherapy (C arm), ABMT with an unpurged graft (U arm), or ABMT with a purged graft (P arm). Due to slow accrual, the study was closed early and no differences were seen between the two ABMT arms. However, when the two BMT arms were compared to the chemotherapy arm superior progression free survival (PFS) and overall survival (OS) were noted in patients who received the high-dose therapy (HDT). For PFS, the hazard ratio (95% CI) for C versus U + P was 0.30 (0.15 to 0.61). Hazard ratios (95% CIs) for OS for C versus U + P was 0.40 (0.18 to 0.89). Kaplan-Meier estimates (95% CIs) of OS at 4 years for C, U, and P were 46% (25% to 67%), 71% (52% to 91%), and 77% (60% to 95%) respectively. The CUP study is the only randomized clinical trial in patients with low-grade lymphoma to demonstrate a survival advantage of any therapy.

1.3   ABMT for Mantle Cell Lymphoma

Although at one time regarded as a low grade non-Hodgkin's lymphoma[14], mantle cell lymphoma is an aggressive disease that is generally considered incurable with conventional chemotherapy. The distinct natural history mandates that mantle cell lymphoma outcomes be studied separately from those of other lymphomas and that the diagnostic criteria are well defined in analyses of treatment outcomes. Relapse often occurs within twelve to eighteen months of first-line therapy, with a median survival typically of three to four years[15,16]. Accordingly there has been recent interest in BMT for this disease. The ability of ABMT to prolong event-free and overall survival in mantle cell lymphoma has been a matter of debate[17-20]. Numerous studies have demonstrated that durable remissions can be achieved, but as in the case with low-grade lymphoma, patients ultimately relapse with their disease. In a recent series of 58 patients with mantle cell lymphoma undergoing autologous or allogeneic BMT, multiple regression analysis revealed transplantation after one or more relapses (HR 2.98, $P = 0.02$), primary induction failure (HR 5.39, $P = 0.002$), and allogeneic transplantation (HR 3.03, $P = 0.007$) were associated with an inferior EFS[21]. However, EFS curves were not statistically different for autologous and allogeneic BMT performed in first remission, with an estimated 3-year EFS approaching or equaling 70%. Primary induction failure and residual bone marrow involvement were the only statistically significant predictors of relapse on multiple regression analysis. The estimated 3-year EFS for the entire cohort following BMT was 51%, probability of relapse 31%, and overall survival 59%. The benefit of autologous or allogeneic BMT for mantle cell lymphoma is thus most apparent when performed in first remission.

1.4   ABMT for Hodgkin's Disease

HDT with ABMT has been widely used for patients with relapsed or refractory Hodgkin's disease (HD) for at least two decades. Randomized and retrospective studies in patients in first relapse have demonstrated the superiority of ABMT to conventional salvage therapies[22,23]. Given the high cure rate in patients with even the poorest prognosis, ABMT has not been used in patients as initial therapy unless as part of a clinical trial. As is true with other types of lymphoma, patients with sensitive disease have a better expected long-term disease-free and OS[24,25]. OS rates of approximately 50% at 5 years have been seen in several studies. Patients with resistant disease or patients failing to respond to primary therapy have worse outcomes with 3 year survival noted between 15-36%[23,25-27]. This wide variation in patients with resistant disease is probably a reflection of different definitions of refractory disease and selection bias of patients who actually receive the ABMT. For instance, many centers will not transplant patients with obvious progression of disease during the pre-transplant evaluation.

Numerous other prognostic factors have been identified[27-32]. These factors include duration of first remission, achieving CR prior to ABMT, number of prior therapies, and bone marrow involvement at the time of ABMT. Most of these prognostic factors reflect the biology of the underlying disease of which there is very little control. However, the superiority of ABMT at first relapse rather than later in the natural history of the disease is an important finding of these studies.

The durable remissions achieved with ABMT increases the importance of the incidence of second malignancies in patients with HD who have had an ABMT as it does with primary therapy. Radiation either as part of the preparative regimen or used before or after ABMT has been implicated in one series, but not in others[24,33]. The durable remissions achieved in patients with relapsed, sensitive disease have lead to the perception of a high cure rate with ABMT. However, late relapses are seen and most survival curves persistent decreases in OS and DFS[25].(see figure 2)

2.   INNOVATIONS IN HIGH DOSE THERAPY

In the most basic sense, there can only be two causes of relapse after ABMT. The causes of relapse include persistent residual neoplastic cells in patients despite HDT and reintroduction of malignant cells into the host with the stem cell graft. While the relative contributions of each factor to relapse are unknown, both have been implicated [34]. Strategies are needed to address both problems.

Attempts have been made to decrease relapse and improve survival by intensifying the preparative regimen. In particular, etoposide has been added to a standard cyclophosphamide regimen. This regimen has resulted in a 33% and 44% three year PFS in patients with relapsed and refractory aggressive non-Hodgkin=s lymphoma [2]. In patients with chemotherapy-sensitive disease the OS and PFS were 55% and 42%. However, given the significant procedure related mortality, 10.6% within 50 days, the upper limit of dose escalation in the preparative regimens has been reached.

An alternative approach to dose escalation involves targeting the high dose therapy to the lymphoma with monoclonal antibodies. Studies with ^{131}I radiolabeled B cell antibodies indicate that significant dose escalation with radioimmunoconjugates is clearly possible with autologous stem cell transplantation. The maximum tolerated dose was found to be 27.25 Gy[35]. The lungs were the most common organ to receive dose-limiting radiation. In a phase II study of ^{131}I tositumomab, 16 of 21 patients achieved complete remissions, two patients achieved partial remissions and one achieved a minor response[36]. In a combined analysis of the phase I and phase II patients, the PFS was 51% at 4 years in patients with indolent lymphomas[37].

[131]I tositumomab has also been used to replace total body irradiation (TBI) in a cyclophosphamide, etoposide TBI preparative regimen. A phase I/II study in fifty-two patients with relapsed B-cell lymphoma combining 131I-tositumomab with etoposide/cytoxan followed by purged auto-graft was conducted[38]. A therapeutic ^{131}I-tositumomab dose-escalation was done from 20 Gy to a maximum of 27 Gy as measured by radiation to normal organs. Patients were monitored and isolated until their total-body radiation was less than 0.07 mSv/h at which time they were given etoposide at 60 mg/m^2 and cytoxan at 100mg/m^2. Interestingly, the investigators found that they could deliver nearly the same dose of radiation to the lungs when the radiolabeled antibody was combined with chemotherapy as they could in their single agent studies (25 Gy vs. 27 Gy respectively). Response rate in the patients with measurable disease was 86%, two year survival of all enrolled patients was 83% and PFS 68%. These numbers compare favorably with historical controls treated with TBI/Cytoxan/Etoposide and auto-BMT.

One approach to reducing or eliminating contamination of the autologous stem cell product involves purging the autologous stem cell graft of tumor cells. There is evidence to suggest that antibody purging of bone marrow with autologous transplantation may be effective in follicular lymphomas. The successful purging of a marrow graft with a monoclonal antibody *in vitro* is associated with improved DFS[39] in one study. The efficacy of the marrow purge was assessed by PCR of marrow specimens before and after the purge. Detection of residual lymphoma cells in marrow after purging was associated with a 39% relapse rate after a median follow-up of 23 months versus a 5% relapse rate in patients whose marrows showed no residual lymphoma (P<0.00001). However, this strong correlation between the efficacy of marrow purging as measured by PCR amplification and clinical outcome might indicate that the ability to purge marrow is a useful prognostic factor rather than an effective therapeutic intervention. Indeed the presence of overt (morphologically detectable) marrow involvement at the time of harvest was also a good predictor of clinical outcome. Among 65 patients with no involvement there were only 11 relapses (17%) and among 11 patients with overt involvement there were 7 relapses (64%).

The use of rituximab as an *in vivo* purging agent is an alternative to *in vitro* purging has recently become popular. Numerous studies have now demonstrated that rituximab does not interfere with stem cell mobilization and can produce a lymphoma free graft in many patients. However its efficacy in terms of improvement in PFS and OS is unclear. Another important aspect of the use of monoclonal antibodies in the transplant setting is when to incorporate them during the transplant procedure. The well-tolerated profile of most of these antibodies allows for their use in the post-transplant setting. In addition, rituximab is efficacious in patients with follicular lymphoma that has relapsed after an ABMT. Horwitz *et al.* have reported the feasibility of using rituximab as an adjuvant therapy in the post transplant setting with minimal toxicity[40]. Thirty-five patients with diffuse large cell (25 patients), mantle cell (3 patients), transformed (3 patients), or other (4 patients) subtypes of B-cell lymphoma received HDT followed by a purged autologous graft. The rituximab schedule was 4 weekly infusions (375 mg/m^2) starting at day 42 after ABMT and, for patients 5 to 35, a second 4-week course 6 months after ABMT. All planned therapy was completed in 29 patients. With 30 months' median follow-up, the 2-year EFS rate was 83% and the OS rate was 88%. For 21 patients with relapsed or refractory large cell lymphoma, the EFS rate was 81% and the OS rate was 85%. While there was not an increase in serious infections observed in this and other trials despite delayed B cell recovery and suppressed immunoglobulin G levels[41,42], unusual infections have been noted in some patients who have undergone ABMT with rituximab[43,44]. The ultimate answer in terms of risks and benefit of the addition of rituximab to ABMT awaits the completion of ongoing phase III trials.

3. ALLOGENEIC BLOOD AND MARROW TRANSPLANTATION

Despite the best efforts offered by current available treatments for lymphoma, over half of intermediate and high-grade lymphomas and nearly all low-grade lymphomas will not be cured. Improvements in supportive care and purging mechanisms in autologous stem cell transplantation have allowed the relatively safe incorporation of this treatment modality in many relapsed intermediate lymphomas and some low-grade lymphomas. However, as discussed in detail earlier, the majority of patients, especially those with low grade lymphomas show a continuous relapsing pattern suggesting that autologous peripheral stem cell transplants may not cure these groups of disorders. Furthermore, autologous stem cell transplantation may not be feasible for patients with poor marrow reserve, significant bone marrow contamination by lymphoma and patients resistant to chemotherapeutic modalities.

Allogeneic blood and marrow transplantation (BMT) has been an intriguing and exciting treatment modality since the original reports of its feasibility in hematologic malignancies appeared in the literature.[45] Allogeneic BMT offers several potential advantages over autologous transplantation including a source of stem cells free of neoplastic cells, and a marrow without exposure to chemotherapy mutagens. But perhaps the most important advantage of allogeneic BMT is the ability of the donor immune system to control and possibly eradicate the clone of interest. This so-called graft versus tumor effect has been well described by multiple investigators.[46-50] Furthermore, the ability of donor lymphocyte infusions (DLI) to induce remission in patients relapsed following allogeneic BMT[51,52] lends further credence to the graft versus tumor hypothesis, proof that at its core, allogeneic BMT is first and foremost a type of immunotherapy.

The use of allogeneic BMT in patients with various types of lymphoma has been tempered by several factors. The ability to cure highly chemosensitive diseases such as Hodgkin's and intermediate/high-grade lymphoma with chemotherapy and or autologous BMT has limited the role of allogeneic BMT in these disorders. Similarly the low-grade lymphomas present alternate issues limiting the use of allogeneic BMT including their long natural history, median survival of 8-10 years, and older median age of this population.[53,54] Despite these obstacles, in patients with high risk disease, resistant to chemotherapy and patients not otherwise candidates for autologous BMT, the role of allogeneic BMT is rapidly expanding.

3.1   Allogeneic stem cell transplantation in low-grade lymphoma and chronic lymphocytic leukemia (CLL)

Low-grade lymphomas comprise a heterogeneous group of disorders with a median survival of 7-10 years.[53,54] The relative indolent course and median older age of the affected population coupled with the high early transplant-related mortality (TRM) of allogeneic BMT have limited the role of this treatment modality in the majority of these patients. Nevertheless, despite this relatively indolent course, the general pattern is that of relapsing disease with most patients eventually succumbing to their disease. Furthermore, advanced stage patients relapsing or progressing following initial treatment have a median survival of only 2-4 years.[54,55] Similarly, the inability of nontransplant modalities to positively impact on survival has prompted some investigators and patients to pursue more aggressive management. A summary of the most prominent reports of allogeneic BMT in patients with low-grade lymphoma and/or CLL is shown in table 1. [56-70] On average, allogeneic BMT are feasible in this patient population. OS and EFS are similar in all series, save one.[63] Excluding this report, OS ranges from 46-80% and EFS ranges from 39-78%. Transplant-related mortality (TRM) ranges from 30-46%, while relapsed disease rates are well below 20% in most published series. The rates of acute and chronic graft-versus-host disease (GVHD) are variable depending on whether T cell depletion is employed or not but range 27-54% and 6-66% respectively, accounting for a large portion of the TRM. Increasing number of previous therapies prior to transplantation and resistance to chemotherapy may adversely affect outcome.[56,64,67] The choice of conditioning regimen remains unclear, although one series reported the use of TBI to correlate with decreased disease relapse but a higher TRM.[56] It appears that careful selection of patients and consideration of transplantation earlier in the course may make this a safe and potentially curative procedure in this patient population.

3.2   Allogeneic stem cell transplantation in intermediate/high-grade lymphoma

Good outcomes following standard chemotherapy and autologous BMT in relapsed patients have delegated the role of allogeneic BMT in this group of disorders largely to the patients who are refractory to chemotherapy or who are ineligible for autologous BMT. Patients with refractory disease benefit little from high dose chemotherapy and autologous stem cell rescue with PFS in the 20% range.[71] Not surprisingly, the outcomes of most series of myeloablative allogeneic BMT reflect this particular high-risk subpopulation. Table 2 summarizes some of the larger series published.[63,65,72-81] Studies with mixed histologies were used if the majority of the patients reported had intermediate or high grade lymphomas. On average, the TRM ranges 23-48% and OS ranges 21-71%. The percentage of patients with resistant lymphoma appeared to correlate with higher TRM and lower survival rates. In general, the majority of studies report that allogeneic BMT is feasible and can induce long-term remissions in a population with a poor prognosis and few treatment options.

3.3 Allogeneic stem cell transplantation in Hodgkin's lymphoma

Standard chemotherapy can induce complete remission in most patients with Hodgkin's lymphoma [82] yet 50% of patients with advanced, bulky disease will relapse.[83] In patients with relapsed or refractory disease conventional chemotherapies yield poor responses. [84] High-dose chemotherapy and autologous stem cell rescue may offer an important treatment option especially in patients with chemosensitive disease.[22,28,85] The role of allogeneic BMT remains controversial. Table 3 lists the outcomes of four large series.[25,65,86,87] The majority of studies report overall and EFS between 20-30%. Furthermore, the TRM rates are higher than those seen with non-Hodgkin's lymphoma and average about 50%. Bulky disease, increasing number of prior treatment regimens and chemoresistant disease may predict for a worse outcome. [25,86] Although the results are disappointing, long term remissions can be induced in a patient population with a poor prognosis and should continue to be investigated.

3.4 Allogeneic versus autologous stem cell transplantation in lymphoma

Several studies have been published reporting outcomes in patients with relapsed, or refractory lymphoma undergoing autologous or allogeneic BMT. Table 4 lists the studies reporting on the largest number of patients or longer follow-ups. [25,56,57,62,76,80,81,86-88] In general, allogeneic BMT is associated with higher TRM and lower relapse rates, while autologous BMT is associated with lower TRM but higher relapse rates. As a result, the overall survival rates between the two modalities are similar in most series. None of these studies is randomized, and the patients on the allogeneic arm were more likely to have poor performance status, advanced disease, increase LDH, bone marrow involvement at the time of transplant, and chemoresistant disease. [57,58] Thus direct comparisons between the two procedures should be interpreted with caution.

3.5   Allogeneic stem cell transplant-specific issues

As is evident from the data summarized, the desired graft versus tumor effect is often accompanied by significant consequences. GVHD, conditioning regimen toxicity and infections continue to result in high transplant-related mortality in many patients. Improvements in GVHD prophylaxis and supportive care have had positive effects on outcome, but means to improve further continue to be explored. This section will address some of these variables that may ultimately render allogeneic BMT safer and more widely acceptable.

4.   CONDITIONING REGIMENS

A variety of myeloablative conditioning regimens have been studied and used in patients with lymphoma. The first and most used regimens incorporate TBI (TBI). The feasibility and effectiveness of the combination of cyclophosphamide and TBI is well described.[5,89,90] An IBMTR survey found the use of TBI containing regimens to confer improved survival in patients with low grade lymphoma.[64] Alternatively, other investigators have reported that the use of TBI containing regimens may adversely affect outcome in patients with Hodgkin's lymphoma.[24] Furthermore the use of radiation as primary or adjunctive treatment in patients with lymphoma may preclude the use of radiation containing conditioning regimens.

As a result, non-TBI containing alternative conditioning regimens were created. The first of its kind used busulfan and cyclophosphamide.[91,92] Since then other regimens include combinations such as cyclophosphamide, carmustine, etoposide (CBV)[93]; carmustine, etoposide, cytarabine, melphalan (BEAM)[94,95]; busulfan, cyclophosphamide and etoposide.[96] The choice of preparative regimen appears to be dependent not only on disease histology, but on patient specific characteristics such as type of prior therapies and baseline organ function. There are no randomized trials comparing the different preparative regimens and thus the superiority of one over the other is still debated.

5.   SOURCE AND TYPE OF STEM CELLS

Several sources of hematopoietic stem cells have been described and studied for use in immune reconstitution following myeloablative therapy. These include bone marrow, [97] peripheral blood, [98] fetal liver [99] and cord blood.[100] The use of bone marrow as a stem cell source has been researched and accepted as the standard for over forty years. [101,102] The identification of hematopoietic stem cells circulating in peripheral blood at low concentrations [103] followed by the observations that the number of cells could greatly be enhanced by the use of cytokines such as recombinant human granulocyte colony-stimulating factor (rhG-CSF) [104] paved the way for the use of peripheral blood derived stem cell transplantations. Reports of safety and feasibility of peripheral hematopoietic stem cell transplantation in the autologous setting [105,106] quickly established this stem cell source as the standard over bone marrow derived stem cells in most centers. In the allogeneic setting however, this conversion has met more resistance. Concerns regarding the composition of the product from peripheral blood versus bone marrow, the safety of use of stem cell stimulants in normal donors, and the fear of inferior outcomes and higher rates of GVHD have been raised.

Several clinical studies have been reported which have helped allay some of the concerns regarding peripheral blood stem cells as a source in allogeneic transplantation. [107-113] In summary, time to neutrophil and platelet recovery is consistently shorter in patients receiving peripheral blood stem cells. Furthermore there appears to be no difference in terms of rates of transplant-related mortality, acute GVHD and DFS. There is discordance regarding the rates of chronic GVHD with some studies reporting higher rates in patients receiving peripheral blood stem cells and others citing similar rates. Finally, although follow-up is still short, there appears to be no long term effects of rhG-CSF use in normal donors. [114] To date the use of peripheral blood or bone marrow as a source of allogeneic hematopoietic stem cells remains largely a center dependent decision.

6.   GRAFT VERSUS HOST PROPHYLAXIS

Graft versus host disease has been the most respected and feared early and late complication of allogeneic stem cell transplantation. Efforts to control acute and chronic GVHD without adversely affecting the graft versus tumor effect have been and continue to be an active area of investigation. The most common prophylaxis involves the use of immunosuppressive medications alone or in combination such as cyclosporine, methotrexate, steroids, and tacrolimus.[110,115-117] The use of these medications is effective but with well known complications including acute renal failure, mucositis, hypertension, delayed immune reconstitution and increased risk of infections. The combinations yielding the lowest rates of graft versus host are still under investigation.

An extremely effective way to reduce graft versus host is the use of T cell depletion. This can be accomplished in several ways including lectin-separation followed by sheep erythrocyte rosetting,[118] *in vitro* or *in vivo* use of anti-T cell monoclonal antibodies including CAMPATH-1G, [119-122] and by counterflow centrifugal elutriation. [123,124] Reported rates and severity of GVHD are significantly lower in centers using T cell depleted grafts. [67,122,125] Unfortunately, higher rates of delayed engraftment, graft failure, post-transplant lymphoproliferative disorders, and disease recurrence have also been reported. [60,89,126] Efforts to address some of these drawbacks of T cell depletion include the add back of CD34+ cells that coseparate with small lymphocytes, [127] identifying and rejecting specific lymphocyte subtypes such as CD6+ lymphocytes, [125] delaying administration of small, graded doses of donor lymphocytes [128] or selecting lymphocyte subsets used for DLI.[129]

Newer immunosuppressive medications such as mycophenolate mofetil and FK506 are being evaluated. Exciting research sorting out immune differences responsible for the graft versus host or graft versus tumor effect will result in important therapeutic implications.[130] Ultimately, the answer to this paradigm will be the most important advance in allogeneic stem cell transplantation.

7.   NONMYELOABLATIVE ALLOGENEIC TRANSPLANTATION

The continued struggle to minimize transplant-related mortality, coupled with the many observations alluding to the graft versus tumor effect as the most potent anti-tumor component in an allogeneic stem cell transplantation paved the way for an alternate approach. The result was the idea of using nonmyeloablative conditioning regimens just strong enough to allow engraftment of allogeneic stem cells, but with much less toxic effects than the traditional myeloablative conditioning regimens. [131,132] Since the first reports by Slavin et al [131] and Khouri et al [132] several investigators have now reported on their clinical outcomes in various hematologic disorders. [131-136] In fact reports of nonmyeloablative BMT in lymphoproliferative disorders alone are now being reported and are summarized in table 5. [137-141]

The results thus far have been promising. Most patients have little conditioning regimen associated toxicity. [131-140,142,143] The median time to neutrophil and platelet engraftment is consistently lower than that seen with myeloablative approaches. Furthermore, the degree of hematotoxicity, judging by the requirement of blood products, is markedly reduced.[137,144] Most series report induction of donor/recipient chimerism with the majority of patients achieving full donor chimerism (>95% cells of donor origin).[134,137,138] The ability and rapidity with which full donor chimerism is achieved appears to be dependent on preparative regimen, the use of T cell depletion for GVHD prophylaxis and the use of DLI and may not be fully evident until an average of three months following BMT. [134,139] The optimal conditioning regimen, as with myeloablative allogeneic BMT, remains an area of active investigation. Most investigators use a combination of fludarabine, melphalan, cyclophosphamide, busulfan, thiotepa, carmustine, BEAM and low-dose TBI. [137-139,141,142,145-150] No randomized studies comparing the different conditioning regimens has been done, although fludarabine based regimens may be associated with higher rates of cytomegalovirus (CMV) reactivation. [150]

Unfortunately, the rates of GVHD in non-T cell depleted nonmyeloablative BMT remain high. This is especially true of chronic GVHD and patients receiving DLI to ensure full donor chimerism. [145,146,148,149] The higher rates of GVHD are not unexpected given the older age and heavy pretreatment of the population thus far studied. Attempts to lower the rates of GVHD are similar to those discussed in the GVHD prophylaxis section earlier. The specific role of *in vivo* T cell depletion using CAMPATH-1H will be covered in more detail.

Attempts to lower the GVHD rates with nonmyeloablative BMT have prompted some investigators to pursue the use of CAMPATH-1H. This has been viewed with skepticism given the therapeutic effect of nonmyeloablative transplantation is due to its graft versus tumor effect likely mediated by alloreactive T cells. Several reports have been conducted using CAMPATH-1H as GVHD prophylaxis with interesting results. [139,140,151] In general, the use of CAMPATH-1H in this setting results in very low rates of both acute and chronic GVHD. Not surprisingly, the rates of full donor chimerism are lower and immunosuppression is prolonged. This often translates into higher disease relapse rates and higher CMV reactivation in patients at risk. [151,152] A study by Perez-Simon et al [139] compared two prospective studies in patients with lymphoproliferative disorders undergoing nonmyeloablative BMT. Each study employed similar conditioning regimens of fludarabine and melphalan. One study employed cyclosporine A and methotrexate while the other used cyclosporine and CAMPATH-1H as GVHD prophylaxis. DLI was given to patients who had relapsed disease or did not achieve full donor chimerism after tapering immunosuppression. The results revealed that the overall transplant-related mortality (TRM) was low in both studies but favored the CAMPATH-1H arm, 10% to 20%. The CAMPATH-1H arm also had a lower rate of both acute and chronic GVHD (20% and 2.5%, respectively) compared with the methotrexate arm (45% and 60%, respectively). As predicted the CAMPATH-1H arm had a higher rate of mixed chimeras and persistent disease following BMT. After DLI however, these differences were no longer evident. Interestingly, the use of DLI in the CAMPATH-1H arm did not increase the rates of GVHD, contrary to observations in other studies.[132,140] The rate of CMV reactivation was significantly higher in the CAMPATH-1H arm but resulted in only one death. Finally, the OS and EFS at two years did not differ, 72% and 34%, respectively, for the CAMPATH-1H group and 66% and 39%, respectively, for the methotrexate.

The feasibility and safety of nonmyeloablative allogeneic stem cell transplant in patients with HLA-identical sibling donors has led to trials using matched and mismatched unrelated donor transplants. Several investigators have reported their results, with outcomes similar to those observed when using HLA-identical sibling donors. [136,153-155] Another approach is to dissociate the conditioning regimen toxicity and the potential GVHD complications seen in many myeloablative allogeneic BMT, yet still capitalize on the chemosensitive nature of most lymphomas and preserve the graft versus tumor effect. This can be accomplished by tandem autologous BMT followed by a nonmyeloablative allogeneic BMT. Reports on the safety and feasibility of this approach in patients with multiple myeloma and refractory lymphoma have now been reported with early good results. [142,156]

Ultimately, the goal of nonmyeloablative allogeneic BMT was to decrease transplant-related mortality and provide enough graft versus tumor effect to eradicated disease. Transplant-related mortality has been consistently lower than that observed in myeloablative BMT.[139,141,146] This despite the fact that many of these patients would not have been considered allogeneic BMT candidates because of age, poor organ function and prior high dose chemotherapy. The high rates of GVHD, however, remain an area of great concern and improved GVHD prophylaxis, as with myeloablative allogeneic BMT, need to be improved upon.

8.   CONCLUSION

BMT is an integral part of the care of patients with lymphoma. ABMT is the standard of care for many patients. Allogeneic BMT remains an important option for many patients. However, the optimal incorporation of allogeneic BMT in the treatment paradigm of lymphoma is still to be determined.   Advances in GVHD prophylaxis and nonmyeloablative modalities continue to make allogeneic BMT a safer alternative. Ultimately, continued investigation and enrollment in clinical trials will best dictate the role each of these modalities will play in the treatment of patients with lymphoma.

Table 1. Summary of Published Reports on Myeloablative Allogenic BMT in Low-Grade Lmphoma and Chronic Lymphocytic Leukemia

Source	Disease	# Pts	OS	EFS	Med F/U	AGVHD	CGVHD	TRM	T Cell Dep
Van Besien[56]	LGL	176	51% 5-yr act	45% 5-yr act	36	37%	26%	30%	16%
Verdonck[57]	LGL	15	70%	70%	36	40%	30%	30%	Partial
Van Besien[58,59]	LGL	10	80%	70%	72	-	-	-	-
Mandigers[50]	LGL	15	59%	39%	36	50%	38%	30%	All
Toze[61]	LGL/CLL	26	58%	54%	17	54%	54%	30%	4 pts
Stein[62]	FSC	15	15% 5-yr act	64% 5-yr act	-	-	-	-	No
Juckett[63]	LGL	16	-	62%	70	34%	35%	-	All
IBMTR[64]	LGL	113	49%	49%	25	27%	66%	40%	22%
EBMT[45]	LGL	231	51% 4-yr act	-	-	-	-	-	-
Forrest[66]	LGL	24	78%	78%	28	-	-	-	-
Berdeja[67]	LGL/CLL	35	-	50%	25	37%	6%	46%	All
Khouri[68]	CLL	28	78%* 31%**	78%* 26%**	66 mos	49%	-	-	-
Michallet[69]	CLL	54	46% 3-yr act	-	-	37%	49%	-	-
Pavletic[70]	CLL	23	61%	61%	26 mos	54%	-	-	-

* Patients with sensitive disease ** Patients with resistant disease

Abbreviations: LGL, low-grade lymphoma; CLL, chronic lymphocytic leukemia; FSC, follicular small cleaved cell lymphoma; FL, follicular lymphoma; OS, overall survival; EFS, event free survival; pt(s), patient(s); aGVHD, acute graft versus host disease; cGVHD, chronic graft versus host disease; TRM, transplant-related mortality; T cell dep, T cell depletion; IBMTR, International Bone Marrow Transplant Registry; EBMT, European Bone Marrow Transplant Registry.

Table 2. Summary of Published Reports on Myeloablative Allogenic BMT in Intermediate and High-Grade Lymphoma

Source	Disease	#Pts	OS	EFS	Med F/U	AGVHD	CGVHD	TRM	Resistant Dz
Dhedin [72]	IGL/HGL	73	41% 5-yr act	40% 5-yract	90 mos	-	-	44%	37%
Van Besien [73]	IGL	14	21%	0%	36 mos	-	-	-	93%
Peniket [65]	IGL	147	38.30% 4-yr act	-	-	-	-	-	-
Juckett [63]	IGL	21	-	33% 5-yr act	39 mos	34%*	35%*	-	29%
Dann [74]	LGL/IGL/HGL	27	22%		56 mos	-	11%	41%	48%
Bernard [75]	LGL/IGL/HGL	13	67%	-	50 mos	69%	15%	-	23%
Chopra [76]	IGL/HGL	43	-	43%	31 mos	54%**	78%**	28%	-

Source	Disease	#Pts	OS	EFS	Med F/U	AGVHD	CGVHD	TRM	Resistant Dz
Lundberg [77]	LGL/ IGL/ HGL/HL	22	-	54.60%	28 mos	-	-	23%	64%
Mendoza [78]	LGL/ IGL/HGL L/HL	23	29%	26%	34 mos	-	-	-	61%
Mitterbauer [79]	LGL/IGL L/HGL	35	35% 5-yr act	-	-	-	-	48%	-
Ratanatharathorn [80]	LGL/IGL L/HGL	40	-	47% 2-yr act	-	52%	35%	-	40%
Schimmer [81]	LGL/IGL L	44	71% 3-yr act	-	-	-	-	23%	-

* Includes patients with low-grade lymphoma as well ** Includes patients with Burkitt's and lymphoblastic lymphoma as well

Abbreviations: LGL, low-grade lymphoma; CLL, chronic lymphocytic leukemia; FSC, follicular small cleaved cell lymphoma; FL, follicular lymphoma; OS, overall survival; EFS, event free survival; pt(s), patient(s); aGVHD, acute graft versus host disease; cGVHD, chronic graft versus host disease; TRM, transplant-related mortality; T cell dep, T cell depletion; IBMTR, International Bone Marrow Transplant Registry; EBMT, European Bone Marrow Transplant Registry.

Table 3. Summary of Published Reports on Myeloablative Allogenic BMT in Hodgkin's Lymphoma

Source	# Pts	Conditioning Regimens	OS	EFS	Med F/U	AGVHD	CGVHD	TRM	Resistant Dz
Akpek [25]	53	Bu/Cy Cy/TBI	30% 10-yr act	26% 10-yr act	60 mos	45%	47%	32%	53%
Anderson [86]	53	Cy/TBI Bu/Cy Cy/Car/Etop	20% 5-yr act	22% 5-yr act	-	55%	-	52.8%	-
Milpied [87]	45	Chemo/TBI Chemo only	25% 4-yr act	15% 4-yr act	31 mos	58%	41%	48%	53%
EBMT [65]	167	Various	24.7% 4-yr act	-	-	-	-	51%	-

Abbreviations: OS, overall survival; EFS, event free survival; pt(s), patient(s); yr act, year actuarial; aGVHD, acute graft versus host disease; cGVHD, chronic graft versus host disease; TRM, transplant-related mortality; Bu, busulfan; Cy, cyclophosphamide; TBI, total body irradiation; Car, carmustine; Etop, etoposide; EBMT, European Bone Marrow Transplant Registry.

Table 4. Summary of Published Reports Comparing Myeloablative Autologous and Allogeneic BMT in Lymphoma

Source	Disease	Autologous BMT				Allogeneic BMT			
		OS	EFS	RR	TRM	OS	EFS	RR	TRM
Van Besien[56]	FL	55% (62%)* 5-yr act	31% (39%)* 5-yr act	58% (43%)*	8% (14%)*	51% 5-yr act	45% 5-yr act	21%	30%
Stein[62]	LGL	56% 5-yr act	71% 5-yr act	-	17%	18% 5-yr act	64% 5-yr act	-	53%
Verdonck[57,88]	LGL	33% 3-yr act	22% 3-yr act	78%	0%	70% 3-yr act	70% 3-yr act	0%	27%
Ratanatharathorn[80]	LGL/IGL/HGL		24% 2-yr act	69%	-	-	47% 2-yr act	20%	-
Chopra[76]	IGL/HGL		49% 31 mos	35%	14%	-	43% 31 mos	29%	28%
Schimmer[81]	LGL/IGL	62% 3-yr act	-	41%	6%	71% 3-yr act	-	6%	23%
Akpek[25]	HL	37% 10-yr act	26% 10-yr act	60%	16%	30% 10-yr act	26% 10-yr act	53%	32%
Anderson[86]	HL	13% 5-yr act	14% 5-yr act	77%	-	20% 5-yr act	22% 5-yr act	48%	-
Milpied[87]	HL	37%	24%	61%	27%	25%	15%	61%	48%

* Results of unpurged grafts, results of purged grafts in parenthesis

Abbreviations: LGL, low-grade lymphoma; FL, follicular lymphoma; IGL, intermediate grade lymphoma; HGL, high grade lymphoma; OS, overall survival; EFS, event free survival; RR, relapsed rate; TRM, transplant-related mortality; yr act, year actuarial.

Table 5. Summary of Published Reports Nonmyeloablative Allogeneic BMT in Lymphoproliferative Disorders

Source	Disease	# Pts	Conditioning Regimen	GVHD Prophylaxis	OS	EFS	Med F/U	AGVHD	CGVHD	TRM
Khouri [137]	LGL	20	Flu/Cy	Tac/Mtx	-	84%	21 mos	20%	64%	-
EBMT [138]	LGL	52	Flu/Cy; Flu/Bu; Flu/Mel/	CSA/MTX; CAM; ALG	65%	54%	2-yr act	37%*	9%*	-
	HGL	62	Flu/Cy; Flu/Bu; Flu/Mel/	CSA/MTX; CAM; ALG	46.7 %	12.9%	2-yr act			
	HD	52	Flu/Cy; Flu/Bu; Flu/Mel/	CSA/MTX; CAM; ALG	56.3 %	42%	2-yr act			
	MCL	22	Flu/Cy; Flu/Bu; Flu/Mel/	CSA/MTX; CAM; ALG	12.8 %	0%	2-yr act			
Perez [139]	LPD	78	Flu/Mel	CSA/CAM	72%	34%	2-yr act	20%	2.5%	10%
Perez [139]	LPD	51	Flu/Mel	CSA/MTX	66%	39%	2-yr act	45%	60%	20%
Branson [140]	LPD	38	Flu/Mel	CSA/CAM	53%	50%	14 mos	21%	15%	20%
Dreger [141]	CLL	77	TBI; Flu/Cy; Flu/Bu; Mel	40% ATG or CAM	72%	56%	24 mos			18%

*Average rates for entire group, includes all histologies

Abbreviations: LGL, low-grade lymphoma; CLL, chronic lymphocytic leukemia; LPD, lymphoproliferative disorders; OS, overall survival; EFS, event free survival; pt(s), patient(s); Med F/U, median follow up; aGVHD, acute graft versus host disease; cGVHD, chronic graft versus host disease; TRM, transplant-related mortality; EBMT, European Bone Marrow Transplant Registry

9.   REFERENCES

1.   Gulati SC, Shank B, Black P, et al: Autologous bone marrow transplantation for patients with poor-prognosis lymphoma. J Clin Oncol 6:1303-13, 1988

2.   Stiff PJ, Dahlberg S, Forman SJ, et al: Autologous bone marrow transplantation for patients with relapsed or refractory diffuse aggressive non-Hodgkin's lymphoma: value of augmented preparative regimens--a Southwest Oncology Group trial. J Clin Oncol 16:48-55, 1998

3.   Bosly A, Coiffier B, Gisselbrecht C, et al: Bone marrow transplantation prolongs survival after relapse in aggressive-lymphoma patients treated with the LNH-84 regimen. J Clin Oncol 10:1615-23, 1992

4.   Philip T, Armitage JO, Spitzer G, et al: High-dose therapy and autologous bone marrow transplantation after failure of conventional chemotherapy in adults with intermediate-grade or high-grade non-Hodgkin's lymphoma. N Engl J Med 316:1493-8, 1987

5.   Petersen FB, Appelbaum FR, Hill R, et al: Autologous marrow transplantation for malignant lymphoma: a report of 101 cases from Seattle. J Clin Oncol 8:638-47, 1990

6.   Vose JM, Anderson JR, Kessinger A, et al: High-dose chemotherapy and autologous hematopoietic stem-cell transplantation for aggressive non-Hodgkin's lymphoma. J Clin Oncol 11:1846-51, 1993

7.   Mills W, Chopra R, McMillan A, et al: BEAM chemotherapy and autologous bone marrow transplantation for patients with relapsed or refractory non-Hodgkin's lymphoma. J Clin Oncol 13:588-95, 1995

8.   Stockerl-Goldstein KE, Horning SJ, Negrin RS, et al: Influence of preparatory regimen and source of hematopoietic cells on outcome of autotransplantation for non-Hodgkin's lymphoma. Biol Blood Marrow Transplant 2:76-85, 1996

9.   Caballero MD, Rubio V, Rifon J, et al: BEAM chemotherapy followed by autologous stem cell support in lymphoma patients: analysis of efficacy, toxicity and prognostic factors. Bone Marrow Transplant 20:451-8, 1997

10.   Rapoport AP, Lifton R, Constine LS, et al: Autotransplantation for relapsed or refractory non-Hodgkin's lymphoma (NHL): long-term follow-up and analysis of prognostic factors. Bone Marrow Transplant 19:883-90, 1997

11.   Popat U, Przepiork D, Champlin R, et al: High-dose chemotherapy for relapsed and refractory diffuse large B-cell lymphoma: mediastinal localization predicts for a favorable outcome. J Clin Oncol 16:63-9, 1998

12.   Philip T, Guglielmi C, Hagenbeek A, et al: Autologous bone marrow transplantation as compared with salvage chemotherapy in relapses of chemotherapy-sensitive non-Hodgkin's lymphoma [see comments]. N.Engl.J.Med. 333:1540-1545, 1995

13.   Bierman PJ, Sweetenham JW, Loberiza FR, Jr., et al: Syngeneic hematopoietic stem-cell transplantation for non-Hodgkin's lymphoma: a comparison with allogeneic and autologous transplantation--The Lymphoma Working Committee of the International Bone Marrow Transplant Registry and the European Group for Blood and Marrow Transplantation. J Clin Oncol 21:3744-53, 2003

14.   Schwonzen M, Pohl C, Steinmetz T, et al: Immunophenotyping of low-grade B-cell lymphoma in blood and bone marrow: poor correlation between immunophenotype and cytological/histological classification. Br J Haematol 83:232-9, 1993

15.   Baidas SM, Cheson BD, Kauh J, et al: Mantle cell lymphoma: clinicopathologic features and treatments. Oncology (Huntingt) 17:879-91, 896; discussion 896-8, 2003

16.   Zucca E, Roggero E, Pinotti G, et al: Patterns of survival in mantle cell lymphoma. Ann Oncol 6:257-62, 1995

17.   Hiddemann W, Dreyling M, Preundschuh M, et al: Myeloablative radiochemotherapy followed by autologous blood stem cell transplantation leads to a significant prolongation of the event-free survival in patients with mantle cell lymphoma (MCL) -- results of a prospective randomized European Intergroup study [abstract]. Blood:abstract 3572, 2001

18.   Freedman AS, Neuberg D, Gribben JG, et al: High-dose chemoradiotherapy and anti-B-cell monoclonal antibody-purged autologous bone marrow transplantation in mantle-cell lymphoma: no evidence for long-term remission. J Clin Oncol 16:13-8, 1998

19.   Sweetenham JW: Stem cell transplantation for mantle cell lymphoma: should it ever be used outside clinical trials? Bone Marrow Transplant 28:813-20, 2001

20.   Ketterer N, Salles G, Espinouse D, et al: Intensive therapy with peripheral stem cell transplantation in 16 patients with mantle cell lymphoma. Ann Oncol 8:701-4, 1997

21.   Kasamon YL, Jones RJ, Diehl LF, et al: Outcomes of autologous and allogeneic blood or marrow transplantation for mantle cell lymphoma. Biol Blood Marrow Transplant 11:39-46, 2005

22.   Yuen AR, Rosenberg SA, Hoppe RT, et al: Comparison between conventional salvage therapy and high-dose therapy with autografting for recurrent or refractory Hodgkin's disease. Blood 89:814-22, 1997

23.   Linch DC, Winfield D, Goldstone AH, et al: Dose intensification with autologous bone-marrow transplantation in relapsed and resistant Hodgkin's disease: results of a BNLI randomised trial. Lancet 341:1051-4, 1993

24.   Sureda A, Arranz R, Iriondo A, et al: Autologous stem-cell transplantation for Hodgkin's disease: results and prognostic factors in 494 patients from the Grupo Espanol de Linfomas/Transplante Autologo de Medula Osea Spanish Cooperative Group. J Clin Oncol 19:1395-404, 2001

25.   Akpek G, Ambinder RF, Piantadosi S, et al: Long-term results of blood and marrow transplantation for Hodgkin's lymphoma. J Clin Oncol 19:4314-21, 2001

26.   Lazarus HM, Rowlings PA, Zhang MJ, et al: Autotransplants for Hodgkin's disease in patients never achieving remission: a report from the Autologous Blood and Marrow Transplant Registry. J Clin Oncol 17:534-45, 1999

27.   Sweetenham JW, Carella AM, Taghipour G, et al: High-dose therapy and autologous stem-cell transplantation for adult patients with Hodgkin's disease who do not enter remission after induction chemotherapy: results in 175 patients reported to the European Group for Blood and Marrow Transplantation. Lymphoma Working Party. J Clin Oncol 17:3101-9, 1999

28.   Horning SJ, Chao NJ, Negrin RS, et al: High-dose therapy and autologous hematopoietic progenitor cell transplantation for recurrent or refractory Hodgkin's disease: analysis of the Stanford University results and prognostic indices. Blood 89:801-13, 1997

29.   Sweetenham JW, Taghipour G, Milligan D, et al: High-dose therapy and autologous stem cell rescue for patients with Hodgkin's disease in first relapse after chemotherapy: results from the EBMT. Lymphoma Working Party of the European Group for Blood and Marrow Transplantation. Bone Marrow Transplant 20:745-52, 1997

30.   Brice P, Bouabdallah R, Moreau P, et al: Prognostic factors for survival after high-dose therapy and autologous stem cell transplantation for patients with relapsing

Hodgkin's disease: analysis of 280 patients from the French registry. Societe Francaise de Greffe de Moelle. Bone Marrow Transplant 20:21-6, 1997

31.   Lancet JE, Rapoport AP, Brasacchio R, et al: Autotransplantation for relapsed or refractory Hodgkin's disease: long-term follow-up and analysis of prognostic factors. Bone Marrow Transplant 22:265-71, 1998

32.   Arranz R, Tomas JF, Gil-Fernandez JJ, et al: Autologous stem cell transplantation (ASCT) for poor prognostic Hodgkin's disease (HD): comparative results with two CBV regimens and importance of disease status at transplant. Bone Marrow Transplant 21:779-86, 1998

33.   Andre M, Henry-Amar M, Blaise D, et al: Treatment-related deaths and second cancer risk after autologous stem-cell transplantation for Hodgkin's disease. Blood 92:1933-40, 1998

34.   Bachier CR, Giles RE, Ellerson D, et al: Hematopoietic retroviral gene marking in patients with follicular non- Hodgkin's lymphoma. Leuk.Lymphoma. 32:279-288, 1999

35.   Press OW, Eary JF, Appelbaum FR, et al: Radiolabeled-antibody therapy of B-cell lymphoma with autologous bone marrow support [see comments]. N.Engl.J.Med. 329:1219-1224, 1993

36.   Press OW, Eary JF, Appelbaum FR, et al: Phase II trial of 131I-B1 (anti-CD20) antibody therapy with autologous stem cell transplantation for relapsed B cell lymphomas. Lancet 346:336-340, 1995

37.   Liu SY, Eary JF, Petersdorf SH, et al: Follow-up of relapsed B-cell lymphoma patients treated with iodine-131- labeled anti-CD20 antibody and autologous stem-cell rescue. J.Clin.Oncol. 16:3270-3278, 1998

38.   Press OW, Eary JF, Gooley T, et al: A phase I/II trial of iodine-131-tositumomab (anti-CD20), etoposide, cyclophosphamide, and autologous stem cell transplantation for relapsed B-cell lymphomas [In Process Citation]. Blood 96:2934-2942, 2000

39.   Gribben JG, Freedman AS, Neuberg D, et al: Immunologic purging of marrow assessed by PCR before autologous bone marrow transplantation for B-cell lymphoma [see comments]. N.Engl.J.Med. 325:1525-1533, 1991

40.   Horwitz SM, Negrin RS, Blume KG, et al: Rituximab as adjuvant to high-dose therapy and autologous hematopoietic cell transplantation for aggressive non-Hodgkin lymphoma. Blood 103:777-83, 2004

41.   Flinn IW, O'Donnell PV, Goodrich A, et al: Immunotherapy with rituximab during peripheral blood stem cell transplantation for non-Hodgkin's lymphoma. Biol Blood Marrow Transplant 6:628-32, 2000

42.   Magni M, Di Nicola M, Devizzi L, et al: Successful in vivo purging of CD34-containing peripheral blood harvests in mantle cell and indolent lymphoma: evidence for a role of both chemotherapy and rituximab infusion [In Process Citation]. Blood 96:864-869, 2000

43.   Flohr T, Hess G, Kolbe K, et al: Rituximab in vivo purging is safe and effective in combination with CD34-positive selected autologous stem cell transplantation for salvage therapy in B-NHL. Bone Marrow Transplant 29:769-75, 2002

44.   Goldberg SL, Pecora AL, Alter RS, et al: Unusual viral infections (progressive multifocal leukoencephalopathy and cytomegalovirus disease) after high-dose chemotherapy with autologous blood stem cell rescue and peritransplantation rituximab. Blood 99:1486-8, 2002

45.   Thomas ED, Buckner CD, Rudolph RH, et al: Allogeneic marrow grafting for hematologic malignancy using HL-A matched donor-recipient sibling pairs. Blood 38:267-87, 1971

46.   Weiden PL, Flournoy N, Thomas ED, et al: Antileukemic effect of graft-versus-host disease in human recipients of allogeneic-marrow grafts. N Engl J Med 300:1068-73, 1979

47.   Jones RJ, Ambinder RF, Piantadosi S, et al: Evidence of graft-versus-lymphoma effect associated with allogeneic bone marrow transplantation. Blood 3:649-653, 1991

48.   van Besien KW, de Lima M, Giralt SA, et al: Management of lymphoma recurrence after allogeneic transplantation: the relevance of graft-versus-lymphoma effect. Bone Marrow Transplant 19:977-82, 1997

49.   Slavin S, Morecki S, Weiss L, et al: Donor lymphocyte infusion: the use of alloreactive and tumor-reactive lymphocytes for immunotherapy of malignant and nonmalignant diseases in conjunction with allogeneic stem cell transplantation. J Hematother Stem Cell Res 11:265-76, 2002

50.   Mandigers CM, Meijerink JP, Raemaekers JM, et al: Graft-versus-lymphoma effect of donor leucocyte infusion shown by real- time quantitative PCR analysis of t(14;18) [letter]. Lancet 352:1522-1523, 1998

51.   Slavin S, Naparstek E, Nagler A, et al: Allogeneic cell therapy for relapsed leukemia after bone marrow transplantation with donor peripheral blood lymphocytes. Exp Hematol 23:1553-62, 1995

52.   Collins RH, Jr., Shpilberg O, Drobyski WR, et al: Donor leukocyte infusions in 140 patients with relapsed malignancy after allogeneic bone marrow transplantation. J Clin Oncol 15:433-44, 1997

53.   Horning SJ, Rosenberg SA: The natural history of initially untreated low-grade non-hodgkin's lymphoma. N Engl J Med 311:1471-1475, 1984

54.   Johnson PW, Rohatiner AZ, Whelan JS, et al: Patterns of survival in patients with recurrent follicular lymphoma: a 20-year study from a single center. J Clin Oncol 13:140-7, 1995

55.   Weisdorf DJ, Andersen JW, Glick JH, et al: Survival after relapse of low-grade non-Hodgkin's lymphoma: implications for marrow transplantation. J Clin Oncol 10:942-7, 1992

56.   Van Besien K, Loberiza FR, Bajorunaite R, et al: Comparison of autologous and allogeneic hematopoietic stem cell transplantation for follicular lymphoma. Blood, 2003

57.   Verdonck LF: Allogeneic versus autologous bone marrow transplantation for refractory and recurrent low-grade non-Hodgkin's lymphoma: updated results of the Utrecht experience. Leuk Lymphoma 34:129-36, 1999

58.   van Besien K, Champlin IK, McCarthy P: Allogeneic transplantation for low-grade lymphoma: long-term follow-up. J Clin Oncol 18:702-3, 2000

59.   van Besien KW, Khouri IF, Giralt SA, et al: Allogeneic bone marrow transplantation for refractory and recurrent low-grade lymphoma: the case for aggressive management. Journal of Clinical Oncology 13:1096-1102, 1995

60.   Mandigers CM, Raemaekers JM, Schattenberg AV, et al: Allogeneic bone marrow transplantation with T-cell-depleted marrow grafts for patients with poor-risk relapsed low-grade non-Hodgkin's lymphoma. Br J Haematol 100:198-206, 1998

61.   Toze CL, Shepherd JD, Connors JM, et al: Allogeneic bone marrow transplantation for low-grade lymphoma and chronic lymphocytic leukemia. Bone Marrow Transplant. 25:605-612, 2000

62.   Stein RS, Greer JP, Goodman S, et al: High-dose therapy with autologous or allogeneic transplantation as salvage therapy for small cleaved cell lymphoma of follicular center cell origin. Bone Marrow Transplant. 23:227-233, 1999

63.   Juckett M, Rowlings P, Hessner M, et al: T cell-depleted allogeneic bone marrow transplantation for high-risk non-Hodgkin's lymphoma: clinical and molecular follow-up. Bone Marrow Transplant. 21:893-899, 1998

64.   van Besien K, Sobocinski KA, Rowlings PA, et al: Allogeneic bone marrow transplantation for low-grade lymphoma. Blood 92:1832-1836, 1998

65.   Peniket AJ, Ruiz de Elvira MC, Taghipour G, et al: An EBMT registry matched study of allogeneic stem cell transplants for lymphoma: allogeneic transplantation is associated with a lower relapse rate but a higher procedure-related mortality rate than autologous transplantation. Bone Marrow Transplant 31:667-78, 2003

66.   Forrest DL, Thompson K, Nevill TJ, et al: Allogeneic hematopoietic stem cell transplantation for progressive follicular lymphoma. Bone Marrow Transplant 29:973-8, 2002

67.   Berdeja JG, Jones RJ, Zahurak ML, et al: Allogeneic bone marrow transplantation in patients with sensitive low-grade lymphoma or mantle cell lymphoma. Biol.Blood Marrow Transplant.2001.:561-567, 2001

68.   Khouri IF, Keating MJ, Saliba RM, et al: Long-term follow-up of patients with CLL treated with allogeneic hematopoietic transplantation. Cytotherapy 4:217-21, 2002

69.   Michallet M, Archimbaud E, Bandini G, et al: HLA-identical sibling bone marrow transplantation in younger patients with chronic lymphocytic leukemia. European Group for Blood and Marrow Transplantation and the International Bone Marrow Transplant Registry. Ann Intern Med 96:311-315, 1996

70.   Pavletic ZS, Arrowsmith ER, Bierman PJ, et al: Outcome of allogeneic stem cell transplantation for B cell chronic lymphocytic leukemia. Bone Marrow Transplant. 25:717-722, 2000

71.   Prince HM, Imrie K, Crump M, et al: The role of intensive therapy and autologous blood and marrow transplantation for chemotherapy-sensitive relapsed and primary refractory non-Hodgkin's lymphoma: identification of major prognostic groups. Br J Haematol 92:880-9, 1996

72.   Dhedin N, Giraudier S, Gaulard P, et al: Allogeneic bone marrow transplantation in aggressive non-Hodgkin's lymphoma (excluding Burkitt and lymphoblastic lymphoma): a series of 73 patients from the SFGM database. Societ Francaise de Greffe de Moelle. Br J Haematol 107:154-61, 1999

73.   van Besien KW, Mehra RC, Giralt SA, et al: Allogeneic bone marrow transplantation for poor-prognosis lymphoma: response, toxicity and survival depend on disease histology. American Journal of Medicine 100:299-307, 1996

74.   Dann EJ, Daugherty CK, Larson RA: Allogeneic bone marrow transplantation for relapsed and refractory Hodgkin's disease and non-Hodgkin's lymphoma. Bone Marrow Transplant 20:369-74, 1997

75.   Bernard M, Dauriac C, Drenou B, et al: Long-term follow-up of allogeneic bone marrow transplantation in patients with poor prognosis non-Hodgkin's lymphoma. Bone Marrow Transplant 23:329-33, 1999

76.   Chopra R, Goldstone AH, Pearce R, et al: Autologous versus allogeneic bone marrow transplantation for non-Hodgkin's lymphoma: a case-controlled analysis of the European Bone Marrow Transplant Group Registry data. J Clin Oncol 10:1690-5, 1992

77.   Lundberg JH, Hansen RM, Chitambar CR, et al: Allogeneic bone marrow transplantation for relapsed and refractory lymphoma using genotypically HLA-identical and alternative donors. J Clin Oncol 9:1848-59, 1991

78.   Mendoza E, Territo M, Schiller G, et al: Allogeneic bone marrow transplantation for Hodgkin's and non-Hodgkin's lymphoma. Bone Marrow Transplant 15:299-303, 1995

79.   Mitterbauer M, Neumeister P, Kalhs P, et al: Long-term clinical and molecular remission after allogeneic stem cell transplantation (SCT) in patients with poor prognosis non-Hodgkin's lymphoma. Leukemia 15:635-41, 2001

80.   Ratanatharathorn V, Uberti J, Karanes C, et al: Prospective comparative trial of autologous versus allogeneic bone marrow transplantation in patients with non-Hodgkin's lymphoma. Blood 84:1050-5, 1994

81.   Schimmer AD, Jamal S, Messner H, et al: Allogeneic or autologous bone marrow transplantation (BMT) for non-Hodgkin's lymphoma (NHL): results of a provincial strategy. Ontario BMT Network, Canada. Bone Marrow Transplant 26:859-64, 2000

82.   Longo DL: The use of chemotherapy in the treatment of Hodgkin's disease. Semin Oncol 17:716-35, 1990

83.   Buzaid AC, Lippman SM, Miller TP: Salvage therapy of advanced Hodgkin's disease. Critical appraisal of curative potential. Am J Med 83:523-32, 1987

84.   Longo DL, Duffey PL, Young RC, et al: Conventional-dose salvage combination chemotherapy in patients relapsing with Hodgkin's disease after combination chemotherapy: the low probability for cure. J Clin Oncol 10:210-8, 1992

85.   Nademanee A, O'Donnell MR, Snyder DS, et al: High-dose chemotherapy with or without total body irradiation followed by autologous bone marrow and/or peripheral blood stem cell transplantation for patients with relapsed and refractory Hodgkin's disease: results in 85 patients with analysis of prognostic factors. Blood 85:1381-90, 1995

86.   Anderson JE, Litzow MR, Appelbaum FR, et al: Allogeneic, syngeneic, and autologous marrow transplantation for Hodgkin's disease: the 21-year Seattle experience. J Clin Oncol 11:2342-50, 1993

87.   Milpied N, Vasseur B, Parquet N, et al: Humanized anti-CD20 monoclonal antibody (Rituximab) in post transplant B-lymphoproliferative disorder: a retrospective analysis on 32 patients. Ann.Oncol. 11 Suppl 1:113-116, 2000

88.   Verdonck LF, Dekker AW, Lokhorst HM, et al: Allogeneic versus autologous bone marrow transplantation for refractory and recurrent low-grade non-Hodgkin's lymphoma. Blood 90:4201-5, 1997

89.   Appelbaum FR, Sullivan KM, Buckner CD, et al: Treatment of malignant lymphoma in 100 patients with chemotherapy, total body irradiation, and marrow transplantation. J Clin Oncol 5:1340-7, 1987

90.   Phillips GL, Wolff SN, Herzig RH, et al: Treatment of progressive Hodgkin's disease with intensive chemoradiotherapy and autologous bone marrow transplantation. Blood 73:2086-92, 1989

91.   Santos GW, Tutschka PJ, Brookmeyer R, et al: Marrow transplantation for acute nonlymphocytic leukemia after treatment with busulfan and cyclophosphamide. N.Engl.J.Med. 309:1347-1353, 1983

92.   Tutschka PJ, Copelan EA, Klein JP: Bone marrow transplantation for leukemia following a new busulfan and cyclophosphamide regimen. Blood 70:1382-8, 1987

93.   Demirer T, Weaver CH, Buckner CD, et al: High-dose cyclophosphamide, carmustine, and etoposide followed by allogeneic bone marrow transplantation in patients with lymphoid malignancies who had received prior dose-limiting radiation therapy. J Clin Oncol 13:596-602, 1995

94.   Przepiorka D, van Besien K, Khouri I, et al: Carmustine, etoposide, cytarabine and melphalan as a preparative regimen for allogeneic transplantation for high-risk malignant lymphoma. Ann Oncol 10:527-32, 1999

95.   Chopra R, McMillan AK, Linch DC, et al: The place of high-dose BEAM therapy and autologous bone marrow transplantation in poor-risk Hodgkin's disease. A single-center eight-year study of 155 patients. Blood 81:1137-45, 1993

96.   Kroger N, Hoffknecht M, Hanel M, et al: Busulfan, cyclophosphamide and etoposide as high-dose conditioning therapy in patients with malignant lymphoma and prior dose-limiting radiation therapy. Bone Marrow Transplant 21:1171-5, 1998

97.   Thomas ED, Storb R: Technique for human marrow grafting. Blood 36:507-15, 1970

98.   Korbling M, Burke P, Braine H, et al: Successful engraftment of blood derived normal hemopoietic stem cells in chronic myelogenous leukemia. Exp Hematol 9:684-90, 1981

99.   Thomas DB: The infusion of human fetal liver cells. Stem Cells 11 Suppl 1:66-71, 1993

100.   Gluckman E, Broxmeyer HA, Auerbach AD, et al: Hematopoietic reconstitution in a patient with Fanconi's anemia by means of umbilical-cord blood from an HLA-identical sibling. N Engl J Med 321:1174-8, 1989

101.   Thomas E, Storb R, Clift RA, et al: Bone-marrow transplantation (first of two parts). N Engl J Med 292:832-43, 1975

102.   Thomas ED, Storb R, Clift RA, et al: Bone-marrow transplantation (second of two parts). N Engl J Med 292:895-902, 1975

103.   McCredie KB, Hersh EM, Freireich EJ: Cells capable of colony formation in the peripheral blood of man. Science 171:293-4, 1971

104.   Korbling M, Huh YO, Durett A, et al: Allogeneic blood stem cell transplantation: peripheralization and yield of donor-derived primitive hematopoietic progenitor cells (CD34+ Thy-1dim) and lymphoid subsets, and possible predictors of engraftment and graft-versus-host disease. Blood 86:2842-8, 1995

105.   Appelbaum FR, Herzig GP, Ziegler JL, et al: Successful engraftment of cryopreserved autologous bone marrow in patients with malignant lymphoma. Blood 52:85-95, 1978

106.   Kessinger A, Armitage JO, Landmark JD, et al: Autologous peripheral hematopoietic stem cell transplantation restores hematopoietic function following marrow ablative therapy. Blood 71:723-7, 1988

107.   Bensinger WI, Martin PJ, Storer B, et al: Transplantation of bone marrow as compared with peripheral-blood cells from HLA-identical relatives in patients with hematologic cancers. N Engl J Med 344:175-81, 2001

108.   Vigorito AC, Azevedo WM, Marques JF, et al: A randomised, prospective comparison of allogeneic bone marrow and peripheral blood progenitor cell transplantation in the treatment of haematological malignancies. Bone Marrow Transplant 22:1145-51, 1998

109.   Blaise D, Kuentz M, Fortanier C, et al: Randomized trial of bone marrow versus lenograstim-primed blood cell allogeneic transplantation in patients with early-stage leukemia: a report from the Societe Francaise de Greffe de Moelle. J Clin Oncol 18:537-46, 2000

110.   Ringden O, Horowitz MM, Sondel P, et al: Methotrexate, cyclosporine, or both to prevent graft-versus-host disease after HLA-identical sibling bone marrow transplants for early leukemia? Blood 81:1094-101, 1993

111.   Heldal D, Tjonnfjord G, Brinch L, et al: A randomised study of allogeneic transplantation with stem cells from blood or bone marrow. Bone Marrow Transplant 25:1129-36, 2000

112.   Powles R, Mehta J, Kulkarni S, et al: Allogeneic blood and bone-marrow stem-cell transplantation in haematological malignant diseases: a randomised trial. Lancet 355:1231-7, 2000

113.   Champlin RE, Schmitz N, Horowitz MM, et al: Blood stem cells compared with bone marrow as a source of hematopoietic cells for allogeneic transplantation.

IBMTR Histocompatibility and Stem Cell Sources Working Committee and the European Group for Blood and Marrow Transplantation (EBMT). Blood 95:3702-9, 2000

114.   Cavallaro AM, Lilleby K, Majolino I, et al: Three to six year follow-up of normal donors who received recombinant human granulocyte colony-stimulating factor. Bone Marrow Transplant 25:85-9, 2000

115.   Deeg HJ, Storb R, Thomas ED, et al: Cyclosporine as prophylaxis for graft-versus-host disease: a randomized study in patients undergoing marrow transplantation for acute nonlymphoblastic leukemia. Blood 65:1325-34, 1985

116.   Storb R, Deeg HJ, Whitehead J, et al: Methotrexate and cyclosporine compared with cyclosporine alone for prophylaxis of acute graft versus host disease after marrow transplantation for leukemia. N Engl J Med 314:729-35, 1986

117.   Ratanatharathorn V, Nash RA, Przepiorka D, et al: Phase III study comparing methotrexate and tacrolimus (prograf, FK506) with methotrexate and cyclosporine for graft-versus-host disease prophylaxis after HLA-identical sibling bone marrow transplantation. Blood 92:2303-14, 1998

118.   Reisner Y, Kapoor N, O'Reilly RJ, et al: Allogeneic bone marrow transplantation using stem cells fractionated by lectins: VI, in vitro analysis of human and monkey bone marrow cells fractionated by sheep red blood cells and soybean agglutinin. Lancet 2:1320-4, 1980

119.   Filipovich AH, McGlave PB, Ramsay NK, et al: Pretreatment of donor bone marrow with monoclonal antibody OKT3 for prevention of acute graft-versus-host disease in allogeneic histocompatible bone-marrow transplantation. Lancet 1:1266-9, 1982

120.   Waldmann H, Polliak A, Hale G, et al: Elimination of graft-versus-host disease by in-vitro depletion of alloreactive lymphocytes with a monoclonal rat anti-human lymphocyte antibody (CAMPATH-1). Lancet 2:483-6, 1984

121.   Heit W, Bunjes D, Wiesneth M, et al: Ex vivo T-cell depletion with the monoclonal antibody Campath-1 plus human complement effectively prevents acute graft-versus-host disease in allogeneic bone marrow transplantation. Br J Haematol 64:479-86, 1986

122.   Cull GM, Haynes AP, Byrne JL, et al: Preliminary experience of allogeneic stem cell transplantation for lymphoproliferative disorders using BEAM-CAMPATH conditioning: an effective regimen with low procedure-related toxicity. Br.J.Haematol. 108:754-760, 2000

123.   Wagner JE, Donnenberg AD, Noga SJ, et al: Lymphocyte depletion of donor bone marrow by counterflow centrifugal elutriation: results of a phase I clinical trial. Blood 72:1168-76, 1988

124.   Noga SJ, Vogelsang GB, Seber A, et al: CD34+ stem cell augmentation of allogeneic, elutriated marrow grafts improves engraftment but cyclosporine A is still required to reduce GVHD and morbidity. Transplant Proc 29:728-32, 1997

125.   Soiffer RJ, Freedman AS, Neuberg D, et al: CD6+ T cell-depleted allogeneic bone marrow transplantation for non-Hodgkin's lymphoma. Bone Marrow Transplant 21:1177-81, 1998

126.   Maraninchi D, Gluckman E, Blaise D, et al: Impact of T-cell depletion on outcome of allogeneic bone-marrow transplantation for standard-risk leukaemias. Lancet 2:175-8, 1987

127.   Nigam A, Yacavone RF, Zahurak ML, et al: Immunomodulatory properties of antineoplastic drugs administered in conjunction with GM-CSF-secreting cancer cell vaccines. Int J Oncol 12:161-70, 1998

128.   Mackinnon S, Papadopoulos EB, Carabasi MH, et al: Adoptive immunotherapy evaluating escalating doses of donor leukocytes relapse of chronic myeloid leukemia after bone marrow transplantation: Separation of graft-versus-leukemia responses from graft-versus-host disease. Blood 86:1261-1268, 1995

129.   Soiffer RJ, Alyea EP, Hochberg E, et al: Randomized trial of CD8+ T-cell depletion in the prevention of graft-versus-host disease associated with donor lymphocyte infusion. Biol Blood Marrow Transplant 8:625-32, 2002

130.   Kim YM, Sachs T, Asavaroengchai W, et al: Graft-versus-host disease can be separated from graft-versus-lymphoma effects by control of lymphocyte trafficking with FTY720. J Clin Invest 111:659-69, 2003

131.   Slavin S, Nagler A, Naparstek E, et al: Nonmyeloablative stem cell transplantation and cell therapy as an alternative to conventional bone marrow transplantation with lethal cytoreduction for the treatment of malignant and nonmalignant hematologic diseases. Blood 91:756-763, 1998

132.   Khouri IF, Keating M, Korbling M, et al: Transplant-lite: induction of graft-versus-malignancy using fludarabine-based nonablative chemotherapy and allogeneic blood progenitor-cell transplantation as treatment for lymphoid malignancies. J Clin Oncol 16:2817-24, 1998

133.   Craddock C, Bardy P, Kreiter S, et al: Short Report: Engraftment of T-cell-depleted allogeneic haematopoietic stem cells using a reduced intensity conditioning regimen. Br J Haematol 111:797-800, 2000

134.   Corradini P, Tarella C, Olivieri A, et al: Reduced-intensity conditioning followed by allografting of hematopoietic cells can produce clinical and molecular remissions in patients with poor-risk hematologic malignancies. Blood 99:75-82, 2002

135.   Champlin R, Khouri I, Shimoni A, et al: Harnessing graft-versus-malignancy: non-myeloablative preparative regimens for allogeneic haematopoietic transplantation, an evolving strategy for adoptive immunotherapy. Br J Haematol 111:18-29, 2000

136.   Bornhauser M, Thiede C, Platzbecker U, et al: Dose-reduced conditioning and allogeneic hematopoietic stem cell transplantation from unrelated donors in 42 patients. Clin Cancer Res 7:2254-62, 2001

137.   Khouri IF, Saliba RM, Giralt SA, et al: Nonablative allogeneic hematopoietic transplantation as adoptive immunotherapy for indolent lymphoma: low incidence of toxicity, acute graft-versus-host disease, and treatment-related mortality. Blood 98:3595-9, 2001

138.   Robinson SP, Goldstone AH, Mackinnon S, et al: Chemoresistant or aggressive lymphoma predicts for a poor outcome following reduced-intensity allogeneic progenitor cell transplantation: an analysis from the Lymphoma Working Party of the European Group for Blood and Bone Marrow Transplantation. Blood 100:4310-6, 2002

139.   Perez-Simon JA, Kottaridis PD, Martino R, et al: Nonmyeloablative transplantation with or without alemtuzumab: comparison between 2 prospective studies in patients with lymphoproliferative disorders. Blood 100:3121-7, 2002

140.   Branson K, Chopra R, Kottaridis PD, et al: Role of nonmyeloablative allogeneic stem-cell transplantation after failure of autologous transplantation in patients with lymphoproliferative malignancies. J Clin Oncol 20:4022-31, 2002

141.   Dreger P, Brand R, Hansz J, et al: Treatment-related mortality and graft-versus-leukemia activity after allogeneic stem cell transplantation for chronic lymphocytic leukemia using intensity-reduced conditioning. Leukemia 17:841-8, 2003

142.   Carella AM, Cavaliere M, Lerma E, et al: Autografting followed by nonmyeloablative immunosuppressive chemotherapy and allogeneic peripheral-blood hematopoietic stem-cell transplantation as treatment of resistant Hodgkin's disease and non-Hodgkin's lymphoma. J Clin Oncol 18:3918-24, 2000

143.   Mohty M, Fegueux N, Exbrayat C, et al: Reduced intensity conditioning: enhanced graft-versus-tumor effect following dose-reduced conditioning and allogeneic transplantation for refractory lymphoid malignancies after high-dose therapy. Bone Marrow Transplant 28:335-9, 2001

144.   Weissinger F, Sandmaier BM, Maloney DG, et al: Decreased transfusion requirements for patients receiving nonmyeloablative compared with conventional peripheral blood stem cell transplants from HLA-identical siblings. Blood 98:3584-8, 2001

145.   Nagler A, Slavin S, Varadi G, et al: Allogeneic peripheral blood stem cell transplantation using a fludarabine-based low intensity conditioning regimen for malignant lymphoma. Bone Marrow Transplant 25:1021-8, 2000

146.   Raiola AM, Van Lint MT, Lamparelli T, et al: Reduced intensity thiotepa-cyclophosphamide conditioning for allogeneic haemopoietic stem cell transplants (HSCT) in patients up to 60 years of age. Br J Haematol 109:716-21, 2000

147.   Alessandrino EP, Bernasconi P, Colombo AA, et al: Thiotepa and fludarabine (TT-FLUDA) as conditioning regimen in poor candidates for conventional allogeneic hemopoietic stem cell transplant. Ann Hematol 80:521-4, 2001

148.   Giralt S, Thall PF, Khouri I, et al: Melphalan and purine analog-containing preparative regimens: reduced-intensity conditioning for patients with hematologic malignancies undergoing allogeneic progenitor cell transplantation. Blood 97:631-7, 2001

149.   Wasch R, Reisser S, Hahn J, et al: Rapid achievement of complete donor chimerism and low regimen-related toxicity after reduced conditioning with fludarabine, carmustine, melphalan and allogeneic transplantation. Bone Marrow Transplant 26:243-50, 2000

150.   Bainton RD, Byrne JL, Davy BJ, et al: CMV infection following nonmyeloablative allogeneic stem cell transplantation using Campath. Blood 100:3843-4, 2002

151.   Kottaridis PD, Milligan DW, Chopra R, et al: In vivo CAMPATH-1H prevents graft-versus-host disease following nonmyeloablative stem cell transplantation. Blood 96:2419-25, 2000

152.   Chakrabarti S, Mackinnon S, Chopra R, et al: High incidence of cytomegalovirus infection after nonmyeloablative stem cell transplantation: potential role of Campath-1H in delaying immune reconstitution. Blood 99:4357-63, 2002

153.   Chakraverty R, Peggs K, Chopra R, et al: Limiting transplantation-related mortality following unrelated donor stem cell transplantation by using a nonmyeloablative conditioning regimen. Blood 99:1071-8, 2002

154.   Niederwieser D, Maris M, Shizuru JA, et al: Low-dose total body irradiation (TBI) and fludarabine followed by hematopoietic cell transplantation (HCT) from HLA-matched or mismatched unrelated donors and postgrafting immunosuppression with cyclosporine and mycophenolate mofetil (MMF) can induce durable complete chimerism and sustained remissions in patients with hematological diseases. Blood 101:1620-9, 2003

155.   Sykes M, Preffer F, McAfee S, et al: Mixed lymphohaemopoietic chimerism and graft-versus-lymphoma effects after non-myeloablative therapy and HLA-mismatched bone-marrow transplantation. Lancet 353:1755-9, 1999

156.   Maloney DG, Molina AJ, Sahebi F, et al: Allografting with non-myeloablative conditioning following cytoreductive autografts for the treatment of patients with multiple myeloma. Blood, 2003

Chapter 9

VACCINE THERAPIES FOR NON-HODGKIN'S LYMPHOMAS

Sarah Montross, MD, and John M. Timmerman, MD

University of California, Los Angeles Center for Health Sciences Department of Medicine and Division of Hematology-Oncology, Los Angeles, CA

1.   INTRODUCTION

Chemotherapy and radiation therapy can slow the progression of indolent non-Hodgkin's lymphoma (NHL), but few if any patients are cured with these modalities. Active immunotherapy, which attempts to harness the host's own immune system to eradicate the malignant clone, has emerged as an important area of investigation in lymphoma. The attractiveness of this approach lies in the remarkable specificity of the adaptive immune system in recognizing tumor-associated or tumor-specific antigens. Even anti-CD20 monoclonal antibodies cannot match the potential specificity of an active host immune response, as these agents deplete both normal and malignant B cells. Many investigators have thus sought to find ways to exploit the host's own immune system to achieve the specific destruction of malignant cells.

The success of a tumor vaccine is predicated on the identification of an antigen that is differentially-expressed between normal and tumor cells, and then overcoming the immune system's existing tolerance to that antigen. For a wide variety of cancers, tumor antigens may include peptide products of genes with mutations unique to tumor cells (i.e, p53), the products of rearranged or dysregulated oncogenes such as bcr-abl or HER2/neu, sequences from viruses including Epstein-Barr virus or human papilloma virus, or genes normally expressed in fetal life such as carcinoembryonic antigen or alpha-fetoprotein. B cells express clonal immunoglobulin, whose molecular structure is uniquely determined by the variable regions of its heavy and light chains. The collection of unique antigenic epitopes formed by the immunoglobulin heavy and light chains is termed the idiotype (Id). Analogously, T cell lymphomas also express T-cell receptors on their cell surface which also possess unique idiotypes. These idiotypes are currently the only well-characterized tumor antigens available as therapeutic vaccine targets in non-Hodgkin's lymphomas. Investigators have now spent more than 16 years studying the immunologic and clinical effects of immunoglobulin Id vaccination for human B cell malignancies. However, at this time, all of these promising approaches remain investigational, as phase I, II, and III clinical trials are ongoing. Therapeutic vaccines have not yet been approved by the U.S. Food and Drug Administration (FDA) for the treatment of any malignancy.

2.   EVOLUTION OF IDIOTYPE AS A THERAPEUTIC TARGET

        Early work in animals demonstrated the therapeutic potential of anti-idiotype approaches in combating lymphoid malignancy. Studies by Lynch *et al* in 1972 revealed that immunization of healthy mice with myeloma (idiotype) proteins could prevent later establishment and growth of injected myeloma cells (1). In 1977, Stevenson *et al* used polyclonal anti-idiotype antisera to successfully treat a B cell leukemia in guinea pigs (2).
        Pioneering studies in humans focused on the production and administration of exogenous monoclonal antibodies against idiotype. In 1978, Ronald Levy and colleagues at Stanford University used the technique of "rescue hybridization" to fuse individual patients' follicular lymphoma cells with immortalized myeloma cells, yielding stable hybridoma cell lines that secreted large amounts of tumor-specific idiotype protein (3). This idiotype protein was then purified and injected into mice, and mouse anti-idiotype monoclonal antibodies were generated that could selectively bind to individual patient's tumor cells. The first patient to receive these antibodies had remarkable regression of widespread, chemotherapy-refractory follicular lymphoma (4). This result caused a sensation in the fledgling field of monoclonal antibody therapy, and led to the founding of IDEC Pharmaceuticals, whose original intent was to produce custom-made anti-idiotype antibodies commercially. Between 1982 and 1993, 45 patients were treated with 52 courses of patient-specific mouse (or rat) anti-idiotype antibodies with a 66% overall response rate and 18% complete response rate (5). Six patients (13%) have had prolonged complete remission, and several have remained in remission without any additional therapy for many years and appear to be cured (5)(R. Levy, personal communications).

However, producing unique monoclonal antibodies against the idiotype expressed by each patient's tumor proved to be prohibitively time-consuming and expensive. In addition, idiotype-negative "escape" variant tumor cells were found to emerge after therapy, arising from the ongoing somatic mutation in the variable regions of the tumor immunoglobulin genes encoding (6). In some cases, production and administration of a second monoclonal anti-idiotype antibody was required to achieve remission (7). Moreover, the murine constant regions of these antibodies are themselves foreign proteins. After repeated injections, patients may develop human anti-mouse antibodies (HAMA). These HAMA may bind to subsequent infused doses of the murine antibody, leading to both decreased efficacy of the therapy as well as the formation of immune complexes that mediate hypersensitivity reactions. Thus, although passive, individualized anti-idiotype monoclonal antibody therapy was highly effective, investigators realized the practicality and potential additional benefits of an active vaccination strategy with patient-specific idiotype.

3. ACTIVE IMMUNIZATION AGAINST IDIOTYPE

3.1 Immunologic Considerations

Immunization with lymphoma idiotype has the advantage of potentially activating both humoral and cellular immune responses in the patient, which may result in superior efficacy over passive administration of a single antibody. In addition, the tumor-specific B cells and T cells evoked by such a vaccine will likely mediate long-term immunological memory, theoretically capable of continuous surveillance and killing of residual tumor cells. It is now possible to collect a sample of patient's lymphoma cells, produce idiotype protein *in vitro* by rescue hybridization or molecular methods, and then use this tumor-specific protein to immunize that patient directly (Figure 1). This strategy has the advantage of potentially inducing a polyclonal anti-idiotype antibody response, along with CD4+ (8-12) and CD8+ (13-20) T cells that recognize idiotype-derived peptides on the cell surface bound to class II and class I major histocompatibility (MHC) molecules, respectively. B cell lymphomas differ from most other cancers in their constitutive expression of class II MHC molecules, thus allowing direct recognition by CD4+ T cells.

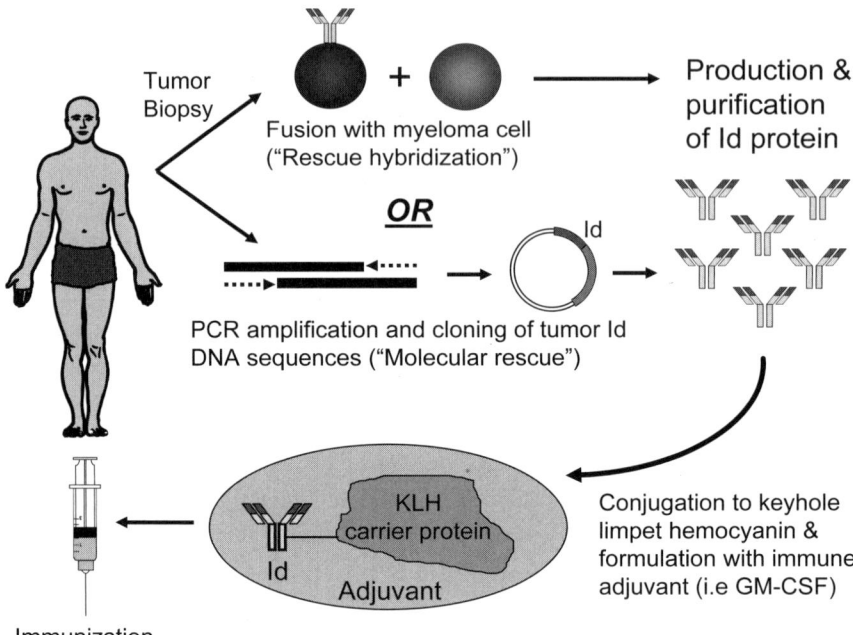

Figure 1.   Schema for production of patient-specific idiotype (Id) vaccines. Idiotype vaccines are custom-made from each patient's own tumor cells either by fusing to an immortal myeloma cell ("rescue hybrid" method), or by genetically engineering techniques ("molecular rescue" method). In each case, an unlimited supply of the vaccine can be made. The Id protein is then chemically linked to the foreign protein keyhole limpet hemocyanin (KLH), combined with an immune stimulant (adjuvant), and injected under the skin. (Timmerman JM. Therapeutic Idiotype Vaccines for Non-Hodgkin's Lymphoma. Reproduced with permission from Elsevier, Inc., Adv. Pharmacol. 51:259-280, 2004.)

However, because a tumor's idiotype is derived from "self" immunoglobulin, it is expected to be only weakly immunogenic. Thus, various strategies have been implemented to increase its immunogenicity in the host. One strategy is to chemically conjugate the idiotype protein to a highly immunogenic carrier protein, which will help overcome immunologic tolerance to the idiotype. The most commonly used carrier protein is called keyhole limpet hemocyanin (KLH), an oxygen-carrying protein from the marine mollusk *Megathura crenulata*. Brief incubation of idiotype and KLH in the presence of 0.1% glutaraldehyde cross-links the two proteins via lysine, cysteine, tyrosine, and histidine residues, yielding Id-KLH. The Id-

KLH complex can then be combined with an immunologic adjuvant that serves to further boost the response to this tumor antigen. In early studies of idiotype vaccination in murine lymphoma models, vaccination with Id-KLH plus a chemical adjuvant was found to evoke protection from lethal tumor challenge (8, 21-23). Anti-idiotype antibodies played a major role in the tumor-protective responses, in being sufficient to provide protection (8, 22, 24-26), although CD4+ and CD8+ T cell also contribute to tumor resistance (8, 22, 27, 28). Importantly, established tumors could be cured in mice using a combination of vaccination plus chemotherapy (29). Also, active vaccination was able to evoke a polyclonal anti-idiotype immune response that covered idiotype-negative variants which had otherwise escaped recognition by a monoclonal anti-idiotype antibody (30). These animal studies helped to shape the early clinical testing of idiotype vaccination in follicular lymphoma.

3.2 Early Trials of Id-KLH Vaccines

The first clinical study of Id vaccination was performed at Stanford University by Ronald Levy and colleagues (9). This study included nine patients with follicular lymphoma either in complete remission or with minimal residual disease after one or more courses of chemotherapy. Lymphoma cells from lymph node biopsy specimens obtained before chemotherapy were used to produce tumor-specific idiotype by the rescue hybridoma method. Idiotype protein was conjugated to KLH using glutaraldehyde. Subcutaneous injections of Id-KLH plus an oil-in-water type chemical adjuvant were administered at 0, 2, 6, 10, and 14 weeks. Seven of the 9 patients developed idiotype-specific humoral (2 patients), T cell proliferative (4 patients), or both (1 patient) immune responses. Two patients with measurable disease at the time of immunization had complete regression of their residual tumor. Toxicity was minimal, and consisted primarily of local injection site reactions attributable to the co-injected adjuvant.

In 1997, long-term follow-up data from this study was reported on 41 patients, including the 9 previously-reported subjects (10). Thirty-two were in their first chemotherapy-induced remission, and 9 in subsequent remissions. All 41 patients developed anti-KLH responses following vaccination, proving their general immune competence. Twenty of the 41 patients (49%) developed idiotype-specific antibody or T cell proliferative responses following vaccination. Antibody responses were detected more often than T cell responses (85% vs. 35%, respectively). However, it should be pointed out that the sensitivity of the assay used was significantly lower than the current techniques which measure cytokine release instead of T cell proliferation (31, 32). Thus, the true level of T cell priming to tumor antigen in these early trials remains unknown. As measured, anti-idiotype immune responses were more frequent among patients in complete remission at the time of vaccination (75%) than in those with residual tumor (25%). Among the 32 first remission patients vaccinated, 44% (14 of 32) mounted anti-idiotype immune responses to the vaccine. In long-term follow-up, the measurement of an anti-idiotype immune response was highly correlated with improved disease-free ($p < 0.0001$) and overall ($p = 0.04$) survival (10). These data support a possible therapeutic benefit for Id-KLH vaccination. However, it is possible that the ability to mount an anti-idiotype immune response was merely a marker for other unknown factors that improve relapse-free survival, such as the level of residual disease. Furthermore, although the vaccinated patients' overall survival was superior to that of historical controls, efficacy could not be proven because most of the patients treated were in clinical remission at the time of vaccination and without easily measurable tumor. Therefore, traditional modes for demonstrating efficacy, such as monitoring tumors for regression, could not be applied. This study nonetheless suggested that induction of anti-idiotype immune responses might have clinically beneficial effects, thus prompting the search for ways to increase the frequency and potency of anti-Id immune responses in vaccinated patients.

3.3   Idiotype-Pulsed Dendritic Cell Vaccination

The success of the protein-based Id-KLH vaccine strategy is dependent on recruitment of antigen presenting cells (APCs) to the vaccine site, where the APCs process the Id-KLH peptide and present it on class I and II major histocompatibility complex (MHC) molecules, initiating the immune response. Dendritic cells, which are highly effective APCs, have been used to improve the potency of idiotype and other cancer vaccines (33). These cells can be isolated directly from the peripheral blood, or generated in vitro from monocytes or CD34+ hematopoietic progenitor cells using granulocyte-macrophage colony-stimulating factor (GM-CSF), interleukin (IL)-4, and tumor necrosis factor (TNF)-alpha. The dendritic cells can be briefly co-cultured with tumor-derived proteins or peptides, thus allowing these antigens to be ingested, processed, and presented on MHC glycoproteins together with abundant costimulatory molecules. These cells can then be injected as a cellular vaccine.

A study performed at Stanford University demonstrated that vaccination with dendritic cells pulsed with lymphoma Id protein could induce immune responses as well as marked tumor regressions (34, 35). The study population included 35 patients with follicular lymphoma, either measurable relapsed disease, or in first remission after chemotherapy. Dendritic cells were isolated from patients' peripheral blood by leukapheresis and a series of complex density gradient separation procedures, and co-cultured for 2 days with Id and KLH separately (22 patients) or with Id-KLH conjugate (13 patients). The dendritic cells were then administered intravenously at week 0, 4, 8, 12, and 20. Patients also received subcutaneous injections of Id and KLH at separate sites or Id-KLH conjugate 2 weeks after each dendritic cell infusion. After completing the series of vaccines, 67% of patients demonstrated idiotype-specific T-cell proliferative and/or humoral immune responses. Anti-Id humoral responses were much more frequent in patients who received dendritic cells co-cultured with Id-KLH (6 of 13 with humoral responses) compared with those who received dendritic cells loaded with Id and KLH separately (3 of 22 with humoral responses).

Tumor regression responses were also observed. Eight of 28 patients (with measurable tumor had demonstrable shrinkage of tumor after vaccination, including 4 durable complete remissions. These clinical responses occurred in both immune responders and non-responders, without a statistically significant difference between the groups. Among those completing vaccination in their first remission after chemotherapy, sixteen of 23 remained progression-free at a median of 43 months post-chemotherapy. Six patients with persistent or relapsed tumors were offered "booster" vaccination with Id-KLH protein and adjuvant, administered without dendritic cells. Three of the 6 had tumor regression responses (2 complete, one partial), each associated with a corresponding boost in measured immune response. These data suggest a strategy in which utilizing Id-KLH-loaded dendritic cells for initial vaccinations, followed by subcutaneous boosters with Id-KLH plus immune adjuvant for patients who do not achieve complete remission.

This approach is the subject of an upcoming phase II clinical trial opening at the University of California, Los Angeles in early 2005. Thirty-two subjects with follicular lymphoma that has relapsed or failed to regress after chemotherapy, local radiotherapy, or rituximab will be enrolled. Dendritic cells will derived from autologous monocytes collected by leukapheresis and cultured in the presence of GM-CSF and IL-4, and then co-cultured with recombinant Id and Id-KLH proteins and a dendritic cell maturation stimulus. The idiotype-loaded cells will be administered intravenously in three monthly doses. All patients will receive booster vaccinations with Id-KLH and GM-CSF (see below). Endpoints will include safety and toxicity, tumor-specific immune responses, and objective tumor regression.

3.4   The Use of GM-CSF to Enhance T Cell Responses

Rather than using dendritic cells loaded *ex vivo* with antigens such as Id-KLH, an alternate strategy is to co-inject cytokines to either attract APCs to the vaccine site, or to enhance the activity of APCs already present at the vaccine site. A study in the 38C13 murine lymphoma model suggested that the ability of the Id-KLH vaccine to prime a T-cell response could be enhanced by co-injection with granulocyte-monocyte colony-stimulating factor (GM-CSF), a potent growth and maturation factor for dendritic cells (27). GM-CSF proved more potent in this model than other cytokines tested, including IL-1β, IL-2, IL-12, and γ-IFN, mirroring the results of earlier gene transfer studies (36).

This strategy was then tested in lymphoma patients in a clinical trial at the National Cancer Institute (NCI) (31). Twenty patients with follicular lymphoma in first clinical CR after a uniform chemotherapy regimen were vaccinated. Each Id-KLH vaccine dose was administered with GM-CSF, and daily doses of GM-CSF were given at the same site for three days thereafter in order to provide potent local immune stimulation. Nineteen of 20 patients mounted tumor-specific T cell responses as measured by cytokine release, and 75% developed serum anti-idiotype antibodies. The investigators sought to demonstrate efficacy by utilizing polymerase chain reaction (PCR) technology to detect molecular residual disease. Prior to vaccination, the patients were analyzed for PCR evidence of the bcl-2/IgH translocation t(14;18) characteristic of follicular lymphoma. Eight out of 11 patients evaluable with this technique converted to PCR negativity in the peripheral blood after completing vaccination. While these results are intriguing, it is possible that loss of the bcl-2 signal signifies only clearance of tumor cells from the bloodstream due to antibody-mediated tumor opsonization within the reticuloendothelial system. Nonetheless, these impressive results served to make GM-CSF a preferred adjuvant in trials of Id-KLH vaccination. At the time of initial publication, 18 of 20 patients remained in continuous first CR at a median of 42 months from the completion of chemotherapy(31). In subsequent follow-up analysis, it was reported that as of August, 2003, at a median follow-up of 7.2 years, 10 of 20 (50%) of subjects remain in continuous first CR (37).

4. MOLECULAR METHODS OF IDIOTYPE PRODUCTION

As an alternative to the rescue hybridoma method of idiotype production, a variety of recombinant DNA techniques have been developed to simplify tumor idiotype manufacture. The traditional rescue hybrid approach requires large numbers of starting tumor cells, can take 6-12 months or longer to complete, and has a failure rate of up to 10-15%, making it less than ideal for industrial-scale production. In the "molecular rescue" approach, a tumor sample is obtained, and PCR is used to amplify the DNA sequences encoding the tumor cells' heavy and light chain variable regions. These sequences are ligated into plasmid or viral vectors under the control of constitutive promoters that direct gene transcription. These vectors are then used to transfect a variety of bacterial, insect, plant, or mammalian cells that then secrete large quantities of idiotype protein.

Genitope, Inc. (Redwood City, CA, USA) utilizes recombinant techniques to express full-length, tetrameric idiotype proteins with an IgG3 backbone in murine lymphoma cells. In a phase I/II study of this recombinant Id-KLH (MyVax™) administered with GM-CSF, the vaccine was found to be safe and to have immunogenicity comparable with that of hybridoma-derived idiotype protein (38). Importantly, antibodies and T-cells reactive to the recombinant idiotype were also reactive toward native, hybridoma-derived idiotype. In addition, the two patients who had PCR evidence of bcl-2 in peripheral blood both converted to bcl-2-negative status following vaccination. Based on these promising results, Genitope initiated a phase III, randomized, controlled clinical trial of recombinant Id-KLH plus GM-CSF (see below).

Favrille Corporation (San Diego, CA, USA) utilizes a baculovirus vector system to express idiotype proteins with a human IgG1 backbone in sf9 insect cells (39). Vaccine proteins can be produced within 8-12 weeks in most cases. This insect-derived recombinant Id-KLH plus GM-CSF has been found to be well-tolerated, immunogenic, and clinically-active. Preliminary results from phase II studies with this agent have been reported (40, 41). Patients received an initial series of 6 monthly immunizations. Those with stable disease after 6 months received additional vaccinations every two months for one year, then every three months until disease progression. Among 27 patients with measurable, relapsed follicular lymphoma, one patient sustained a complete remission and three patients achieved partial remissions, for an overall response rate of 15%. An additional four patients had minor responses with tumor shrinkage of at least 25%, for an overall tumor regression rate of 30%.

Favrille has also investigated the efficacy of FavId™ and GM-CSF in follicular lymphoma after treatment with rituximab (42). Prior rituximab therapy had not been allowed in earlier idiotype vaccine studies given that it rapidly depletes normal B-cells (43), markedly impairing the host's ability to mount primary and secondary humoral immune responses to vaccines (44, 45). Anti-idiotype antibodies are believed to be important in mediating anti-tumor effects in B cell lymphoma (5, 8, 24, 46). However, T-cell mediated anti-tumor immunity in B-cell deficient mice can be enhanced in response to tumor antigen vaccination (47). Given this, it is hypothesized that cytoreduction of B-cells with rituximab prior to idiotype vaccination might enhance anti-idiotype T-cell responses. Moreover, with continued boosting throughout B-cell recovery (6 to 9 months following rituximab(43)), the humoral anti-idiotype response should eventually be recruited. Eighty-eight patients began FavId™ two months after completing a standard 4-week course of rituximab and having at least stable disease. Among 45 patients with relapsed/refractory disease at study entry, 32 (72%) had not progressed at a median follow-up of 12 months, compared with 40% progression among historical control patients treated with rituximab alone(48). Among 43 treatment-naive patients, 82% had not progressed after a median follow-up of 9 months. Twelve patients improved from stable disease to PR and 9 patients improved from PR to CR following FavId™ immunization. T-cell immune responses to both tumor idiotype and KLH were observed in 3 of 3 patients tested, although anti-KLH antibody responses were generally not seen until B-cell recovery. Patients receiving FavId™ following cytoreduction with rituximab thus appeared to have favorable outcome compared to historical subjects treated with rituximab alone, setting the stage for the current phase III trial of FavId™ following rituximab.

CellGenix (Freiberg, Germany) is now producing recombinant lymphoma idiotype proteins in *E. coli* as Fab fragments (IdioVax®)(49). Idiotype proteins made in this manner have been shown capable of inducing tumor-specific cytotoxic T lymphocytes *in vitro* using idiotype-loaded dendritic cells (17). A recent phase I trial enrolled a heterogeneous group of NHL patients relapsing after anthracycline-based chemotherapy (50, 51). Fab production was successful in thirteen of 18 patients (89%). The Fab idiotype protein was not conjugated to KLH as in other clinical studies. Half of subjects developed T cell and/or humoral anti-idiotype immune responses, and two complete tumor regressions have been observed (one follicular, one diffuse large B cell lymphoma). Additional phase II testing of this product is underway.

Large Scale Biology (Vacaville, CA) has produced idiotype proteins in the form of single chain variable region immunoglobulin (scFv) fragments in tobacco plants employing recombinant tobacco mosaic virus. This product has undergone phase I testing in follicular lymphoma patients in first remission after CVP chemotherapy (52). Although T cell and humoral immune responses were reported in 10 of 16 subjects, the relevance of these immune responses to native tumor idiotype protein or autologous tumor cells was not verified, and no clinical responses were reported. There are no known plans for continued testing of this vaccine formulation.

5. PHASE III CLINICAL TRIALS OF IDIOTYPE VACCINATION

The favorable results of phase II clinical trials of Id-KLH plus GM-CSF vaccines have now spawned three large, multi-center, randomized, phase III clinical trials of idiotype vaccination for follicular lymphoma (see Table 3 for comparison). In each trial, a tumor biopsy is performed to production of the patient–specific vaccine while cytoreduction is carried out using multi-agent chemotherapy (2 trials) or rituximab (1 trial). Patients achieving adequate remissions are then randomized to receive either Id-KLH or KLH alone plus GM-CSF in double-blind fashion. The primary endpoint in these studies is progression-free survival, an endpoint deemed sufficient for FDA approval of idiotype vaccines in follicular lymphoma.

5.1 Id-KLH plus GM-CSF after Chemotherapy

Based on the phase II trials cited above, the NCI and Genitope each initiated phase III trials of Id-KLH plus GM-CSF in 1999 and 2000, respectively (See Table 3 for comparison). Eligible patients are those with previously-untreated follicular lymphoma (prior local radiotherapy permitted), WHO grades 1-3. After collection of tumor for vaccine production, patients are treated with a uniform chemotherapy regimen. Those who achieve remission and do not progress during a 6 month immunologic recovery period following completion of chemotherapy are randomized 2:1 to receive Id-KLH plus GM-CSF versus KLH plus GM-CSF. The principal endpoint for both studies is prolongation of progression-free survival after chemotherapy.

The NCI-sponsored trial was initiated at 8 U.S. medical centers including the NCI Clinical Center. Patients are treated with the PACE regimen (prednisone, doxorubicin, cyclophosphamide, and etoposide) to their best clinical response, and only those with complete clinical remissions

(CR or CRu) are eligible for vaccination. The study has a target enrollment of 563 patients, and assumes that at least two-thirds of patients will achieve clinical complete remission to meet an accrual goal of 375 randomized patients. At interim analysis in August 2003, of 124 patients completing chemotherapy, 105 (85%) had achieved a CR or CRu, and 50 subjects had initiated or completed immunization (37). In this study, idiotype proteins are produced using the traditional rescue hybridoma method (9). A total of 5 vaccinations are administered as previously described (31). Vaccines were manufactured at the NCI for the initial patients on this trial. However, in 2003 Biovest International partnered with the NCI to carry out the manufacture of vaccines for the remainder of the study, and in 2004 the number of participating sites was increased to 20 in order to speed accrual.

The Genitope study (Genitope 2000-03) completed accrual of 676 patients at 35 centers throughout the U.S. and Canada in April of 2004. Accrual to the Genitope study has outpaced that of the NCI study in large part due to the greater number of clinical sites. Following tissue collection, patients receive 8 cycles of cyclophosphamide, vincristine, and prednisone, and are then evaluated for clinical response. This study differs from that of the NCI in that all patients achieving (and maintaining for 6 months) at least a PR will be eligible to proceed to randomization and vaccination. This design offers the opportunity to observe regression of gross residual tumor after vaccination, unlike the NCI study. However, it is still unclear whether the greater tumor burdens permissible in this study might interfere with the host's ability to mount an effective immune response to Id-KLH (10). Recombinant idiotype proteins are produced by the "molecular rescue" method described above. Patients receive seven monthly vaccinations rather than the traditional five. A preliminary analysis of time to progression by the data safety monitoring board is planned for mid-2005, though announcement of results is not anticipated until 2006. Clinical results for the NCI trial are not expected until well after 2007, given the study's longer accrual period and more infrequent events with the selection of only better prognosis (i.e. CR) patients for vaccination.

Another notable feature of the phase III Genitope study is that patients who fail to achieve complete or partial remission after chemotherapy (and who are therefore ineligible for randomization) will be offered enrollment into a new phase II clinical trial of rituximab followed by Id-KLH vaccination. Those having a CR or PR after rituximab will be randomized to receive recombinant Id-KLH vaccine and GM-CSF, either 13 or 26 weeks after completing rituximab.

5.2   Id-KLH plus GM-CSF after Rituximab

Based on the phase II results described above, Favrille has initiated a phase III randomized, double blind, placebo-controlled multi-center trial to assess the efficacy of FavId™ after rituximab cytoreduction (**Table 3**). Eligible patients are those with grade 1-3 follicular lymphoma, previously untreated or relapsed/refractory after no more than 2 prior chemotherapy regimens. Patients who relapsed after a prior complete or partial response to rituximab lasting at least 6 months are also eligible. However, more than two years must have passed since receiving combination chemotherapy with rituximab. Prior stem cell transplantation, vaccines containing KLH, idiotype immunotherapy, fludarabine within 9 months, or radioimmunoconjugates are not permitted.

Treatment begins with a standard 4 week course of rituximab, just as in the phase II (FavId™ 04) trial described above. Patients without progressive disease 2 months later are randomized 1:1 to receive FavId™ plus GM-CSF or placebo plus GM-CSF. Treatment is continued monthly for six months in the absence of clinically significant progressive disease. After the first six months, patients without progression may continue therapy every two months for one year and then every three months thereafter until disease progression, the study's primary endpoint. Accrual of 342 evaluable patients is planned, with over 60 U.S. sites participating. It is expected that patients will be accrued over 18 months, with results available as early as mid-2006.

6.   PHASE I/II TRIALS OF ID-KLH VACCINES IN OTHER SETTINGS

6.1   Untreated Follicular Lymphoma during the "Watch and Wait" Period

Follicular lymphoma patients are often asymptomatic at the time of diagnosis, and initial chemotherapy is sometimes deferred for months or years, which is known as a "watch-and-wait approach." It was hypothesized that Id-KLH vaccines may be efficacious in patients with untreated follicular lymphoma during this "watch and wait" period, before the administration of immunosuppressive chemotherapy. A phase II trial was initiated to evaluate the efficacy of recombinant Id-KLH and GM-CSF in this setting (53). Thirteen of 16 patients developed specific immune responses: 6 humoral only, 4 cellular only, and 3 with both humoral and cellular immune responses. Clinical efficacy was difficult to assess, with only one of 16 patients having a partial response, 1 mixed response, and 8 demonstrating stable disease. Furthermore, four of the 16 patients had waxing and waning lymphadenopathy even before the vaccination, and it was thus unclear whether the lone partial response resulted from vaccination or was merely incidental. These data suggest that Id-KLH plus GM-CSF is not an optimal strategy for untreated follicular lymphoma during the watch-and-wait period, and rather supports the strategies described above in applying vaccination in the setting of residual disease following conventional treatments. Current first generation Id-KLH vaccines will likely be more effective in the complete remission or minimal residual disease setting than in patients with bulky, untreated disease. Nonetheless, the regression of measurable tumor after idiotype-pulsed dendritic cell vaccination (34, 35) suggests that a more potent vaccine formulation might have efficacy in this setting.

6.2   Id-KLH for Minimal Residual Disease after Hematopoietic Stem Cell Transplant

Idiotype vaccines have been administered in several trials after autologous peripheral blood stem cell transplantation, which may be an attractive setting in which minimal residual disease status is obtained. Davis *et al* reported that idiotype-specific immune responses could be measured in 10 of 12 subjects with follicular or diffuse large B cell lymphoma, indicating that post-transplant immunosuppression may not be a barrier to effective vaccination (54). Indeed, the preclinical studies of Borrello *et al* suggest that this setting may in fact be highly favorable for breaking immune tolerance to self tumor antigens (55). An ongoing phase II clinical trial at the University of Nebraska will examine the efficacy of recombinant Id-KLH and GM-CSF vaccination in patients with follicular lymphoma after autologous stem cell transplantation. Investigators at the University of California, San Diego are carrying out a Phase II study to evaluate the immunogenicity and safety of FavId™ plus GM-CSF after autologous peripheral blood stem cell transplantation (ASCT) in patients with indolent lymphoma (IL) or mantle cell lymphoma (MCL). Preliminary data were presented in 2003 (56). Six patients (four with MCL, two with IL) received five monthly vaccinations with FavId™ plus GM-CSF starting a median of 5 months post-ASCT. At the time of transplant, 3 of 4 patients with MCL had CR or CRu and 1 had partial remission (PR). Of the 2 patients with IL, 1 had a PR and 1 had stable disease (SD) at the time of transplantation. Vaccination was well-tolerated, and T-cell anti-KLH and anti-Id responses were demonstrated in 4 of 4 patients tested. Four of five patients tested developed anti-KLH humoral responses, and 2 of these had Id-specific humoral responses. The great majority of these patients had maintained complete remissions. To date however, in none of the above trials can favorable outcomes be attributed to vaccinations given the preceding transplantation and lack of a control group.

6.3   Id-KLH for Aggressive Lymphomas

Genitope has sponsored a study of Id-KLH vaccination in patients with aggressive lymphomas (diffuse large B cell and mantle cell). Recombinant Id-KLH was administered with GM-CSF in first remission after chemotherapy, usually cyclophosphamide, doxorubicin, vincristine, and prednisone (CHOP). Fourteen patients with aggressive lymphomas were enrolled: 6 diffuse large cell, 5 mantle cell, and 3 follicular large cell. Half of patients mounted idiotype-specific immune responses: 7 of 14 with a humoral response and 1 of 7 evaluable with a cellular response (57). Eleven additional patients with mantle cell lymphoma have been accrued to this study using an accelerated (biweekly) vaccination schedule, and at a median follow-up of 522 days post CHOP induction (range 133-944), median time to progression has not been reached (58). Further immune response and long term clinical outcome data are pending.

Wilson and colleagues at the NCI have treated 25 mantle cell lymphoma patients in first remission after dose-adjusted EPOCH-R (etoposide, prednisone, vincristine, cyclophosphamide, doxorubicin, and rituximab) with idiotype vaccination (59). Therapy consisted of 5 monthly doses rescue hybrid-derived Id-KLH plus GM-CSF starting 12 weeks after chemotherapy. Due to the inclusion of rituximab in the induction regimen, B cells were markedly suppressed at the initiation of vaccinations. Accordingly, humoral anti-KLH responses were measurable in only 65% of subjects and were delayed and of lower titer that those found almost uniformly in patients cytoreduced with chemotherapy only (10, 31). Anti-idiotype humoral responses have not been reported on. Nonetheless, 73% mounted tumor-specific T cell responses as measured by cytokine secretion. The event-free survival of 24 months reported appears similar to that expected after chemotherapy alone, and leaves open the question of whether the B cell depletion just prior to vaccination blunted the anti-idiotype antibody response, partially negating the potentially beneficial effects of vaccination.

7.   NOVEL IDIOTYPE VACCINE FORMULATIONS

7.1   DNA Vaccines

The potential of idiotype as a vaccine target has been demonstrated by the above studies, but the task of individualized vaccine production remains complex and costly. The process would be greatly simplified if patients could be directly immunized with DNA encoding their tumor idiotype, allowing *in vivo* production of idiotype protein in a pro-inflammatory milieu. Antigen-encoding plasmid DNA has been shown to be immunogenic in a number of murine models (60). Bacterial plasmid DNA has inherent immunostimulatory capacity due to content of unmethylated cytidine-phosphate-guanosine (CpG) oligonucleotide sequences, which are underrepresented in vertebrates (61). These CpG sequences activate the innate immune system and induce production of IFN-gamma, IL-12, and other cytokines that direct a T-helper 1 (Th1)-type immune response.

Indeed, vaccination with idiotype-encoding plasmid DNA has shown promising preclinical efficacy in B cell and T cell lymphoma models (62-65). However, the first trial of idiotype DNA vaccination yielded disappointing results (66). In patients with follicular lymphoma, inoculation with plasmid DNA encoding tumor idiotype linked to xenogeneic (murine) immunoglobulin constant region sequences was found to induce a detectable anti-idiotype immune response in only one of 12 patients, and no clinical activity was observed. Nonetheless, DNA vaccination remains a potentially attractive platform for the further development of idiotype vaccines, offering opportunities to manipulate antigen sequences to include additional "helper" epitopes, intracellular targeting sequences, and immunostimulatory (i.e. cytokine, chemokine, or CpG) motifs. Preclinical studies have demonstrated the powerful effects of linking carrier protein (tetanus toxoid) (67) or chemokine (65) sequences to the tumor antigen-encoding DNA. Freda Stevenson and colleagues in England are currently conducting a phase II clinical trial in relapsed follicular lymphoma using idiotype DNA linked to fragment C of tetanus toxoid as a carrier protein (67), and the immunologic and clinical results are anxiously awaited. In murine lymphoma and myeloma models, this strategy has shown potent anti-tumor effects (63).

7.2 Recombinant Viral Vaccines

Perhaps the most potent of all recombinant nucleic acid vaccines are those employing replication-defective viral vectors as antigen delivery vehicles. We have previously reported that immunization with adenoviral vectors encoding idiotype induced high titers of anti-idiotypic antibodies and provided protection against tumor challenge in two B cell lymphoma models (38C13 and BCL-1) that was equal or superior to that obtained with Id-KLH (68). The adenovirus vaccine even provided a survival advantage in mice with established tumor, when given in conjunction with systemic chemotherapy. However, concerns about the safety of adenovirus vaccines in human subjects dampened enthusiasm for translation of this approach into the clinic. More recently, Muraro *et al* have utilized recombinant vaccinia viruses encoding idiotype linked to a lysosomal targeting signal (28). Immunization with virus-infected dendritic cells elicited immunity to the murine 38C13 lymphoma dependent on CD8+ effector T cells, in contrast to numerous prior studies in which tumor protection was not affected by *in vivo* depletion of effector CD8+ T cells (25, 26, 68).

8. TUMOR CELL-BASED VACCINE STRATEGIES

Other vaccine approaches seek to stimulate immune responses to the entire spectrum of tumor antigens, not just to a single protein such as idiotype. Using whole tumor cells in a vaccine may allow stimulation of immune responses to a large number of putative (and largely unknown) tumor antigens. As with idiotype, these approaches all involve production of customized vaccines from each patient's own tumor cells. Whole tumor cell-based strategies generally seek to make tumor cells, which have previously been ignored by the patient's immune system, more immunogenic. This may be accomplished by expressing co-stimulatory molecules on the tumor cells surface, or by engineering the tumor cells to secrete immunostimulatory cytokines such as GM-CSF. Alternatively, killed tumor cells may be co-administered with GM-CSF, or with bystander cells that produce GM-CSF. These latter approaches obviate the need to transduce each patient's tumor cells with genes encoding GM-CSF.

Such a strategy has been shown to be effective in a murine lymphoma model (55), and is now being explored for the treatment of multiple myeloma in a phase I/II clinical trial at Johns Hopkins University(69). Tumor cells obtained by bone marrow harvest are irradiated and co-injected with allogeneic, GM-CSF-secreting, bystander cells (K562; GVAX®Vaccine; Cell Genesys; South San Francisco, CA)(70) prior to and following autologous stem cell transplantation. In preliminary data, the vaccine was well-tolerated and immunogenic, but clinical efficacy could not be assessed given the concurrent stem cell transplant.

Ligation of CD40, a cell surface receptor expressed on both normal and malignant B-cells, by CD154 (CD40 ligand) results in up-regulation of antigen presentation machinery such as MHC, costimulatory, and adhesion molecules. This approach has undergone initial phase I/II testing in patients with chronic lymphocytic leukemia(71). Circulating leukemic cells were collected by leukapheresis, transduced with a replication-defective adenovirus vector encoding CD154, and re-infused intravenously. The therapy was found to be safe, and tumor cell-specific immune responses were noted, along with transient improvement in lymphocyte counts and lymphadenopathy. This approach has been applied to B cell lymphoma in preclinical studies. Investigators at Baylor College of Medicine transduced human B lymphoma cells with adenoviruses encoding CD154 and interleukin-2 (72). Transduced tumor cells were able to activate a cytotoxic T lymphocyte response against unmodified tumor cells *in vitro*. Briones *et al* demonstrated similar results *in vivo* in a murine model(73). Murine lymphoma cells were transduced with an adenovirus encoding CD154, irradiated and injected as a cellular vaccine. Vaccinated mice demonstrated strikingly improved survival after challenge with wild-type, unmodified tumor cells.

Briones *et al* also used a nonreplicating fowlpox virus encoding a *tri*ad of *co*stimulatory *mo*lecules (TRICOM™, Therion Biologics, Cambridge, MA) to transduce murine lymphoma cells and render them more immunogenic(74). After transduction, the lymphoma cells expressed the costimulatory molecules B7.1/CD80, intracellular adhesion molecule (ICAM)-1/CD54, and leukocyte functional antigen (LFA)-3/CD58. Immunization with irradiated, transduced cells elicited resistance to tumor challenge with live lymphoma cells. This approach has yet to be tested against human lymphomas, but phase I/II studies are underway in other malignancies.

Yet another vaccination approach utilizes heat shock proteins (HSPs), the ubiquitous cellular chaperones that shuttle peptides to class I MHC molecules. HSP96 purified from tumor cells carry bound tumor antigen-derived peptides. Injection of HSP-peptide complexes leads to uptake by host APCs via the CD91 receptor for presentation on MHC class I, stimulating a cytotoxic T cell response. This strategy has been employed in a phase II clinical trial for patients with untreated or relapsed low grade lymphomas (75). Preliminary results show that among 10 patients, vaccination with autologous tumor-derived HSP96 complex induced one partial and two minor responses, and 3 instances of stable disease.

In our own laboratory we have recently sought to combine the *ex vivo*-loaded dendritic cell approach with a whole tumor cell antigen strategy. Several investigators have shown that the *in vitro* priming of tumor-specific T cells by dendritic cells phagocytosing killed tumor cells is augmented in the presence of anti-tumor antibodies (76, 77). This approach was tested in an *in vivo* murine lymphoma model, in which irradiated lymphoma cells coated with a tumor-specific antibody were fed to dendritic cells to promote uptake via Fc receptors (78). This opsonized tumor cell-dendritic cell vaccine was potent in eliciting protective anti-lymphoma immunity. Importantly, this immunity was mediated by T cells and directed at non-idiotype antigens. This suggests that idiotype vaccines and whole cell-based approaches may target distinct antigens, and thereby be complementary in their efficacy. While the clinical development of whole lymphoma cell-based vaccine strategies lags well behind that of idiotype vaccines, it is hoped that the many promising strategies cited above will soon be adapted for clinical trials in lymphoma.

9. PHARMACOLOGIC CONSIDERATIONS FOR INTEGRATION WITH STANDARD THERAPIES

Although idiotype vaccines have reached an advanced the optimal biochemical formulation for achieving clinical potency remains unknown. For instance, the influence of the idiotype's molecular form (whole immunoglobulins vs. single chain Fv fragment vs. Fab fragment, etc), glycosylation patterns (expected to differ among recombinant proteins), and KLH conjugation on the ability to elicit humoral and T cell-medicated immunity have not been subjected to controlled studies in preclinical model systems, let alone human trials. Moreover, GM-CSF, the favorite adjuvant for idiotype vaccines, was chosen for clinical testing based on limited data in a single murine lymphoma model study (27), and many additional immune adjuvants are now available (79). It is not known currently whether other adjuvant formulations, combinations of adjuvants, or delivery with dendritic cells might provide superior immunologic potency (26).

As for all immunizations, therapeutic idiotype vaccines depend on an intact host immune system for their optimal activity. Thus, integration of vaccine therapies with standard lymphoma treatments must take into account the latter's potential immunosuppressive influences. Immune effector mechanisms operative after idiotype vaccination likely involve antibodies as well as CD8+ and CD4+ T cells (46). While anti-idiotypic antibodies may not be necessary for clinical anti-tumor effects in all patients (31, 35), available evidence suggests their recruitment should be an important goal of vaccination. In a recent analysis of 136 patients with follicular lymphoma who had received Id vaccines demonstrated that those mounting Id-specific humoral immune responses had a significantly longer progression-free survival (PFS) than those who did not (8.21 v 3.38 years, p = 0.018) (46). Moreover, patients possessing the Fcγ-receptor (FcγR) IIIA V/V polymorphism genotype, previously shown to predict response to rituximab(80, 81), also had a longer PFS than those with other genotypes. Humoral immune response and FcγR genotype were independent positive predictors for PFS. These results suggest that antibodies induced following Id vaccination are important effectors, and that FcγR-bearing effector cells can participate in the killing of antibody-coated tumor cells *in vivo*.

The relative contributions of antibody versus T cell effectors will likely differ among individual patients successfully vaccinated against Id. For some, anti-idiotype antibodies may be critical to vaccine efficacy, though in others, it may be dispensable. Given that rituximab rapidly depletes normal B cells (43) and markedly impairs the host's ability to mount primary and secondary humoral immune responses (44, 45), its use was excluded in the first two phase III Id vaccine trials. Although B cells often begin to recover within 6-9 months of completing rituximab therapy, B cell depletion can persist for several years in some cases (J.Timmerman and R. Levy, unpublished observations). To preserve the host's ability to mount humoral responses to Id vaccines, it has been suggested that rituximab be held until after vaccinations are completed and the anti-idiotype humoral response is well-established. However, as mentioned above, augmentation of T cell-mediated anti-tumor immunity has been described in B cell deficient mice (47). This has led to the hypothesis that cytoreduction with anti-CD20 monoclonal antibodies prior to idiotype vaccination may augment anti-idiotype T cell responses. Should this approach be taken, it is imperative that vaccinations continue throughout the period of B cell recovery, as now done in the Favrille trials. Purine analogs such as fludarabine profoundly suppress T cell immunity (82), and their use is generally not advised prior to vaccine therapy.

10.   CONCLUSIONS AND FUTURE PROSPECTS

Given the rapid advances in tumor immunology research, it is likely that the full potential for active lymphoma immunotherapy is only beginning to be realized. Results of the three ongoing phase III trials of idiotype vaccinations for follicular lymphoma are eagerly anticipated. It is hoped that these studies will show a progression-free survival benefit for patients vaccinated with Id-KLH versus those receiving KLH alone. This should lead to FDA approval, and the availability of these agents for appropriate patients and additional clinical trials. Further studies could then serve to improve clinical potency through combination with additional immune stimulants (cytokines, chemokines, toll-like receptor ligands, and chemical adjuvants), and to define the optimal integration of vaccination with standard therapies for follicular lymphoma such as chemotherapy and anti-CD20 monoclonal antibodies.

Studies of Id-KLH vaccines would then likely be further tested in controlled trials for other NHL histologies, such as diffuse large B cell lymphoma, mantle cell lymphoma, and small lymphocytic lymphoma/CLL. However, from current data, it appears that idiotype vaccine strategies appear to be less successful in multiple myeloma than in follicular lymphoma (83). Additional maneuvers to improve vaccine potency may be successful in overcoming this resistance. Extension of the tumor-specific idiotype vaccination approach to T cell receptor (TCR) idiotypes remains a potential therapy for T cell lymphomas, as shown in a murine T cell lymphoma model (84, 85). Interestingly, tumor protection from a TCR-Id-KLH vaccine has been found to rely on cytotoxic antibodies rather than T cell effectors, once again pointing to the critical importance of humoral immunity in targeting lymphoma idiotype.

Although recombinant DNA methodologies have overcome some of the practical and technical hurdles for the mass production of patient-specific idiotype protein vaccines, the availability of "shared" lymphoma antigens appropriate for the active immunotherapy of lymphoid cancers would be welcome. It is possible that such antigens may be identified using genomic or proteomic technologies (86), or using patient-derived T-cell clones (20, 87). Recently, the protein survivin, involved in tumor cell resistance to apoptosis has been studied as potential lymphoma antigen target (88, 89), and clinical studies to validate this potential may be forthcoming. Nonetheless, patient-specific idiotype will likely remain an attractive target for the active immunotherapy of lymphomas owing to its high degree of tumor specificity and safety. Given the promise now held by lymphoma vaccines, it is anticipated that patient-specific tumor vaccinations will one day become an important therapeutic option in the treatment of lymphoid malignancies.

Table 1. Active Vaccination Approaches against Lymphoid Malignancies

Vaccine	Properties	Clinical results	Current status	References
I. Idiotype (Id) vaccines				
Id-KLH + chemical adjuvant	Target tumor-specific immunoglobulin. Custom-made for each patient. Elicit T cells (CD4+, CD8+) & antibodies.	Tested in NHL (follicular, diffuse large B cell, mantle cell) and multiple myeloma		7
Id-KLH + chemical adjuvant	First formulation tested in humans. Id produced by hybridoma method.	Immune responses correlated with improved survival	Completed	9, 10
Id-loaded dendritic cells	Autologous antigen presenting cells, loaded ex vivo with Id protein.	Tumor regressions observed, elicits T cells & antibodies	Phase II trials	33-35
Hybridoma-derived Id-KLH + GM-CSF	Co-injected with GM-CSF, a cytokine adjuvant.	Molecular complete remissions	Phase III trial	31
Recombinant Id-KLH + GM-CSF	Id produced in genetically-engineered mammalian or insect cells	Immunogenicity demonstrated	Phase II, and III trials	38-42, 49-52
Naked DNA vaccines	Plasmid DNA encoding Id injected directly into host, eliminates need to make protein. Convenient platform for linkage to other immunostimulatory molecules.	1st generation vectors only weakly immunogenic.	Phase I/II with 2nd generation vector	62-67
Recombinant Id-encoding viruses	Highly immunogenic platform	Preclinical only	Preclinical	28, 68

Vaccine	Properties	Clinical results	Current status	References
II. Whole tumor cell-derived vaccines	Prepared directly from patient's own tumors. Elicit primarily cell-mediated immune responses.			
GM-CSF gene-transduced tumor cells	Retrovirus or adenoviral gene transduction, or co-injection with GM-CSF-secreting cell line	Modest activity in melanoma, renal cell and lung carcinomas	Phase I/II in myeloma	69, 70
CD40 ligand-transduced tumor cells	CLL cells transduced with adenoviral vector	Clinical and immune responses	Phase II in CLL	71
Tumor-derived heat shock proteins	Purified from patient's own tumor cells	Some clinical responses	Phase I/II	75
Tumor cell-loaded dendritic cells	Load with tumor cell lysates, killed tumor cells, antibody-coated tumor cells	Promising pre-clinical results	Preclinical	76-78

Abbreviations: CLL, chronic lymphocytic leukemia; GM -CSF, granulocyte-macrophage colony stimulating factor; HSPs, heat shock proteins; Id-KLH, Idiotype coupled to keyhole limpet hemocyanin; NHL, non-Hodgkin's lymphoma

Table 2. Current and Published Idiotype Vaccine Trials for Lymphoma

Sponsor & Type	Disease / Situation	Vaccine	Current Status	Refs.
NCI / Biovest, Inc. Phase III randomized	Follicular lymphoma 1st remission after PACE	Id-KLH vs. KLH plus GM-CSF	Open for accrual: www.ncilymphomavaccine.gov	31
Genitope, Inc. Phase III randomized	Follicular lymphoma 1st remission after CVP	Id-KLH vs. KLH plus GM-CSF	Accrual complete www.genitope.com	38
Favrille, Inc. Phase III	Follicular lymphoma Previously untreated, or relapsed /measurable	Rituximab, then Id-KLH vs. placebo plus GM-CSF	Open for accrual: www.favrille.com	40-42
Genitope Phase II	Follicular lymphoma 1st remission after CVP	Id-KLH plus GM-CSF	Accrual complete	38
Genitope Phase II	Aggressive lymphomas 1st remission after CHOP	Id-KLH plus GM-CSF	Accrual complete	57, 58
Genitope Phase II	Follicular lymphoma Untreated "watch & wait"	Id-KLH plus GM-CSF	Accrual complete	53
Favrille, Inc. Phase II	Follicular lymphoma Previously untreated, or relapsed /measurable	Rituximab, then Id-KLH plus GM-CSF	Accrual complete Favorable TTP among rituximab responders	41, 42
Favrille, Inc. Phase II	Recurrent indolent, measurable lymphoma	Id-KLH plus GM-CSF	Accrual complete	40
UCSD Phase II	Indolent or mantle cell NHL, after HDC+HSCT	Id-KLH plus GM-CSF	Open for accrual	56

UCLA Phase II	Follicular lymphoma Relapsed / measurable	Id-loaded dendritic cells, then boost with Id-KLH plus GM-CSF	Open for accrual	33-35
Large Scale Biology Phase I/II	Follicular lymphoma 1st remission after CVP	Tobacco plant-derived Id +/- GM-CSF	Accrual complete No clinical responses	52
NCI Phase I/II	Mantle cell lymphoma 1st remission after EPOCH plus rituximab	Id-KLH plus GM-CSF	Accrual complete Impaired humoral responses to Id and KLH	59
U. of Navarra, Spain Phase II	Follicular lymphoma 1st relapse, measurable	CHOP, then Id-KLH plus GM-CSF	Open for accrual	31
CellGenix Freiburg, Germany Phase I	NHL Relapse or progression after anthracycline chemotherapy	Recombinant Id Fab fragment plus MF59 and GM-CSF	Open for accrual Some clinical responses	49-51
Tenovus Laboratory Southampton, England Phase I/II	Follicular lymphoma CR after chemotherapy, radiation, or HDC+HSCT	Plasmid DNA vaccine: scFv-FrC	Accrual complete	63, 67

Abbreviations: CHOP, cyclophosphamide, doxorubicin, vincristine, prednisone; CR, complete remission; CVP, cyclophosphamide, vincristine, and prednisone; EPOCH, VP-16, prednisone, vincristine, cyclophosphamide, doxorubicin; Fab, antigen binding fragment; GM-CSF, granulocyte-macrophage colony stimulating factor; HDC+HSCT, high-dose chemotherapy and hematopoietic stem cell transplantation; Id-KLH, Idiotype coupled to keyhole limpet hemocyanin; MF59, adjuvant; NCI, U.S. National Cancer Institute; PACE, prednisone, doxorubicin, cyclophosphamide, VP-16; PR, partial remission; scFv-FrC, single chain variable fragment of idiotype coupled to fragment C of tetanus toxin; UCLA, University of California, Los Angeles; UCSD, University of California, San Diego; U. Neb, University of Nebraska.

Table 3. Phase III Clinical Trials of Idiotype Vaccination for Follicular Lymphoma

	Genitope	NCI/Biovest	Favrille
Year opened:	2000	1999	2004
Target Enrollment:	n=676 (reached 4/04)	n=563	342
Results Expected:	2005-2006	2007 or later	2006 or later
Eligibility:			
Histology	Grades 1-3	Grades 1-2	Grades 1-3
Stages	III, IV	bulky II, III, IV	III, IV
Prior therapy	Local XRT only	Local XRT only	2 or fewer regimens
Tumor sample required	LN, FNA, blood, BM	LN, FNA, blood, BM	LN, FNA, blood, BM
Production of Id protein:	Molecular rescue, in mammalian cells	Rescue hybridoma	Molecular rescue, in insect cells
Pre-vaccine cytoreduction:	CVP x 8	PACE to best response	Rituximab x 4

	Genitope	NCI/Biovest	Favrille
Response requirement:	CR, CRu, or PR (Non-responders eligible for rituximab followed by Id-KLH vaccination)	CR or CRu	CR, CRu, PR, or SD
Randomization:	2:1 (Id-KLH vs. KLH)	2:1 (Id-KLH vs. KLH)	1:1 (Id-KLH vs. placebo)
Vaccines (monthly):	Id-KLH+GM-CSFx7	Id-KLH+GM-CSFx5	Id-KLH+GM-CSFx6, every 2 months x6, then every 3 months until progression.

Abbreviations: NCI, U.S. National Cancer Institute; XRT, radiotherapy; LN, lymph node; FNA, fine needle aspiration; BM, bone marrow; CVP, cyclophosphamide, vincristine, and prednisone; PACE, prednisone, doxorubicin, cyclophosphamide, and etoposide; CR, complete response; CRu, complete response unconfirmed; PR, partial response; SD, stable disease; Id-KLH, Idiotype coupled to keyhole limpet hemocyanin; GM-CSF, granulocyte-macrophage colony stimulating factor.

11.   REFERENCES

1.   Lynch, R. G., Graff, R. J., Sirisinha, S., Simms, E. S., and Eisen, H. N. Myeloma proteins as tumor-specific transplantation antigens. Proc Natl Acad Sci U S A, *69:* 1540-1544, 1972.

2.   Stevenson, F. K., Elliott, E. V., and Stevenson, G. T. Some effects on leukaemic B lymphocytes of antibodies to defined regions of their surface immunoglobulin. Immunology, *32:* 549-557, 1977.

3.   Levy, R. and Dilley, J. Rescue of immunoglobulin secretion from human neoplastic lymphoid cells by somatic cell hybridization. Proc Natl Acad Sci U S A, *75:* 2411-2415, 1978.

4.   Miller, R. A., Maloney, D. G., Warnke, R., and Levy, R. Treatment of B-cell lymphoma with monoclonal anti-idiotype antibody. N Engl J Med, *306:* 517-522, 1982.

5.   Davis, T. A., Maloney, D. G., Czerwinski, D. K., Liles, T. M., and Levy, R. Anti-idiotype antibodies can induce long-term complete remissions in non-Hodgkin's lymphoma without eradicating the malignant clone. Blood, *92:* 1184-1190, 1998.

6.   Meeker, T., Lowder, J., Cleary, M. L., Stewart, S., Warnke, R., Sklar, J., and Levy, R. Emergence of idiotype variants during treatment of B-cell lymphoma with anti-idiotype antibodies. N Engl J Med, *312:* 1658-1665, 1985.

7.   Timmerman, J. M. and Levy, R. L. The history of the development of vaccines for lymphoma. Clinical Lymphoma, *1:* 129-139, 2000.

8.   Campbell, M. J., Carroll, W., Kon, S., Thielemans, K., Rothbard, J. B., Levy, S., and Levy, R. Idiotype vaccination against murine B cell lymphoma. Humoral and cellular responses elicited by tumor-derived immunoglobulin M and its molecular subunits. J Immunol, *139:* 2825-2833, 1987.

9.   Kwak, L. W., Campbell, M. J., Czerwinski, D. K., Hart, S., Miller, R. A., and Levy, R. Induction of immune responses in patients with B-cell lymphoma against the surface-immunoglobulin idiotype expressed by their tumors. N Engl J Med, *327:* 1209-1215, 1992.

10.   Hsu, F. J., Caspar, C. B., Czerwinski, D., Kwak, L. W., Liles, T. M., Syrengelas, A., Taidi-Laskowski, B., and Levy, R. Tumor-specific idiotype vaccines in the treatment of patients with B- cell lymphoma--long-term results of a clinical trial. Blood, *89:* 3129-3135, 1997.

11.   Lauritzsen, G. F., Weiss, S., Dembic, Z., and Bogen, B. Naive idiotype-specific CD4+ T cells and immunosurveillance of B-cell tumors. Proc Natl Acad Sci U S A, *91:* 5700-5704, 1994.

12.   Lundin, K. U., Hofgaard, P. O., Omholt, H., Munthe, L. A., Corthay, A., and Bogen, B. Therapeutic effect of idiotype-specific CD4+ T cells against B-cell lymphoma in the absence of anti-idiotypic antibodies. Blood, *102:* 605-612, 2003.

13.   Cao, W., Myers-Powell, B. A., and Braciale, T. J. Recognition of an immunoglobulin VH epitope by influenza virus-specific class I major histocompatibility complex-restricted cytolytic T lymphocytes. J Exp Med, *179:* 195-202, 1994.

14.   Chakrabarti, D. and Ghosh, S. K. Induction of syngeneic cytotoxic T lymphocytes against a B cell tumor. II. Characterization of anti-idiotypic CTL lines and clones. Cell Immunol, *144:* 443-454, 1992.

15.   Chakrabarti, D. and Ghosh, S. K. Induction of syngeneic cytotoxic T lymphocytes against a B cell tumor. III. MHC class I-restricted CTL recognizes the processed form(s) of idiotype. Cell Immunol, *144:* 455-464, 1992.

16. Abe, A., Emi, N., Taji, H., Kasai, M., Kohno, A., and Saito, H. Induction of humoral and cellular anti-idiotypic immunity by intradermal injection of naked DNA encoding a human variable region gene sequence of an immunoglobulin heavy chain in a B cell malignancy. Gene Ther, *3:* 988-993, 1996.

17. Osterroth, F., Garbe, A., Fisch, P., and Veelken, H. Stimulation of cytotoxic T cells against idiotype immunoglobulin of malignant lymphoma with protein-pulsed or idiotype-transduced dendritic cells. Blood, *95:* 1342-1349, 2000.

18. Trojan, A., Schultze, J. L., Witzens, M., Vonderheide, R. H., Ladetto, M., Donovan, J. W., and Gribben, J. G. Immunoglobulin framework-derived peptides function as cytotoxic T-cell epitopes commonly expressed in B-cell malignancies. Nat Med, *6:* 667-672, 2000.

19. Wen, Y. J., Barlogie, B., and Yi, Q. Idiotype-specific cytotoxic T lymphocytes in multiple myeloma: evidence for their capacity to lyse autologous primary tumor cells. Blood, *97:* 1750-1755., 2001.

20. Baskar, S., Kobrin, C. B., and Kwak, L. W. Autologous lymphoma vaccines induce human T cell responses against multiple, unique epitopes. J Clin Invest, *113:* 1498-1510, 2004.

21. Kaminski, M. S., Kitamura, K., Maloney, D. G., and Levy, R. Idiotype vaccination against murine B cell lymphoma. Inhibition of tumor immunity by free idiotype protein. J Immunol, *138:* 1289-1296, 1987.

22. Campbell, M. J., Esserman, L., Byars, N. E., Allison, A. C., and Levy, R. Idiotype vaccination against murine B cell lymphoma. Humoral and cellular requirements for the full expression of antitumor immunity. J Immunol, *145:* 1029-1036, 1990.

23. George, A. J., Folkard, S. G., Hamblin, T. J., and Stevenson, F. K. Idiotypic vaccination as a treatment for a B cell lymphoma. J Immunol, *141:* 2168-2174, 1988.

24. George, A. J., Tutt, A. L., and Stevenson, F. K. Anti-idiotypic mechanisms involved in suppression of a mouse B cell lymphoma, BCL1. J Immunol, *138:* 628-634, 1987.

25. Syrengelas, A. D. and Levy, R. DNA vaccination against the idiotype of a murine B cell lymphoma: mechanism of tumor protection. J Immunol, *162:* 4790-4795, 1999.

26. Timmerman, J. M. and Levy, R. Linkage of foreign carrier protein to a self-tumor antigen enhances the immunogenicity of a pulsed dendritic cell vaccine. J Immunol, *164:* 4797-4803, 2000.

27. Kwak, L. W., Young, H. A., Pennington, R. W., and Weeks, S. D. Vaccination with syngeneic, lymphoma-derived immunoglobulin idiotype combined with granulocyte/macrophage colony-stimulating factor primes mice for a protective T-cell response. Proc Natl Acad Sci U S A, *93:* 10972-10977, 1996.

28. Muraro, S., Bondanza, A., Bellone, M., Greenberg, P. D., and Bonini, C. Molecular modification of idiotypes from B cell lymphomas for expression in mature dendritic cells as a strategy to induce tumor-reactive CD4+ and CD8+ T cell responses. Blood, 2005.

29. Campbell, M. J., Esserman, L., and Levy, R. Immunotherapy of established murine B cell lymphoma. Combination of idiotype immunization and cyclophosphamide. J Immunol, *141:* 3227-3233, 1988.

30. Caspar, C. B., Levy, S., and Levy, R. Idiotype vaccines for non-Hodgkin's lymphoma induce polyclonal immune responses that cover mutated tumor idiotypes: comparison of different vaccine formulations. Blood, *90:* 3699-3706, 1997.

31. Bendandi, M., Gocke, C. D., Kobrin, C. B., Benko, F. A., Sternas, L. A., Pennington, R., Watson, T. M., Reynolds, C. W., Gause, B. L., Duffey, P. L., Jaffe, E. S., Creekmore, S. P., Longo, D. L., and Kwak, L. W. Complete molecular remissions induced by patient-specific vaccination plus granulocyte-monocyte colony-stimulating factor against lymphoma [see comments]. Nat Med, *5:* 1171-1177, 1999.

32. Keilholz, U., Weber, J., Finke, J. H., Gabrilovich, D. I., Kast, W. M., Disis, M. L., Kirkwood, J. M., Scheibenbogen, C., Schlom, J., Maino, V. C., Lyerly, H. K., Lee, P. P., Storkus, W., Marincola, F., Worobec, A., and Atkins, M. B. Immunologic monitoring of

cancer vaccine therapy: results of a workshop sponsored by the Society for Biological Therapy. J Immunother, *25:* 97-138, 2002.

33.   Timmerman, J. M. and Levy, R. Dendritic cell vaccines for cancer immunotherapy. Annu Rev Med, *50:* 507-529, 1999.

34.   Hsu, F. J., Benike, C., Fagnoni, F., Liles, T. M., Czerwinski, D., and et al. Vaccination of patients with B-cell lymphoma using autologous antigen-pulsed dendritic cells. Nat Med, *2:* 52-58, 1996.

35.   Timmerman, J. M., Czerwinski, D. K., Davis, T. A., Hsu, F. J., Benike, C., Hao, Z. M., Taidi, B., Rajapaksa, R., Caspar, C. B., Okada, C. Y., van Beckhoven, A., Liles, T. M., Engleman, E. G., and Levy, R. Idiotype-pulsed dendritic cell vaccination for B-cell lymphoma: clinical and immune responses in 35 patients. Blood, *99:* 1517-1526., 2002.

36.   Dranoff, G., Jaffee, E., Lazenby, A., Golumbek, P., Levitsky, H., and et al. Vaccination with irradiated tumor cells engineered to secrete murine granulocyte-macrophage colony-stimulating factor stimulates potent, specific, and long-lasting anti-tumor immunity. Proc Natl Acad Sci U S A, *90:* 3539-3543, 1993.

37.   Neelapu, S. S., Gause, B. L., Nikcevich, D., Schuster, S., Winter, J., Gockerman, J., Sotomayor, E., Inghirahimi, G., Muggia, F., Watson, T. M., Snow, S., Kubovic, P., Ferraro, M., Jaffe, E. S., Reynolds, C., and Kwak, L. W. Vaccine therapy of follicular lymphoma in first remission: Long-term follow-up of phase II results and high rate of chemotherapy-induced complete remissions in a controlled, randomized phase III trial. Blood, *102:* 307b (abstract #4953), 2003.

38.   Timmerman, J. M., Czerwinski, D., Taid, B., Van Beckhoven, A., Vose, J., Ingolia, D., Kunkel, L., Denney, D., and Levy, R. A phase I/II trial to evaluate the immunogenicity of recombinant Idiotype protein vaccines for the treatment of non-Hodgkin's lymphoma (NHL). Blood, *96:* 578a, 2000.

39.   Jones, I. and Morikawa, Y. Baculovirus vectors for expression in insect cells. Curr Opin Biotechnol, *7:* 512-516, 1996.

40.   Redfern, C., Guthrie, T. H., Adler, M., Holman, P., Smith, M. R., Levy, R., Janakiramaan, N., Leonard, J. P., Rosenfelt, F., Wiernik, P. H., Just, R., Densmore, J., Gold, D., Gutheil, J., and Bender, J. F. Single agent activity of FavId [Id-KLH vaccine] for indolent NHL. Blood, *102:* 898a (abstract #3341), 2003.

41.   Redfern, C., Guthrie, T. H., Adler, M., Holman, P., Smith, M. R., Levy, R., Janakiramaan, N., Leonard, J. P., Rosenfelt, F., Wiernik, P. H., Just, R., Densmore, J., Gold, D., Gutheil, J., and Bender, J. F. FavId [Id-KLH vaccine] following rituximab for patients with indolent NHL. Blood, *102:* 899a (abstract#3347), 2003.

42.   Koc, O., Redfern, C., Wiernik, P. H., Rosenfelt, F., Winter, J., Guthrie, T. H., Kaplan, L., Holman, P., Densmore, J., Hainsworth, J., Lin, T., Castillo, R., Janakiraman, N., and Bender, J. F. Id/KLH vaccine (FavId TM) following treatment with rituximab: An analysis of response rate immprovement (RRI) and time-to-progression (TTP) in follicular lymphoma (FL). Blood, *104:* 170a (abstract #587), 2004.

43.   McLaughlin, P., Grillo-Lopez, A. J., Link, B. K., Levy, R., Czuczman, M. S., Williams, M. E., Heyman, M. R., Bence-Bruckler, I., White, C. A., Cabanillas, F., Jain, V., Ho, A. D., Lister, J., Wey, K., Shen, D., and Dallaire, B. K. Rituximab chimeric anti-CD20 monoclonal antibody therapy for relapsed indolent lymphoma: half of patients respond to a four-dose treatment program. J Clin Oncol, *16:* 2825-2833, 1998.

44.   van der Kolk, L. E., Baars, J. W., Prins, M. H., and van Oers, M. H. Rituximab treatment results in impaired secondary humoral immune responsiveness. Blood, *100:* 2257-2259., 2002.

45.   Gonzalez-Stawinski, G. V., Yu, P. B., Love, S. D., Parker, W., and Davis, R. D., Jr. Hapten-induced primary and memory humoral responses are inhibited by the infusion of anti-CD20 monoclonal antibody (IDEC-C2B8, Rituximab). Clin Immunol, *98:* 175-179., 2001.

46. Weng, W. K., Czerwinski, D., Timmerman, J., Hsu, F. J., and Levy, R. Clinical outcome of lymphoma patients after idiotype vaccination is correlated with humoral immune response and immunoglobulin G Fc receptor genotype. J Clin Oncol, *22:* 4717-4724, 2004.

47. Qin, Z., Richter, G., Schuler, T., Ibe, S., Cao, X., and Blankenstein, T. B cells inhibit induction of T cell-dependent tumor immunity. Nat Med, *4:* 627-630., 1998.

48. Witzig, T. E., Gordon, L. I., Cabanillas, F., Czuczman, M. S., Emmanouilides, C., Joyce, R., Pohlman, B. L., Bartlett, N. L., Wiseman, G. A., Padre, N., Grillo-Lopez, A. J., Multani, P., and White, C. A. Randomized controlled trial of yttrium-90-labeled ibritumomab tiuxetan radioimmunotherapy versus rituximab immunotherapy for patients with relapsed or refractory low-grade, follicular, or transformed B-cell non-Hodgkin's lymphoma. J Clin Oncol, *20:* 2453-2463, 2002.

49. Osterroth, F., Alkan, O., Mackensen, A., Lindemann, A., Fisch, P., Skerra, A., and Veelken, H. Rapid expression cloning of human immunoglobulin Fab fragments for the analysis of antigen specificity of B cell lymphomas and anti-idiotype lymphoma vaccination. J Immunol Methods, *229:* 141-153, 1999.

50. Veelken, H., Mauerer, K., Mikesch, K., Osterroth, F., Rosenthal, F., Thomas, A.-K., and Bertinetti, C. Immune responses and clinical outcome of patients with advanced non-Hodgkin's lymphoma after immunization with a novel recombinant idiotype vaccine. Blood, *102:* 898a (abstract#3342), 2003.

51. Bertinetti, C. and Veelken, H. Characterization of cellular immune responses to a recombinant idiotype vaccine by ELISPOT and identification of MHC class I-restricted T cell epitopes by peptide mapping. Blood, *104:* 395a (abstract #1409), 2004.

52. Reddy, S. A., Czerwinski, D. K., Rajapaksa, R., Reinl, S., Garger, S. J., Cameron, T., Barrett, J., Novak, J., Holtz, R. B., and Levy, R. Plant derived single chain Fv Idiotype vaccines are safe and immunogenic in patients with follicular lymphoma: Results of a Phase I study. Blood, *100:* 163a (abstract #609), 2002.

53. Timmerman, J. M., Levy, R., Czerwinski, D. K., Ingolia, D., Denney, D., and Kunkel, L. A phase 2 trial to evaluate the efficacy of recombinant idiotype vaccines in untreated follicular lymphoma in the "watch-and-wait" period. Proc. Amer. Soc. Clin. Oncol., *21:* 4a, abstract 13 (Full manuscript in preparation), 2002.

54. Davis, T. A., Hsu, F. J., Caspar, C. B., van Beckhoven, A., Czerwinsk, D. K., Liles, T. M., Taidi, B., Benike, C. J., Engleman, E. G., and Levy, R. Idiotype vaccination following ABMT can stimulate specific anti-idiotype immune responses in patients with B-cell lymphoma. Biol Blood Marrow Transplant, *7:* 517-522, 2001.

55. Borrello, I., Sotomayor, E. M., Rattis, F. M., Cooke, S. K., Gu, L., and Levitsky, H. I. Sustaining the graft-versus-tumor effect through posttransplant immunization with granulocyte-macrophage colony-stimulating factor (GM-CSF)-producing tumor vaccines [In Process Citation]. Blood, *95:* 3011-3019, 2000.

56. Holman, P., Corringham, S., Bashey, A., Carrier, E., Mu, X., Gold, D., and Ball, E. D. Early and Robust Immune Responses to Idiotype (Id) Vaccination Occur in Mantle Cell Lymphoma (MCL) and Indolent Lymphoma (IL) Patients Following Autologous Stem Cell Transplantation (ASCT). Blood, *102:* 899a (abstract 3345), 2003.

57. Timmerman, J., Vose, J., Kunkel, L., Bierman, P., Czerwinski, D., Hohenstein, M., Ingolia, D., Denney, D., and Levy, R. A phase 2 study demonstrating recombinant Idiotype vaccine elicits specific anti-Idiotype immune responses in aggressive non-Hodgkin's lymphoma. Blood, *98:* 341a (abstract#1440), 2001.

58. Leonard, J. P., Vose, J. M., Timmerman, J. M., Levy, R., Coleman, M., King, S., Ingolia, D., and Denney, D. Recombinant idiotype-KLH vaccination (MyVax™) following CHOP chemotherapy in mantle cell lymphoma. Blood, *102:* 105a (abstract #357). 2003.

59. Wilson, W. H., Neelapu, S., Rosenwald, A., White, T., Dunleavy, K., Pittaluga, S., Hakim, F., Stetler-Stevenson, M., Steinberg, S. M., Jaffe, E. S., Gress, R., Wright, G., Staudt, L. M., Janik, J., and Kwak, L. Idiotype vaccine and dose-adjusted EPOCH-Rituximab

treatment in untreated mantle cell lymphoma: Preliminary report on clinical outcome and analysis of immune response. Blood, *102:* 105a (abstract #358), 2003.

60.   Restifo, N. P., Ying, H., Hwang, L., and Leitner, W. W. The promise of nucleic acid vaccines. Gene Ther, *7:* 89-92., 2000.

61.   Krieg, A. M. Antitumor applications of stimulating toll-like receptor 9 with CpG oligodeoxynucleotides. Curr Oncol Rep, *6:* 88-95, 2004.

62.   Syrengelas, A. D., Chen, T. T., and Levy, R. DNA immunization induces protective immunity against B-cell lymphoma. Nat Med, *2:* 1038-1041, 1996.

63.   King, C. A., Spellerberg, M. B., Zhu, D., Rice, J., Sahota, S. S., Thompsett, A. R., Hamblin, T. J., Radl, J., and Stevenson, F. K. DNA vaccines with single-chain Fv fused to fragment C of tetanus toxin induce protective immunity against lymphoma and myeloma. Nat Med, *4:* 1281-1286, 1998.

64.   Biragyn, A., Tani, K., Grimm, M. C., Weeks, S., and Kwak, L. W. Genetic fusion of chemokines to a self tumor antigen induces protective, T-cell dependent antitumor immunity [see comments]. Nat Biotechnol, *17:* 253-258, 1999.

65.   Biragyn, A., Surenhu, M., Yang, D., Ruffini, P. A., Haines, B. A., Klyushnenkova, E., Oppenheim, J. J., and Kwak, L. W. Mediators of innate immunity that target immature, but not mature, dendritic cells induce antitumor immunity when genetically fused with nonimmunogenic tumor antigens. J Immunol, *167:* 6644-6653., 2001.

66.   Timmerman, J. M., Singh, G., Hermanson, G., Hobart, P., Czerwinski, D. K., Taidi, B., Rajapaksa, R., Caspar, C. B., Van Beckhoven, A., and Levy, R. Immunogenicity of a plasmid DNA vaccine encoding chimeric idiotype in patients with B-cell lymphoma. Cancer Res, *62:* 5845-5852., 2002.

67.   Zhu, D., Rice, J., Savelyeva, N., and Stevenson, F. K. DNA fusion vaccines against B-cell tumors. Trends Mol Med, *7:* 566-572., 2001.

68.   Timmerman, J. M., Caspar, C. B., Lambert, S. L., Syrengelas, A. D., and Levy, R. Idiotype-encoding recombinant adenoviruses provide protective immunity against murine B-cell lymphomas. Blood, *97:* 1370-1377., 2001.

69.   Borrello, I., Biedryzcki, B., Sheets, N., Racke, F., Loper, K., Lemas, V., Noonan, K., Nelson, L., Hege, K., and Levitsky, H. I. Autologous tumor combined with a GM-CSF-secreting cell line vaccine (GVAX) following autologous stem cell transplant (ASCT) in multiple myeloma. Blood, *102:* 493a (abstract # 1794), 2003.

70.   Borrello, I., Sotomayor, E. M., Cooke, S., and Levitsky, H. I. A universal granulocyte-macrophage colony-stimulating factor-producing bystander cell line for use in the formulation of autologous tumor cell-based vaccines. Hum Gene Ther, *10:* 1983-1991, 1999.

71.   Wierda, W. G., Cantwell, M. J., Woods, S. J., Rassenti, L. Z., Prussak, C. E., and Kipps, T. J. CD40-ligand (CD154) gene therapy for chronic lymphocytic leukemia. Blood, *96:* 2917-2924., 2000.

72.   Takahashi, S., Yotnda, P., Rousseau, R. F., Mei, Z., Smith, S., Rill, D., Younes, A., and Brenner, M. K. Transgenic expression of CD40L and interleukin-2 induces an autologous antitumor immune response in patients with non-Hodgkin's lymphoma. Cancer Gene Ther, *8:* 378-387, 2001.

73.   Briones, J., Timmerman, J., and Levy, R. In vivo antitumor effect of CD40L-transduced tumor cells as a vaccine for B-cell lymphoma. Cancer Res, *62:* 3195-3199., 2002.

74.   Briones, J., Timmerman, J. M., Panicalli, D. L., and Levy, R. Antitumor immunity after vaccination with B lymphoma cells overexpressing a triad of costimulatory molecules. J Natl Cancer Inst, *95:* 548-555, 2003.

75.   Younes, A., Fayad, L. E., Pro, B., McLaughlin, P., Hagemeister, F. B., Mansfield, P., Clayman, G., Medeiros, L. J., Manning, J., Lewis, J., and Srivastava, P. Safety and efficacy of heat shock protein-peptide 96 complex (HSPPC-96) vaccine therapy in patients with relapsed or previously untreated in low-grade non-Hodgkin's lymphoma. Blood, *102:* 898-899a (abstract#3343), 2003.

76. Selenko, N., Maidic, O., Draxier, S., Berer, A., Jager, U., Knapp, W., and Stockl, J. CD20 antibody (C2B8)-induced apoptosis of lymphoma cells promotes phagocytosis by dendritic cells and cross-priming of CD8+ cytotoxic T cells. Leukemia, *15:* 1619-1626., 2001.

77. Dhodapkar, K. M., Krasovsky, J., Williamson, B., and Dhodapkar, M. V. Antitumor monoclonal antibodies enhance cross-presentation of cellular antigens and the generation of myeloma-specific killer T cells by dendritic cells. J Exp Med, *195:* 125-133., 2002.

78. Franki, S., Levy, R., and Timmerman, J. M. Dendritic cells co-cultured with antibody-coated tumor cells provide protective immunity against B cell lymphoma in vivo. Blood, *102:* 107a (abstract#361), 2003.

79. Marciani, D. J. Vaccine adjuvants: role and mechanisms of action in vaccine immunogenicity. Drug Discov Today, *8:* 934-943, 2003.

80. Cartron, G., Dacheux, L., Salles, G., Solal-Celigny, P., Bardos, P., Colombat, P., and Watier, H. Therapeutic activity of humanized anti-CD20 monoclonal antibody and polymorphism in IgG Fc receptor FcgammaRIIIa gene. Blood, *99:* 754-758., 2002.

81. Weng, W. K. and Levy, R. Two immunoglobulin G fragment C receptor polymorphisms independently predict response to rituximab in patients with follicular lymphoma. J Clin Oncol, *21:* 3940-3947, 2003.

82. McLaughlin, P., Robertson, L. E., and Keating, M. J. Fludarabine phosphate in lymphoma: an important new therapeutic agent. Cancer Treat Res, *85:* 3-14, 1996.

83. Ruffini, P. A., Neelapu, S. S., Kwak, L. W., and Biragyn, A. Idiotypic vaccination for B-cell malignancies as a model for therapeutic cancer vaccines: from prototype protein to second generation vaccines. Haematologica, *87:* 989-1001., 2002.

84. Okada, C. Y., Wong, C. P., Denney, D. W., and Levy, R. TCR vaccines for active immunotherapy of T cell malignancies. J Immunol, *159:* 5516-5527, 1997.

85. Lambert, S. L., Okada, C. Y., and Levy, R. TCR vaccines against a murine T cell lymphoma: a primary role for antibodies of the IgG2c class in tumor protection. J Immunol, *172:* 929-936, 2004.

86. Schultze, J. L. and Vonderheide, R. H. From cancer genomics to cancer immunotherapy: toward second-generation tumor antigens. Trends Immunol, *22:* 516-523, 2001.

87. Rosenberg, S. A. A new era for cancer immunotherapy based on the genes that encode cancer antigens. Immunity, *10:* 281-287, 1999.

88. Zeis, M., Siegel, S., Wagner, A., Schmitz, M., Marget, M., Kuhl-Burmeister, R., Adamzik, I., Kabelitz, D., Dreger, P., Schmitz, N., and Heiser, A. Generation of cytotoxic responses in mice and human individuals against hematological malignancies using survivin-RNA-transfected dendritic cells. J Immunol, *170:* 5391-5397, 2003.

89. Siegel, S., Wagner, A., Schmitz, N., and Zeis, M. Induction of antitumour immunity using survivin peptide-pulsed dendritic cells in a murine lymphoma model. Br J Haematol, *122:* 911-914, 2003.

Chapter 10

MANAGEMENT OF EARLY STAGE HODGKIN'S LYMPHOMA

David J. Straus, MD

Memorial Sloan-Kettering Cancer Center, Lymphoma Service, Department of Medicine
Weill Medical College of Cornell University, New York, NY

1. INTRODUCTION

The best treatment of early stage Hodgkin lymphoma has been controversial because of the success achieve with several approaches. These include large field radiation therapy alone, the combined modalities of chemotherapy and radiation therapy, and more recently, chemotherapy alone. Current clinical trials are attempting to reduce toxicity while continuing to achieve excellent results. This chapter will review the evolution of treatment for early stage Hodgkin lymphoma and will describe different the different approaches that have been developed.

2. STAGING

Advances in the treatment of early stage Hodgkin lymphoma were greatly aided by the development of precise definition of the sites of involvement. This was particularly important when the extended field radiation therapy approach was developed, the systemic use of what is essentially a regional treatment, which will be described. The current staging classification was established by the Ann Arbor Workshop in 1971. There is both clinical staging (CS), which consists of all staging procedures short of staging laparotomy, and pathologic staging (PS), which refers to the findings at staging laparotomy during which liver biopsies, splenectomy and excisional biopsies of retroperitoneal nodes are performed. The surgeon makes an attempt to biopsy nodes that are suspicious on lymphangiogram. Some centers have also performed open bone marrow biopsies from the iliac crest. Staging laparotomies are performed infrequently at the present time, since fewer patients are treated with radiation therapy alone and more with systemic treatment with chemotherapy alone or in combination with radiation therapy.

The Ann Arbor classification divides Hodgkin lymphoma into four stages: Stage I refers to disease limited to a single lymph node or lymph node group. Stage II refers to disease in two or more noncontiguous lymph node groups and/or spleen on the same side of the diaphragm. Stage III refers to disease in two or more lymph node groups and/or spleen on both sides of the diaphragm. Stage IV refers to disease in extranodal sites, usually lung, liver, bone or bone marrow, and more rarely other sites. Extranodal involvement by extension from lymph node disease to such sites as the lung, bone, pleura or skin may occur in stages IE and is not considered to increase the stage to IV. Such disease is designated by a subscript E (IE, IIE, IIIE). For each stage the absence of systemic symptoms is designated by the subscript "A," while the presence of unexplained fevers to 38° C or higher, night sweats and/or weight loss or greater than 10% over 6 months are designated by a "B" subscript. In general the prognosis worsens with higher stage, and, within each stage, the presence of B symptoms carries a worse prognosis than absence of such symptoms (A). A mediastinal mass >1/3rd of the thoracic diameter on chest x-ray or lymph node disease greater than 10 cm. is defined as "bulky;" a suffix X is added to the numerical stage if such disease is present (e.g., IxA, IxB, IIxA, IIxB, IIIxA, IIIxB)[1].

Staging procedures include chest x-ray, computerized tomography (CT) of the chest, abdomen and pelvis with oral and intravenous contrast, complete blood counts with platelet and differential counts, bone marrow aspiration and biopsy, serum liver biochemistries including alkaline phosphatase and 5' nucleotidase, and erythrocyte sedimentation rate. The latter test has been shown to carry prognostic significance. Computerized tomography of the abdomen and pelvis will show enlarged retroperitoneal and pelvic lymph nodes that are involved by disease. Occasionally, there may be nodes involved by disease, which are not enlarged. A bipedal lymphangiogram may show an abnormal filling pattern of contrast in lymph nodes that are involved but are only borderline or not enlarged. Lymphangiograms are labor intensive and require skilled, dedicated personnel and are infrequently necessary today with modern imaging procedures. Mesenteric nodal involvement at presentation in Hodgkin lymphoma is much less common than in the non-Hodgkin lymphoma.

If there are masses in the liver on CT scan or liver-spleen scintigram or gross abnormalities of serum liver biochemical studies, a liver biopsy should be performed under CT-guided or laparoscopic visualization if the masses are accessible. Slight elevations of serum alkaline phosphatase may be seen without liver involvement.

Gallium 67 scanning is a useful imaging procedure for following mediastinal disease, but it can be associated with false negatives and false positives. It is of value in the decision of whether or not to biopsy a residual mass following treatment to determine the presence or absence of residual disease. Positron emission tomography (PET) may provide similar and even more detailed information. [18F]FDG PET scanning has been found to be useful in predicting recurrences in residual masses following treatment for Hodgkin's disease. False negative studies are less common (negative predictive value 95%) than false positives (positive predictive value 60%)[2].

Computerized tomography of the chest may show disease, particularly retrosternal disease, missed by plain chest x-ray. Also, some patients with bulky mediastinal and hilar nodal disease will have peripheral lung nodules that can only be detected by chest CT. Although traditional radiotherapy treatment seems rarely affected by these findings, computerized tomography does allow for refinements in radiotherapy treatment planning.

The major finding at staging laparotomy has been that 10%-30% of patients who are CS IA or CS IIA will have occult disease in the spleen and will hence increase their stage to PS IIIAS. Some patients with splenic involvement will also have liver or retroperitoneal nodal involvement, although such involvement is unusual without splenic involvement. A review of the laparotomy experience at Stanford demonstrated that some subgroups of early stage patients have an even lower risk of having subdiaphragmatic disease: CS I female patients with mediastinal disease only, CS I males with lymphocyte predominant or interfollicular histologies and CS II woman less than 27 years of age and with only 2 or 3 sites of disease have a risk of having disease below the diaphragm of less than 10%[3].

Surgical staging has been largely abandoned. It was always agreed that it is not necessary when treatment of even early stage patients involves combination chemotherapy. However, it was controversial as to whether or not it is necessary when the treatment planned for supradiaphragmatic stage I or II disease will be RT including the mantle port (cervical, supraclavicular, mediastinal and axillary regions) and para-aortic nodes including the spleen or splenic pedicle (if the spleen has been removed), a field known as "subtotal lymphoid or nodal irradiation (STLI, STNI)." A large study using this type of treatment with either surgical or clinical staging showed no difference in overall survival, relapse-free survival or pelvic recurrence rate between patients clinically and those surgically staged[4]. The problems associated with staging laparotomy have also contributed to its abandonment. The overall mortality is 1.5% and has been as high as 3%. The morbidity is in the range of 6% including wound infection, subphrenic abscess, intestinal obstruction from adhesions and pulmonary embolus. Late sepsis with pneumococcus or *Haemophilus influenzae* has also been reported, but pneumococcal vaccine may reduce the risk of pneumococcal sepsis. The discomfort caused by the surgery to the patient and its expense are additional problems.

Whether disease in spleen or high para-aortic nodes is associated with a better prognosis than disease in the lower para-aortic nodes or pelvis following treatment with RT only has been a subject of controversy. The Stanford and Harvard groups found that minimal disease in the spleen (four or less tumor nodules) carries a more favorable prognosis than more extensive disease in the spleen (five or more tumor nodules) following treatment with RT only. This suggests that patients with extensive splenic involvement should be treated with chemotherapy or combined modality therapy.

3.   EXTENDED FIELD RADIATION THERAPY

The work of Gilbert, Peters and later Kaplan[5] demonstrated that recurrences rarely occur within the treated lymph node areas with doses of RT to 3500-4500 cGy. The use of the linear accelerator made it possible to deliver these doses to large fields. The "mantle" port (cervical, supraclavicular, mediastinal, and axillary regions – an area like the mantle on a suit of armor) and the "inverted Y" port (para-aortic nodes, spleen [if not removed] splenic pedicle and iliac, inguinal and femoral nodes) and combinations of the 2 were developed in the 1960s. Total lymphoid or nodal irradiation (TLI, TNI) refers to combinations of the two that has also at times included low dose irradiation of liver and lung. Subtotal lymphoid or nodal irradiation (STLI, STNI) includes the mantle port with irradiation of para-aortic nodes, splenic pedicle and spleen if it was not removed.

Extended field radiation therapy (EF RT) was the first dramatically successful treatment of early stage Hodgkin lymphoma, both in surgically staged and more recently in clinically staged patients. Subtotal lymphoid irradiation, which can include the spleen, to doses of at least 3500 cGy in 3 1/2 weeks has resulted in complete remission (CR) percentage in excess of 90% with a 20%-40% relapse rate in pathologically-staged patients, probably depending upon radiotherapy technique and/or patient selection[5]. The likelihood of "salvage" of these patients into a second durable CR may be in excess of 50%. The risks of leukemia and sterility are less than with combination chemotherapy. Long term potential side effects of radiotherapy include radiation lung fibrosis, pericarditis, premature coronary artery disease, carotid and peripheral artery disease, neuromuscular problems including muscle wasting and peripheral nerve plexopathies, lymphedema and second solid tumor malignancies, including breast carcinoma, lung carcinoma and sarcomas. The actuarial risk of second malignancies following treatment for Hodgkin lymphoma that is mostly attributable to RT has been reported to be 22-27% at 25-30 years[6-9].

Local irradiation (involved field radiation therapy, IF RT) is probably adequate for high cervical stage IA disease and lymphocyte predominant or nodular sclerosis histology in a young patient. Lymphocyte-predominant Hodgkin lymphoma is often clinically localized, is usually effectively treated with irradiation alone, expresses CD20, a mature B-cell marker, and may relapse late (a clinical feature reminiscent of non-aggressive B-cell non-Hodgkin lymphomas). The 15-year disease-specific survival is excellent (>90%).

There is also general agreement that bulky mediastinal disease with a mediastinal mass diameter over 1/3 of the chest diameter should be treated with combined modality treatment with chemotherapy and RT[10]. Recently some groups have treated selected patients with bulky mediastinal masses whose disease is well defined on CT scan with RT only using ports designed with the aid of the CT scan.

The prognostic importance of contiguous extension of disease from hilar nodes into the lung parenchyma is controversial. Some centers employing radiotherapy only report good results using low dose irradiation also administered to the entire affected lung aided by thin lung blocks. Others have had better success with combined modality treatment.

The European Organization for Research and Treatment of Cancer (EORTC) found elevations of erythrocyte sedimentation rate (ESR) (>50 mm/hr for stages IA and IIA, >30 mm/hr for stages IB and IIB) to be a powerful adverse prognostic factor among patients treated with RT only[11]. This does not appear to be an adverse prognostic factor for patients treated with combined modality treatment[12].

Combined modality treatment with chemotherapy and radiation therapy

Superior results have been achieved with combined modality treatment (CMT) as compared with EF RT alone. Combined modality treatment has resulted in a CR percentage of greater than 90% with a relapse rate of approximately 10% or less. This was achieved in the past with 6 cycles of chemotherapy with the MOPP (nitrogen mustard, vincristine, procarbazine and prednisone) or similar regimens.

When radiotherapy is also used, fewer cycles of chemotherapy may give similar results. A protocol at Memorial Hospital randomized CS IA, IIA and IIIA patients to 4 cycles of either MOPP or TBV (thioTEPA, bleomycin, and vinblastine). An interruption was made between the second and third cycle of chemotherapy in both arms for radiotherapy to involved regions to 3500 cGy over 3 1/2 weeks. The treated regions consisted of the mantle port, para-aortic nodes, spleen and pelvic and inguinal/femoral nodes. Every effort was made to try to avoid or limit radiotherapy to the pelvis, since it may be associated with considerable morbidity. The results with a median follow-up time of 65 mo (7 mo-96 mo) were similar in both arms of this trial and also similar to the results achieved with 6 cycles of MOPP and involved region radiotherapy[12]. Two French studies suggested that 3 cycles of MOPP may be sufficient in combination with radiotherapy[13, 14]

A number of recent randomized studies have established combined modality treatment as the new standard. These have focused on reducing the chemotherapy and or limiting the RT. The H8-F trial of the European Organization for Research and Treatment of Cancer (EORTC) demonstrated the superiority of three cycles of MOPP/ABV hybrid (MOPP/doxorubicin, bleomycin and vinblastine) + IF RT (36-40 Gy) (four-year treatment failure-free survival [TTFS] rate 99%) to EFRT at the same dose (TTFS rate 77%, p<0.001) in favorable early stage Hodgkin lymphoma [15]. The Southwest Oncology Group demonstrated a superior failure-free survival for three cycles of doxorubicin and vinblastine + STNI (94%) as compared to STNI alone (81%, p<.001) for patients with supradiaphragmatic CS IA or IIA Hodgkin lymphoma[16]. The German Hodgkin's Lymphoma Study Group HD-7 study compared 2 cycles of ABVD (doxorubicin, bleomycin vinblastine and dacarbazine) + EF RT (30 Gy) / IF RT boost (10 Gy) to EF RT (30 Gy)/ IF RT boost (10 Gy) in favorable stages I and II patients. The freedom from treatment failure was 96% for combine modality treatment as compared to 84% for EF RT alone [17].

Azoospermia occurs in approximately 80% of men treated with 6 cycles of MOPP, and another 10% are rendered oligospermic. Sperm banking with cryopreservation is encouraged for male patients who may wish to have children in the future. Female patients under 30 years of age are less likely to become permanently infertile than those over the age of 30. The risk of acute leukemia or myelodysplastic syndrome following MOPP-type chemotherapy is 9 times greater than with radiation therapy only[18]. The risk may be further increased approximately 2 times in patients who underwent prior splenectomy. As described below, the ABVD regimen seems to have less potential for secondary leukemia and sterility than MOPP. Other less potentially leukemogenic and sterilizing regimens have also been investigated. The results of a randomized trial of extended field RT alone or involved field RT followed by 6 cycles of vinblastine, bleomycin and methotrexate showed no significant difference in 5-year freedom from progression or survival[19].

Reduction in the size of the RT fields has also been possible, even with a reduction in the number of cycles of chemotherapy. The group at the Istituto Nazionale Tumori recently reported excellent long-term excellent equivalent results in a randomized trial of four cycles of ABVD + IF RT (30-40 Gy) compared to ABVD + STNI (30-40 Gy) in CS I and II Hodgkin lymphoma at a median followup of 116 months [20]. Among 136 assessable "unfavorable" stage I and stage IIA patients, the 12-year rates of freedom from progression rates were 93%, event-free survival 87% and overall survival 96% for ABVD + STLI and 94%, 91% and 94% for IF RT, respectively. This study was not highly powered to prove equivalence and 95% confidence intervals were up to 17%. With the exception of pulmonary toxicity, the ABVD regimen appeared to have less toxicity than regimens with alkylating agents of the nitrogen mustard class and procarbazine. Pulmonary toxicity occurred acutely with ABVD. Fourteen patients developed pulmonary symptoms and 22% had asymptomatic drops in lung diffusing capacity (DLCO) of $\geq 20\%$. Three second malignancies were seen; one was an acute leukemia. Only 1 premenopausal woman became amenorrheic and 6% of men developed persistent azoospermia. Many physicians in the U.S.A. now use four cycles of ABVD + IF RT as standard treatment for stages I and IIA Hodgkin lymphoma.

4.   CHEMOTHERAPY ONLY

A small non-randomized study from Spain demonstrated a progression free survival of 86% and an OS of 92% at 56 months for six cycles of ABVD without RT for stages I and II Hodgkin's disease, results similar to our experience as described below [21,22]. There have been several randomized trials of chemotherapy alone vs. combined modality treatment in early stage Hodgkin lymphoma, and none are definitive.

A variant of MOPP chemotherapy with low-dose cyclophosphamide, vinblastine, procarbazine and prednisone (CVPP) alone for six cycles was compared to six cycles of CVPP and involved field RT for 277 clinical stage (CS) IA and IIA patients in a trial of GATLA and GLATHEM groups in Argentina. At seven years of followup, differences in the disease-free and overall survival for CVPP alone and CVPP+RT were not statistically significant in a subgroup analysis of 177 "favorable" patients. However, patients with "unfavorable" early-stage Hodgkin's disease (age>45 years, >2 sites, bulky disease), treatment with CVPP and IFRT produced a longer disease-free and overall survival than with CVPP alone. Some have argued that the low-dose chemotherapy may have been suboptimal [23].

Two multi-institutional randomized trials have recently been closed to accrual of patients on chemotherapy alone. The results of a randomized phase II trial conducted by the National Cancer Institute of Canada (NCIC) and the Eastern Cooperative Oncology Group was recently reported[24] . It was closed to accrual slightly before completing the accrual target because the investigators were unwilling to continue to treat patients with combined modality therapy that included EF RT in view of the results of the EORTC-GELA H8-F trial mentioned above. In this trial, patients with CS IA and IIA Hodgkin lymphoma without tumor bulk or other poor prognosis features were randomized to "standard" treatment (STNI) for more favorable; 2 cycles of ABVD + STNI for less favorable or "experimental" treatment (4-6 cycles of ABVD alone). Somewhat less than 30% of patients on the "experimental" arm received only 4 cycles of ABVD, although it is not clear that excessive relapses were seen in this subgroup. At a median duration of follow-up of 4.2 years, the estimated 5-year progression-free survival was 93% for patients in the "standard" arm and 87% for those in the "experimental" arm, a difference that was statistically significant. There was no difference in overall survival. In view of the salvageability of the small excess for patients who might relapse after chemotherapy alone and the late morbidity of treatment that is mostly attributable to RT, the clinical meaning of a 6% difference in PFS is unclear. Six cycles of ABVD alone has been more commonly used for Hodgkin's disease patients than 4 cycles for which this will be the first reported experience. Also, neither STNI nor 2 cycles of ABVD + STNI are currently the most commonly used "standard" treatments for early stage Hodgkin lymphoma. Thus the results of this trial are not conclusive.

The EORTC H9-F trial randomized favorable patients with CS I and II to six cycles of chemotherapy with epirubicin, bleomycin vinblastine and prednisone (EBVP) for six cycles alone, EBVP x 6 + IF RT (20 Gy) or EVBP x 6 + IF RT (36 Gy). The EBVP alone arm was closed because an excess of relapses were seen while the CMT arms continue to accrue. There is concern that the EBVP alone may be suboptimal chemotherapy (Dr. Patrice Carde, personal communication). In "unfavorable" stage I and II patients, EBVP + IF RT was inferior to MOPP/ABV hybrid + IF RT. (EORTC H7-U trial) [15]. Recently, ABVD has been demonstrated to have equivalent treatment results with less toxicity as compared to MOPP/ABV hybrid in advanced stage Hodgkin lymphoma [25].

Results of two randomized trials of patients in all stages comparing combined modality treatment with chemotherapy alone have been recently reported. A randomized trial from India comparing ABVD + RT vs. ABVD alone in all stages of Hodgkin lymphoma found a significant difference in event-free and overall survival in favor of ABVD + RT, but there was no significant difference in either outcome in a subset analysis of patients with stages I and II disease[26]. The population of patients reported in this trial was different from those typically reported in trials from Europe and North America. The Children's Cancer Group reported on trials on 829 pediatric Hodgkin lymphoma patients with all stages. The 501 patients who achieved a CR with chemotherapy were randomized to low-dose IF RT or no further treatment. An analysis by "intent-to-treat" demonstrated a borderline significant increase in 3-year EFS (P=0.057) in the group receiving CMT, and the increase was significant by an "as-treated" analysis (P=.0024). There was no difference in OS [27].

More definitive results have been recently reported from a trial comparing chemotherapy alone with combined modality treatment for patients with advanced stages of Hodgkin lymphoma. In stages III and IV Hodgkin lymphoma the EORTC has reported the results of a large trial 739 patients treated with 6-8 cycles of MOPP/ABV hybrid chemotherapy with a randomization of patients achieving a CR (421 patients) to IF RT or no RT. Of the 739 patients, 421 achieved a CR. The median followup time was 79 months. The 5-year event-free survival was 84% for the arm without RT and 79% for the RT group (P=0.35). The 5-year overall survival rates were 91% and 85%, respectively (P=0.07). This trend toward a worse survival in the combined modality arm was due to an excess of deaths not directly due to Hodgkin lymphoma, in particular second cancers. A probable benefit of RT was seen in the 250 patients who achieved a partial remission (PR) and were irradiated with 5-year event-free and overall survival rates of 79% and 87%, respectively[28].

To determine whether combined modality therapy (CMT) is superior to chemotherapy alone (CT), 152 untreated Hodgkin lymphoma patients with CS IA, IB, IIA, IIB, and IIIA without bulk disease were prospectively randomized to 6 cycles of doxorubicin, bleomycin, vinblastine and dacarbazine (ABVD) alone or 6 cycles of ABVD followed by RT (3600 cGy: involved field for 11 patients, modified extended field for the rest). The trial was conducted at Memorial Sloan-Kettering Cancer Center. Sixty-five of 76 patients randomized to receive RT actually received it and 11 did not (4 progressed, 1 bleomycin toxicity, 6 refused). For ABVD+RT, the complete remission (CR) percentage was 94% and no major response 6%. For ABVD alone, 94% achieved a CR, 1.5 % a partial response (PR) and no major response 4.5%. At 60 months CR duration, freedom from progression (FFP), and overall survival (OS) for ABVD+ RT vs. ABVD alone are 91% vs. 87% (P=0.61), 86% vs. 81% (P=0.61) and 97% vs. 90% (P=0.08), respectively (logrank). The 95% confidence intervals for CR duration, FFP and OS differences at 5 years were (-8%, 15%), (-8%, 18%) and (-4%, 12%), respectively. Although significant differences were not seen, it is possible that a benefit in outcome of < 20% for CMT might be seen in a larger trial. Thirty-three patients (22%) discontinued bleomycin because of a decrease in DLCO. Ten of the symptomatic patients received brief courses of corticosteroids, and there was one death due to bleomycin during treatment in a 65-year-old woman[29].

5.   NEW STRATEGIES

The challenge in early stage Hodgkin lymphoma treatment is unusual in medical oncology. Excellent treatment results have been achieved for decades. It would be difficult to improve upon them. The challenge is to continue to achieve excellent results, but with less toxicity, particularly less long-term morbidity. There are two different directions in the current investigation of the treatment of early stage Hodgkin lymphoma.

One is to attempt to reduce the chemotherapy and RT fields and doses. The German Hodgkin Study Group HD10 protocol has been closed to accrual. Patients with favorable clinical stages I and II were randomized to 4 cycles of ABVD + 30 Gy IF RT, 4 cycles of ABVD + 20 Gy IF RT, 2 cycles of ABVD + 30 Gy IF RT or 2 cycles of ABVD + 20 Gy IF RT. The early results for all arms are excellent and equivalent[30]. As described above, most of the long-term morbidity has been related to RT, and it is possible that less extensive fields and doses will result in lower rates of long-term treatment-related morbidity and mortality. Further followup time is clearly necessary to determine whether or not this will be true.

The second direction is the use of chemotherapy alone as primary treatment of favorable early stage Hodgkin lymphoma. CALGB 50203 has recently been activated. In this trial patients with clinical stages IA and IIA Hodgkin lymphoma will be treated with 6 cycles of a new regimen, doxorubicin, vinblastine and gemcitabine (AVG). As described below, this regimen may be less toxic than ABVD. This trial will also use PET scanning prospectively to determine completeness of response after 2 and after completion of 6 cycles of treatment. There is data suggesting that early resolution of PET avidity of lymphoma patients on chemotherapy may be even more predictive of a favorable outcome than the resolution of PET avidity at the completion of chemotherapy.

Gemcitabine is a highly effective and potentially less toxic drug that could be substituted for bleomycin. In 22 assessable patients with refractory Hodgkin lymphoma treated with gemcitabine at a dose of 1250 mg/m^2 on days 1, 8, and 15 of a 28 day cycle, the overall response rate was 39% (CR 9%, PR 30%). Toxicity was mild, not fatal and mostly hematologic [31]. There was one patient who experienced grade 4 thrombocytopenia with hemorrhage. Grade 3 thrombocytopenia was seen in 3, decreased hemoglobin in 2 and neutropenia in 6 of 20 assessable patients. An overall response rate of 43% (CR 14%, PR 29%) was seen in 14 pretreated Hodgkin lymphoma patients with gemcitabine at a dose of 1200 mg/m^2 on days 1, 8 and 15 of a 28 day cycle for 6 cycles. Grades 3-4 neutropenia was seen in 6% and thrombocytopenia in 3% of administered cycles (Haematologica 85: 926-9, 2000).

Recently experience with gemcitabine in combination with doxorubicin and vinca alkaloids in patients with Hodgkin lymphoma has been reported. Bartlett and colleagues described the preliminary results of CALGB 59804, a phase I/II study of gemcitabine, vinorelbine and pegylated liposomal doxorubicin (Doxil®) in relapsed Hodgkin lymphoma)(Proc Am. Soc. Clin Oncol. 22: 566, 2003, abs.#2275). For patients who had not received prior stem cell transplants, the phase II doses were gemcitabine 1000 mg/m^2 on day 1 and day 8; vinorelbine 20 mg/m^2 on day 1 and day 8; and pegylated liposomal doxorubicin 15 mg/m^2 on day 1 and day 8 administered every 21 days. In 47 patients with relapsed Hodgkin lymphoma without prior transplant, the overall response rate was 66% with 19% CR and 47% PR. Grade 3/4 neutropenia was seen in 59% of patients in the phase II trial. There were no treatment related deaths [32].

Mild reversible dyspnea, often not requiring cessation of drug, has been reported overall in approximately 25% of patients treated with gemcitabine. It was highest in (40%) the registration trial for lung carcinoma and lower in pancreas cancer (10%). Severe pulmonary toxicity has been reported in less than 1% of patients (data supplied by Eli Lilly and Company). The combination of gemcitabine with chemotherapy including bleomycin has caused unacceptable pulmonary toxicity[33]. Bredenfeld and colleagues reported that 8 of 27 patients with stages IIB, II or IV Hodgkin's disease developed significant pulmonary toxicity with a combination of gemcitabine with bleomycin, doxorubicin, cyclophosphamide, vincristine, procarbazine and prednisone. With a median followup of 27 months, 25 patients are in continuing CR[33]. Significant pulmonary toxicity of the bleomycin type was also reported by Friedberg and colleagues in 5 of 12 patients with newly diagnosed bulky or advanced stage Hodgkin lymphoma with doxorubicin, bleomycin, vinblastine and gemcitabine, although all patients completing 6 cycles of treatment responded[34]. The use of gemcitabine with doxorubicin and vinca alkaloids appears to be effective and safe as long as the drugs are not combined with bleomycin.

Doxorubicin, vinblastine and gemcitabine (AVG) is a new combination of 3 of the most active chemotherapeutic drugs in the treatment of Hodgkin lymphoma. It follows up on the excellent results with pegylated liposomal doxorubicin (Doxil®), vinorelbine and gemcitabine in relapsed Hodgkin lymphoma (CALGB 59804). Radiation therapy has been omitted based on our own results with ABVD chemotherapy alone, the potential long-term morbidity of radiation therapy and likelihood of successful salvage of patients with persistent or relapsed disease in this population following chemotherapy only. It eliminates bleomycin, the drug with the most problematic toxicity. Stringent early stopping rules are in place if the CR rate from this regimen is not optimal during the course of the trial.

6.   CONCLUSIONS AND FUTURE DIRECTIONS

For the present, trials will be directed to achieving excellent results while reducing the short and particularly long-term toxicities of the current treatment modalities of chemotherapy and radiation therapy. In the future, applications of new approaches may find their way into the treatment regimens for Hodgkin lymphoma. One of these is the use of small molecule chemotherapy agents with novel mechanisms of action. The proteosome inhibitor, bortezomib is a new agent that has recently been introduced into the treatment of multiple myeloma. Promising results have been recently reported in non-Hodgkin lymphomas, particularly mantle cell lymphoma[35,36]. It is a very interesting drug for Hodgkin lymphoma because of its activity against NF-κB, a transcription factor that is overexpressed in Hodgkin lymphoma and may be an important mechanism in the malignant process by its blockage of apoptosis. CALGB 50206 is a phase II trial of bortezomib in relapsed and refractory Hodgkin lymphoma.

Monoclonal antibodies have also been recently used in Hodgkin lymphoma. Rituximab, and anti-CD20 chimeric mouse-human monoclonal antibody, widely used in B-cell non-Hodgkin lymphoma, has also demonstrated activity in lymphocyte-predominant Hodgkin lymphoma. This type has been recently separated from classical Hodgkin lymphoma by expression of a mature B-cell phenotype, including CD20 on the variant Reed-Sternberg cells. In contrast, the Reed-Sternberg cells in classical Hodgkin lymphoma universally express CD30 and rarely CD20. In a phase II trial of rituximab in lymphocyte predominant Hodgkin lymphoma conducted at Stanford all 22 patients treated responded (9 CR, 1 CR undetermined [CRu], 12 PR), although estimated freedom from progression was only 10.2 months[37]. Similar results were reported by the German Hodgkin Study Group in a phase II trial of rituximab for lymphocyte predominant Hodgkin lymphoma in which the overall response rate was 86% in 14 patients with 8 patients achieving a CR, 4 a PR and 2 demonstrating progressive disease. The median duration of response (20+ months) had not been reached in this report[38]. In a trial of rituximab treatment for classical Hodgkin lymphoma at M. D. Anderson, 5 of 22 patients demonstrated a response (22%, 1 CR, 4 PR) for a brief median duration of response of 7.8 months[39].

A phase I/II trial of MDX-060, a fully human IgGI antibody against CD30[40], is in progress for in CD30-expressing lymphomas including classical Hodgkin lymphoma. Phase I trials of anti-CD30 ricin A-chain (Ki-4.dgA) and anti-CD-25 ricin A-chain (RFT5.dgA) immunotoxins have also been reported in Hodgkin lymphoma, and suggestions of clinical activity were observed[41,42]. A further phase I trial with a suggestion of clinical activity in Hodgkin lymphoma has been reported with a novel bispecific molecule H22xKi-4. This molecule consists of F(ab') fragments derived from the murine anti-CD30 monoclonal antibody Ki-4 and the humanized anti-CD64 monoclonal antibody H22. CD64, as a part of the FcγRI, triggers cytotoxic effector cells expressing this receptor, resulting in increased cytotoxic activity[43].

In the more distant future treatments based on such applications and others of the new cancer biology may compliment or even replace the older effective but toxic treatment modalities of chemotherapy and RT in early stage Hodgkin lymphoma.

7. REFERENCES

1. Lister TA, Crowther D, Sutcliffe SB, et al: Report of a committee convened to discuss the evaluation and staging of patients with Hodgkin's disease: Cotswolds meeting. J Clin Oncol 7:1630-6, 1989

2. Weihrauch MR, Re D, Scheidhauer K, et al: Thoracic positron emission tomography using 18F-fluorodeoxyglucose for the evaluation of residual mediastinal Hodgkin disease. Blood 98:2930-4, 2001

3. Leibenhaut MH, Hoppe RT, Efron B, et al: Prognostic indicators of laparotomy findings in clinical stage I-II supradiaphragmatic Hodgkin's disease. J Clin Oncol 7:81-91, 1989

4. Tubiana M, Hayat M, Henry-Amar M, et al: Five-year results of the E.O.R.T.C. randomized study of splenectomy and spleen irradiation in clinical stages I and II of Hodgkin's disease. Eur J Cancer 17:355-63, 1981

5. Kaplan HS: Hodgkin's disease (ed 2d). Cambridge, Mass., Harvard University Press, 1980

6. van Leeuwen FE, Klokman WJ, Veer MB, et al: Long-term risk of second malignancy in survivors of Hodgkin's disease treated during adolescence or young adulthood. J Clin Oncol 18:487-97, 2000

7. Swerdlow AJ, Barber JA, Hudson GV, et al: Risk of second malignancy after Hodgkin's disease in a collaborative British cohort: the relation to age at treatment. J Clin Oncol 18:498-509, 2000

8. Green DM, Hyland A, Barcos MP, et al: Second malignant neoplasms after treatment for Hodgkin's disease in childhood or adolescence. J Clin Oncol 18:1492-9, 2000

9. Dores GM, Metayer C, Curtis RE, et al: Second malignant neoplasms among long-term survivors of Hodgkin's disease: a population-based evaluation over 25 years. J Clin Oncol 20:3484-94, 2002

10. Mauch P, Gorshein D, Cunningham J, et al: Influence of mediastinal adenopathy on site and frequency of relapse in patients with Hodgkin's disease. Cancer Treat Rep 66:809-17, 1982

11. Henry-Amar M, Friedman S, Hayat M, et al: Erythrocyte sedimentation rate predicts early relapse and survival in early-stage Hodgkin disease. The EORTC Lymphoma Cooperative Group. Ann Intern Med 114:361-5, 1991

12. Straus DJ, Yahalom J, Gaynor J, et al: Four cycles of chemotherapy and regional radiation therapy for clinical early-stage and intermediate-stage Hodgkin's disease. Cancer 69:1052-60, 1992

13. Ferme C, Teillet F, d'Agay MF, et al: Combined modality in Hodgkin's disease. Comparison of six versus three courses of MOPP with clinical and surgical restaging. Cancer 54:2324-9, 1984

14. Andrieu JM, Montagnon B, Asselain B, et al: Chemotherapy--radiotherapy association in Hodgkin's disease, clinical stages IA, II2A: results of a prospective clinical trial with 166 patients. Cancer 46:2126-30, 1980

15. Hagenbeek A EH, Ferme C, Meerwaldt JH, Divine M, Raemaekers JMM, Reman O, Zagonel V, Ferrant A, Gabarre J, Berger F, Rieux C Henry-Amar M: Three cycles of MOPP/ABV (M/A) hybrid and involved-field irradiation is more effective than subtotal nodal irradiation (STNI) in favorable supradiaphragmatic clinical stages (CS) I-II Hodgkin's disease (HD): Preliminary results of the EORTC-GELA H8F randomized trial in 543 patients. Blood 96 (#11, Part 1):575a, 2000

16. Press OW, LeBlanc M, Lichter AS, et al: Phase III randomized intergroup trial of subtotal lymphoid irradiation versus doxorubicin, vinblastine, and subtotal lymphoid irradiation for stage IA to IIA Hodgkin's disease. J Clin Oncol 19:4238-44, 2001

17. Wiedenmann S, Schiller P, Paulus U, et al: Treatment of early and intermediate stage Hodgkin's lymphoma in the German Hodgkin's Lymphoma Study Group. Ann Oncol 13 Suppl 1:84-5, 2002

18. Kaldor JM, Day NE, Clarke EA, et al: Leukemia following Hodgkin's disease. N Engl J Med 322:7-13, 1990

19. Horning SJ, Hoppe RT, Mason J, et al: Stanford-Kaiser Permanente G1 study for clinical stage I to IIA Hodgkin's disease: subtotal lymphoid irradiation versus vinblastine, methotrexate, and bleomycin chemotherapy and regional irradiation. J Clin Oncol 15:1736-44, 1997

20. Bonadonna G, Bonfante V, Viviani S, et al: ABVD Plus Subtotal Nodal Versus Involved-Field Radiotherapy in Early-Stage Hodgkin's Disease: Long-Term Results. J Clin Oncol 22:2835-41, 2004

21. Rueda A, Alba E, Ribelles N, et al: Six cycles of ABVD in the treatment of stage I and II Hodgkin's lymphoma: a pilot study. J Clin Oncol 15:1118-22, 1997

22. Rueda A, Ribelles N, Sevilla I, et al.: Six cycles of ABVD for stage I and II Hodgkin's lymphoma (HL). Proc Annu Meet Am Soc Clin Oncol 17:139a, 1998

23. Pavlovsky S, Maschio M, Santarelli MT, et al: Randomized trial of chemotherapy versus chemotherapy plus radiotherapy for stage I-II Hodgkin's disease. J Natl Cancer Inst 80:1466-73, 1988

24. Meyer R, Gospodarowicz M, Connors J, et al: A Randomized Phase II Trial Comparison of Single-Modality ABVD with a Strategy that Includes Radiation Therapy in Patients with Early-Stage Hodgkin's Disease: The HD-6 Trial of the National Cancer Institute of Canada Clinical Trials Group (Eastern Cooperative Oncology Group JHD06). Blood 102:26a, 2003

25. Duggan DB, Petroni GR, Johnson JL, et al: Randomized comparison of ABVD and MOPP/ABV hybrid for the treatment of advanced Hodgkin's disease: report of an intergroup trial. J Clin Oncol 21:607-14, 2003

26. Laskar S, Gupta T, Vimal S, et al: Consolidation radiation after complete remission in Hodgkin's disease following six cycles of doxorubicin, bleomycin, vinblastine, and dacarbazine chemotherapy: is there a need? J Clin Oncol 22:62-8, 2004

27. Nachman JB, Sposto R, Herzog P, et al: Randomized comparison of low-dose involved-field radiotherapy and no radiotherapy for children with Hodgkin's disease who achieve a complete response to chemotherapy. J Clin Oncol 20:3765-71, 2002

28. Aleman BM, Raemaekers JM, Tirelli U, et al: Involved-field radiotherapy for advanced Hodgkin's lymphoma. N Engl J Med 348:2396-406, 2003

29. Straus DJ, Portlock CS, Qin J, et al: Results of a prospective randomized cinical trial of doxorubicin, bleomycin, vinblastine and dacarbazine (ABVD) followed by radiation therapy (RT) vs. ABVD alone for stages I, II and IIA non bulky Hodgkin's disease. Blood (In Press0, 2004

30. Diehl V, Stein H, Hummel M, et al: Hodgkin's lymphoma: biology and treatment strategies for primary, refractory, and relapsed disease. Hematology (Am Soc Hematol Educ Program):225-47, 2003

31. Santoro A, Bredenfeld H, Devizzi L, et al: Gemcitabine in the treatment of refractory Hodgkin's disease: results of a multicenter phase II study. J Clin Oncol 18:2615-9, 2000

32. Bartlett N, al. e: A phase I/II study of gemcitabine, vinorelbine, and liposomal doxorubicin for relapsed Hodgkin's disease: Preliminary results of CALGB 59804. Proc Am Soc Clin Oncol 22:566, 2003

33. Bredenfeld H, Franklin J, Nogova L, et al: Severe pulmonary toxicity in patients with advanced-stage Hodgkin's disease treated with a modified bleomycin, doxorubicin, cyclophosphamide, vincristine, procarbazine, prednisone, and gemcitabine (BEACOPP) regimen is probably related to the combination of gemcitabine and bleomycin: a report of the German Hodgkin's Lymphoma Study Group. J Clin Oncol 22:2424-9, 2004

34. Friedberg JW, al. e: Gemcitabine added to doxorubicin, bleomycin, and vinblastine for the treatment of de novo Hodgkin's disease. Unacceptable acute pulmonary toxicity. Cancer 98:978-82, 2003

35. Goy A, Hart S, Pro B, et al: Report of a phase II Study of Proteosome Inhibitor Bortezomib (VELCADE) in Patients with Relapsed or Refractory Indolent or Aggressive Lymphomas. Blood 102:108a, 2003

36. O'Connor O: Marked Clinical Activity of the Novel Proteosome Inhibitor Bortezomib in Patients with Relapsed Follicular (RL) and Mantle Cell Lymphoma (MCL). Proc Am Soc Clin Oncol 23:567, 2004

37. Ekstrand BC, Lucas JB, Horwitz SM, et al: Rituximab in lymphocyte-predominant Hodgkin disease: results of a phase 2 trial. Blood 101:4285-9, 2003

38. Rehwald U, Schulz H, Reiser M, et al: Treatment of relapsed CD20+ Hodgkin lymphoma with the monoclonal antibody rituximab is effective and well tolerated: results of a phase 2 trial of the German Hodgkin Lymphoma Study Group. Blood 101:420-4, 2003

39. Younes A, Romaguera J, Hagemeister F, et al: A pilot study of rituximab in patients with recurrent, classic Hodgkin disease. Cancer 98:310-4, 2003

40. Borchmann P, Treml JF, Hansen H, et al: The human anti-CD30 antibody 5F11 shows in vitro and in vivo activity against malignant lymphoma. Blood 102:3737-42, 2003

41. Schnell R, Staak O, Borchmann P, et al: A Phase I study with an anti-CD30 ricin A-chain immunotoxin (Ki-4.dgA) in patients with refractory CD30+ Hodgkin's and non-Hodgkin's lymphoma. Clin Cancer Res 8:1779-86, 2002

42. Schnell R, Borchmann P, Staak JO, et al: Clinical evaluation of ricin A-chain immunotoxins in patients with Hodgkin's lymphoma. Ann Oncol 14:729-36, 2003

43. Borchmann P, Schnell R, Fuss I, et al: Phase 1 trial of the novel bispecific molecule H22xKi-4 in patients with refractory Hodgkin lymphoma. Blood 100:3101-7, 2002

Chapter 11

MANAGEMENT OF ADVANCED STAGE HODGKIN'S LYMPHOMA

Nancy L. Bartlett, MD and Avram J. Smukler, MD

Washington University, Siteman Cancer Center, Division of Medical Oncology
660 South Euclid Street, St. Louis, MO 63110

1. INTRODUCTION

Hodgkin's lymphoma (HL) is an uncommon malignancy of unknown etiology with an annual incidence in Western populations of 2-3 per 100,000 (1). On average there are 7000 new cases reported in the United States each year, distributed in a bimodal pattern with a first peak in the third decade and a second peak after the age of 50 (1, 2).

Although the trigger for malignant proliferation is poorly understood, it has become increasingly clear that most cases of HL represent a clonal proliferation of B cells (1, 3). As a result, the WHO has since classified "Hodgkin's disease" as a lymphoma, allowing the two terms to be used interchangeably (4). According to this classification, two subtypes of HL with distinct immunohistochemical profiles, natural histories and prognoses have emerged: classical HL and nodular lymphocyte predominant HL. Pathologists further subdivided classical HL into nodular sclerosis, mixed cellularity, lymphocyte-rich and lymphocyte-depleted, however, these different entities have no known clinical significance and will be discussed only as classical HL (1).

Since the original discovery of HL in 1834, management of the disease has undergone a paradigm shift. By the 1960's it had become apparent that, in most cases, extended field radiotherapy was curative in patients with localized disease at presentation. At that time, advanced HL was invariably fatal with a median survival of 2 years or less, and virtually no patient survived beyond 5 years. The development of combination chemotherapy with MOPP (nitrogen mustard, vincristine, procarbazine, prednisone) was a milestone, as this regimen demonstrated the curative potential of polychemotherapy in patients with advanced HL (5). The full impact of MOPP and the other drug regimens subsequently introduced was soon appreciated. Mortality data revealed that in 1950, HL accounted for 30% of the total lymphoma associated deaths, by the 1990's it accounted for only 6% (6).

It soon became apparent that the principle factor dictating the success of the therapy introduced for HL was accurate staging of the patients underlying disease. From this observation, the Ann Arbor staging system emerged in 1971 (7). This system created a distinction between early stage (stage I-II) and advanced HL (stage III-IV) that has both prognostic and therapeutic implications. Current therapies for early stage HL result in long-term survival rates approximating 90%, compared with advanced disease where long-term survival rates are 50-60% (8).

Development of an accurate prognostic model was an important step in evaluating new therapies for advanced stage disease. Hasenclever et al. collected data on 5141 patients with advanced stage HL and identified seven adverse prognostic factors (Table 1) (9). The International Prognostic Score

Table 1: Prognostic factors in advanced stage Hodgkin's lymphoma.

1. Male gender.
2. Age of 45 years or older.
3. Stage IV (according to the Ann Arbor classification).
4. Hemaglobin < 10.5g/dl.
5. Serum albumin < 4g/dl.
6. Leukocytosis (WBC > 15000/mm^3).
7. Lymphocytopenia (ALC < 600/mm^3 or lymphocyte count < 8% of WBC).

No. of risk factors	Freedom from progression at 5 years
0	84%
1	77%
2	67%
3	60%
4	51%
> 5	42%

(IPS) predicted a 5-year freedom from progression (FFP) ranging from 84% in patients with no risk factors to 42% in those with 5 or more factors present. Most notably, no IPS score predicted a 5-year FFP of less than 42%. Identification of other poor prognostic factors, particularly biologic factors, may allow a more tailored approach to therapy.

This chapter will concentrate on the contemporary management of advanced HL, highlighting the current standard chemotherapy regimens, the role of radiotherapy, new approaches under investigation for initial therapy, and therapy of relapsed disease.

2.   STANDARD THERAPY

The development of a combination chemotherapy program, MOPP (mechlorethamine, vincristine, procarbazine, prednisone) in the 1960's was associated with a dramatic improvement in the prognosis of patients with advanced HL. The initial excitement surrounding the discovery of MOPP, however, was soon tempered with the emergence of an increased risk of acute leukemia, sterility in nearly all men and a majority of women, primary treatment failure in 20% of patients, and relapse following complete response in 10-40% (10). These limitations spurred efforts to search for alternative therapies and led to the development of the ABVD (adriamycin, bleomycin, vinblastine, dacarbazine) regimen (Table 2).

Table 2. ABVD Regimen

DRUG	Dose	Schedule*
Adriamycin	25 mg/m^2	D1, 15
Bleomycin	10 u/m^2	D1, 15
Vinblastine	6 mg/m^2	D1, 15
DTIC	375 mg/m^2	D1, 15

*Repeat every 28 days

Bonadonna et al. at the Milan Cancer Institute introduced ABVD in 1974 (11). This regimen contained none of the agents included in MOPP and non-cross resistance was suggested based on preliminary observations of its efficacy in MOPP-resistant patients (11). Based on these observations, the Milan group conducted a prospective, randomized trial comparing MOPP to a program combining the 2 non-cross resistant regimens in an alternating sequence, MOPP/ABVD (10). Eight year follow up of this trial revealed superiority for MOPP/ABVD both in relapse-free and overall survival (OS) in patients with stage IV HL (10).

In an attempt to confirm these observations, CALGB designed a randomized phase III trial (CALGB 8251) comparing ABVD, MOPP/ABVD and MOPP in stage III-IV HL patients and included patients who had failed previous radiation (12). The results of this landmark study dictated the contemporary management of advanced HL. At 5 years, failure-free survival (FFS) rates were superior for ABVD (61%) and MOPP/ABVD (65%) when compared with MOPP monotherapy (50%) (P=0.02 for the comparison of MOPP to the other regimens). Overall survival was not statistically different among the three arms. There was significantly less myelotoxicity in patients treated with ABVD with only 2% of patients experiencing grade 3 or 4 infection compared with 12-15% in the MOPP-containing arms. The long-term follow up of this trial has recently been published (13). At a median follow up of 14.1 years, the superiority of ABVD and MOPP/ABVD over MOPP in terms of FFS is maintained. OS was not significantly different among the three treatment groups. The advantage of ABVD over MOPP-containing regimens was again confirmed by an intergroup trial comparing ABVD to the MOPP/ABV hybrid regimen (14). These regimens showed equal efficacy but significantly fewer short and long-term toxicities with ABVD.

The efficacy and favorable toxicity profile of 6-8 cycles of ABVD, established this regimen as the current gold standard for the treatment of advanced HL. However, both the efficacy and toxicity data also point out the need for further improvement. The long-term follow-up of patients with advanced stage HL treated with ABVD shows a 14-yr FFS rate of 48% and OS of 58% (13). With less than half the patients alive and in remission, better therapies are needed. In addition, nearly all series of patients treated with ABVD include both acute and delayed cardiopulmonary deaths. In the initial CALGB trial, Canellos et al. reported "clinically important severe pulmonary toxicity" in 6% of patients with 3 of 115 patients treated with ABVD dying from pulmonary toxicity (12). In the more recent CALGB trial, Duggan et al. reported Grade 2 or greater pulmonary toxicity in 24.5% of patients during ABVD treatment and 8.3% after completion of treatment (14). Eight of 433 patients treated with ABVD died of respiratory failure either on or after therapy. Interestingly, Canellos and Duggan reviewed the outcome of patients with advanced HL treated with ABVD in whom bleomycin was discontinued and found no difference in 10-yr relapse rates among the 40 pts who received less than 6 cycles of bleomycin compared to the 323 patients who received all doses of bleomycin (15). "This analysis suggests that bleomycin may have a limited role in the ABVD regimen and can be discontinued with impunity in the event of pulmonary complications" (15).

3. NEW APPROACHES TO INITIAL THERAPY

Combining MOPP and ABVD, either as alternating cycles or in a hybrid fashion based on the Goldie-Coldman hypothesis that therapeutic efficacy is enhanced by introducing all effective agents within each treatment cycle instead of in an alternating fashion, showed no benefit in efficacy and was more toxic compared to ABVD(13, 14, 16). Due to a lack of new agents, recent efforts have continued to emphasize new ways to give old drugs, including alterations in both dose and schedule. The German Hodgkin Study Group (GHSG) has published favorable results with dose-intense BEACOPP (bleomycin, etoposide, doxorubicin, cyclophosphamide, vincristine, procarbazine, and prednisone) and investigators from Stanford as part of a national trial are currently evaluating the Stanford V regimen, which alternates myelosuppressive and non-myelosuppressive drugs weekly to provide continuous exposure to active chemotherapy while limiting cumulative doses (17, 18). Results of randomized trials of both regimens compared to ABVD are not yet available.

3.1 BEACOPP

Based on observations in several animal models that a clear relationship between chemotherapy dose and tumor response exist, the GHSG developed a mathematical model which predicted that moderate dose escalation would increase tumor control by 10-15% at five years (19). Based on this model, the BEACOPP regimen was developed with a 21-day drug administration schedule and additional local RT to sites of bulky disease and those with residual disease after chemotherapy (20).

A pilot study of 30 advanced HL patients treated with 8 cycles of the regimen, confirmed both its safety and efficacy (20). This was followed by a dose-finding study with granulocyte colony stimulating factor support, in which the respective doses of cyclophosphamide, doxorubicin and etoposide were escalated to 190%, 200% and 140% of baseline BEACOPP (21). The escalated BEACOPP regimen (Table 3) was both tolerable and efficacious, providing an estimated freedom from treatment failure (FFTF) rate of 89% at 5 years.

Table 3. Escalated BEACOPP Regimen

Drug	Dose	Schedule*
Bleomycin	10 u/m^2	D8
Etoposide	200 mg/m^2	D1, 2, 3
Doxorubicin	35 mg/m^2	D1
Cyclophosphamide	1200 mg/m^2	D1
Vincristine	1.4 mg/m^{2**}	D8
Procarbazine	100 mg	D1 – 7
Prednisone	40 mg	D1 – 14

* Repeat every 21 days
** Maximum dose 2 mg

The preliminary data gathered in these two studies provided the basis for the GHSG three arm randomized HD9 study comparing COPP/ABVD, baseline BEACOPP and escalated BEACOPP (25). Additional RT was provided for initial bulky disease at diagnosis or for residual disease after chemotherapy. Accrual to the COPP/ABVD arm was halted in 1996 due to inferior FFTF in this arm compared with the pooled BEACOPP arms. Results of this trial demonstrate 5-year FFTF rates of 69% for COPP/ABVD, 76% for BEACOPP and 87% for escalated BEACOPP ($P<0.05$ for each 2-arm comparison) (22). Furthermore, escalated BEACOPP had a significantly superior 5-year OS rate compared with COPP/ABVD (91% vs. 83%, p=0.002).

The toxicities of escalated BEACOPP are substantial, including grade 4 leukopenia in 90%, grade 3-4 thrombocytopenia in 70%, and grade 3-4 infections in 22% of patients (22). Fatal acute toxicities were <2% and were due primarily to sepsis and pneumonia. The 5-year actuarial rate of secondary acute leukemia was 2.5% in the escalated BEACOPP arm. Infertility is frequent with this regimen and sperm banking is recommended for all males interested in fathering children. Escalated BEACOPP is not appropriate for patients 65 years or older due to unacceptable toxicity (23).

The GHSG is continuing to explore ways to improve therapy for patients with advanced HL. Preliminary results of HD12, a randomized trial of eight cycles of escalated BEACOPP vs. four cycles of escalated BEACOPP followed by four doses of standard BEACOPP showed no difference on toxicity between the two arms (3.3% early death rate) and a slight advantage for escalated BEACOPP in 2-yr FFTF rates (92% vs. 87%) (24). Results of a second randomization ± RT showed no advantage to RT following either regimen. A pilot study of the BEACOPP-14 regimen (standard dose BEACOPP given every 14 days instead of 21 days) showed 34-mo FFTF and OS rates of 90% and 97% respectively, results similar to those seen with escalated BEACOPP, despite lower cumulative doses of cyclophosphamide, etoposide, and doxorubicin (25). The GHSG is currently comparing escalated BEACOPP (8 cycles), escalated BEACOPP (6 cycles) and BEACOPP-14 (8 cycles).

The European Organization for Research and Treatment of Cancer (EORTC) conducted a randomized trial (20012) comparing eight cycles of ABVD to four cycles of escalated BEACOPP plus four cycles of standard BEACOPP (26). Eligibility was limited to patients with IPS of greater than three. RT was not given in either arm. Results of this study are not yet available, but may establish a new standard of care for high-risk advanced stage HL.

3.2   Stanford V

Concerns regarding the risk of sterility and leukemia associated with MOPP-containing regimens and theoretical concerns of cardiopulmonary toxicity with ABVD led to the development of the Stanford V regimen (doxorubicin, vinblastine, nitrogen mustard, vincristine, bleomycin, etoposide and prednisone) in 1988 by investigators at Stanford University (18, 27). In an attempt to minimize these toxicities without compromising efficacy, they proposed shortening the duration of chemotherapy by a combination of dose intensification and sophisticated consolidative RT. Treatment is administered weekly over 12 weeks and is characterized by a reduction in the cumulative doses of doxorubicin (150 mg/m^2) and bleomycin (30 units/m^2) compared with ABVD, marked reduction of total dose of nitrogen mustard (18 mg/m^2) compared to MOPP and omission of procarbazine (Table 4). Upon completion of chemotherapy, patients receive consolidative RT of 36Gy, restricted to sites of bulky disease ($\geq$ 5cm) or macroscopic splenic disease at presentation.

Data on the first 142 patients with stage I/II disease with bulky mediastinal nodes or stage III/IV HL treated at Stanford showed 5-yr FFP (freedom from progression) and OS rates of 89% and 96%, respectively (27). Ninety percent of patients received RT. Results by IPS showed a 5-yr

FFP rate of 100% in patients with no risk factors, 91% for 1 risk factor, 95% for 2 risk factors, 86% for 3 risk factors and 65% for 4 or more risk factors. In the short-term, toxicity appears primarily to be limited to myelosuppression, constipation, fatigue and peripheral neuropathy with preservation of fertility.

Table 4. Stanford V Regimen

Drug	Dose	Schedule*
Nitrogen Mustard	6 mg/m^2	Week 1, 5, 9
Doxorubicin	25 mg/m^2	Week 1, 3, 5, 7, 9, 11
Vinblastine	6 mg/m^2	Week 1, 3, 5, 7, 9, 11
Bleomycin	5 mg/m^2	Week 2, 4, 6, 8, 10, 12
Vincristine	1.4 mg/m^{2**}	Week 2, 4, 6, 8, 10, 12
VP-16	60 mg/m^2 D1, 2	Week 3, 7, 11
Prednisone	40 mg/m^2	Daily, weeks 1 – 10§

* Repeat every 21 days
** Maximum dose 2 mg
§ Taper weeks 11 – 12

Although the Stanford V regimen appears effective, its role in the contemporary management of advanced HL is unclear. A recently updated Italian study of 332 patients with advanced HL shows the regimen to be significantly inferior to both ABVD and MEC (meclorethamine, CCNU, vindesine, alkeran, prednisone, epidoxorubicin, vincristine, procarbazine, vinblastine, bleomycin) in terms of response, FFS and FFP (28, 29). At a median follow-up of 56 months, the 5-yr FFP was 86%, 93% and 76% for ABVD, MEC and Stanford V respectively (p<0.01) (29). Only 66% of the patients in the Stanford V arm received RT and may explain the discrepancy between this data and that obtained at Stanford University. This is concerning and lends credence to the theory that the chemotherapy phase of Stanford V only reduces tumor bulk to a point and that consolidative RT, which is not without significant long-term risk, is necessary to effect a CR (30).

The ongoing United States Intergroup trial in which patients with bulky stage II and stage III-IV HL, are randomized to ABVD or Stanford V (with involved field RT), will hopefully clearly define the precise role of the Stanford V regimen in the management of advanced HL.

3.3 Stem Cell Transplant

In an effort to decrease relapse rates, several investigators have evaluated the use of autologous stem cell transplantation (ASCT) in first remission for high-risk patients. Carella et al. was the first to report a significant survival advantage for patients with advanced stage HL undergoing ASCT in first remission compared to historical controls with similar risk factors (31, 32). Based on this encouraging preliminary data, two large randomized trials were initiated in Europe. Unfortunately, both of these studies demonstrated no benefit from early intensification with high-dose therapy and ASCT compared with conventional chemotherapy in patients with advanced unfavorable HL who initially responded to front line chemotherapy (33, 34). Frederico et al. randomized 163 patients to ABVD x 8 cycles vs. ABVD x 4 cycles + ASCT (33). The 5-yr FFS rates were 82% for ABVD and 75% for ABVD + ASCT (P=NS) with no difference in the 5-yr OS (88%). The GEOLAMS randomized 122 patients to ABVD x 4 cycles + ASCT vs. ABVD x 4 cycles + 3 cycles of "intermediate dose chemotherapy"(34). The 4-yr FFP rates were 55% for ASCT and 85% for the intermediate chemotherapy arm (P=0.16). Based on these results, there is no indication for ASCT in first remission.

3.4 New Agents

While limited new agents are available for HL, investigators have attempted to incorporate the pyrimidine metabolite, gemcitabine into regimens for untreated advanced stage HL. Response rates of 39-43% were noted with single agent gemcitabine in relapsed or refractory HL (35, 36). Bredenfeld et al. replaced etoposide in the BEACOPP regimen with gemcitabine (37). Eight of 27 patients treated with BAGCOPP experienced severe pulmonary toxicity, mainly pneumonitis. The authors hypothesized that the lung toxicity was related to the concomitant application of gemcitabine and bleomycin and concluded the combination was not feasible. Friedberg et al. treated 12 patients on a pilot study of ABVG (doxorubicin, bleomycin, vinblastine, gemcitabine) replacing dacarbazine with gemcitabine 800 mg/m^2 on day 1 and 15 (38). Five of the 12 patients developed clinically significant pulmonary toxicity resulting in early closure of the study. Again, the authors concluded that bleomycin and gemcitabine should not be combined in the treatment of HL. New regimens, eliminating bleomycin and incorporating gemcitabine into first-line treatment for HL, are in development.

3.5   Radiotherapy

RT remains the most effective single agent for the treatment of HL and the curative potential of this modality in early-stage disease has been extensively documented. The rationale for the use of adjuvant RT in patients with advanced HL was the initial observation that relapse after MOPP occurred, in the majority of cases, primarily in previously involved or non-irradiated sites (39). Early studies clearly demonstrated reduction in the frequency of recurrence and improvement in both the rate of CR and disease-free survival with the addition of well-tolerated adjuvant RT (40). This encouraging preliminary data provided the initial impetus for the routine use of combined modality regimens in the treatment of advanced HL.

Several large, prospective randomized trials were subsequently undertaken to more clearly delineate the role of consolidative RT and to quantify the potential benefit, if any, of combined modality therapy (41-43). These studies, although small and underpowered, have consistently failed to show any benefit to RT. A Southwest Oncology Group (SWOG) multi-institutional study of 278 patients with stage III and stage IV HL, who achieved a CR with MOP-BAP (nitrogen mustard, vincristine, prednisone, bleomycin, doxorubicin and procarbazine), were randomized to receive low dose RT or no further therapy (41). No extended remission duration or OS advantage was noted with consolidative low dose RT, although significantly better outcomes were seen in a subset analyses of patients who actually received RT. There was a significantly higher relapse-free survival rate in the patients with bulky, mediastinal nodular sclerosing HL following RT. Two subsequent European studies in which further chemotherapy was compared to consolidative RT after CR with chemotherapy, also failed to detect any disease-free or overall survival benefit in the irradiated cohorts (42, 43).

In 2003, the EORTC published results of a trial which randomized 333 patients with stage III/IV HL in CR following MOPP/ABV hybrid to observation vs. radiotherapy with 24 Gy to all initially involved nodal areas and 16-24 Gy to all initially involved extranodal sites (44). The 5-yr event-free survival (EFS) rates were 84% in the group that did not receive radiotherapy and 79% in the group that received radiotherapy (P=0.035). 5-yr OS rates were 91% and 85% respectively (P=0.07). With a median follow-up of 79 months, second cancers developed in 6 patients in the chemotherapy group and 15 pts in the chemotherapy plus involved field radiotherapy group. The 5-yr cumulative rates of second cancer were 4% and 7.8%, respectively (P=0.05). Of the 15 cases of acute leukemia or myelodysplasia, 13 were in patients who were irradiated.

Accurate interpretation of individual studies is often limited by both small sample size and deviations from assigned treatment (intent to treat analysis) inviting the possibility of potential false negative outcomes. In an attempt to overcome these limitations, Loeffler et al. performed a meta-analysis on 1740 patients from 14 randomized adjuvant radiation trials (45). Two separate designs were compared. In the additional design, RT was added to the same chemotherapy (MOPP–like regimens in majority of studies) while in the parallel design; RT was substituted in the control (chemotherapy) arm with further chemotherapy. In the additional RT design, there was an 11% overall improvement in tumor control rate after 10 years but OS was unchanged. In contrast, the parallel design trials demonstrated no difference in tumor control rates in the two arms but OS was significantly better after 10 years in those patients who did not receive RT.

Stanford V and BEACOPP both include involved field RT. While these regimens both demonstrated enhanced FFP and OS, no data is available yet comparing them with ABVD. It is possible that the encouraging data observed with these two newer regimens may in fact be a function of the additional RT given, rather than the chemotherapy agents used. Furthermore, it will be at least two decades before the second malignancy risk resulting from the additional RT can be fully appreciated. How this may ultimately impact on the long-term survival of patients treated with these regimens is currently unknown. The results of multiple randomized trials indicate that RT should not be administered as consolidative therapy in patients with advanced stage HL treated with standard therapy regimens.

4. RELAPSED/REFRACTORY DISEASE

Approximately 40% of patients with advanced stage HL will eventually relapse. Cytoreduction with a standard salvage regimen (re-treatment with the primary regimen or use of non-cross resistant regimen) followed by ASCT is the most effective treatment for patients with relapsed or refractory HL.

Poor prognostic factors at relapse include first remission duration less than 12 months, stage III/IV disease, B symptoms, anemia, poor performance status, and elevated ESR (46-50). In a report of 280 patients with relapsed HL treated with ASCT, remission duration of less than 12 months and extranodal relapse were identified as poor prognostic features (50). Four-year OS rates were 93%, 59%, and 43% (P<0.0001) respectively, for patients with none, one, or both of these factors. In 119 patients with relapsed HL transplanted at Stanford University, lung or marrow involvement at time of transplant, B symptoms at relapse, and more than minimal residual disease at transplant were independent predictors of worse FFP and OS (48). Four-year FFP was 82% for patients with none of these risk factors, versus 41% for one or more. Patients with all three risk factors had a 12% FFP rate. Patients with initial remission duration longer than 12 months may have a long-term remission with additional standard chemotherapy without transplantation (47, 51). These patients are also the ones with the best outcome following ASCT. In a randomized trial of the GHSG comparing standard chemotherapy to ASCT, patients with early and late relapse both benefited from transplant (52). Three-yr FFTF rates were 12% and 44% with standard chemotherapy and 41% and 75% for ASCT, for patients with early and late relapse respectively.

4.1   Standard Salvage Regimens

A wide variety of salvage regimens have been used with reported response rates of 40-80% (53-56). These programs are predominantly etoposide or cisplatin based, in an effort to provide non-cross resistant drugs to patients previously failing ABVD. The most commonly used salvage regimens are ESHAP (etoposide, solumedrol, high-dose cytarabine and cisplatin), ICE (ifosfamide, carboplatin, and etoposide), MINE (mitoguazone, ifosfamide, vinorelbine, and etoposide), and ASHAP (doxorubicin, solumedrol, high-dose cytarabine, and cisplatin) (53-56). In single institution series, CR rates of 30-40% have been documented with these regimens in refractory/relapsed HL. Response to standard salvage chemotherapy is an important predictor of outcome following ASCT. Although there are no clear guidelines, the use of these regimens is generally limited to 2-4 cycles pre-transplant to maximize cytoreduction and minimize stem cell injury prior to apheresis.

4.2   Autologous Stem Cell Transplantation

The role of high dose chemotherapy and stem cell transplantation in the management of patients with relapsed or refractory HL has been extensively evaluated since its introduction 15 years ago. The early literature was characterized by unacceptably high relapse rates, in excess of 60% in some studies, and transplant related mortality rates of 20% or greater. The introduction of growth factors, improvement of antimicrobial therapy, refinement of conditioning regimens and a movement to earlier transplantation have led to both a significant reduction in mortality and improved survival rates. Most centers now perform ASCT with less than a 5% early mortality and with relapse rates of 40-50% (52).

Two randomized trials have confirmed the benefit of ASCT over conventional salvage chemotherapy for relapsed HL. The British National Lymphoma Study Group compared high-dose BEAM (carmustine, etoposide, cytarabine, melphalan) followed by ASCT with a dose-reduced variation of BEAM, mini-BEAM, for patients who failed front-line therapy (57). This study closed prematurely after accruing only 40 patients because of patient refusal to enter the dose-reduced arm. At 36 months, the progression-free survival rate was 53% in the transplant arm compared with only 10% in the mini-BEAM arm (p=0.025). In a subsequent study in a similar population group conducted by the GHSG, 161 patients with relapsed disease were randomized to 4 cycles of DexaBEAM (aggressive conventional chemotherapy) versus 2 cycles of DexaBEAM and high dose chemotherapy with BEAM followed by ASCT (52). Only pts with chemosensitive disease following 2 cycles of DexaBEAM proceeded to further treatment (n-117). The 3-yr FFTF rates were 34% and 55% for DexaBEAM and ASCT respectively (P=0.019). There was no difference in overall survival. 3-year FFTF with ASCT was 75% for patients with late relapse (>12 months) and 41% for patients with early relapse.

4.3   Allogeneic Stem cell Transplantation

The role of allogeneic stem cell transplantation for patients with relapsed or refractory HL is uncertain. Until the introduction of non-myeloablative preparative regimens, allogeneic transplantation was considered only for patients with inadequate autologous stem cell collection or relapse after ASCT. Based on review of 90 "matched" patients undergoing allogeneic or autologous transplantation reported to the European Bone Marrow Transplant (EBMT) registry, Milpied et al. reported better OS rates for patients undergoing ASCT compared to allogeneic transplantation (58). Four-year procedure related mortality was 48% versus 27% for allogeneic versus autologous transplantation, and for patients with chemosensitive relapse, 65% vs. 12%, respectively. The EBMT also published results of 167 patients with relapsed or refractory HL who received allogeneic transplant as their first transplant procedure (59). Four-year OS was 24.7% and the procedure related mortality was 51.7%. Interestingly, in this series, relapse rate was also worse in the allogeneic group.

Current efforts are focused on evaluation of non-myeloablative allogeneic transplantation, primarily for patients who relapse after ASCT or have inadequate marrow reserve for successful ASCT. Anderlini et al.

reported a 100-day transplant related mortality of 8% in 25 patients with heavily pre-treated HL treated with a fludarabine-based reduced-intensity conditioning regimen and matched related or unrelated donor stem cells (60). Tandem transplants with a non-myeloablative allogeneic transplant following ASCT are also under investigation in patients with refractory HL, again with acceptable treatment-related mortality rates (61).

5.   NON-TRANSPLANT APPROACHES

Treatment choices for patients ineligible for transplant because of advanced age, comorbidity, or inadequate stem cell reserve or those relapsing after transplant, is often limited by the cumulative toxicity of their prior therapy. These patients are often good candidates for clinical trials testing new agents.   Alternatively, sequential single-agents are often reasonable options. Many patients will respond to previously administered agents, especially if the remission following such agents was greater than a year.

In this setting, the goals of therapy are largely palliative and primarily include symptom control with a major emphasis placed on limiting treatment-related toxicity (62). Several agents have been successfully used in a sequential fashion. Examples of agents, which are usually well tolerated for an extended period of time, include vinorelbine, vinblastine, gemcitabine, etoposide, chlorambucil, and cyclophosphamide (35, 36, 62-65).

Vinorelbine, used as single-agent therapy, had a response rate of 50% (complete 14%; partial 36%) in 22 extensively pre-treated HL patients (63). The median duration of response for a weekly dose of 30 mg/m^2 was 6 months and treatment related toxicity including neurological, was mild and reversible. Furthermore, myelosuppression, which was the dose-limiting toxicity, was not cumulative. Vinblastine, which has a similar mode of action to vinorelbine, has also been successfully used in extensively pre-treated patients (62). Using a dose of 4-6 mg/m^2 every 1-2 weeks, Little et al. reported a response rate of 59% (complete12%; partial 47%). Hematological, gastrointestinal, and neurological toxicities were mild and there were no treatment-related deaths. Gemcitabine has also been used in the salvage setting. Two recent phase II trials reported response rates of 39-43% in relapsed HL (35, 36).

It is clear that several well-tolerated chemotherapy agents used as monotherapy, demonstrate activity in extensively pre-treated patients with advanced HL. The challenge for the future is to possibly combine these agents, without increasing toxicity, to maximize the benefit to relapsed or refractory patients. In a Phase I/II study, CALGB evaluated GVD (gemcitabine, vinorelbine, and liposomal doxorubicin) in patients with relapsed or refractory HL. Overall response rates were 58% for patients not previously transplanted and 68% for patients failing a prior transplant (66). The regimen was well tolerated with no treatment-related deaths. This regimen may be useful in both the salvage setting prior to transplant as well as for patients failing transplant or ineligible for transplant.

6.   CONCLUSIONS

The treatment of advanced HL represents a success story for medical oncology. Over the past 50 years, a universally fatal disease is now potentially curable with the contemporary standard of care, ABVD, effecting cure in 65% of patients treated. Several challenges remain and include defining the pathogenesis of HL at the cellular level, identifying patients at increased risk of treatment failure and improving therapies for patients with high risk or relapsed disease. The results of several ongoing clinical trials evaluating new agents are eagerly awaited.

7.   REFERENCES

1. Thomas RK, Re D, Zander T, Wolf J, Diehl V. Epidemiology and etiology of Hodgkin's lymphoma. Annals of Oncology. 2002; 13 Suppl 4:147-52.
2. Fung HC, Nademanee AP. Approach to Hodgkin's lymphoma in the new millennium. Hematological Oncology 2002; 20(1):1-15.
3. Kuppers R, Klein U, Hansmann ML, Rajewsky K. Cellular origin of human B-cell lymphomas. New England Journal of Medicine 1999; 341(20): 1520-1529.
4. Jaffe ES, Harris NL, Diebold J, Muller-Hermelink HK. World Health Organization classification of neoplastic diseases of the hematopoietic and lymphoid tissues. A progress report. Am J Clin Pathol. 1999; 111(Suppl 1): S8-12.
5. DeVita VT Jr, Simon RM, Hubbard SM, Young RC, Berard CW, Moxley JH 3rd, Frei E 3rd, Carbone PP, Canellos GP. Curability of advanced Hodgkin's disease with chemotherapy. Long-term follow-up of MOPP-treated patients at the National Cancer Institute. Ann Intern Med. 1980; 92(5): 587-95.
6. Aisenberg AC. Problems in Hodgkin's disease management. Blood 1999; 93(3): 761-779.
7. Carbone PP, Kaplan HS, Musshoff K, Smithers DW, Tubiana M. Report of the Committee on Hodgkin's Disease Staging Classification. Cancer Res. 1971; 31(11):1860-1861.
8. Glossman JP, Josting A, Diehl V. New treatments for Hodgkin's disease. Current Treatment Options in Oncology 2002; 3: 283-290.
9. Hasenclever D, Diehl V. A prognostic score for advanced Hodgkin's disease. International Prognostic Factors Project on Advanced Hodgkin's Disease. N Engl J Med 1998; 339(21):1506-14.

10. Bonadonna G, Valagussa P, Santoro A. Alternating non-cross-resistant combination chemotherapy or MOPP in stage IV Hodgkin's disease. A report of 8-year results. Ann Intern Med. 1986;104(6): 739-46.

11. Bonadonna G, Zucali R, Monfardini S, De Lena M, Uslenghi C. Combination chemotherapy of Hodgkin's disease with adriamycin, bleomycin, vinblastine, and imidazole carboxamide versus MOPP. Cancer 1975; 36(1): 252-9.

12. Canellos GP, Anderson JR, Propert KJ, Nissen N, Cooper MR, Henderson ES, Green MR, Gottlieb A, Peterson BA. Chemotherapy of advanced Hodgkin's disease with MOPP, ABVD, or MOPP alternating with ABVD. N Engl J Med. 1992; 327(21):1478-84.

13. Canellos GP, Niedzwiecki D. Long-term follow-up of Hodgkin's disease trial. N Engl J Med 2002; 346(18):1417-1418.

14. Duggan DB, Petroni GR, Johnson JL, Glick JH, Fisher RI, Connors JM, Canellos GP, Peterson BA. Randomized comparison of ABVD and MOPP/ABV hybrid for the treatment of advanced Hodgkin's disease: report of an intergroup trial. J Clin Oncol. 2003; 21(4): 607-14.

15. Canellos GP, Duggan D. How important is Bleomycin in the Adriamycin + Bleomycin + Vinblastine + Dacarbazine. J Clin Oncol. 2004; 22(8): 1532-1533.

16. Goldie JH, Coldman AJ. A mathematic model for relating the drug sensitivity of tumors to their spontaneous mutation rate. Cancer Treat Rep. 1979; 63(11-12): 1727-33.

17. Diehl V, Franklin J, Hasenclever D, Tesch H, Pfreundschuh M, Lathan B, Paulus U, Sieber M, Rueffer JU, Sextro M, Engert A, Wolf J, Hermann R, Holmer L, Stappert-Jahn U, Winnerlein-Trump E, Wulf G, Krause S, Glunz A, von Kalle K, Bischoff H, Haedicke C, Duehmke E, Georgii A, Loeffler M. BEACOPP, a new dose-escalated and accelerated regimen, is at least as effective as COPP/ABVD in patients with advanced-stage Hodgkin's lymphoma: interim report from a trial of the German Hodgkin's Lymphoma Study Group. J Clin Oncol. 1998;16(12): 3810-21.

18. Bartlett NL, Rosenberg SA, Hoppe RT, Hancock SL, Horning SJ. Brief chemotherapy, Stanford V, and adjuvant radiotherapy for bulky or advanced-stage Hodgkin's disease: a preliminary report. J Clin Oncol. 1995; 13(5):1080-88.

19. Hasenclever D, Loeffler M, Diehl V. Rationale for dose escalation of first line conventional chemotherapy in advanced Hodgkin's disease. German Hodgkin's Lymphoma Study Group. Ann Oncol. 1996; 7 Suppl 4: 95-98.

20. Diehl V, Sieber M, Ruffer U, Lathan B, Hasenclever D, Pfreundschuh M, Loeffler M, Lieberz D, Koch P, Adler M, Tesch H. BEACOPP: an intensified chemotherapy regimen in advanced Hodgkin's disease. The German Hodgkin's Lymphoma Study Group. Ann Oncol. 1997; 8(2):143-148.

21. Tesch H, Diehl V, Lathan B, Hasenclever D, Sieber M, Ruffer U, Engert A, Franklin J, Pfreundschuh M, Schalk KP, Schwieder G, Wulf G, Dolken G, Worst P, Koch P, Schmitz N, Bruntsch U, Tirier C, Muller U, Loeffler M. Moderate dose escalation for advanced stage Hodgkin's disease using the bleomycin, etoposide, adriamycin, cyclophosphamide, vincristine, procarbazine, and prednisone scheme and adjuvant radiotherapy: a study of the German Hodgkin's Lymphoma Study Group. Blood. 1998; 92(12): 4560-67.

22. Diehl V, Franklin J, Pfreundschuh M, Lathan B, Paulus U, Hasenclever D, Tesch H, Herrmann R, Dorken B, Muller-Hermelink HK, Duhmke E, Loeffler M. Standard and increased-dose BEACOPP chemotherapy compared with COPP-ABVD for advanced Hodgkin's disease. N Engl J Med. 2003; 348(24):2386-2395.

23. Ballova V, et al. BEACOPP chemotherapy in elderly patients with advanced Hodgkin's disease: analysis of the randomized trial HD9 for elderly patients of the German Hodgkin Lymphoma Study Group. Blood. 2003; 103: 40a. Abstract.

24. Diehl V, et al. Results of the third interim analysis of the HD12 trial of the GHSG: 8 courses of the escalated BEACOPP versus 4 escalated and 4 baseline courses of

BEACOPP with or without additive radiotherapy for advanced stage Hodgkin's lymphoma. Blood. 2003; 102:27a. Abstract.

25. Sieber M, Bredenfeld H, Josting A, et al. 14-day variant of the bleomycin, etoposide, doxorubicin, cyclophosphamide, vincristine, procarbazine, and prednisone regimen in advanced-stage Hodgkin's lymphoma: results of a pilot study of the German Hodgkin's Lymphoma Study Group. J Clin Oncol. 2003; 21: 1734-1739.

26. Franklin J, Diehl V. Current clinical trials for the treatment of advanced-stage Hodgkin's disease: BEACOPP. Ann Oncol. 2002; 13 Suppl 1:98-101.

27. Horning SJ, Hoppe RT, Breslin S, Bartlett NL, Brown BW, Rosenberg SA. Stanford V and radiotherapy for locally extensive and advanced Hodgkin's disease: mature results of a prospective clinical trial. J Clin Oncol. 2002; 20(3): 630-637.

28. Chisesi T, Federico M, Levis A, Lambertenghi G, Gobbi PG, Santini G, Luminari S, Brugiatelli M. ABVD versus Stanford V versus MEC in unfavorable Hodgkin's lymphoma: results of a randomized trial. Annals of Oncology. 2002; 13 Suppl 1: 102-106.

29. Federico M, Levis A, Luminari S, Chisesi T, Marcheselli L, Goldaniga M, Vitolo U, Neri S, Brugiatelli M, Gobbi PG. ABVD vs Stanford V vs MOPP-EBV-CAD (MEC) in advanced Hodgkins lymphoma. Final results of the IIL HD9601 randomized trial. Proc ASCO. 2004; 6507 (abstract).

30. Canellos GP. New treatments for advanced Hodgkin's disease: an uphill fight beginning close to the top. J Clin Oncol. 2002; 20(3): 607-609.

31. Carella AM, Carlier P, Congiu A, Occhini D, Nati S, Santini G, Pierluigi D, Giordano D, Bacigalupo A, Damasio E. Autologous bone marrow transplantation as adjuvant treatment for high-risk Hodgkin's disease in first complete remission after MOPP/ABVD protocol. Bone Marrow Transplant. 1991; 8(2): 99-103.

32. Carella AM, Prencipe E, Pungolino E, Lerma E, Frassoni F, Rossi E, Giordano D, Occhini D, Gatti AM, Bruni R, Spriano M, Nati S, Pierluigi D, Congiu M, Vimercati R, Ravetti JL, Federico M. Twelve years experience with high-dose therapy and autologous stem cell transplantation for high-risk Hodgkin's disease patients in first remission after MOPP/ABVD chemotherapy. Leuk Lymphoma. 1996; 21(1-2): 63-70.

33. Federico M, Bellei M, Brice P, Brugiatelli M, Nagler A, Gisselbrecht C, Moretti L, Colombat P, Luminari S, Fabbiano F, Di Renzo N, Goldstone A, Carella AM. High-dose therapy and autologous stem-cell transplantation versus conventional therapy for patients with advanced Hodgkin's lymphoma responding to front-line therapy. J Clin Oncol. 2003; 21(12): 2320-2325.

34. Saghatchian M, Djeridane M, Escoffre-Barbe M, Desablens B, Foussard C, Lacotte-Thierry L, Lamy T, Vigier M, Lucas V, Casassus P, Legouffe E, Ghandour C, Dugay J, Flesch M, Le Tortorec S, Maigre M, Jardel H, Audhuy B, Colombat P, Colonna P, Andrieu JM. Very high risk Hodgkin's disease (HD): ABVd (4 cycles) plus BEAM followed by autologous stem cell transplantation (ASCT) and radiotherapy (RT) versus intensive chemotherapy (3 cycles) (INT-CT) and RT. Four-year results of the GOELAMS H97-GM multicentric randomized trial. Proceedings of ASCO. 2002; 263a. Abstract 1051.

35. Santoro A, Bredenfeld H, Devizzi L, Tesch H, Bonfante V, Viviani S, Fiedler F, Parra HS, Benoehr C, Pacini M, Bonadonna G, Diehl V. Gemcitabine in the treatment of refractory Hodgkin's disease: results of a multicenter phase II study. J Clin Oncol. 2000;18(13): 2615-2619.

36. Zinzani PL, Bendandi M, Stefoni V, Albertini P, Gherlinzoni F, Tani M, Piccaluga PP, Tura S. Value of Gemcitabine treatment in heavily pretreated Hodgkin's disease patients. Haematologica, 2000; 85(9): 926-9.

37. Bredenfeld H, Franklin J, Nogova L, Josting A, Fries S, Mailander V, Oertel J, Diehl V, Engert A. Severe pulmonary toxicity in patients with advanced-stage Hodgkin's disease

treated with a modified Bleomycin, Doxorubicin, Cyclophosphamide, Vincristine, Procarbazine, Prednisone, and Gemcitabine (BEACOPP) regimen is probably related to the combination of Gemcitabine and Bleomycin: A report of the German Hodgkin's Lymphoma Study Group. J Clin Oncol. 2004; 22(12); 2424-2429.

38. Friedberg JW, Nurberg D, Bendell C, Miyata S, McCauley M, Fisher DC, Takvorian T, Canellos GP. Phase I study of Gemcitabine added to Doxorubicin, Bleomycin, and Vinblastine for the treatment of De Novo Hodgkin's disease (HD): Increased pulmonary toxicity compared with ABVD. Proceedings of ASH. 2002; 159a. Abstract 596.

39. Young RC, Canellos GP, Chabner BA, Hubbard SM, DeVita VT. Patterns of relapse in advanced Hodgkin's disease treated with combination chemotherapy. Cancer. 1978; 42(2 Suppl):1001-1007.

40. Yahalom J, Ryu J, Straus DJ, Gaynor JJ, Myers J, Caravelli J, Clarkson BD, Fuks Z. Impact of adjuvant radiation on the patterns and rate of relapse in advanced-stage Hodgkin's disease treated with alternating chemotherapy combinations. J Clin Oncol. 1991; 9(12): 2193-2201.

41. Fabian CJ, Mansfield CM, Dahlberg S, Jones SE, Miller TP, Van Slyck E, Grozea PN, Morrison FS, Coltman CA Jr, Fisher RI. Low-dose involved field radiation after chemotherapy in advanced Hodgkin disease. A Southwest Oncology Group randomized study. Ann Intern Med. 1994;120(11): 903-912.

42. Diehl V, Loeffler M, Pfreundschuh M, Ruehl U, Hasenclever D, Nisters-Backes H, Sieber M, Smith K, Tesch H, Geilen W, et al. Further chemotherapy versus low-dose involved-field radiotherapy as consolidation of complete remission after six cycles of alternating chemotherapy in patients with advance Hodgkin's disease. German Hodgkins' Study Group (GHSG). Ann Oncol. 1995; 6(9): 901-910.

43. Ferme C, Sebban C, Hennequin C, Divine M, Lederlin P, Gabarre J, Ferrant A, Caillot D, Bordessoule D, Brice P, Moullet I, Berger F, Lepage E. Comparison of chemotherapy to radiotherapy as consolidation of complete or good partial response after six cycles of chemotherapy for patients with advanced Hodgkin's disease: results of the groupe d'etudes des lymphomes de l'Adulte H89 trial. Blood. 2000 ;95(7): 2246-2252.

44. Aleman BM, Räemaekers JM, Tirelli U, Bortolus R, van 't Veer MB, Lybeert ML, Keuning JJ, Carde P, Girinsky T, van der Maazen RW, Tomsic R, Vovk M, van Hoof A, Demeestere G, Lugtenburg PJ, Thomas J, Schroyens W, De Boeck K, Baars JW, Kluin-Nelemans JC, Carrie C, Aoudjhane M, Bron D, Eghbali H, Smit WG, Meerwaldt JH, Hagenbeek A, Pinna A, Henry-Amar M; European Organization for Research and Treatment of Cancer Lymphoma Group. Involved-field radiotherapy for advanced Hodgkin's lymphoma. N Engl J Med. 2003; 348(24): 2396-2406.

45. Loeffler M, Brosteanu O, Hasenclever D, Sextro M, Assouline D, Bartolucci AA, Cassileth PA, Crowther D, Diehl V, Fisher RI, Hoppe RT, Jacobs P, Pater JL, Pavlovsky S, Thompson E, Wiernik P. Meta-analysis of chemotherapy versus combined modality treatment trials in Hodgkin's disease. International Database on Hodgkin's Disease Overview Study Group. J Clin Oncol. 1998;16(3): 818-829.

46. Bonfante V, Santoro A, Viviani S, Devizzi L, Balzarotti M, Soncini F, Zanini M, Valagussa P, Bonadonna G. Outcome of patients with Hodgkin's disease failing after primary MOPP-ABVD. J Clin Oncol. 1997;15(2)528-534.

47. Josting A, Franklin J, May M, Koch P, Beykirch MK, Heinz J, Rudolph C, Diehl V, Engert A. New prognostic score based on treatment outcome of patients with relapsed Hodgkin's lymphoma registered in the database of the German Hodgkin's lymphoma study group. J Clin Oncol. 2002; 20(1):221-230.

48. Horning SJ, Chao NJ, Negrin RS, Hoppe RT, Long GD, Hu WW, Wong RM, Brown BW, Blume KG. High-dose therapy and autologous hematopoietic progenitor cell transplantation for recurrent or refractory Hodgkin's disease: analysis of the Stanford University results and prognostic indices. Blood. 1997; 89(3): 801-813.

49. Brice P, Bastion Y, Divine M, et al. Analysis of prognostic factors after the first relapse of Hodgkin's disease in 187 patients. Cancer. 1996; 78: 1293-1299.
50. Brice P, Bouabdallah R, Moreau P, et al. Prognostic factors for survival after high-dose therapy and autologous stem cell transplantation for patients with relapsing Hodgkin's disease: Analysis of 280 patients from the French registry. Bone Marrow Transplant. 1997; 20: 21-26.
51. Yuen AR, Rosenberg SA, Hoppe RT, Halpern JD, Horning SJ. Comparison between conventional salvage therapy and high-dose therapy with autografting for recurrent or refractory Hodgkin's disease. Blood. 1997; 89(3): 814-822.
52. Schmitz N, Pfistner B, Sextro M, Sieber M, Carella AM, Haenel M, Boissevain F, Zschaber R, Muller P, Kirchner H, Lohri A, Decker S, Koch B, Hasenclever D, Goldstone AH, Diehl V. Aggressive conventional chemotherapy compared with high-dose chemotherapy with autologous haemopoietic stem-cell transplantation for relapsed chemosensitive Hodgkin's disease: A randomized trial. The Lancet. 2002; 359: 2065-2071.
53. Aparicio J, Segura A, Garcera S, Oltra A, Santaballa A, Yuste A, Pastor M. ESHAP is an active regimen for relapsing Hodgkin's disease. Ann Oncol. 1999; 10(5): 593-595.
54. Moskowitz CH, Bertino JR, Glassman JR, Hedrick EE, Hunte S, Coady-Lyons N, Agus DB, Goy A, Jurcic J, Noy A, O'Brien J, Portlock CS, Straus DS, Childs B, Frank R, Yahalom J, Filippa D, Louie D, Nimer SD, Zelenetz AD. Ifosfamide, carboplatin, and etoposide: a highly effective cytoreduction and peripheral-blood progenitor-cell mobilization regimen for transplant-eligible patients with non-Hodgkin's lymphoma. J Clin Oncol. 1999; 17(12): 3776-3785.
55. Ferme C, Bastion Y, Lepage E, Berger F, Brice P, Morel P, Gabarre J, Nedellec G, Reman O, Cheron N, et al. The MINE regimen as intensive salvage chemotherapy for relapsed and refractory Hodgkin's disease. Ann Oncol. 1995; 6(6): 543-549.
56. Rodriguez J, Rodriguez MA, Fayad L, McLaughlin P, Swan F, Sarris A, Romaguera J, Andersson B, Cabanillas F, Hagemeister FB. ASHAP: a regimen for cytoreduction of refractory or recurrent Hodgkin's disease. Blood. 1999; 93(11): 3632-3636.
57. Linch DC, Winfield D, Goldstone AH, Moir D, Hancock B, McMillan A, Chopra R, Milligan D, Hudson GV. Dose intensification with autologous bone-marrow transplantation in relapsed and resistant Hodgkin's disease: results of a BNLI randomised trial. Lancet. 1993; 341(8852): 1051-1054.
58. Milpied N, Fielding AK, Pearce RM, Ernst P, Goldston AH. Allogeneic Bone Marrow Transplant is not better than autologous transplant for patients with relapsed Hodgkin's disease. J Clin Oncol. 1996; 14(4): 1291-1296.
59. Peniket AJ, Ruiz de Elvira MC, Taghipour G, Cordonnier C, Gluckman E, de Witte T, Santini G, Blaise D, Greinix H, Ferrant A, Cornelissen J, Schmitz N, Goldstone AH. An EBMT registry matched study of allogeneic stem cell transplants for lymphoma: allogeneic transplantation is associated with a lower relapse rate but a higher procedure-related mortality rate than autologous transplantation. 2003; 31(8): 667-78.
60. Anderlini P, Acholonu S, Okoroji GJ, Giralt S, Ueno N, Donato M, Andersson BS, Khouri I, Couriel D, Ippoliti C, Valverde RB, Champlin RE. Reduced early transplant-related mortality following allogeneic stem cell transplantation (SCT) with Fludarabine-based, reduced-intensity conditioning from matched related and unrelated donors in advanced Hodgkin's disease (HD). Blood. 2002; 620a. Abstract 2444.
61. Carella AM, Cavaliere M, Lerma E, Ferrara R, Tedeschi L, Romanelli A, Vinci M, Pinotti G, Lambelet P, Loni C, Verdiani S, De Stefano F, Valbonesi M, Corsetti MT. J Clin Oncol. 2000; 18(23): 3918-24.
62. Little R, Wittes RE, Longo DL, Wilson WH. Vinblastine for recurrent Hodgkin's disease following autologous bone marrow transplant. J Clin Oncol. 1998; 16(2): 584-588.

63. Devizzi L, Santoro A, Bonfante V, Viviani S, Balzarini L, Valagussa P, Bonadonna G. Vinorelbine: an active drug for the management of patients with heavily pretreated Hodgkin's disease. Ann Oncol. 1994; 5(9): 817-820.
64. Borchmann P, Schnell R, Diehl V, Engert A. New drugs in the treatment of Hodgkin's disease. Ann Oncol. 1998; 9 (Suppl 5) : S103-108.
65. Younes A, Cabanillas F, McLaughlin PW, Hagemeister FB, Farber C, Sarris A, Pate O, Myers J, Portlock C. Preliminary experience with paclitaxel for the treatment of relapsed and refractory Hodgkin's disease. Ann Oncol. 1996; 7(10): 1083-1085.
66. Bartlett N, Niedzwiecki D, Johnson J, Friedberg JW, Zelenetz AD, Canellos GP. A phase I/II study of gemcitabine, vinorelbine and liposomal doxorubicin for relapsed Hodgkin's disease: Preliminary results of CALGB 59804. Proc ASCO. 2003; 2275 (abstract).

Chapter 12

NODULAR LYMPHOCYTE PREDOMINANT HODGKIN'S DISEASE

Carol S. Portlock, MD

Memorial Sloan-Kettering Cancer Center New York, New York 10021

1. INTRODUCTION

The WHO Classification for Hodgkin's disease (HD) has made an important step by separating nodular lymphocyte predominant HD, NLPHD, from classical HD subtypes.[1,2] Although uncommon, approximately 5% of all HD, NLPHD is important because of its unique morphologic/immunophenotypic features, as well as its clinical characteristics and evolving recommendations for therapy.

2. PATHOLOGY

The morphologic diagnosis of lymphocyte predominant Hodgkin's disease is inadequate by itself and must always be supplemented by immunohistochemistry (IHC). As demonstrated by the European Task Force Study[3] in which 388 cases were retrospectively reviewed and further classified with IHC, only 56% were later confirmed as NLPHD. The remainder were: 35% Lymphocyte-Rich classical Hodgkin's disease (LRCHD) and 9% other histologies (including 12 with non-Hodgkin's lymphomas). Each of these histologic entities is managed differently thus it is essential that the initial diagnosis be accurate.

LPHD is characterized by a nodular pattern at least in part and is now referred to as nodular LPHD in all instances (NLPHD).[4] When the pattern is entirely diffuse, it is more likely to be LRCHD or rarely a non-Hodgkin's lymphoma (T cell rich B-cell lymphoma, TCR-BCL). The NLPHD tumor cells, termed L & H or "popcorn" cells, have a B-cell (CD20) immunophenotype and are negative for the classical HD markers (CD15 and/or CD30). Epithelial membrane antigen (EMA) is positive in approximately half the cases. The background cells are composed of predominantly small lymphocytes and some histiocytes. Polyclonal small B-cells are the majority. Fibrosis is rare in the lymph node of NLPHD in contrast to cHD where this is common.

In LRCHD the tumor cells (Reed-Sternberg cells and variants) are CD15 and/or CD 30 positive, CD20 and EMA negative with a background cellular infiltrate of lymphocytes, histiocytes, eosinophils, and plasma cells. The small lymphoid population is predominantly T-cell. Unlike NLPHD, approximately half of classical HD is associated with Epstein-Barr virus (EBV).

TCR-BCL is a subtype of diffuse large B cell lymphoma. The large B cells are CD20 positive, CD15 and 30 negative. Like NLPHD, the large cells are the minority population and small lymphoid cells predominate. Importantly however, the small cells of TCR-BCL are T cells rather than polyclonal B cells, as in NLPHD. Recently Lin et al[5] have reported that the IHC pattern of the background T-cells may assist in distinguishing NLPHD (CD134 positive in 94%; CD38 positive in 14% where CD 38 is in association with diffuse areas of involvement) from TCR-BCL where there is uniform expression of CD38 in background T cells. Future research will clarify this interesting observation.

The relationship between TCR-BCL and NLPHD is best considered a spectrum. Each is a distinct pathologic entity, however there are cases in which NLPHD is associated with TCR-BCL at initial presentation or sequentially. The finding or later development of TCR-BCL in NLPHD heralds an aggressive clinical behavior and is managed as DLBCL (de novo or with transformation). In some instances, single cell studies have demonstrated the clonal relationship of such cases.[6]

3.   CLINICAL PRESENTATION

3.1   NLPHD

The classical characteristics of NLPHD include male predominance (65 - 85% of cases), median age of approximately 35 years but occurring at all ages, non-bulky peripheral adenopathy which spares the mediastinum and upper abdomen, and no B symptoms. The majority of patients have regional disease presentations (70 – 80% stages I and II) while advanced stage is uncommon (stage III, 15 – 20%; stage IV, <10%), and when present may indicate another histology.

The European Task Force compared the clinical presentation of NLPHD with that of LRCHD.[7] Significant differences more common in LRCHD included age >50 (32% vs. 18%); presence of a mediastinal mass (15% vs. 7%); and splenic involvement (15% vs. 8%). Although limited disease below the diaphragm is more common in NLPHD (24% in stages I and II) as compared to LRCHD (15%), this was not significantly different.

3.2   TCR-BCL

Clinical features which may distinguish TCR-BCL from NLPHD[8] include: presence of B symptoms (29% vs. 10%), mediastinal involvement (18% vs. 7%), splenic involvement (42% vs. 8%), stage IV presentation (40% vs. 6%), presence of extranodal involvement (60% vs. 8%), and bone marrow disease (31% vs. 1%). As pointed out by Khoury et al[9], bone marrow involvement in NLPHD is exceptionally rare (7 of 275 patients) and in all instances was involved by large B cells.

4.   TREATMENT

4.1   NLPHD

The standard treatment options for NLPHD include radiation therapy alone, combined modality therapy and even deferral of initial therapy. Primary chemotherapy experience is anecdotal.

Miettinen et al[10] reported 51 patients accrued from 1961 – 1978, all but 3 of whom had CS I presentations. Twenty patients received therapy: 11 involved field RT (2000 – 4000 rads), 6 chemotherapy, and 3 combined modality therapy. Among the 31 untreated patients, 23 progressed: 13 with local recurrence (6 mos – 9 years after diagnosis), 2 with classical HD, 5 with non-Hodgkin's lymphomas (4 – 11 years later, presenting in new sites), and one with composite NLPHD/NHL at the original biopsy site 5 years after diagnosis.

In this large series, there were 15 deaths: 6 of HD, 3 of DLCL, 3 with second cancers and 3 due to other causes. The actuarial survival was 88% at 5 years and 70% at 10 years. Most importantly there appeared to be no significant differences in the number of fatalities between previously treated and untreated groups. These data have raised the question of whether patients with NLPHD should receive any initial therapy, similar to the management strategy utilized in indolent non-Hodgkin's lymphoma.

More contemporary series in children have addressed this question further. Pellegrino et al[11] reported 27 patients diagnosed from 1988 – 1998, ages 4 – 16 years (median, 10 years), stages I (22 patients), II (2), and III (3). Thirteen were monitored after initial node resection, 10 received combined modality therapy, 1 involved field RT, and 3 chemotherapy only. At 70 months median followup (32 – 214 months range), overall survival was 100%. Among 12 patients in complete remission after initial biopsy, event free survival was not significantly different from those initially treated. If residual disease was present after diagnostic biopsy, the EFS was inferior in those monitored as compared to patients treated at diagnosis, but without impact on survival. The authors concluded that no initial treatment was valid for patients in CR after initial diagnostic surgery.

Murphy et al[12] reported similar findings among 11 patients with stage I NLPHD. None progressed whether receiving initial therapy or not. One patient with stage II disease relapsed after chemotherapy, however all patients remained alive 2 – 13+ years after diagnosis.

The EORTC examined their retrospective experience in treatment of 48 patients, aged 16 – 49 years (median 28 years) with NLPHD.[13] All had regional disease (30 stage I; 18 stage II) and were treated with radiotherapy alone (37) or combined modality therapy (11). Median followup was 9.3 years (2.7 – 34 years).

There was no significant difference in relapse-free survival at 10 years, comparing radiotherapy alone (primarily regional irradiation), 77% vs. combined modality therapy, 68%. Likewise, overall survival at 10 years was similar: 90% vs. 100%. The authors concluded that adjuvant chemotherapy provided no additional benefit to RT alone in NLPHD and did not reduce the relapse risk outside the radiated field. Again the authors asked the pivotal question of whether treatment may be delayed or further reduced.

4.2   LRCHD

Approximately one-third of cases signed out morphologically as LPHD will be reclassified as LRCHD with immunostaining for CD15 and CD30. The European Task Force[7] demonstrated the clinical importance of this distinction in their series utilizing conventional radiotherapy, chemotherapy, and combined modality regimens. Complete response was achieved in 96% of patients with either NLPHD or LRCHD. Overall relapse rates were similar as well (21% vs. 17%). However, patients with NLPHD were much more likely to experience more than one relapse (27% of relapsers) as compared to LRCHD (5%). Moreover, patients with NLPHD, even when experiencing multiple relapses had a lesser frequency of death 14% vs. 26%.

The event free survival curve for NLPHD revealed a continuous fall, reminiscent of the curve seen in indolent lymphoma, and unlike that for LRCHD in which late events were absent after 10 years. Causes of death were likewise different. In NLPHD second solid tumors were most frequent (4.6% vs. 3.5% LRCHD) yet death from cardiac complications secondary to mediastinal RT were uncommon in NLPHD (1.8%) in contrast to LRCHD (6.1%). Remembering the clinical presentation of NLPHD, sparing mediastinal nodes, this is not surprising, as mediastinal late effects would not be expected since these lymph node sites are not irradiated.

In NLPHD, death from lymphoma or secondary non-Hodgkin's lymphomas was less frequent (4.6%) than deaths attributable to side effects of therapy (6.4%). This is in contrast to LRCHD in which lymphoma related deaths (HD, 8.7% and NHL, 1.7%) were more frequent than secondary complications (9.6%).

In sum, these data emphasize the importance of accurate pathologic diagnosis in identifying appropriate therapy and expected prognosis. Further, the fact that NLPHD patients experienced fatal secondary effects of treatment more frequently than life-threatening events due to lymphoma, underscores the emphasis on reducing therapy when appropriate.

4.3   TCR-BCL

Although rare, TCR-BCL is also an important histology to distinguish from NLPHD. In the European Task Force study[3], 388 patients had morphologic features of LPHD, but were reclassified as NHL in 12 (3.1%). More frequently TCR-BCL may be identified concurrently or subsequent to a diagnosis of NLPHD. In single cell studies of such cases, it has been possible to demonstrate that the large B cells of both histologies are clonally related.[6]

Several groups have reported the superiority of disease-free or progression-free survival when patients with TCR-BCL are treated with NHL-directed therapies (such as CHOP or R-CHOP) in comparison to HD-directed approaches. Greer et al[14] reported an overall disease-free survival of 29% at 3 years among 44 patients with TCR-BCL. This DFS was improved to 42% among those receiving NHL-directed regimens. Moreover, as reviewed by Ripp et al,[8] TCR-BCL patients treated with HD-directed chemotherapy regimens (18 patients reported in 3 series) achieved CR in only 8 patients (44%) and only one of these experienced a durable CR. Likewise RT alone for early stage TCR-BCL presentations resulted in only transient CR in the majority (3 of 10 sustained CR).

Whether treated initially for HD or NHL, overall survival of patients with TCR-BCL was similar in these reports. Salvage autologous transplantation may result in secondary curative outcome when required. As pointed out by Ripp et al,[8] if a patient with NLPHD fails to achieve initial CR with HD-directed therapy, one must seriously consider an underlying non-Hodgkin's lymphoma diagnosis.

4.4   DLBCL

Recently Huang et al[15] have retrospectively reviewed the concurrent (7 patients) or subsequent occurrence (14 patients) of DLBCL in NLPHD. This histologic development is generally referred to as transformation (applied in a similar manner to indolent lymphoma). In their series, only one-third of DLBCL cases were concurrent with NLPHD, and just one-quarter fulfilled criteria for a TCR-BCL histology. Most importantly, a retrospective comparison with a similarly treated de novo DLBCL cohort suggested a comparable failure-free and overall survival.

These authors further emphasized the importance of treating the aggressive histology, even if it appears in the context of a composite lymphoma with NLPHD. The most important prognostic factor in their 21 patients was the ability to achieve complete remission at the time of DLBCL diagnosis and they advocated the use of NHL-directed regimens in this context. Less aggressive regimens or HD-directed therapies were found to be ineffective.

5.   NEW THERAPIES

As a B-cell malignancy, NLPHD is a candidate for treatment with the anti-CD 20 antibody Rituximab. The largest experience is from a phase II study reported from Stanford.[16] There were 22 patients enrolled, ten previously treated for LPHD and 12 previously untreated. Rituximab was administered at standard dose and schedule (375 mg/m2 IV weekly x 4 doses). The overall response rate was 100% with 10 of 22 achieving CR/CRu (46%). Median progression-free survival was 10.2 months. Three patients were re-treated and 1 achieved CR and 2 had stable disease with second antibody therapy.

Biopsies were obtained in 5 of 9 patients who experienced relapse after Rituximab: 3 biopsies revealed recurrent LPHD; however, 2 revealed large B cell lymphomas (DLBCL and TCR-BCL, respectively). In the two patients with transformation, one had been previously treated, but one was initially untreated prior to Rituximab. The authors retrospectively reviewed these two cases carefully and found no evidence of transformation prior to the antibody therapy. They emphasized that because of this concern about transformation and the role, if any, antibody therapy might play, Rituximab should be considered investigational in LPHD.

In contrast, Rituximab has become a standard component in the combination chemotherapy of DLBCL and TCR-BCL. Thus, a patient with composite NLPHD/DLBCL or TCR-BCL, should certainly be treated with a Rituximab-containing regimen such as R-CHOP when indicated.

6. RECOMMENDATIONS FOR MANAGEMENT

Since the management of NLPHD is far different from the "look-alike" histologies of LRCHD and TCR-BCL, it is key that the histologic diagnosis be firm. This requires expert morphologic interpretation, coupled with immunohistochemistry.

Staging studies may alert the clinician to a histology other than NLPHD when, for example, there is mediastinal adenopathy, splenomegaly, or bone marrow involvement. These sites suggest LRCHD or TCR-BCL/DLBCL.

Although randomized studies are not available, most authors agree that stage I NLPHD which has been surgically excised may be monitored expectantly. Whether other presentations of limited stage NLPHD can also be monitored is less certain and ideally requires a prospective clinical trial. Such a study is ongoing within the EORTC and GELA.

Involved field irradiation is the treatment of choice for regional presentations. More extensive irradiation has not been shown to reduce relapse rate in retrospective studies, and may increase the late toxicities experienced with radiation therapy.[17]

Chemotherapy is rarely indicated at initial diagnosis of NLPHD, as the vast majority of patients have limited stage at diagnosis and are candidates for involved field RT. When utilized adjunctively with RT, chemotherapy does not appear to improve the relapse-free survival, and is therefore not recommended at initial diagnosis. If the patient has an advanced stage presentation, by far the most important question is that of histologic diagnosis. NLPHD is very rare with stage III and IV presentations, raising the possibility of LRCHD (in which ABVD chemotherapy would be standard) or TCR-BCL (in which R-CHOP would be standard). Embarking upon chemotherapy without confidence in the pathology is a serious mistake.

If response to treatment is poor, or relapse occurs quickly after initial therapy, one must seriously consider histologic transformation. Biopsy is key, remembering that a mixed picture of composite NLPHD with DLBCL or one of its subtypes is expected.

Anti-CD 20 antibody therapy holds promise in NLPHD, however, the potential emergence of transformation is problematic. One must be circumspect in the use of Rituximab alone in the previously untreated patient and ideally administer the drug in the context of a clinical trial.

Table 1: NLPHD AND ITS "LOOK ALIKES"

- Lymphocyte Predominant Hodgkin's Disease (LPHD) by Morphology,
- **AFTER** Immunohistochemistry:
- Nodular Lymphocyte Predominant Hodgkin's Disease (NLPHD) in 56%
- Lymphocyte-Rich Classical Hodgkin's Disease (LRCHD) in 35%
- T cell rich-B cell Lymphoma (TCR-BCL) in 3.1%

**According to data of the European Task Force[3]

Table 2. NLPHD, CLINICAL CHARACTERISTICS

- 5% of all Hodgkin's disease
- Male predominance, 65-85% of all cases
- Median age approximately 35 years, but occurs at all ages
- Usually non-bulky and peripheral adenopathy
- Spares the mediastinum and upper abdomen
- No B symptoms in greater than 85%
- Early Stage disease
  - o Stages I and II: 70-80%
  - o Stage III: 15-20%
  - o Stage IV: << 10%

Table 3. FEATURES SUGGESTING A "LOOK ALIKE"
HISTOLOGY, LRCHD AND/OR TCR-BCL*

- Age greater than 50 years
- B symptoms
- Mediastinal adenopathy
- Splenic involvement
- Advanced stage
- Extranodal involvement
- Bone marrow involvement

*see Text

Table 4: NLPHD, SHOULD TREATMENT BE REDUCED?

- Consider treatment deferral in Stage I patients with surgical CR
  and in other selected Stage I and II patients
- Involved Field Radiotherapy
- Short course ABVD + IF-RT or ABVD in selected patients
- Rituximab: ? At relapse, and in clinical trials

7.   REFERENCES

1.   Harris NL, Jaffe ES, Diebold J, Flandrin G, Muller-Hermelink HK, Vardiman J, Lister TA, Bloomfield CD. The World Health Organization classification of neoplasms of the hematopoietic and lymphoid tissues: report of the Clinical Advisory Committee meeting--Airlie House, Virginia, November, 1997. Hematol J. 2000;**1**(1):53-66.

2.   Harris NL. Hodgkin's lymphomas: Classification, diagnosis, and grading. Semin Hematol. 1999; **36**: 220-232.

3.   Anagnostopoulos I, Hansmann ML, Franssila K, Harris M, Harris NL, Jaffe ES, Han J, van Krieken JM, Poppema S, Marafioti T, Franklin J, Sextro M, Diehl V, Stein H. European Task Force on Lymphoma project on lymphocyte predominance Hodgkin disease: histologic and immunohistologic analysis of submitted cases reveals 2 types of Hodgkin disease with a nodular growth pattern and abundant lymphocytes. Blood. 2000 Sep 1;**96**(5):1889-99.

4.   Ekstrand BC, Horning SJ. Lymphocyte predominant Hodgkin's disease. Curr Oncol Rep. 2002 Sep;**4**(5):424-33.

5.   Lin P, Medeiros LJ, Wilder RB, Abruzzo LV, Manning JT, Jones D. The activation profile of tumour-associated reactive T-cells differs in the nodular and diffuse patterns of lymphocyte predominant Hodgkin's disease. Histopathology. 2004 Jun;44(6):561-9.

6.   Ohno T, Huang JZ, Wu G, Park KH, Weisenburger DD, Chan WC. The tumor cells in nodular lymphocyte-predominant Hodgkin disease are clonally related to the large cell lymphoma occurring in the same individual. Direct demonstration by single cell analysis. Am J Clin Pathol. 2001 Oct;116(4):506-11.

7.   Diehl V, Sextro M, Franklin J, Hansmann ML, Harris N, Jaffe E, Poppema S, Harris M, Franssila K, van Krieken J, Marafioti T, Anagnostopoulos I, Stein H. Clinical presentation, course, and prognostic factors in lymphocyte-predominant Hodgkin's disease and lymphocyte-rich classical Hodgkin's disease: report from the European Task Force on Lymphoma Project on Lymphocyte-Predominant Hodgkin's Disease. J Clin Oncol. 1999 Mar;17(3):776-83.

8.   Ripp JA, Loiue DC, Chan W, Nawaz H, Portlock CS. T-cell rich B-cell lymphoma: clinical distinctiveness and response to treatment in 45 patients. Leuk Lymphoma. 2002 Aug;43(8):1573-80.

9.   Khoury JD, Jones D, Yared MA, Manning JT Jr, Abruzzo LV, Hagemeister FB, Medeiros LJ. Bone marrow involvement in patients with nodular lymphocyte predominant Hodgkin lymphoma. Am J Surg Pathol. 2004 Apr;28(4):489-95.

10.   Miettinen M, Franssila KO, Saxen E. Hodgkin's disease, lymphocytic predominance nodular. Increased risk for subsequent non-Hodgkin's lymphomas. Cancer. 1983 Jun 15;51(12):2293-300.

11.   Pellegrino B, Terrier-Lacombe MJ, Oberlin O, Leblanc T, Perel Y, Bertrand Y, Beard C, Edan C, Schmitt C, Plantaz D, Pacquement H, Vannier JP, Lambilliote C, Couillault G, Babin-Boilletot A, Thuret I, Demeocq F, Leverger G, Delsol G, Landman-Parker J; Study of the French Society of Pediatric Oncology. Lymphocyte-predominant Hodgkin's lymphoma in children: therapeutic abstention after initial lymph node resection--a Study of the French Society of Pediatric Oncology. J Clin Oncol. 2003 Aug 1;21(15):2948-52.

12.   Murphy SB, Morgan ER, Katzenstein HM, Kletzel M. Results of little or no treatment for lymphocyte-predominant Hodgkin disease in children and adolescents. J Pediatr Hematol Oncol. 2003 Sep;25(9):684-7.

13.   Wilder RB, Schlembach PJ, Jones D, Chronowski GM, Ha CS, Younes A, Hagemeister FB, Barista I, Cabanillas F, Cox JD. European Organization for Research and Treatment of Cancer and Groupe d'Etude des Lymphomes de l'Adulte very favorable and favorable, lymphocyte-predominant Hodgkin disease. Cancer. 2002 Mar 15;94(6):1731-8.

14.   Greer JP, Macon WR, Lamar RE, Wolff SN, Stein RS, Flexner JM, Collins RD, Cousar JB. T-cell-rich B-cell lymphomas: diagnosis and response to therapy of 44 patients. J Clin Oncol. 1995 Jul;13(7):1742-50.

15.   Huang JZ, Weisenburger DD, Vose JM, Greiner TC, Aoun P, Chan WC, Lynch JC, Bierman PJ, Armitage JO; Nebraska Lymphoma Study Group. Diffuse large B-cell lymphoma arising in nodular lymphocyte predominant hodgkin lymphoma. A report of 21 cases from the Nebraska Lymphoma Study Group. Leuk Lymphoma. 2003 Nov;44(11):1903-10.

16.   Ekstrand BC, Lucas JB, Horwitz SM, Fan Z, Breslin S, Hoppe RT, Natkunam Y, Bartlett NL, Horning SJ. Rituximab in lymphocyte-predominant Hodgkin disease: results of a phase 2 trial. Blood. 2003 Jun 1;101(11):4285-9.

17.   Bodis S, Kraus MD, Pinkus G, Silver B, Kadin ME, Canellos GP, Shulman LN, Tarbell NJ, Mauch PM. Clinical presentation and outcome in lymphocyte-predominant Hodgkin's disease. J Clin Oncol. 1997 Sep;15(9):3060-6.

Chapter 13

LYMPHOMA IMAGING: NUCLEAR MEDICINE

Lale Kostakoglu, MD, and Stanley J. Goldsmith, MD

Department of Radiology, Division of Nuclear Medicine, The New York Presbyterian Hospital Weill Medical College of Cornell University, New York, NY

1. INTRODUCTION

Careful staging and treatment planning using a multidisciplinary approach is required to determine optimal treatment of patients with Hodgkin's disease (HD) and aggressive subtypes of non-Hodgkin's lymphoma (NHL). The advent of more sensitive imaging modalities have increased staging and restaging accuracy and provided more effective means to evaluate response to therapy. In the post-therapy setting, the unnecessary use of aggressive chemotherapy and external beam radiation could lead to development of secondary malignancies and various organ toxicity. Poor prognosis associated with some second malignancies warrants better and less harmful screening strategies (1). Hence, the early identification of high-risk and low-risk patients can effectively select subpopulations that would benefit from more intensive chemotherapy protocols and can avoid unwarranted further therapy.

Anatomic imaging modalities, primarily computed tomography (CT) and magnetic resonance imaging (MRI), are dependent on size criteria, thus, they provide limited information regarding lymphoma involvement in normal size lymph nodes. Additionally, CT or MRI cannot differentiate lymphadenopathy due to benign or therapy-related causes from that due to lymphoma infiltration (2). Accordingly, at initial staging all disease sites may not be detected and following therapy progression-free survivals may not significantly differ between patients with partial resolution (residual masses) and those with complete resolution based on post-therapy CT scans

(3-6). MRI is reported to be helpful in distinguishing recurrent tumor from fibrosis or normal tissue on T2-weighted images. MRI findings, however, are not specific for tumor recurrence and cannot differentiate tumor from acute radiation pneumonitis, infection, hemorrhage or radiation fibrosis (7-9). MRI detects active lymphoma 6 months following completion of therapy more accurately than during the course of, or early after chemotherapy (6). Nevertheless, MRI offers advantages over CT in the evaluation of disease process in the bone marrow and central nervous system.

Ga-67 imaging has been the imaging modality of choice along with CT in the staging of lymphomas. However, the niche for Ga-67 imaging is in the assessment of therapy response in HD and aggressive NHL (5, 6, 10-12). At initial presentation, Ga-67 scintigraphy does not contribute significantly to the staging process due to its inherently low resolution, although a pre-therapy baseline scan is necessary for proper comparison purposes in the assessment of response to therapy. Ga-67 scintigraphy also lacks sensitivity in the assessment of abdominal lymphoma and for identifying lesion sites in indolent subtypes (13, 14). Thallium-201 thallous chloride (Tl-201) or Tc-99m-Sestamibi (MIBI) imaging have been proposed as alternative or complementary studies in patients with low-grade lymphomas, nonetheless, similar restrictions apply to both of these radiotracers in the identification of infradiaphragmatic disease (14, 15).

Positron emission tomography (PET) imaging using [F-18] fluorodeoxyglucose (FDG) has recently become a valuable part of the staging and restaging algorithm. FDG uptake in tumors is proportional to the glycolytic metabolic rate of viable tumor cells representing increased metabolic demand for glucose (16). A multitude of studies have reported that FDG-PET is a consistently reliable imaging modality in the staging and restaging as well as in the assessment of therapy response in malignant lymphomas (17-29). With the advent of the state-of-the-art dedicated PET scanners, a resolution of approximately 5 mm can be achieved. In the post-therapy setting, changes in tumor metabolic activity between pre- and post-therapy FDG-PET scans provide useful information on response to anti-tumor therapy. Recently, the accuracy of FDG-PET imaging has significantly improved with the introduction of iterative reconstruction algorithms and image fusion of PET data with simultaneously acquired CT (PET-CT). PET-CT imaging improves specificity in staging and re-staging of lymphoma and offers advantages over separate FDG-PET and CT imaging.

This chapter will focus on mainly on applications of FDG-PET in staging, restaging and evaluating response to therapy of lymphomas which has recently been integrated into the management algorithm of lymphomas. The use of traditional radiotracers such as Ga-67 citrate, Tl-201, MIBI will also be discussed in the scope of lymphoma imaging as alternative imaging options (Table 1).

Table 1. Suggested Imaging Parameters

Scintigraphy	Radiotracer Dose	NPO prior to imaging	Suggested Parameters
FDG-PET	10-15 mCi	4-6 hrs	Acquisition starts at 1-2 hrs after injection. Oral contrast can be given 30 min prior to imaging. Patient's blood glucose level should be measured prior to FDG injection to assure a level <200u/dL.
Ga-67 citrate	8-10 mCi	Not applicable	Acquisition starts at 48-72 hrs following injection. Whole body and SPECT images (usually chest) acquired using a medium energy collimator with energy peaks of 93, 185 and 300 keV with setting 20% windows. Additional views can be obtained up to 7 days, especially for abdominal lesions.
Thallium-201	3-4 mCi	4 hrs	Acquisition starts at 20-30min following injection. Whole body and SPECT images acquired using a low energy collimator with energy peaks of 80 and 167 keV with 20% windows. Additional views can be obtained up to 4 hrs.
Tc-99m Sestamibi	20-25 mCi	4 hrs	Acquisition starts at 20-30min following injection. Whole body and SPECT images acquired using a low energy collimator with an energy peak of 140keV with 15-20% windows. Additional views can be obtained up to 4 hrs.
In-111 Ocreotide	5-6 mCi	Not applicable	Suspend therapy with octreotide acetate during this procedure, if applicable. Whole body images obtained at 4 and 24 hrs. SPECT is obtained at 24 hrs. Whole body and SPECT images are acquired using a medium energy collimator with energy peaks of 173 and 246 keV with 15-20% windows. Additional views can be obtained at 48-72 hrs.

2.   ANATOMIC IMAGING MODAILITIES

2.1   Primarily Nodal Presentation

2.1.1   Neck/Chest/Abdomen/Pelvis

Both CT and MRI can be used in the diagnosis and pre-therapy evaluation of nodal lymphomas of the neck and chest.   CT is more commonly used because of its widespread availability, rapid imaging time; lower relative cost in comparison to MRI, excellent spatial resolution, and excellent evaluation of the lung parenchyma, but has inherent drawbacks consisting of patient exposure to ionizing radiation and iodinated contrast material (30, 31). MRI is generally considered somewhat superior to CT in evaluation for lymphadenopathy of the neck, but its use in evaluation of lymphadenopathy of the chest and abdomen is often compromised by artifact resulting from patient respiratory motion, although this factor is becoming less of an issue with the adoption of faster, non-breath hold imaging sequences (32). In those patients with either allergy to iodinated contrast material or with limited renal function, MRI can serve as a substitute to CT for evaluation of lymphadenopathy. The role of ultrasound in evaluation of the lymphadenopathy associated with lymphoma is limited, particularly outside the neck and other superficial sites such as the axilla or groin. However, ultrasound can be very useful in directing biopsy of lymph nodes in more superficial locations.

All lymph node stations in the neck, chest, abdomen, and pelvis can be affected by both Hodgkin's and non-Hodgkin's lymphomas, usually as evidenced by increase in both the number of lymph nodes and a change in lymph node morphology with loss of the normal fatty hilum, increase in size, and loss of distinctness of nodal margins (33-35). Often times the enlarged lymph nodes form bulky, confluent masses in which the distinction of individual lymph nodes becomes impossible. Calcification within lymph nodes affected by non-treated lymphoma is extremely uncommon, and should alert the radiologist to the possibility of an alternative diagnosis, usually of infectious or inflammatory etiology, while calcification within lymph nodes after treatment of lymphoma is seen, although rarely (34-36). Central low attenuation within lymph nodes is usually a sign of central necrosis, a factor not shown to correlate with patient outcome. Given the large size that nodal masses of both Hodgkin's and non-Hodgkin's lymphomas can attain, symptoms as a result of mass effect from these large nodal conglomerates, such as bowel obstruction or airway compromise, are relatively rare, presumably from the tendency of lymphoma to typically grow in a non infiltrative pattern and displace, rather than encase neighboring structures (37, 38). Hodgkin's lymphomas more commonly tend to spread contiguously from nodal station to adjacent nodal station, while non-Hodgkin's lymphomas are much more likely to skip over neighboring nodal stations (33, 37).

2.2   Primarily Extra-Nodal Presentation

2.2.1   CNS

MRI is the primary modality in the evaluation of lymphoma of the central nervous system. Parenchymal involvement of the brain and spinal cord by lymphoma was once thought to be exceedingly rare, but the recent increase in patients who are immunocompromised has caused a concomitant increase in the number of parenchymal lymphomas of the brain and spinal cord. These lymphomas are almost always of the non-Hodgkin's type and are frequently seen in the deep white matter of the brain in a periventricular location (39, 40). Unfortunately, infection of the brain is also common in these patients, and differentiation between infection and lymphoma is oftentimes difficult based solely on anatomic imaging. Another common presentation of CNS lymphoma is infiltration of the meninges, usually of the spine and the skull base, sometimes to the extent that dural-based masses can cause compression of neighboring structures (41). In addition to MRI, evaluation of spinal fluid in these patients often yields positive cytology.

2.2.2   Head and Neck

Non-nodal lymphomas of the head and neck are often difficult to diagnose due to the wide variety of presentations, including, but not limited to, masses arising from the skull and scalp, the orbits, the sinuses, the salivary glands, the tonsils, and the soft tissues of the neck. These masses lack features that would distinguish them as lymphoma based on anatomic imaging alone, and diagnosis typically rests on biopsy. MRI is the most useful modality in the diagnosis and evaluation of these masses because of its excellent soft tissue resolution and inherent multi-planar imaging characteristics, but CT can also provide useful information, particularly about the integrity of adjacent bony structures (42, 43).

2.2.3   Chest

Outside of the lymph node stations of the chest, lymphoma can also affect the lung parenchyma. Usually this occurs in the presence of concomitant lymphadenopathy of the mediastinum and hilum, with gradual loss of sharp distinction between lymph node masses and the adjacent lung with ill defined, sometimes nodular, increase in density of the adjacent lung. Presumably this represents local spread to adjacent lung and can be seen in both non-Hodgkin's and Hodgkin's lymphomas (44). A different pattern of involvement occurs with nodules of the lung parenchyma at a site distant from nodal involvement, or occasionally in the absence of nodal involvement. This pattern is most commonly associated with non-Hodgkin's lymphomas and the nodules typically have poorly defined, irregular margins and are not as dense as the nodules seen from other causes (45). Isolated nodules can also arise from the mucosal associated lympoid tissue of the lungs. Lastly, the rich lymphatic supply radiating outward from the hila can also be a site of lymphomatous involvement, typically seen as either smooth or nodular thickening of the bronchovascular structures.

Pleural effusions and pericardial effusions are a common finding in lymphoma of the chest and can be a result of central lymphadenopathy causing obstruction of lymphatic drainage or direct lymphomatous involvement of the pleura or pericardium (46). CT is typically most useful for the evaluation of the lung parenchyma, while the role of MRI is limited in this setting.

2.2.4   Abdomen-Solid Organs

Of the solid abdominal organs, the spleen and liver are most commonly affected by lymphoma. Involvement typically manifests more commonly as diffuse infiltration or, less frequently, as focal deposits. Diffuse infiltration nearly always preserves the appearance of the organ with its sole identifying characteristic being either splenomegaly or hepatomegaly (47-49, Avlonitis, Gazelle). Unfortunately the use of various size measurements of the liver and spleen to determine lymphomatous involvement in the setting of diffuse infiltration has been shown to be unreliable, unless massive organomegaly is present. Focal deposits manifest as focal regions of hypo attenuation on CT scanning or regions of T1 and T2 signal abnormality on MR imaging. Although seen less commonly, lymphoma can involve the kidneys, adrenals, pancreas, ureters, bladder, prostate, uterus, and cervix (50-52). Involvement of these organs usually presents as local infiltration from neighboring nodal masses, while intrinsic involvement of these organs is very rare. When seen, intrinsic involvement of these organs usually presents as a focal soft tissue mass, although diffuse infiltration can be seen as well. For the reasons discussed above, CT is more commonly used in the evaluation of the solid abdominal organs, with MRI being a satisfactory alternative.

2.2.5   Abdomen-GI Tract

As seen in the solid abdominal organs, bulky adenopathy of the abdomen and pelvis can cause local invasion of any segment of the GI tract, a finding frequently identified on CT images. In addition, intrinsic involvement of the GI tract, usually by the non-Hodgkin's lymphomas, is a common finding. The stomach and colon are the sites of most frequent involvement, although lesions of the esophagus and small bowel are also seen (53-55). Lymphoma arising from the GI tract has a wide range of presentations, including thickening of the bowel wall or bowel folds, narrowing of the lumen, marked dilation of the lumen, or polyp-like lesions. Also lymphoma, more commonly than other cancers of the GI tract, is multifocal in its presentation. Often, evaluation of lymphoma of the GI tract is challenging, and a combination of cross-sectional imaging, with either CT or MRI, and fluoroscopic barium techniques, such as barium enema or upper GI, are employed (56). Increasingly, the use of modified CT techniques, such as CT-enteroclysis and VC-virtual colonoscopy, are finding a place in the evaluation of tumors of the GI tract.

2.2.6   Musculoskeletal

Infiltration of bones and muscles by neighboring lymph node masses is seen in both Hodgkin's lymphomas and non-Hodgkin's lymphomas (57, 58). Involvement of bone is typically identified on CT imaging or plain radiography as disruption of the normal trabecular pattern by an adjacent lymph node mass. On MR imaging there is loss of cortical integrity as well as signal abnormality of the underlying bone marrow (59). Involvement of adjacent muscle groups is more difficult with CT imaging. When a fat plane exists between the lymphomatous mass and adjacent muscle group, then typically the muscle group is uninvolved, while the absence of a fat plane suggests, but does not prove, involvement. Loss of the normal muscle striation and other morphologic changes usually indicate muscle involvement. MRI imaging is more reliable in the assessment of muscular involvement, with a typical change in the signal characteristics of the involved muscle. Intrinsic involvement of musculoskeletal structures by lymphoma, usually seen in the non-Hodgkin's lymphomas, is evaluated in a similar manner, with MRI more useful for evaluation of the soft tissues and both CT and MRI useful in the evaluation of skeletal structures.

2.2.7   Bone Marrow

Replacement of the normal fatty marrow in adults and older children by lymphomatous involvement is readily demonstrated on MRI imaging. Patchy involvement is more readily identified, while diffuse involvement can occasionally pose a diagnostic challenge, particularly in younger age groups. CT and radiography have not proven useful in the identification of bone marrow involvement, since typically the normal trabecular structure of bone is preserved with bone marrow involvement.

3.   CT AND MRI IN THE EVALUATION OF RESPONSE TO THERAPY

Following therapy, the size of nodal and extranodal masses is expected to decrease, indicating response to therapy. However, using size criteria has limitations, as fibrosis and inflammation may also have effect upon the size of a mass. In addition, lymphoma originating in lymph nodes will decrease in size but the underlying node will nevertheless remain (60-62). Furthermore, there is significant difficulty in accurately measuring masses involved by lymphoma, as these masses are often irregular and complex in three dimensions. Further compounding this difficulty is the interobserver variability that exists in measuring complex lesions which change in shape and size between patient visits. This can be minimized by having the same observer perform all measurements at one time. The use of CT attenuation values in differentiating tumor from fibrosis is not accurate. Overall, CT remains unreliable in differentiating residual tumor from fibrosis.

In addition to allowing for changes in size measurement, changes in the signal characteristics of a mass can also be assessed by MR and inferences about the degree of active of tumor versus fibrosis/necrosis made (62). In general active tumor is lower in signal on T1 weighted images and higher on

T2 weighted images, while fibrosis tends to be of lower signal on T2 weighted images. However, this technique of evaluation is hampered by false positive areas of increased T2 signal caused by edema or inflammation. The degree and pattern of enhancement following intravenous gadolinium-DTPA administration can add further information. Although MRI may perform better than CT in differentiating residual tumor from fibrosis, it is also currently less than ideal. Future advances in MRI pulse sequences and/or spectroscopy may improve its reliability in this respect.

4. NUCLEAR MEDICINE IMAGING MODALITIES

4.1 FDG-PET Imaging

FDG-PET in the initial staging and at restaging following therapy has proven to be an accurate and cost-effective technique compared to anatomic imaging modalities and Ga-67 scintigraphy in the detection of nodal and extranodal disease (24-29). Consequently, FDG-PET has now an established function in the staging algorithm as well as in the post-therapy evaluation of lymphoma.

Mechanism of Uptake: FDG accumulation in malignant cells is a function of combination of increased hypoxia that results in increased glycolysis, overexpression of glucose transporters (Glut-1), and increase in the levels of the enzyme that plays a significant role in glycolysis, hexokinase (63, 64). FDG follows similar metabolic pathways to those in involved in glucose utilization, following transportation into the cell by glucose transporter proteins, mainly GLUT-1, FDG is then phosphorylated to FDG 6-phosphate in the cytosol. As FDG 6-phosphate is not a substrate for the enzyme, glucose-6-phosphate isomerase, the following steps do not occur. Additionally, since the dephosphorylating enzyme, glucose 6 phosphatase, is expressed at low concentrations in malignant tissues, FDG-6-phosphate is not catabolized further and thus, biochemically trapped within metabolizing cancer cells. Although not consistently in every tumor system, FDG uptake is related to the proliferation rate of some tumors including lymphoma as evidenced by the proliferating cell nuclear antigen labeling index (65). This issue is definitively established; however, as there are conflicting data demonstrating that FDG accumulation correlates with the number of viable cells not with their proliferative rate (66, 67).

4.1.1   Clinical Applications

Histologic Subtypes of Lymphoma and FDG-PET Imaging

FDG accumulates in both NHL and HD regardless of the histological grade or subtype except in small lymphocytic lymphoma (CLL/SLL) and mucosa-associated lymphoid tissue-associated lymphoma (MALT). It should be emphasized that standardized uptake values (SUV) may be significantly lower in low-grade NHL's when compared to high grade NHL's and HD (17, 20, 23, 29, 68, 69) (Figures 1, 2). Although there is always an overlap, especially in small size lesions, the SUV's vary greatly between high-grade and low-grade lymphomas with low-grade NHL demonstrating an SUV range of 1.5 – 11.0, an aggressive NHL an SUV range of 3.0 - 32 (70). Additionally, using SUV's as an objective reference to differentiate between various lymphomas may be problematic in lesions with a necrotic component (rare occasion), lesions smaller than 1 cm and in patients with high glucose or insulin levels. More recently, in a comparatively larger patient population with low grade lymphoma, FDG-PET detected 40% more involved lymph nodes than did conventional imaging modalities in the follicular lymphoma subtype, however, it detected less than 58% of nodal disease sites in the small lymphocytic subtype (CLL/SLL) (71). Low-grade lymphoma is a rare lymphoma subtype and gathering sufficient data may take a long period of time, but more data are necessary to establish the role of FDG-PET in low-grade lymphoma. Another crucial issue that FDG-PET may help clinicians significantly is that low-grade lymphomas undergo transformation to a more aggressive subtype, at a rate of 5-10% per year (72). In cases with transformation, FDG uptake characteristics are usually indistinguishable from those of high-grade lymphomas (Figure 3). Hence, FDG-PET may provide a means to determine the sites of high-grade transformation which serves as a useful tool for clinicians to obtain tissue confirmation at these particular locations. In our experience, lesions sites demonstrating SUV's higher than 12 has probably had transformation to an aggressive subtype (73). Nonetheless, these data still have to be expanded and confirmed with further studies.

Although available data are not sufficient for a firm conclusion, the sensitivity of FDG-PET appears to be less reliable in extranodal marginal zone B-cell lymphoma of the mucosa-associated lymphoid tissue (MALT) (74, 75) (Figure 4). Interestingly enough, the detection sensitivity of FDG-PET is reported to be higher in nodal marginal zone lymphoma compared to that in extranodal marginal zone lymphoma of MALT (74). These findings confirm the current concept that nodal marginal lymphoma is a more aggressive disease entity than MALT.

The role FDG-PET in mantle cell lymphoma follows more or less that in follicular lymphoma as the glucose metabolism of these disease entities are similar. Thus, FDG-PET should be able to detect all disease sites in patients with mantle cell lymphoma with high sensitivity. Similarly, FDG-PET is usually positive in T-cell lymphomas including cutaneous T-cell lymphomas.

Staging of Lymphoma
Initial staging of lymphomas is important for proper therapeutic management and prognostic factors. Advanced stage lymphoma may be curable with combination chemotherapy, whereas early stage disease can be cured by local radiotherapy only. FDG-PET is an established staging modality for both nodal and extranodal lymphoma (Table 2).

Nodal Disease
At initial staging, FDG-PET findings are usually in agreement with clinical and morphologic imaging findings. Moreover, the diagnostic efficiency of FDG-PET is superior to CT by detecting additional disease sites in up to 30% of patients with reported sensitivities of 83% and 100% (19-26) (Table 2).

The accuracy of FDG-PET was also found to be higher than CT in evaluating the involvement of the hilar and mediastinal regions at initial staging and follow-up. The reported sensitivity and specificity for FDG-PET in these locations were 96% and 94%, respectively (Figure 5) (26).

The change in staging and thereby patient management is the ultimate alteration that would drive the improvement of prognosis and survival. The superior sensitivity of FDG-PET has been reported to lead to a change in disease stage in up to 40% of patients with untreated NHL and HD (25, 76-79) by virtue of revealing additional disease sites that were confirmed by either biopsy or long-term clinical follow-up. However, the stage category is usually altered within the same risk category (i.e., early stage vs. advanced stage) with the use of FDG-PET although in some cases, early stage disease can be upstaged to advanced disease or downstaged to early stage disease which naturally results in significant management alterations (77).

Table 2. FDG-PET Studies at Initial Staging of Lymphoma: Comparison with Morphological Imaging Modalities

Authors	Study	Patient no	Patient Group	Modality	Sensitivity (%)	Specificity (%)
Hoh (19)	Retrospective	18	NHL+HD	FDG-PET CM*	94 83	NA NA
Thill (20)	Retrospective	27	NHL+HD	FDG-PET CT	100 77	NA NA
Mainolfi (21)	Prospective	98	NHL+HD	FDG-PET CM	†	†
Stumpe (23)	Prospective	50	HD vs NHL HD vs NHL	FDG-PET CT	86 vs 89 81 vs 86	96 vs 100 41 vs 67
Bangerter (26)	Retrospective	89	NHL+HD	FDG-PET CT	96 †	94 †
Wiedmann (27)	Prospective	20	HD	FDG-PET CM	†	†
Bangerter (76)	Prospective	44	HD	FDG-PET CT	†	†
Buchmann (77)	Prospective	52	NHL+HD	FDG-PET CT	99 83	100 100
Partridge (78)	Retrospective	44	HD	FDG-PET CT	†	†
Weihrauch (79)	Prospective	22	HD	FDG-PET CT	88 74	100 100
Kostakoglu (95)	Prospective	62	NHL+HD	FDG-PET Ga-67	100 81	NA NA
Wirth (96)	Prospective	50	NHL+HD	FDG Ga-67 CM*	95 88 90	† † †
Shen (97)	Prospective	30	NHL+HD	FDG Ga-67	96 72	† †

* conventional modalities: CT, ultrasound, MRI, endoscopy or laparoscopy   HD: Hodgkin's disease   NHL:Non-Hodgkin's lymphoma
† FDG Sensitivity and specificity not given but FDG-PET detected more sites than CT or Ga-67 scan

Based on the level of change in disease stage, FDG-PET findings may result in major treatment modifications in up to 10-25% of patients (76-79).

Extranodal Disease

A multitude of studies have reported that FDG-PET may provide more information about the extent of disease regarding extranodal lymphoma compared to CT (20, 24, 27, 80). In up to 30% of patients diagnosed with supradiaphragmatic disease, infradiaphragmatic disease is found at restaging laparotomy (81-83). In NHL, hepatic and splenic involvement occurs in 15% and 22% of patients, respectively while in HD corresponding values are 3.2% and 23%, respectively (3, 24). The involvement of the liver, spleen, and bone marrow cannot be accurately detected on conventional imaging which relies on size criteria, as organ size is a poor predictor of tumor involvement. Ga-67 is also limited in the evaluation of extranodal disease in the abdomen while FDG-PET has been shown to be more sensitive, identifying 23% more hepatic and splenic lesions than CT (20).

FDG-PET can differentiate primary lymphomas of the central nervous system (CNS) from infectious processes with a reported accuracy of 89% (84, 85) (Figure 6). Distinguishing infectious etiology such as toxoplasmosis can be a challenge for morphological imaging studies including CT and MRI, in particular, in patients with AIDS. Essentially, a lesion with an FDG uptake higher than the adjacent gray matter indicates a malignant process which should be biopsied for confirmation rather than treated as infectious.

As bone marrow (BM) involvement in lymphoma confers advanced-stage, accurate evaluation of BM is of crucial importance in patient management. BM involvement at diagnosis is observed in 50-70% of low-grade, 25-40% of high-grade NHL and 5-14 % of HD patients (86). BM biopsy is associated with a high rate of false-negative findings due to sampling errors. Overall, MRI is more sensitive than BM biopsy; however, its routine application to evaluate the entire BM is costly and not practical. Additionally, false negative results can also be obtained with MRI in BM hyperplasia, diffuse lymphoma infiltration as well as with infectious processes. Although physiologic BM uptake is observed on FDG-PET images, focal uptake is usually suggestive of pathological BM activity (Figure 7). Diffusely increased FDG uptake is commonly observed in reactive BM, particularly following administration of colony stimulating factors (e.g. G-CSF) (87, 88) (Figure 8). The reported sensitivity and specificity for FDG-PET are 81% and 100%, respectively in the detection of BM involvement in lymphoma patients (89, 90). In patients with negative BM biopsy, FDG-PET may still reveal focal lymphoma involvement distal from the biopsy site. Overall the negative predictive value for FDG-PET in the detection of BM involvement is higher than the positive predictive value in both pre- and post-therapy patient population. Nevertheless, a minimal degree of BM involvement can result in false negative findings due to the resolution limits of FDG-PET imaging (27, 89-91).

Bone marrow involvement of lymphoma should not be confused with primary bone lymphoma which accounts for less than 5% of all primary bone tumors. MR imaging is most useful for early identification and also depicting the extent of soft-tissue involvement (92). Although there is no series of cases performed using FDG-PET, our experience is that FDG avidly accumulates in bone lesions unlike bone marrow disease (Figure 9).

Consequently, FDG-PET is an accurate and cost-effective staging method that allows simultaneous assessment of the extent of nodal and extranodal lymphoma in patients with HD and NHL. Nevertheless, at pre-therapy staging, FDG-PET should be complemented with CT for better anatomic definition, especially in the evaluation of extranodal disease.

Comparison of FDG-PET and Ga-67 Imaging at Initial Staging

Findings in several comparative studies using dual-head camera-based FDG PET and Ga-67 scintigraphy indicate a higher site and patient sensitivity for FDG-PET (93-97) (Table 2). In aggressive lymphoma and HD, the patient sensitivity for FDG-PET and Ga-67 scintigraphy is 87-100% and 63-80%, respectively (93-95). FDG-PET is usually positive at the majority of disease sites while Ga-67 SPECT may fail to demonstrate uptake in up to 23% of lesion sites regardless of the size, disease location and histology in both nodal and extranodal disease (95). FDG-PET also excluded active lymphoma in patients with Ga-67 positive benign parahilar sites (93).

Although there is a paucity of comparative data, the results obtained using dedicated PET cameras also demonstrate that FDG-PET has a higher sensitivity and detects more disease sites when compared with Ga-67 scintigraphy at initial staging of lymphoma. The site sensitivity for FDG-PET and Ga-67 scintigraphy is reported to be significantly different at 82-96% vs. 69-72%. However, this difference may not translate to major therapeutic strategy changes as FDG-PET findings may not lead to significant stage changes (96, 97).

In light of these data, the disparities in imaging characteristics of these two modalities may indicate dynamic differences in the uptake mechanisms of Ga-67 and FDG by tumor cells. Ga-67 accumulation may require a set of circumstances (as discussed in the "Ga-67 citrate imaging" section) to be fulfilled while hypermetabolism as evidenced by increased glycolysis by the tumor cells is sufficient for FDG uptake. In summary, FDG-PET should supersede Ga-67 imaging for staging of patients with HD or NHL as FDG-

PET may prompt a change in therapeutic management by altering disease stage.

Post-Therapy Evaluation of Lymphoma with FDG-PET

In the post-therapy setting, there are two main questions to which the clinicians need an immediate and accurate answer: whether or not there is residual or recurrent lymphoma during follow-up and there is sufficient therapy response immediately after completion of chemotherapy. We will address these two important issues in this section. In early stage lymphoma, 75-90% of patients respond to therapy regardless of the histological subtype, however, in advanced stage lymphoma, less than 50% of newly diagnosed patients are curable with standard treatments (98, 99). Hence, evaluation of response to therapy is imperative in advanced stage patients.

FDG-PET performs favorably as compared to CT in the differentiation of fibrotic changes from active residual disease as well as monitoring response to therapy (Table 3). Although the available data are scarce, FDG-PET appears to be better than Ga-67 imaging (93-97).

Residual Lymphoma vs. Post-therapy Changes

In the post-therapy setting, FDG-PET correctly identifies majority of patients with residual disease or relapse during follow-up (21-23, 100, 101). Compared to CT, FDG-PET has a significantly higher specificity (89-92% vs. 17-39%) and accuracy (91-96% vs. 54-63%) in the differentiation of residual viable disease from post-therapy fibrosis. FDG-PET could therefore help to identify patients who need additional treatment after the completion of first-line therapy and more importantly could avoid unwarranted further therapy. The negative predictive value for FDG-PET, however, may not be reliable due to microscopic residual disease owing to spatial resolution limitations of PET systems (100).

In summary, in the post-therapy assessment of lymphoma, incongruent results demonstrating negative FDG-PET findings despite the persistence of radiological abnormalities usually indicate post-treatment fibrosis (21-23, 100, 101). Nevertheless, lesions that are below the detection limits of PET systems (<0.5 cm) may give rise to false negative results. Notwithstanding the false positive results occasionally obtained in infectious or inflammatory processes, the positive predictive value of FDG-PET is quite high (> 90%) in the detection of residual or recurrent lymphoma (Table 4).

Prediction of Response to Therapy Response after Completion of Treatment

In the post-therapy setting, residual masses are found in 60- 88% of patients with mediastinal HD, and up to 20-40 % of the patients with bulky aggressive NHL although less than 20% of these masses represent viable persistent lymphoma (102, 103). This is mostly because of post-therapy fibrosis and necrosis that replaces the tumor mass in some cases without a significant size or volume change giving rise to false positive CT readings. FDG PET is a reliable imaging modality in the assessment of response to therapy with a proven superiority to anatomic imaging techniques *(4, 9, 10, 24, 25, 101, 104-107)* (Table 3) (Figures 10 and 11). The relapse free survival rates range from 85 to 100% for patients who have a negative post-therapy FDG-PET compared to 0 to 15% for those with a positive post-therapy FDG-PET.

Table 3. Post-Therapy FDG-PET Studies in the Detection of Residual or Recurrent Lymphoma

Authors	Study	Patient no	Patient Group	PPV (%)	NPV (%)
Cremerius (101)	Retrospective	72	NHL+HD	†	90 vs 67*
Mainolfi (21)	Prospective	32	NHL+HD	†	†
Jerusalem (25)	Prospective	54	NHL+HD	100	90
Hueltenschmidt (100)	Prospective	63	NHL+HD	†	96
Weihrauch (112)	Prospective	28	HD	60	95
Mikhaeel (108)	Retrospective	49	NHL	100	83
De Wit (111)	Prospective	37	HD	46	96
Spaepen (104)	Prospective	93	NHL	100	83.5
Zinzani (109)	Prospective	44	NHL+HD‡	100	96
Becherer (119)	Prospective	16	NHL+HD	87.5	100
Spaepen (117)	Prospective	70	NHL+HD	84	100
Kostakoglu (118)	Prospective	27	NHL+HD	90	100

PPV: positive predictive value   NPV: Negative predictive value
NHL: non-Hodgkin's lymphoma   HD: Hodgkin's disease
* Low-risk vs high-risk patients
† either PPV or NPV or both not given
‡ all patients had intraabdominal lymphoma

Jerusalem et al compared FDG PET and CT in the evaluation of therapy response in 54 patients with HD or aggressive NHL following first-line therapy. They reported a relapse rate of 100% in all (6 patients) patients with a positive FDG PET result while the relapse rate was only 26% in patients with a CT-documented residual mass and a negative companion FDG PET study. A positive FDG PET study was consistently associated with poorer survival than those with a negative FDG PET study, with a one-year median PFS of 0% versus 86%, respectively. The corresponding median survival values for positive and negative CT were 62% and 88%, respectively (25). Mikhaeel et al reported similar results with a relapse rate of 100% for positive PET and only 18% for negative PET, compared to 41% and 25% for patients with positive and negative CT respectively (108). These 2 studies highlight the importance of FDG-PET imaging in assessment of residual masses seen on CT scan.

Zinzani et al evaluated 44 patients with HD and aggressive NHL presenting with abdominal involvement, at the end of chemotherapy with or without RT for bulky lymphoma (109): All PET positive cases eventually succumbed to disease relapse (100%). By contrast, there was only 4% relapse among the 24 patients who were positive at CT but negative at PET. The two-year actuarial relapse-free survival rate was 95% for those with negative PET compared with 0% for positive PET patients: Based on these encouraging results the authors concluded that FDG-PET should be considered the noninvasive imaging modality of choice for differentiating early recurrences or residual disease from fibrosis in patients with abdominal lymphoma

In 93 patients with aggressive lymphoma, Spaepen et al evaluated potential of FDG PET in the prediction of remission or relapse after completion of first line chemotherapy *(104)*. Among patients with negative post-therapy FDG-PET results, 83.5% remained in complete remission with a median follow-up of 653 days. There was persistent FDG uptake at the original site of disease in 26 patients and all patients in this group relapsed with a median progression-free survival of 73 days. The PFS was the shortest in the positive PET group and longest in the negative PET group. Interestingly enough those patients with false negative PET results had a longer PFS than those with positive PET results which is indicative of residual microscopic disease which takes a relatively long period to have a full blown clinical presentation than those with macroscopic residual disease.

In HD, FDG-PET may be of particular help to avoid RT and associated late complications such as second malignancies or cardiovascular disease. If these patients can be accurately risk stratified, avoidance of radiotherapy or lower radiation dose and abbreviated chemotherapy strategies may help mitigate the treatment-related complications (110). In several studies, the predictive value of FDG-PET was evaluated exclusively in patients with HD. In these studies, negative predictive values ranged from 85% to 100%. Nonetheless, positive predictive values were not as high (<70%) (101, 107, 111, 112).

In a study by Cremerius et al, FDG PET was found to predict complete remission better in the moderate risk group (stage I-III, no relapse, no more than two different prior therapy regimens) than in high-risk group with negative predictive values of 90% vs. 50-67% *(102)*. Weihrauch et al studied prognostic value of FDG PET performed at least 3 months after therapy in 28 HD patients with residual mediastinal masses determined by CT *(112)*. Their results indicate that patients with negative FDG PET after therapy are unlikely to relapse within a year. Similarly, Spaepen et al reported a 2-year actuarial PFS rate of 91% for PET negative patients compared with 0% for positive patients after first line therapy in 60 patients with HD. Spaepen (107). Although these results were derived from small patient populations, there is evidence that negative FDG-PET is highly predictive of good prognosis. However, the presence of minimal residual disease cannot be excluded, and may lead to a later relapse. Additionally, these studies underscore the high false positive rates obtained in HD. One explanation to this finding is the frequent occurrences of thymic rebond in this younger age group.

In summary, based on these published results further treatment is appropriate in patients with residual FDG uptake in the region of original disease. The new foci of uptake outside the original disease site/s that appears after therapy should be interpreted with caution and should be histologically verified, especially in the superior anterior mediastinum before further treatment.

Prediction of Response to Therapy Early During the Course of Treatment

Early prediction of response may be clinically more relevant in NHL than in HD, as there is more individual variation in response to specific chemotherapeutic agents in NHL. Furthermore, particularly in aggressive NHL, the rapidity of response has prognostic implications as the patients who experience a partial response or who respond slowly to front-line therapy have a poorer prognosis than those with rapid complete response, (113,114).

Preliminary studies suggest that FDG PET can discriminate responders from nonresponders early during chemotherapy in aggressive NHL and HD. A pilot study demonstrated tat at 6 weeks, there was a significant difference in all parameters of FDG uptake between patients who developed recurrence and those who remained in complete remission. Not surprisingly, anatomic imaging had no value in predicting response to therapy (115).

Jerusalem et al. studied 28 patients before and after three cycles of chemotherapy to predict ultimate response (116). The investigators found that the positive predictive value was 100% but the negative predictive value for prediction of subsequent remission was lower at 67%. Consequently, the PFS at 2 years were 0% for PET positive patients and 62% for PET negative patients. This finding highlights the importance of recognizing false negative findings that may arise from microscopic tumor foci that evade detection by metabolic FDG-PET imaging due to the resolution limits of current PET systems.

Mikhaeel et al reported that the interim FDG-PET obtained after 2-3 cycles provided valuable information regarding early assessment of response and long-term prognosis, revealing no relapses in patients with no or minimal residual uptake compared to a 87.5% relapse rate in patients with persistent FDG uptake *(108)*. Likewise, Spaepen et al found that none of the patients with persistent FDG uptake at mid-treatment achieved a durable complete remission, while in those with a negative scan 84% remained in CR with a median follow-up of 1107 days. In a multivariate analysis, FDG-PET, at midtreatment was a stronger prognostic factor for PFS and OS than the IPI (117).

In a comprehensive literature review, the data revealed that BMT performed immediately after a partial response to induction therapy, before progressive disease occurred has a better chance of resulting in a high CR rate (114). Hence, if therapy response could be predicted as early as one month into therapy, it would effectively direct partial responders to an alternative therapy such as BMT without delay in the course. Additionally, identification of non-complete responders would avoid unwanted side-effects and negative impact on the eligibility for future therapies. Kostakoglu et al demonstrated that FDG PET has a high prognostic value as early as after one cycle in aggressive NHL and HD *(105)*. Ninety percent of patients with a positive FDG PET after one cycle relapsed with a median progression-free survival of 5 months while 85% of patients who had negative FDG PET findings remained in complete remission with a minimum follow-up of 18 months. Recently, in a study by the same investigators, using a dedicated PET system, similar results were obtained. All patients (17 patients) with no appreciable FDG uptake after one cycle of chemotherapy remained in complete remission after a follow-up of 12 months whereas 90% patients with a positive FDG-PET result had a relapse or persistent disease requiring further therapy including bone marrow transplantation (118) (Figures 12, 13). Nonetheless, these data should be interpreted with caution until larger, multiinstitutional studies with a longer follow-up period are executed as both the sample size and follow up periods are not sufficient to arrive at a firm conclusion. If further studies confirm that persistent positive FDG-PET results during therapy, preferably after one cycle, indicate a poor prognosis, one could consider an early change in therapy to a more aggressive approach early during the course of treatment. However, the clinical benefit of such an approach, and whether this early change in therapy would improve upon a predicted outcome would require prospective testing in a randomized clinical trial.

Evaluation of Therapy Response in Patients Undergoing SCT or BMT

High-dose chemotherapy (HDT) with autologous stem cell transplantation (SCT) is the recommended treatment for first chemotherapy-sensitive relapse. The response to HDT/SCT is favorable in patients with chemosensitive disease compared to chemoresistant disease. Consequently in a small group of patients, FDG-PET data demonstrated that none of the patients with a negative PET before HDT/SCT (chemosensitive group) relapsed while the relapse rate was 87.5% in those with a positive FDG-PET result (119, 1209). After 12 months, in the PET-negative and positive groups, the relapse-free survival was 100% and 18%, respectively. In another study, the patients with less than 25% decrease in SUV's after HDT had a progressive disease course while among those who had more than 25% decrease in SUV's, 86% remained in complete remission (119). In another study, the patients with less than 25% decrease in SUV's after HDT had disease progression while in those with more than 25% decrease in SUV's, 86% remained in complete remission (120).

Further studies in larger patient groups are needed to confirm these findings, before they can be applied routinely in clinical management.

Comparison of FDG-PET and Ga-67 Imaging in Post-therapy Evaluation

Only limited data are available in terms of direct comparison of Ga-67 scintigraphy with FDG-PET in lymphoma. In a preliminary study, Hoekstra et al compared planar FDG imaging performed with a conventional gamma-camera equipped with a 511-keV collimator with Ga-67 planar scintigraphy in 26 patients with lymphoma during chemotherapy (121). In patients achieving durable complete remission, tracer distribution had normalized after two courses of chemotherapy; persistent uptake was compatible with treatment failure. More recently, Bar-Shalom et al evaluated the performance of Ga-67 scintigraphy and FDG PET using a dual-head system was retrospectively evaluated in the detection of lymphoma in 84 patients; the majority of the evaluations performed during or after treatment (93). FDG-PET had a significantly higher detection rate compared to Ga-67 scintigraphy for both nodal and extranodal lymphoma sites. Sensitivity and specificity, of Ga-67 scintigraphy were 73% and 51%, respectively. The corresponding values for camera-based FDG PET were 93% and 72%, respectively. Ga-67 scintigraphy accurately defined disease state in 63% of patients and in 33% of sites, compared with 83% and 87%, respectively, for camera-based FDG PET. For discordant findings between the two modalities, camera-based FDG PET findings were confirmed as true-positive in 71% and as true-negative in 92% of patients. FDG-PET was more accurate in the assessment of bone lymphoma compared with Ga-67 scintigraphy in (93% vs. 29%).

4.2 Integrated PET-CT Imaging

With the recent introduction of integrated PET-CT systems a combined method of metabolic and morphologic imaging is available. The main advantage of PET-CT fusion technology is the ability to correlate two contemporaneous imaging modalities for a comprehensive examination that combines anatomic data with functional/metabolic information in the same imaging session (122). This technique provides important information particularly in the post-therapy setting; metabolic findings that are overlooked due to the subtlety of metabolic changes on FDG-PET may result in the detection of residual disease after correlation with the simultaneously acquired CT data. Furthermore, equivocal CT findings which are suggestive of either recurrent tumor or post-therapy changes can now be distinguished with the guidance of the additional information obtained from FDG-PET data. In a recent study, PET-CT performed with nonenhanced CT was found more sensitive and specific than was contrast-enhanced CT for evaluation of lymph node and organ involvement in HD and NHL (123). The diagnostic value of coregistered PET-CT scans obtained with low-dose nonenhanced CT was compared with those routinely obtained with contrast-enhanced CT for staging and restaging of disease in HD and NHL. For evaluation of lymph node involvement, sensitivity of PET-CT and contrast-enhanced CT was 94% and 88%, and specificity was 100% and 86%, respectively. For evaluation of organ involvement, sensitivity of PET/CT and contrast-enhanced CT was 88% and 50%, and specificity was 100% and 90%, respectively. In addition to the application of fusion technology in the diagnosis and staging and restaging of malignant disease, it is useful in planning radiation therapy and determining the optimum approach for CT-guided biopsy (122). Consequently, the addition of metabolic imaging can have a great effect on treatment in patients with a residual mass at post treatment evaluation.

4.3   Ga-67 Citrate Imaging

Carrier-free Ga-67 citrate concentrates in certain viable primary and metastatic tumors as well as focal sites of infection. Ga-67 scintigraphy is particularly an important imaging tool in lymphoma, primarily in the post-therapy setting.

Mechanism of Uptake: Investigational studies have shown that Ga-67 accumulates in lysosomes bound to a soluble intracellular protein. Ga-67 is a ferric ion (Fe+3) analogue and binds to iron-binding proteins, mainly transferrin in the serum. The Ga-67 accumulation in tumors is mediated by various factors associated with tumor composition and physiology such as tumor-associated transferrin receptors (CD-71), anaerobic tumor metabolism that leads to the dissociation of Ga-transferrin complex in low-pH conditions, increased tumor perfusion and vascular permeability (124-126). Several studies demonstrated that expression of transferrin receptors, especially in large cell subtype, correlated with Ga-67 uptake (127). The presence of large cell component in low-grade lymphoma may explain the varying Ga-67 uptake among low-grade lymphomas. Ga-67 biodistribution may be altered in patients with iron overload through diet, iron administration and blood transfusion as Ga-67 competes with iron for transferring binding.

A proper imaging protocol is the key to increase the sensitivity of Ga-67 scintigraphy. In addition to whole body images, SPECT of the chest and abdomen should be routinely obtained in all patients to minimize false negative results (128, 129) (Table 1).

Clinical Applications: Ga-67 imaging has been an integral component of diagnostic algorithm in the pre- and post-treatment evaluation of HD and aggressive lymphomas. Its use at initial diagnosis prior to treatment is not necessary for accurate staging but to obtain a baseline study to subsequently assess response to therapy.

4.3.1 Histologic Subtypes of Lymphoma and Ga-67 Imaging

The sensitivity of Ga-67 is affected by the histologic subtype of lymphoma. Ga-67 scintigraphy is highly sensitive in aggressive NHL [intermediate (~85%) and high grade ~95%], and HD (~95%) (14, 129, 130). Among aggressive lymphomas, Ga-67 has been reported to be more sensitive in histiocytic NHL (~70%) than in lymphocytic NHL (~50%) (131). The sensitivity of Ga-67 for low-grade lymphoma is significantly low at 41-56%, particularly in the lymphocytic subtype (14, 132, 133) (Figure 14). More recently, using a large field-of-view dual-head gamma camera, encouraging results have been reported in low-grade NHL patients with an overall patient sensitivity of 79% (134). The site sensitivity (69%), however, was lower than the patient sensitivity. In this study, the sensitivity of Ga-67 was higher in follicular small cleaved cell at 84%, follicular mixed lymphomas at 91% and lower in small lymphocytic lymphomas at 67% and in mucosa-associated lymphoid tissue lymphoma (MALT) at 25%. One issue that warrants emphasis is the transformation of low-grade lymphomas to a higher grade lymphoma in as much as 50% of patients (135). In these cases, positive lesions detected on Ga-67 imaging may, in fact, indicate transformation to high-grade lymphoma which may guide biopsy sites. Tl-201, Tc-99m Sestamibi and In-111-octreotide have been reported to detect low-grade lymphoma with a higher sensitivity. The role of these radiotracers will be discussed in relevant sections.

4.3.2 Staging of Lymphoma

Nodal Lymphoma: Ga-67 imaging is highly in the mediastinum in both NHL and HD. The overall sensitivity for nodal disease is 75%-90% in NHL and 85%-95% in HD (136). Ga-67 imaging is more sensitive for the detection of disease in the mediastinum, cervical lymph nodes and other superficial sites than in the abdomen. Consequently, Ga-67 was reported to have a sensitivity of 96% and 83% for mediastinal and cervical disease, respectively (137). The sensitivity for the detection of retroperitoneal or intra-abdominal nodal lymphoma, however, is not favorable. In a comparative study of 53 patients with HD, Ga-67 was found to show lower sensitivity than CT and MRI (90% vs. 96% and 100%, respectively) with high number of false-negative results (138). Nevertheless, by using both CT and Ga-67, the sensitivity was equal to that obtained with MRI (100%). Hence, as a single technique, Ga-67 scintigraphy does not replace CT scan or MRI in staging patients with lymphoma and should be complemented by either imaging technique. Ultrasonography is also reported to superior to Ga-

67 scintigraphy in identifying intra-abdominal lymphoma sites with a reported accuracy of 87.5% compared to 82% for Ga-67 scanning (139).

Extranodal Lymphoma: The sensitivity of Ga-67 scintigraphy in the detection of aggressive extranodal lymphoma, primarily located in the stomach and nasopharyngeal region is similar to that obtained with nodal NHL (140). The sensitivity of Ga-67 is lower, however, in those with the involvement of the skin, intestine and testis (0%-25%). In one series, the overall Ga-67 scan sensitivity was 70% for the detection of extranodal lymphoma in 92 patients. In 65% of patients, Ga-67 and CT scans produced similar results while in 18% of patients Ga-67 showed more lesion sites than CT and CT revealed more extensive disease in 17% of patients. Ga-67 findings in patients with hepatic lymphoma vary between focal increased uptake or grossly non-uniform hepatic uptake (134). Hepatomegaly alone is nonspecific as only 15% of patients with hepatomegaly are reported to have hepatic involvement (141). Ga-67 and CT have a complimentary role in diagnosing lymphoma in the liver, although Ga-67 may be preferable in monitoring response to therapy.

Ga-67 scintigraphy can be used to monitor response to treatment in patients with primary bone lymphoma while its role in the detection of bone lymphoma at initial staging is not well defined. Tc-99m-MDP scintigraphy is slightly better than Ga-67 in the detection of bone lymphoma in therapy naïve patients with a reported sensitivity and specificity of 93%, and 91%, respectively (142)

In summary, Ga-67 scintigraphy lacks sensitivity required of a diagnostic imaging modality at initial staging. Many centers utilize Ga-67 study at initial presentation as a baseline to accurately determine response to therapy. Additional sites of disease, however, can be detected by Ga-67 imaging when staging CT does not demonstrate lymphoma in disease harboring normal sized lymph nodes.

4.3.3   Post-Therapy Evaluation of Lymphoma

Residual Lymphoma vs. Post-therapy Changes: Ga-67 accumulates in proportion to the degree viable tumor after therapy. Thus, it is most useful in the post-therapy setting, either to evaluate residual or recurrent disease or to monitor therapy response during the course or at completion of therapy (Table 4).

Early diagnosis of recurrence during follow-up is crucial in patient management.

Ga-67 scintigraphy at completion of therapy has a sensitivity of 76%-100% and a specificity of 75%-96% in the differentiation of residual lymphoma from post-therapy fibrosis (76, 77). The sensitivity and specificity of Ga-67 imaging to identify recurrent lymphoma is approximately 95% and 89%, respectively (143, 144).

Ga-67 imaging is particularly useful in detecting residual disease at restaging when CT depicts a subtle focus or a mass indistinguishable from active disease, especially in cases where further therapy may be necessary. In a retrospective study, during restaging of HD after therapy, Ga-67 imaging and CT correctly identified active disease sites in 96% and 68%, respectively; in patients with histopathologically proven recurrent HD. Ga-67 imaging identified recurrent disease in 87.5% of patients who had equivocal findings on CT studies (128). In a similar study, when post-therapy spiral CT and Ga-67 were compared in patients with HD or aggressive NHL, Ga-67-SPECT proved superior to spiral CT for identifying residual nodal disease with a sensitivity of 94% vs. 83% and a specificity of 100% vs. 92.5% (145). Failure free survivals are better in majority of patients with negative Ga-67 findings compared to those with positive results after therapy (142). No statistically significant difference in failure-free survival has been reported, however, between patients with positive and negative CT findings.

In particular, in patients with HD, for whom treatment with a combined modality (chemotherapy and radiotherapy) is planned, the role of Ga-67 imaging to detect active disease after chemotherapy is useful to plan the subsequent radiotherapeutic strategy. In a group of 53 HD patients, at restaging after therapy, Ga-67 was superior to CT scan and equivalent to MR in identifying true negative cases (specificity: 98% vs. 45% vs. 92%, respectively) (146).

Detection of minimal residual disease admixed with a fibrotic tissue change is challenging with current Ga-67 SPECT systems, particularly if the viable tumor measures less than one cm in diameter. Thus, it is notable that the patients with negative post-therapy Ga-67 scans still have a moderate chance of disease recurrence. The pretreatment agreement between CT and Ga-67 scintigraphy ranges from 75% to 100% in the detection of HD while a greater variation in agreement is observed once chemotherapy is initiated due to the common occurrence of residual mediastinal masses (147).

One well-known dilemma with Ga-67 scintigraphy is the non-specific and persistent hilar uptake following therapy which can be observed in up to 79% of patients in the absence of corresponding CT evidence of lymphoma (148). When the hilar uptake is symmetric and less intense than the uptake within the original disease site, it is deemed to be of benign etiology with a negative predictive value higher than 95%. Asymmetric hilar uptake equal in intensity to the original disease, however, is usually indicative of viable disease with a positive predictive value higher than 85% (13).

4.3.4   Monitoring Response to Therapy and Prediction of Therapy Outcome

Ga-67 imaging after induction chemotherapy has the ability to differentiate chemosensitive patients from those with poor prognosis (Table 4). In one study, in patients with HD, Ga-67 imaging identified residual disease with a negative and positive predictive value of up to 86% and 81%, respectively. In patients with NHL, the corresponding values were 84% and 73%, respectively (148). The 5-year overall survival rate was significantly different between groups with negative (91%) and positive (25%) Ga-67 results (149).

Table 4. Post-Therapy Ga-67 Studies in the Detection of Residual Lymphoma and Evaluation of Response to Therapy

Authors	Patient no	Patient Group	ChemoRx Cycles	PPV (%)	NPV (%)
Janicek (5)	30	NHL	2 cycles	82	94
Front (6)	31	HD	1 cycle	57	92
Hagemeister (10)	46	HD	3 cycles‡	30	97
Salloum (11)	101	HD	Completion	†	83.5
Front (12)	51	NHL	1 cycle	71	81
			3 cycles	74	63
Front (82)	43	HD	Completion	80	84
	56	aNHL	Completion	73	84
Ionescu (150)	53	HD	3-4 cycles	81	86
Bogart (152)	60	HD	Completion	¶	78
Vose (153)	66	aNHL	Completion*	75	47
	77	LGL	Completion*	76	45
Kaplan (154)	37	NHL	4 cycles	76	70

PPV: positive predictive value   NPV: negative predictive value
NHL: non-Hodgkin's lymphoma including low-grade lymphoma
HD: Hodgkin's disease   LGL: Low-grade lymphoma   aNHL: aggressive NHL
* patients were evaluated after high-dose chemotherapy and bone marrow transplant
† inadequate number of patients to determine PPV
‡ patients were evaluated after three cycles of NOVP (Novantrone, vincristine, vinblastine, prednisone) prior to radiotherapy
¶ PPV not given but there was no difference in overall survivals between Ga positive or negative patient

A positive post-therapy Ga-67 scintigraphy is consistently predictive of therapy failure and poor outcome. Hence, patient management can be directly affected by Ga-67 scintigraphy in those with positive post-therapy findings. The risk of recurrence, however, is not a mere function of post-therapy imaging findings, prognostic risk factors such as histology, stage, initial tumor burden, prior therapy and various host factors also contribute to the rate of recurrence. Approximately 20% of patients with mediastinal HD relapse at the original disease site despite a negative post-therapy Ga-67 study (150). Accordingly, the negative predictive value of Ga-67 imaging may vary greatly among patients with various stages of lymphoma. Based on the stage of disease, negative predictive value of a post-therapy Ga-67 can be as high as 97% in early stage lymphoma while the corresponding value can be significantly lower (64.5%) for advanced stage disease (10, 11) (Figures 15, 16). Briefly, a negative Ga-67 imaging scan after therapy, therefore, may have a lower predictive value in advanced stage disease compared with early stage lymphoma (11, 151, 152).

4.3.5 Early Prediction of Response during Therapy

Early during the course of chemotherapy, restaging Ga-67 scans can delineate patients who are likely to fail to respond to intensive induction therapy from those who will have prolonged disease-free survival. Patients whose tumors remain Ga-67 positive during chemotherapy have a poor outcome and may be candidates for alternative treatment protocols. The time span for a positive Ga-67 study to convert to negative during or immediately after chemotherapy may be predictive of complete remission and treatment outcome (6, 7, 12, 152, 153). In an earlier study, following 2-4 cycles of chemotherapy, 46% of patients showed persistent pathological Ga-67 uptake. Of these, during follow-up, 59% had died of disease progression and 12% were alive with active lymphoma and 6% relapsed but survived following bone marrow transplantation. Of the patients who were Ga-67-negative halfway through therapy, 70% were alive without disease, 25% have died and 5% were alive with disease at a median of 34 months from presentation (154). In a similar study, the recurrence rates were similar between early Ga-67 imaging (four cycles of chemotherapy) and late Ga-67 imaging (five or more cycles of chemotherapy) indicating that Ga-67 imaging may predict outcome early during the course of therapy (152).

Other investigators reported that early restaging Ga-67 scans are more predictive of failure-free survival than final restaging Ga-67 scans. The patients who need more cycles of therapy to become Ga-67 negative are found to be more prone to develop recurrent disease (6). CT-documented rates of response and residual mass sizes were indistinguishable in complete responders who remained disease-free, complete responders who subsequently relapsed, and partial responders who then progressed. In marked contrast, early restaging (after two cycles of chemotherapy) Ga-67 scans accurately delineated these three categories of patients: At a median follow-up duration of 31 months, 94% of patients who had negative early restaging Ga-67 scans remained free from progression whereas only 18% of patients who had positive early restaging Ga-67 scans remained progression-free.

Furthermore, in both aggressive NHL and HD, Ga-67 imaging is also a good predictor of outcome after one cycle of chemotherapy (7, 12). In HD, failure-free survival differed significantly between patients with positive and patients with negative Ga-67 imaging after one cycle of chemotherapy but not at midtreatment. Failure-free survival was not significantly different between patients with positive and patients with negative CT scans at midtreatment. In patients with negative Ga-67 imaging, 92% after one cycle and 82% at midtreatment remained in complete remission. Among patients with positive Ga-67 studies after one cycle, 57% relapsed (7). In aggressive NHL, Ga-67 findings after one cycle of chemotherapy and at midtreatment were predictive of outcome in patients with aggressive NHL. There was no significant difference in failure-free survival between patients with positive and negative CT findings during treatment (12). Thus, early Ga-67 imaging during the course of chemotherapy identifies patients who may benefit from more aggressive treatment.

Ga-67 SPECT imaging obtained after high-dose chemotherapy and autologous stem-cell transplantation may be useful for the evaluation of disease activity and to predict the eventual outcome. In one study, the one-year failure free survival for patients with a positive post-therapy Ga-67 scintigraphy was 15% compared with a 3-year failure free survival of 47% for those with a negative scan. The corresponding values for CT scan were not significantly different (36% vs. 39%) (153).

The international prognostic index (IPI) was designed to further clarify lymphoma staging. The IPI predicts the risk of recurrence and overall survival by taking into account factors such as age, stage of disease, performance status, number of extranodal disease sites, and the lactate dehydrogenase (LDH) levels (155). Ga-67 scintigraphy has been reported to be a better predictor than IPI for both response rate and failure-free survival. Thus, positive Ga-67 early during treatment may be used as an independent procedure to select patients who will not respond favorably to current treatment regimens (156).

5. THALLIUM 201 AND TC-99M SESTAMIBI IMAGING IN LYMPHOMA

Tl-201 is primarily a myocardial perfusion agent, however it has been demonstrated that Tl-201 has oncologic applications in the assessment of tumor detection and viability (157).

Mechanism of Uptake: The mechanisms regulating the Tl-201 uptake in tumor cells is multifactoral and related to blood flow, tumor viability, the sodium-potassium adenosinetriphosphatase system (Na-K-ATPase), the non-energy dependent co-transport system, calcium ion channel mechanisms, and increased cell membrane permeability (158) Because of the physical and biological similarity of thallium and potassium, tumor cells with high Na-K-ATPase activity can accumulate Tl-201. Radiotherapy or chemotherapy impacts the activity of Na-K-ATPase on tumor cells, thus decrease the uptake of Tl-201 (159, 160).

Tc-99m Sestamibi (MIBI) is a lipophilic monovalent action and accumulates within the mitochondria through electrical potentials generated across the membrane bilayers. MIBI accumulates preferentially in malignant cells, owing to a higher transmembrane electric potential that results from a higher metabolic rate in malignant cells. Nonetheless, the retention of MIBI within the cell is also related to the energy (ATP) dependent transmembrane transporter proteins including the P-glycoprotein pump system (Pgp) and the multidrug resistance protein (MRP) (161-163). Consequently, MIBI accumulation is reduced in cells expressing MDR or MRP phenotype owing to the ATP-dependent Pgp efflux pump. MIBI tumor washout rate can aid in identification of tumors expressing multi-drug resistance proteins and may provide prognostic information. The imaging parameters are shown in Table 1.

The optimal time for both Tl-201 and MIBI tumor imaging is 20 to 60 minutes post injection. Delayed images at 3-4 hours are recommended when imaging lymphoma because of an improved lesion to background ratio over time. In addition to the whole body images, a SPECT study of the area of interest significantly helps determine the anatomic location of the lesion, particularly with SPECT-CT systems.

Clinical Applications: The role of Tl-201 in the evaluation of lymphomas is limited to low-grade lymphomas and the differentiation of CNS lymphoma from infectious processes. The clinical benefit that could be derived from the use of Tl-201 scintigraphy is not significant in aggressive NHL and HD (14, 164). The results of several studies have demonstrated a disparity between Ga-67 and Tl-201 accumulation in patients with low-grade lymphoma with Ga-67 showing low or absent uptake and Tl-201 moderate to marked accumulation. For practical purposes, Ga-67 and Tl-201 should complement one another in the follow-up of indolent lymphoma. If a patient who used to be negative on Ga-67 scintigraphy and positive on Tl-201 converts to a positive status on Ga-67, one might assume that the indolent tumor biology has transformed to an aggressive pattern. This may have an impact in therapeutic strategy and management.

At initial staging, the overall sensitivity of Tl-201 is reported to be 64% in the follicular subtype of indolent lymphomas. Unlike Ga-67, Tl-201 rarely accumulates in inflammatory sites, accordingly, after radiotherapy, Tl-201 is deemed to be successful in determining complete or partial remission in patients who have a positive baseline Tl-201 (165).

Tl-201 scintigraphy is also useful the evaluation of CNS lesions, especially in the differentiation of toxoplasmosis from CNS lymphoma in patients with AIDS (166) (Figures 17, 18). The patients with lymphoma have significantly higher lesion/contralateral scalp Tl-201 ratios compared to patients without lymphoma. Using a cut-off of 0.90 for the lesion/scalp uptake ratios the sensitivity and specificity for the diagnosis of lymphoma were 86% and 83%, respectively. Furthermore, combining Tl-201 scintigraphy with serum toxoplasma IgG, diagnostic accuracy can be improved in those with either false positive or false negative results.

Several studies report the usefulness of MIBI scintigraphy in the prediction of chemotherapy response in untreated adult lymphomas exploiting the characteristics of MIBI as a transport substrate for the Pgp and MRP pump related drug resistance mechanisms (167-170). The patients with negative or decreased MIBI activity tend to have unfavorable response to chemotherapy compared to those with sufficient MIBI accumulation irrespective of the lymphoma type. These findings are consistent with the inverse relationship between the levels of Pgp and the magnitude of MIBI uptake and washout in the tumor cells. Discrepancies, however, have been observed which could be attributed to the presence of subsets of cells with varying degrees Pgp expression and co-existence of multiple drug resistance mechanisms or poor penetration of MIBI due to reduced blood flow in tumors.

6.   IN-111 OCTREOTIDE IMAGING IN LYMPHOMA

Mechanism of Uptake: Indium-111 pentetreotide is a [In-111 DTPA-D-Phe] conjugate of octreotide, a somatostatin analog that binds to somatostatin receptors (predominantly somatostatin receptor subtypes 2 and

5). The uptake of In-111 octreotide is dependent on somatostatin receptor-mediated internalization of the radioligand by the tumor cells. Somatostatin receptor imaging (SRI) with this octapeptide can be performed in both neuroendrocrine and some non-neuroendrocrine tumors. The presence of cellular somatostatin receptors, particularly of subtype 2, has been reported in a large number of human primary non-neuroendocrine tumours, such as breast cancer, colon cancer and lymphoma.

Clinical Applications: The uptake of In-111-Octreotide is generally lower in lymphomas compared to neuroendocrine tumors (171). In-111-Octreotide imaging is not highly sensitive in patients with NHL as receptor negative lesions can occur in a substantial number of NHL's (172). The sensitivity of In-111-Octreotide for detecting HD is reportedly 70-95% and varies between 98% for supradiaphragmatic lesions and 67% for infradiaphragmatic lesions (173, 174). The sensitivity for NHL, however, is determined to be significantly low at 35%.

In low-grade lymphoma, although SRI findings are positive in a large proportion of patients, in most patients only part of the lesions can be visualized due to the limited sensitivity. The sensitivity of SRI scintigraphy in low grade lymphoma can vary from 62% for supradiaphragmatic lesions to 44% for infradiaphragmatic lesions (171).

SRI imaging lacks superior sensitivity for lymphomas but may be necessary in those patients who would undergo radionuclide-labeled SS analog-based therapy. In a recent study, a selective expression of sst_2 and sst_3 receptors was demonstrated in lymphomas; however the magnitude of expression was relatively low. Although these findings do not appear to be promising, lymphomas are highly radiosensitive tumors and further clinical studies should be performed to evaluate whether the low receptor density is sufficient for targeting treatment in these tumors (175).

7. CONCLUSION

Ga-67 scintigraphy is still a useful modality in the absence of PET imaging. Nevertheless, Ga-67 imaging is more useful in the post-therapy setting than at initial staging as it lacks sensitivity in specific types of lymphomas, particularly in low-grade and abdominal lymphoma. However, a baseline study prior to therapy is necessary to fully assess residual or recurrent disease. Ga-67 imaging after induction chemotherapy has the ability to differentiate chemosensitive patients from those with poor prognosis. A positive post-therapy Ga-67 scintigraphy is consistently associated with poor prognosis while a negative result suggests a favorable prognosis. False negative results, however, may arise due to resolution limitations.

Tl-201 scintigraphy is primarily used in the diagnosis and follow-up of low-grade lymphomas. Although superior to Ga-67, it still lacks sensitivity in low-grade lymphomas. Currently the strength of Tl-201 imaging lies in its ability to differentiate CNS lymphoma from toxoplasmosis in immunocompromised patients. However, FDG-PET imaging appears to be more reliable in the differentiation of infectious process from a malignant process due to its superior resolution although the number of cases are not sufficient for a firm conclusion.

Because of its close association with multidrug resistance, MIBI scintigraphy can provide information in the prediction of chemotherapy response and could guide the design of the most effective therapy protocols. Nevertheless, evaluation of multidrug resistance is a controversial issue because of the multifaceted problems that stem from non-specificity of MIBI imaging, tumor heterogeneity, co-existence of various resistance mechanisms, and in clinical practice lack of effective reversal agents.

Generally, SRI has limited detection sensitivity in lymphoma, thus SRI should not be used as a routine test as part of the initial staging of lymphoma. Overall radiolabeled octreotide scintigraphy is better suited to characterize somatostatin receptor expressing lymphomas than to localize lesion sites. Thus, it may be useful to determine the patient population that would benefit from therapy with radiolabeled somatostatin receptor analogues.

FDG-PET is currently the most sensitive and specific metabolic imaging modality in the staging and restaging of lymphomas. FDG-PET has proven to be more accurate than CT at initial staging and also has higher specificity in the differentiation of active disease from residual inert masses compared with anatomic imaging modalities. FDG-PET is also more sensitive and accurate than Ga-67 imaging at initial diagnosis and post-therapy restaging of lymphoma. FDG-PET has a distinct role in the evaluation of post-therapy abnormalities that fall under the category of unconfirmed/uncertain complete remission. Non-invasive metabolic imaging methods allow significant reduction in the utilization of more costly and invasive methods for staging and treatment monitoring in patients with lymphoma. FDG-PET is an accurate method of assessing remission and predicting prognosis following treatment of aggressive NHL and HD with high positive and negative predictive values, although multicenter trials are necessary for establishing its role in this regard.

ACKNOWLEDGEMENTS

We thank Dr. Roman Mirsky for his contribution to this chapter.

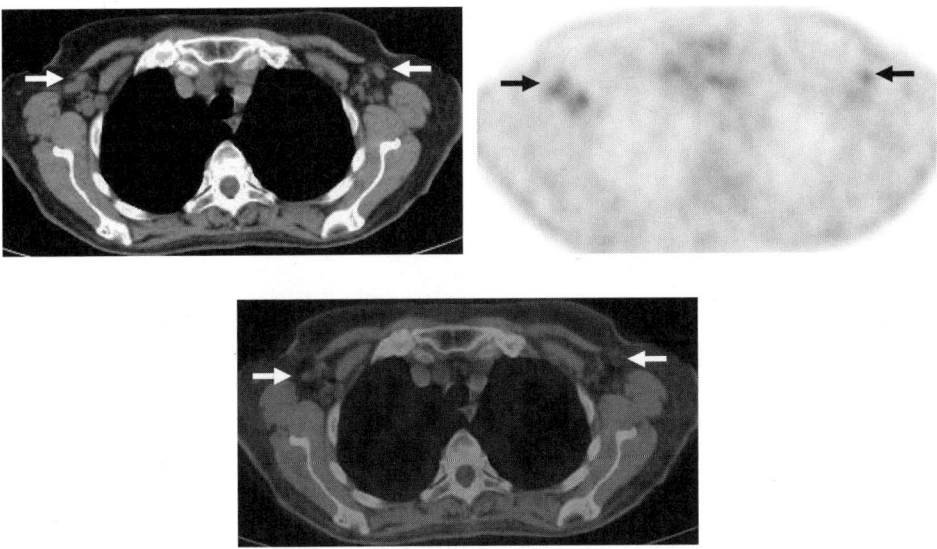

Figure 1. Patient recently diagnosed with small lymphocytic non-Hodgkin's lymphoma (CLL/SLL) underwent a pre-therapy FDG-PET imaging study simultaneously acquired with a CT scan, to evaluate the extent of disease. Axial images of CT (upper left), PET (upper right) and PET-CT fusion (bottom) demonstrate minimal FDG uptake in multiple nodal sites involving the bilateral axillary lymph nodes (arrows) consistent with low grade lymphoma (SUVmax: 1.8).

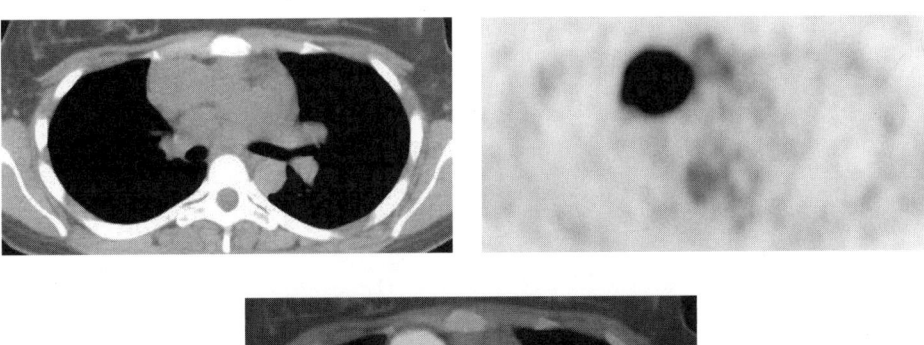

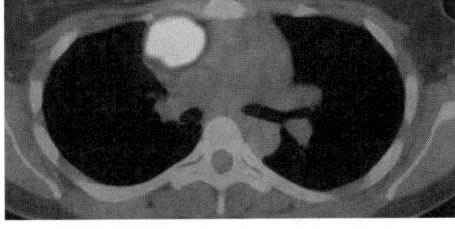

Figure 2. Patient with a diagnosis of diffuse large cell lymphoma underwent a pre-therapy FDG-PET imaging study simultaneously acquired with a CT scan, to evaluate for staging. Axial images of CT (left), PET (middle) and PET-CT fusion (right) demonstrate intense increased FDG uptake in the anterior mediastinum adjacent to the base of the heart, consistent active disease (SUVmax: 24). Note the difference in the degree of FDG uptake from the patient presented in Figure 1.

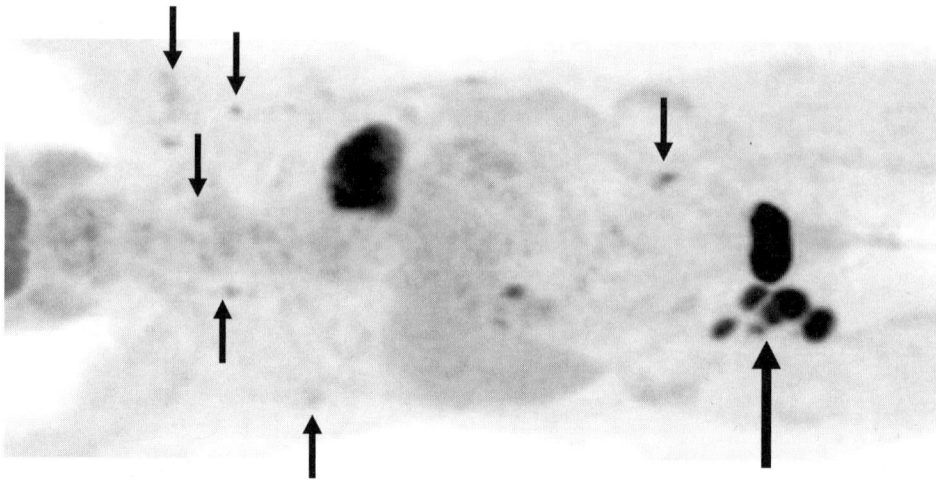

Figure 3. Patient with a history of follicular lymphoma presents with an enlarged right inguinal lymph node. The patient underwent a pre-therapy FDG-PET imaging study simultaneously acquired with a CT scan, to evaluate for extent of disease. Volumetric FDG-PET image demonstrates multiple small foci of abnormal FDG uptake distributed in various lymph node stations in both the infra- and supra-diaphragmatic sites, including bilateral axillary, paratracheal and pelvic lymph nodes (small arrows). There is avid FDG uptake in the right external iliac and inguinal lymph node chains (large arrow) which shows a more intense pattern compared to the rest of the lymph nodes (mean SUVmax: 18 vs. 3.5). This difference in FDG avidity suggests higher metabolic activity, thus transformation to an aggressive subtype in the right inguinal lymph nodes. Subsequent biopsy of a right inguinal lymph node revealed diffuse large cell lymphoma.

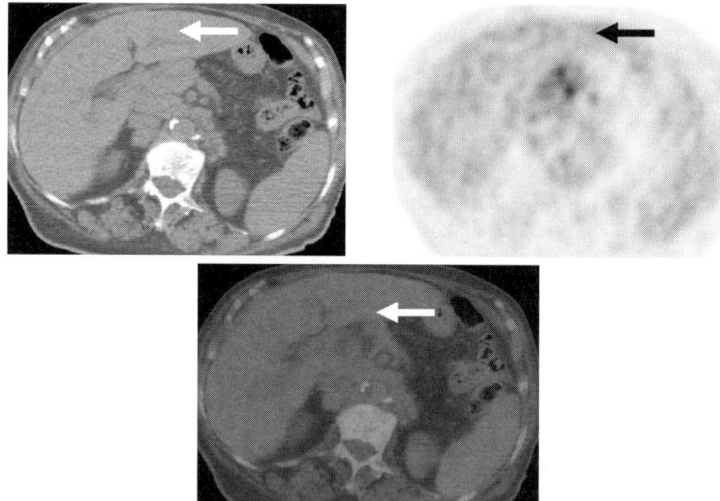

Figure 4. Patient with a diagnosis of MALT of the stomach underwent a pre-therapy FDG-PET imaging study simultaneously acquired with a CT scan, to evaluate for staging. Axial images of CT (left), PET (middle) and PET-CT fusion (right) demonstrate minimally increased FDG uptake in the distal stomach consistent with MALT.

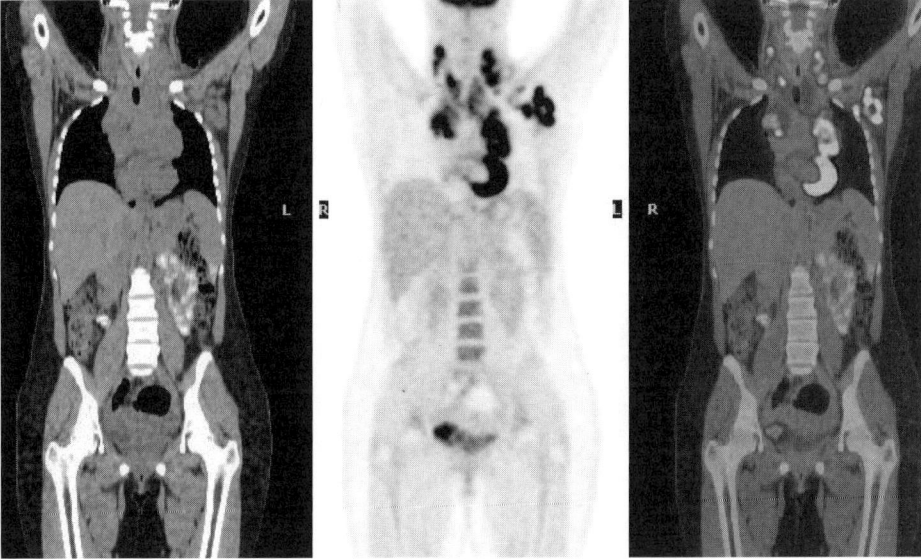

Figure 5. The patient with a recent diagnosis of HD referred for evaluation of extent of disease, staging prior to chemo-therapy. Coronal images of CT (left), PET (middle) and PET-CT fusion (right) demonstrate intense increased FDG uptake in the bilateral supraclavicular, paratracheal, right axillary and mediastinal lymph nodes. The disease is confined to one side of the diaphragm consistent active lymphoma. Note the uptake in the pelvis that corresponds to the superior aspect of the bladder which represents physiologic FDG uptake.

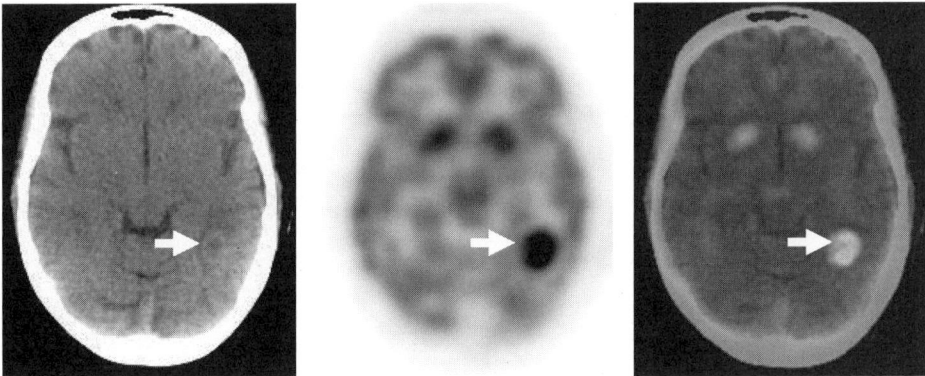

Figure 6. The patient with a history of AIDS recently found to have a brain lesion in the left parietooccipital lobe, referred for FDG-PET imaging to differentiate between toxoplasmosis from CNS lymphoma. There is intense FDG uptake in a lesion corresponding to the left posterior parietooccipital cortex consistent with CNS lymphoma (arrows). The patient was subsequently started on proper therapy.

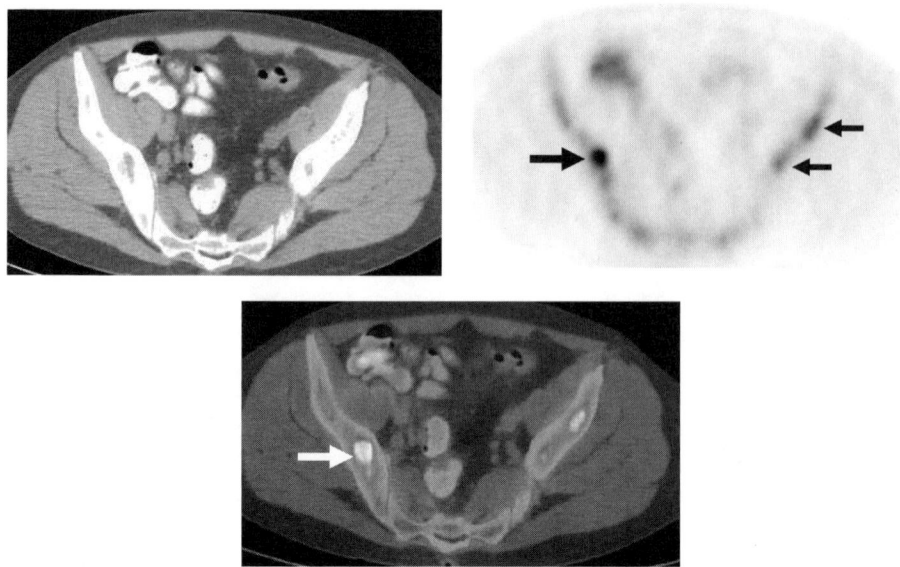

Figure 7. The patient with recently diagnosed non-Hodgkin's lymphoma underwent a pre-therapy FDG-PET imaging study simultaneously acquired with a CT scan, to evaluate the extent of disease. Axial images of CT (upper left), PET (upper right) and PET-CT fusion (bottom) demonstrate focal FDG uptake in the right iliac bone as well as heterogeneous uptake in the remainder of the pelvic bones highly suspicious for bone or bone marrow involvement (arrows). Subsequent biopsy revealed bone marrow involvement.

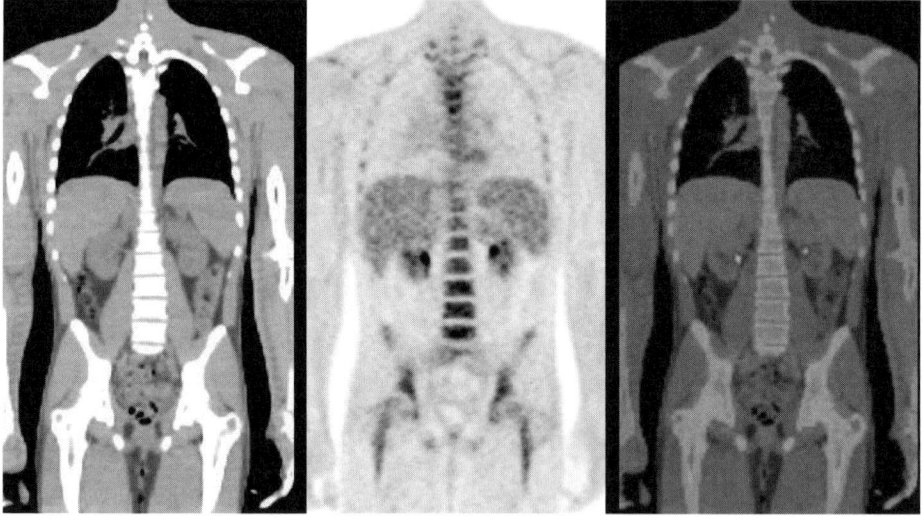

Figure 8. Coronal images of CT (left), PET (middle) and PET-CT fusion (right) demonstrate irregularly diffusely increased FDG uptake most obvious in the entire vertebral column, ribs, pelvis and proximal femora, consistent with reactive bone marrow changes secondary to administration of colony stimulators (G-CSF). Due to the reactive changes in the bone marrow, possible involvement of the bone marrow cannot be evaluated with certainty.

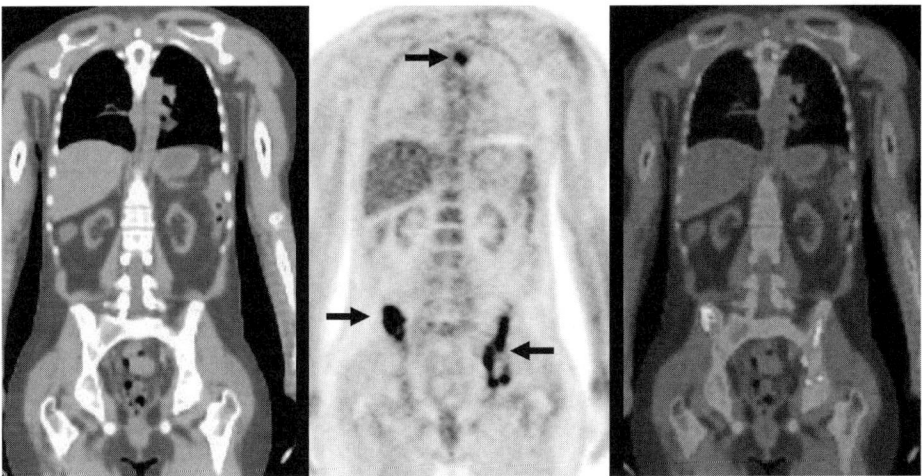

Figure 9. Patient with a recently diagnosed with diffuse large cell lymphoma underwent a FDG-PET imaging study simultaneously acquired with a CT scan, to evaluate extent of disease prior to therapy. Coronal images of CT (left), PET (middle) and PET-CT fusion (right) demonstrate foci of intense increased FDG uptake in the upper thoracic spine, left and right iliac bones (arrows), consistent with lymphoma of the bone.

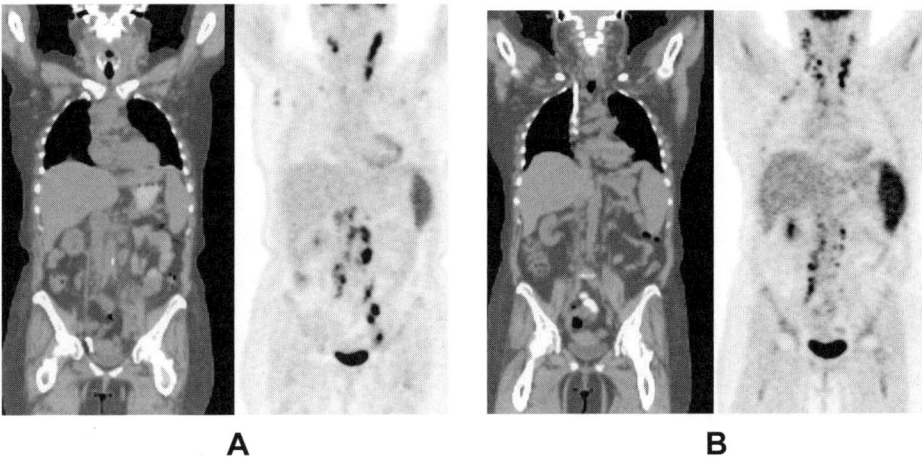

A   B

Figure 10. Patient with non-Hodgkin's lymphoma underwent a PET-CT study prior to and immediately following completion of therapy to evaluate response to therapy. **A.** Pre-therapy coronal images of CT (left), PET (right) demonstrate increased FDG uptake in the bilateral cervical, axillary, paraaortic, left iliac lymph node stations as well as in the spleen. These findings are consistent with advanced stage lymphoma. **B.** Post-therapy coronal images of CT (left), PET (right) demonstrate persistent FDG uptake in the bilateral cervical, right axillary, paraaortic, and iliac lymph node stations as well as in the spleen. There are also additional disease sites in the paratracheal regions. These findings are consistent with unfavorable response to therapy. The patient was subsequently placed on an alternative therapy. Note the increased bone marrow uptake due to recently administered colony stimulators in the post-therapy images.

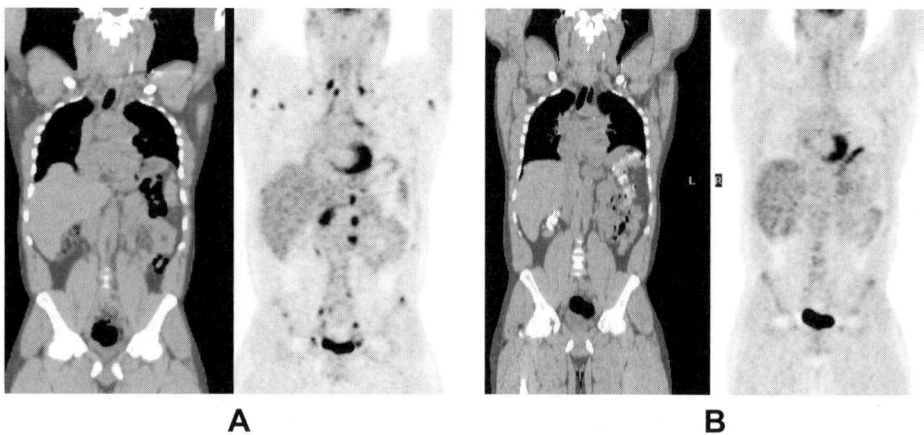

A   B

Figure 11. Patient with non-Hodgkin's lymphoma underwent a PET-CT study prior to and immediately following completion of therapy to evaluate response to therapy. **A.** Pre-therapy coronal images of CT (left), PET (right) demonstrate increased FDG uptake in the bilateral cervical, suraclavicular, paratracheal, axillary, paraaortic, iliac lymph node stations as well as in the bone/bone marrow in the iliac bones. These findings are consistent with advanced stage lymphoma. **B.** Post-therapy coronal images of CT (left), PET (right) demonstrate complete disappearance of FDG uptake in the disease locations noted on the pre-therapy FDG-PET study, consistent with complete metabolic response. The PFS on this patient has bee > 18 months.

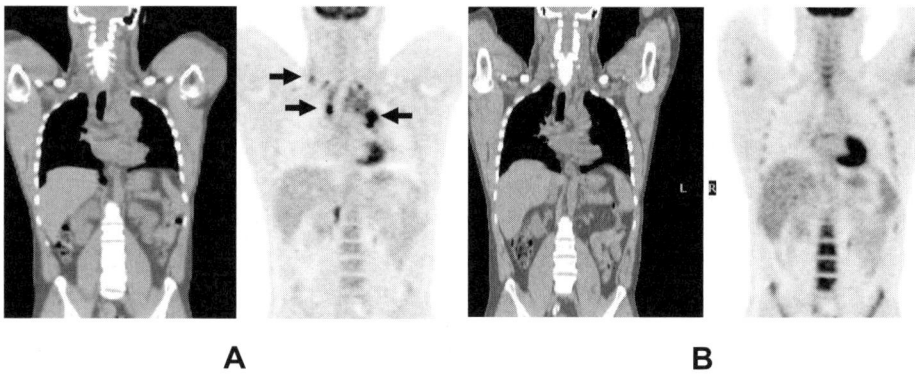

A   B

Figure 12. Patient with a recently diagnosed Hodgkin's lymphoma underwent a PET-CT study prior to, after one cycle of chemotherapy. **A.** Pre-therapy coronal images of CT (left), PET (right) demonstrate increased FDG uptake in the left supraclavicular, paratracheal, anterior medistinal lymph node stations (arrows) consistent with stage II disease. **B.** Post-one cycle coronal images of CT (left), PET (right) demonstrate complete disappearance of FDG uptake in the disease locations noted on the pre-therapy FDG-PET study, consistent with complete metabolic response. The PFS on this patient has been > 24 months. Note the increased bone marrow uptake in the humeri, ribs, lumbar spine and pelvis due to recently administered colony stimulators in the post-therapy images.

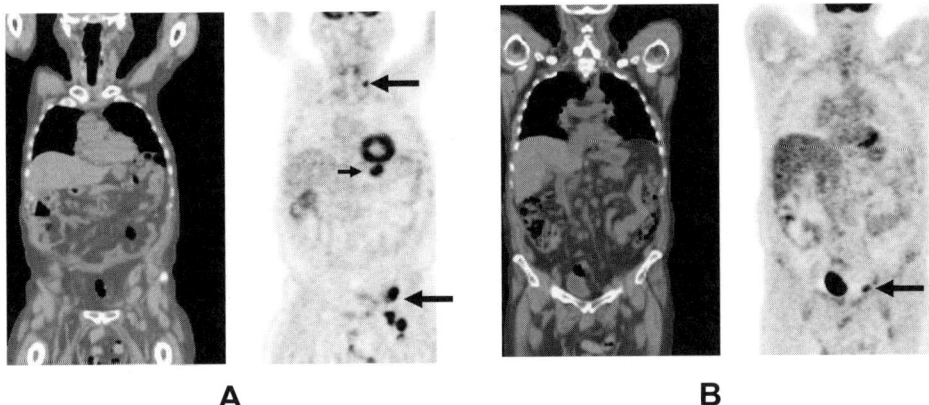

A   B

Figure 13. Patient with non-Hodgkin's lymphoma underwent a PET-CT study prior to and immediately following one cycle of chemotherapy to evaluate response to therapy. **A.** Pre-therapy coronal images of CT (left), PET (right) demonstrate increased FDG uptake in the left supraclavicular and left inguinal lymph nodes (large arrows). These findings are consistent with advanced stage lymphoma. Note the physiologic uptake in the stomach (small arrow) **B.** Post-therapy coronal images of CT (left), PET (right) demonstrate persistent FDG uptake in the left inguinal lymph node station (arrow) although the FDG uptake has resolved in the left supraclavicular region. These findings are consistent with unfavorable response to therapy. The patient had a relapse at 7 months after completion of therapy.

Ga-67 Scintigraphy   **FDG-PET**

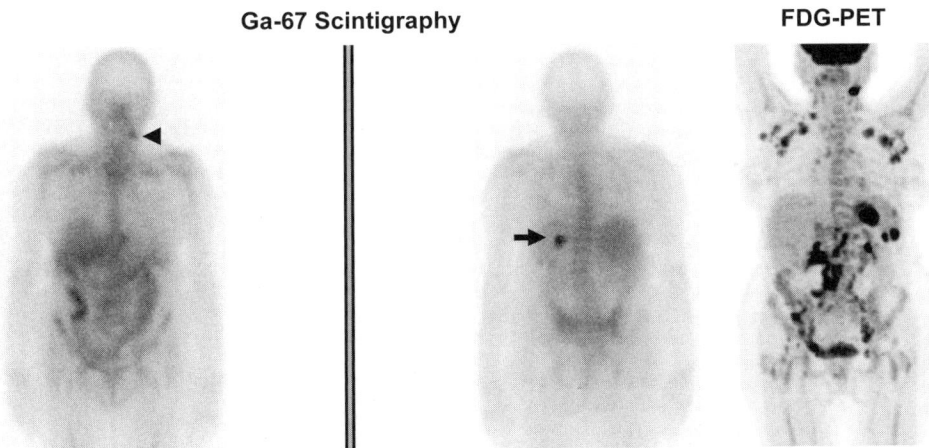

Figure 14. Patient with small lymphocytic non-Hodgkin's lymphoma underwent a Ga-67 scintigraphy prior to therapy to evaluate extent of disease. Anterior and posterior images reveal minimal Ga-67 uptake in the left cervical region and in a region probably corresponding to the spleen (arrows). However, a contemporaneous FDG-PET study reveals that the patient has extensive disease involving bilateral, cervical, axillary, mediastinal, retroperitoneal, inguinal regions as well as multiple sites in the spleen and probably in the bone marrow which are not visualized on the Ga-67 study.

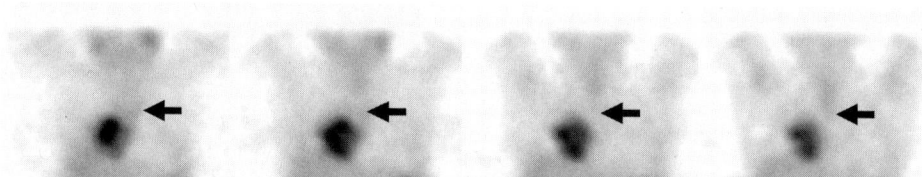

Figure 15. Patient with a history of non-Hodgkin's lymphoma underwent a Ga-67 scintigraphy with SPECT prior to therapy to evaluate extent of disease. Coronal slices on the SPECT study reveal a highly Ga-67 avid mass in the anterior mediastinum, consistent with active lymphoma (arrows).

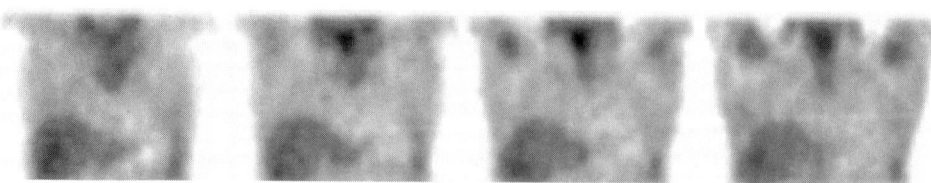

Figure 16. Same patient in Figure 15 underwent a Ga-67 scintigraphy with SPECT after completion of therapy to evaluate response to therapy. Coronal slices on the SPECT study reveal complete resolution of Ga-67 uptake seen on the pre-therapy study in the mediastinal mass, consistent with favorable response to therapy. The PFS on this patient was >18 months.

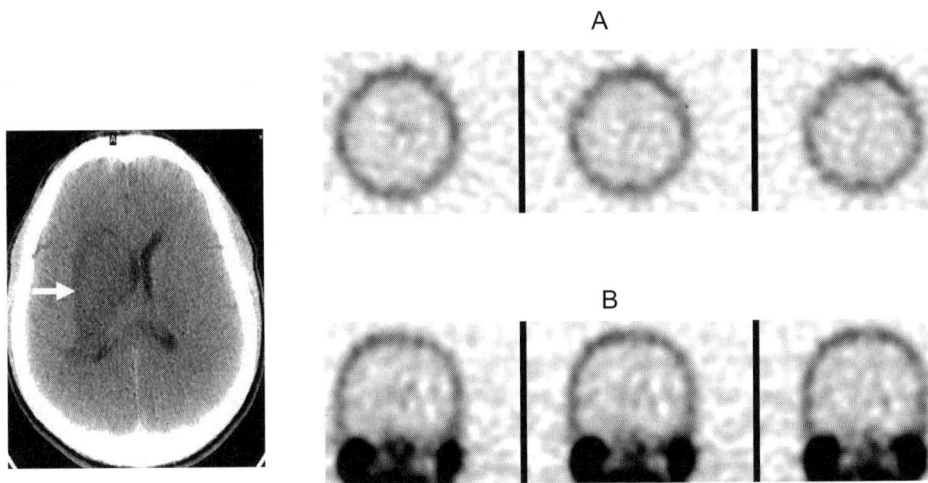

Figure 17. Patient with a history of HIV+ serology, recently diagnosed with a brain lesion, referred for Tl-201 study to differentiate between toxoplasmosis from CNS lymphoma. The axial slice of the CT scan shows a periventricular hypointense lesion on the right side (arrow). The corresponding axial (A) and coronal (B) slices on the Tl-201 study reveal no abnormal Tl-201 uptake in the region of abnormality, consistent with a diagnosis of toxoplasmosis rather than lymphoma. The patient was continued on his antibiotic therapy.

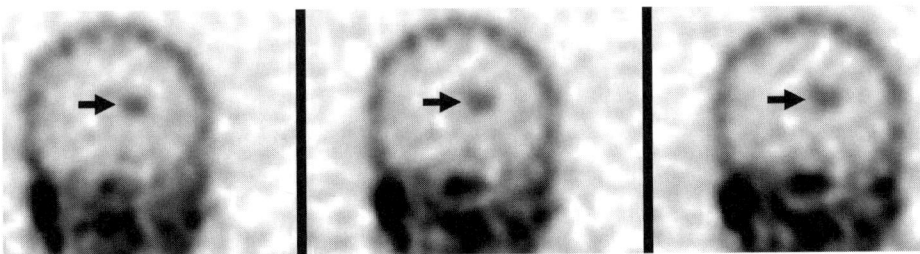

Figure 18. Patient with a history of HIV+ serology, recently diagnosed with a brain lesion, referred for FDG-PET imaging to differentiate between toxoplasmosis from CNS lymphoma. The CT scan shows a left parietal cortex (not shown). The corresponding coronal slices on the Tl-201 study reveal increased uptake in the left parietal cortex (arrows) corresponding to the exact location on the CT scan, consistent with lymphoma rather than toxoplasmosis. The patient was subsequently started on lymphoma therapy.

8.   REFERENCES

1. Yasuda S, Ide M, Fujii H, et al. Application of positron emission tomography imaging to cancer screening. Br J Cancer. 2000;83:1607-1611.

2. Marshall WH Jr, Breiman RS, Harell GS, Glatstein E, Kaplan HS. Computed tomography of abdominal para-aortic lymph node disease:preliminary observation with a 6 second scanner. *AJR Am J Roentgenol*, 1977;128:759-764.

3. Karimjee S, Brada M, Husband J, McCready VR. A comparison of gallium-67 single photon emission computed tomography and computed tomography in mediastinal Hodgkin's disease. *Eur J Cancer*, 1992;28A:1856-1857.

4. Castellino RA, Hopper RT, Blank N et al. Computed tomography, lymphography and staging laparotomy:correlations in initial staging of Hodgkin's disease. *Am J Roentgenol*, 1984:143:37-41.

5. Janicek M, Kaplan W, Neuberg D, et al: Early restaging gallium scans predict outcome in poor-prognosis patients with aggressive non-Hodgkin's lymphoma treated with high-dose CHOP chemotherapy. *J Clin Oncol*, 1997:15:1631-1637.

6. Front D, Bar-Shalom R, Mor M, et al. Hodgkin's disease: prediction of outcome with ^{67}Ga scintigraphy after one cycle of chemotherapy. *Radiology*, 1999:210:487-491.

7. Bendini M, Zuiani C, Bazzocchi M, Dalpiaz G, Zaja F, Englaro E. Magnetic resonance imaging and 67Ga scan versus computed tomography in the staging and in the monitoring of mediastinal malignant lymphoma: a prospective pilot study. *MAGMA*, 1996;4:213-224.

8. Nyman R, Forsgren G, Glimelius B. Long-term follow-up of residual mediastinal masses in treated Hodgkin's disease using MR imaging. *Acta Radiol*, 1996: 37:323-326.

9. Zinzani PL. Lymphoma: Diagnosis, staging, natural history, and treatment strategies. Semin Oncol. 2005;32:4-10.

10. Hagemeister FB, Purugganan R, Podoloff DA, et al: The gallium scan predicts relapse in patients with Hodgkin's disease treated with combined modality therapy. *Ann Oncol*, 1994;5:59-63.

11. Salloum E, Brandt DS, Caride VJ, et al: Gallium scans in the management of patients with Hodgkin's disease: a study of 101 patients. *J Clin Oncol*,1997;15:518-527.

12. Front D, Bar-Shalom R, Mor M, et al. Aggressive non-Hodgkin lymphoma: early prediction of outcome with ^{67}Ga scintigraphy. *Radiology*, 2000;214:253-257.

13. Frohlich DE, Chen JL, Neuberg D, Kehoe KM, Van den Abbeele AD . When is hilar uptake of 67Ga-citrate indicative of residual disease after CHOP chemotherapy? *J Nucl Med,* 2000, 41: 269-274.

14. Waxman AD, Eller D, Ashook G, et al. Comparison of gallium-67-citrate and thallium-201 scintigraphy in peripheral and intrathoracic lymphoma. *J Nucl Med*,1996:37:46-50.

15. Ohta M; Isobe K; Kuyama J et al. Clinical role of Tc-99m-MIBI scintigraphy in non-Hodgkin's lymphoma. Oncol Rep 2001, 8:841-845

16. Som P, Atkins HL, Bandophadhyah D. A fluorinated glucose analog, 2-fluoro-2deoxy-D-glucose (F-18). *J Nucl Med*, 1980;21:670-675.

17. Rodriguez M, Rehn S, Ahlstrom H, Sundstrom C, Glimelius B. Predicting malignancy grade with PET in non-Hodgkin's lymphoma. *J Nucl Med,* 1995, 36:1790-1796 .

18. Jerusalem G, Warland V, Najjar F, Paulus P, Fassotte MF, Fillet G, Rigo P. Whole-body 18F-FDG PET for the evaluation of patients with Hodgkin's disease and non-Hodgkin's lymphoma. *Nucl Med Commun*, 1999:20:13-20.

19. Hoh CK, Glaspy J, Rosen P, et al. Whole-body FDG-PET imaging for staging of Hodgkin's disease and lymphoma. *J Nucl Med*, 1997, 38:343-348.

20. Thill R, Neuerburg J, Fabry U, et al. Comparison of findings with 18-FDG PET and CT in pretherapeutic staging of malignant lymphoma. *Nuklearmedizin*, 1997:36:234-239.

21. Mainolfi C, Maurea S, Varrella P, Alaia C, Imparato C, Alfano B, Aate G, Bazzicalupo L. Positron emission tomography with fluorine-18-deoxyglucose in the staging and control of patients with lymphoma. Comparison with clinico-radiologic assessment. *Radiol Med*, 1998:95:98-104.

22. Cremerius U, Fabry U, Neuerburg J, Zimny M, Osieka R, Buell. Positron emission tomography with 18F-FDG to detect residual disease after therapy for malignant lymphoma. *Nucl Med Commun*, 1998:19:1055-1063.

23. Stumpe KD, Urbinelli M, Steinert HC, Glanzmann C, Buck A, von Schulthess GK. Whole-body positron emission tomography using fluorodeoxyglucose for staging of lymphoma:effectiveness and comparison with computed tomography. *Eur J Nucl Med*, 1998:25:721-728.

24. Moog F, Bangerter M, Diederichs CG, Guhlmann A, Merkle E, Frickhofen N, Reske SN. Extranodal malignant lymphoma: detection with FDG PET versus CT. *Radiology*, 1998:206: 475-481

25. Jerusalem G, Beguin Y, Fassotte MF, Najjar F, Paulus P, Rigo P, Fillet G. Whole-body positron emission tomography using 18F-fluorodeoxyglucose for post-treatment evaluation in Hodgkin's disease and non-Hodgkin's lymphoma has higher diagnostic and prognostic value than classical computed tomography scan imaging. *Blood*, 1999:94:429-433.

26. Bangerter M, Kotzerke J, Griesshammer M, Elsner K, Reske SN, Bergmann L. Positron emission tomography with 18-fluorodeoxyglucose in the staging and follow-up of lymphoma in the chest. *Acta Oncol*, 1999:38:799-804.

27. Wiedmann E, Baican B, Hertel A, et al. Positron emission tomography (PET) for staging and evaluation of response to treatment in patients with Hodgkin's disease. *Leuk Lymphoma*, 1999, 34:545-551.

28. Hany TF, Steinert HC, Goerres GW, Buck A, von Schulthess GK. PET diagnostic accuracy: improvement with in-line PET-CT system: initial results. *Radiology*, 2002;225:575-581.

29. Kostakoglu L, Leonard JP, Kuji I, et al: Comparison of fluorine-18 fluorodeoxyglucose positron emission tomography and Ga-67 scintigraphy in evaluation of lymphoma. *Cancer* 2002;94:879-888.

30. Bragg DG. Radiology of the lymphomas.Curr Probl Diagn Radiol. 1987;16:177-206.

31. Golding SJ. .Use of imaging in the management of lymphoma.Br J Hosp Med. 1989;41:152-154.

32. Musumeci R, Tesoro-Tess JD. New imaging techniques in staging lymphomas. Curr Opin Oncol. 1994 Sep;6:464-469.

33. Halliday T, Baxter G. Lymphoma: pictorial review. Eur Radiol. 2003;13(6):1224-1234.

34. Vinnicombe SJ, Reznek RH. Computerised tomography in the staging of Hodgkin's disease and non-Hodgkin's lymphoma. Eur J Nucl Med Mol Imaging. 2003 Jun;30 Suppl 1:S42-55.

35. Hopper KD, Diehl LF, Lesar M, Barnes M, Granger E, Baumann J. Hodgkin disease: clinical utility of CT in initial staging and treatment. Radiology. 1988;169:17-22

36. Castellino RA. The non-Hodgkin lymphomas: practical concepts for the diagnostic radiologist. Radiology 1991; 178:315-321.

37. Chim CS, Shek T, Ooi GC, Liang R. Unusual features of Hodgkin's disease. J Clin Oncol 2000;18:1153-1155

38. Fishman EK, Kuhlman JE, Jones RJ. CT of lymphoma: spectrum of disease. Radiographics. 1991;11:647-669.

39. Erdag N, Rajeev MB, Alberico RA, Yousuf N, Patel MR. Primary lymphoma of the central nervous system: typical and atypical CT and MR imaging appearances.Am J Roentgenol 2001;176:1319-1326.

40. Gutman J, Kendall B. Unusual appearances of primary central nervous system non-Hodgkin's lymphoma. Clin Radiol 1994;49:292-702.

41. Guermazi A, Brice P, de Kerviler EE, Ferme C, Hannequin C, Meignin V. Extranodal Hodgkin's disease: spectrum of disease. Radiographics 2001; 21:161-179.

42. Takashima S, Ikezoe J, Morimoto S, Arisawa J, Hamada S, Ikeda H et al. (1988) Primary thyroid lymphoma: evaluation with CT. Radiology 168:756-768

43. Kondo M, Hashimoto T, Shinga H et al. (1984) Computed tomography of sinonasal non-Hodgkin's lymphoma. J Comput Assist Tomogr 8:216-219

44. Diehl LF, Hopper KD, Giguere J, Granger E, Lesar M.The pattern of intrathoracic Hodgkin's disease assessed by computed tomography.J Clin Oncol. 1991 Mar;9(3):438-43.

45. Ooi GC, Chim CS, Lie AKW, Tsang KWT (1999) Computed tomography features of primary pulmonary non-Hodgkin's lymphoma. Clin Radiol 54:438-443

46. Aquino SL, Chen MYM, Kuo WT, Chiles C (1999) The CT appearance of pleural and extrapleural disease in lymphoma. Clin Radiol 54:647-650

47. Jung G, Heindel W, Bergwelt-Baildon M, Bredenfeld H, Gossmann A,Zahringer M, Tesch H (2000). Abdominal lymphoma staging: Is MR imaging with T2-weighted turbo-spin-echo sequence a diagnostic alternative to contrast-enhanced spiral CT? J Comput Assist Tomogr 24:783-787

48. Gazelle GS, Lee MJ, Hahn PF, Goldberg MA, Rafaat N, Mueller PR (1994) US, CT and MRI of primary and secondary liver lymphoma. J Assist Comput Tomogr 18:412-415

49. Avlonitis VS, Linos D. Primary hepatic lymphoma: a review.Eur J Surg. 1999 Aug;165(8):725-9.

50. Urban BA, Fishman EK. Renal lymphoma: CT patterns with emphasis on helical CT. Radiographics. 2000 Jan-Feb;20(1):197-212

51 Chen HH, Panella JS, Rochester D, Ignatoff JM, McVary KT (1988) Non-Hodgkin lymphoma of the ureteral wall: findings. J Comput Assist Tomogr 12:157-158

52. Neville A, Herts BR. CT characteristics of primary retroperitoneal neoplasms. Crit Rev Comput Tomogr. 2004;45(4):247-70.

53. Turowski GA, Basson MD (1995) Primary malignant lymphoma of the intestine. Am J Surg 169:433-441

54. Libson E, Mapp E, Dachman AH (1994) Hodgkin's disease of the gastrointestinal tract. Clin Radiol 49:166-169

55. Gossios K, Katsimbri P, Tsianos E (2000) CT features of gastric lymphoma. Eur Radiol 10:425-430

56. Yoo CC, Levine MS, McLarney JK, Rubesin SE, Herlinger H (2000) Value of barium studies for predicting primary versus secondary non-Hodgkin's gastrointestinal lymphoma.Abdom Imaging 25:368-372

57. Chew FS, Schellingerhout D, Kee SB (1999) Primary lymphoma of skeletal muscle. Am J Roentgenol 172:1370

58. Malloy PC, Fishman EK, Magid D (1992) Lymphoma of bone, muscle, and skin: CT findings. Am J Roentgenol 159:805-809

59. Edeiken-Monroe B, Edeiken J, Kim EE. Radiologic concepts of lymphoma of bone. Radiol Clin North Am. 1990 Jul;28(4):841-64.

60. Rehn SM, Nyman RS, Glimelius BL, Hagberg HE, Sundstrom JC. Non-Hodgkin lymphoma: predicting prognostic grade with MR imaging.Radiology. 1990;176:249-53.

61. Rankin SC.Assessment of response to therapy using conventional imaging. Eur J Nucl Med Mol Imaging. 2003 Jun;30 Suppl 1:S56-64.

62. Nyman RS, Rehn SM, Glimelius BL, Hagberg HE, Hemmingsson AL, Sundstrom CJ. Residual mediastinal masses in Hodgkin disease: prediction of size with MR imaging.Radiology. 1989;170:435- 440.

63. McGowan KM, Long SD, Pekala PH. Glucose transporter gene expression: regulation of transcription and mRNA stability. *Pharmacol Ther,* 1995:66:465-505.

64. Flier JS, Mueckler MM, Usher P, Lodish HF. Elevated levels of glucose transport and transporter messenger RNA are induced by ras or src oncogenes. Science,1987: 235:1492-1495.

65. Higashi K; Ueda Y; Sakuma T et al. Comparison of [(18)F]FDG PET and (201)Tl SPECT in evaluation of pulmonary nodules. J Nucl Med, 2001;42:1489-1496.

66. Buck AC, Schirrmeister HH, Guhlmann CA, et al. Ki-67 immunostaining in pancreatic cancer and chronic active pancreatitis: does in vivo FDG uptake correlate with proliferative activity? *J Nucl Med*, 2001; 42:721-725.

67. Brown RS, Leung JY, Kison PV, Zasadny KR, Flint A, Wahl RL. Glucose transporters and FDG uptake in untreated primary human non-small cell lung cancer. J Nucl Med, 1999;40:556-565.

68. Newman JS, Francis IR, Kaminski MS, et al. Imaging of lymphoma with PET with 2-[^{18}F] fluoro-2-deoxy-D-glucose: correlation with CT. *Radiology,* 1994:190:111-116.

69. Leskinen-Kallio S, Ruotsalainen U, Nagren K, et al. Uptake of carbon-11-methionine and fluorodeoxyglucose in non-Hodgkin's lymphoma: A PET study. *J Nucl Med,* 1991:32:1211-1218.

70. JNM abstract

71. Jerusalem G *Ann Oncol*, 2001:12:825

72. Bastion Y, Berger F, Bryon PA, Felman P, Ffrench M, Coiffier B. Follicular lymphomas: assessment of prognostic factors in 127 patients followed for 10 years. *Ann Oncol,* 1991:2 Suppl 2:123-129.

73. JNM abst

74. Hoffmann M, Kletter K, Becherer A, et al: 18F-fluorodeoxyglucose positron emission tomography (18F-FDG-PET) for staging and follow-up of marginal zone B-cell lymphoma. *Oncology*, 2003;64:336-340.

75. Najjar F, Hustinx R, Jerusalem G, et al: Positron emission tomography (PET) for staging low-grade non-Hodgkin's lymphomas (NHL). *Cancer Biother Radiopharm* 2001;16:297-304.

76. Bangerter M, Moog F, Buchmann I, et al. Whole-body 2-[18F]-fluoro-2-deoxy-D-glucose positron emission tomography (FDG-PET) for accurate staging of Hodgkin's disease. *Ann Oncol,* 1998: 9:1117-1122.

77. Buchmann I, Reinhardt M, Elsner K, et al. 2-(fluorine-18)fluoro-2-deoxy-D-glucose positron emission tomography in the detection and staging of malignant lymphoma. A bicenter trial. *Cancer,* 2001: 91:889-899.

78. Partridge S, Timothy A, O'doherty MJ, et al. 2-fluorine-18-fluoro-2-deoxy-D glucose positron emission tomography in the pretreatment staging ofHodgkin's disease:Influenceon paients management in a single institution. *Ann Oncol,* 2000:11:1273-1279.

79. Weihrauch MR; Re D; Bischoff S; et al Whole-body positron emission tomography using 18F-fluorodeoxyglucose for initial staging of patients with Hodgkin's disease. *Ann Hematol,* 2002, 81:20-25.

80. Rodriguez M, Ahlstrom H, Sundin A, Rehn S, Sundstrom C, Hagberg H, Glimelius B. 18F FDG PET in gastric non-Hodgkin's lymphoma. *Acta Oncol,* 1997:36:577-584.

81. Mauch P, Larson D, Osteen R, et al. Prognostic factors for positive surgical staging in patients with Hodgkin's disease. *J Clin Oncol*, 1990;8:257-265.

82. Leibenhaut MH, Hoppe RT, Efron B, et al. Prognostic indicators of laparotomy findings in clinical stage III supradiaphragmatic Hodgkin's disease. *J Clin Oncol*, 1989;7:81-91.

83. Neumann CH, Robert NJ, Canellos G, et al. Computed tomography of the abdomen and pelvis in non-Hodgkin lymphoma. *J Comput Assist Tomogr*, 1983;7:846-850.

84. Hoffman JM, Waskin HA, Schifter T, et al. FDG-PET in differentiating lymphoma from non-malignant central nervous system lesions in patients with AIDS. *J Nucl Med,* 1993:34:567-575.

85. Heald AE, Hoffman JM, Bartlett JA, Waskin HA. Differentiation of central nervous system lesions in AIDS patients using positron emission tomography (PET). *Int J STD AIDS* 1996:7:337-346.

86. Shipp M, Mauch PM, Harris NL. Non-Hodgkin's lymphomas. In: Devita VT, Hellman S, Rosenberg SA, eds. *Cancer principles and practice of oncology.* Philadelphia, PA: Lippincott; 1997:2165-2220.

87. Abdel-Dayem HM, Rosen G, El-Zeftawy H, Naddaf S, Kumar M, Atay S, Cacavio A. Fluorine-18 fluorodeoxyglucose splenic uptake from extramedullary hematopoiesis after granulocyte colony-stimulating factor stimulation. *Clin Nucl Med,* 1999, 24:319-322.

88. Gundlapalli S; Ojha B; Mountz JM. Granulocyte colony-stimulating factor: confounding F-18 FDG uptake in outpatient positron emission tomographic facilities for patients receiving ongoing treatment of lymphoma. *Clin Nucl Med,* 2002, 27:140-141.

89. Carr R, Barrington SF, Madan B, O'Doherty MJ, Saunders CA, van der Walt J, Timothy AR. Detection of lymphoma in bone marrow by whole-body positron emission tomography. *Blood,* 1998:91:3340-3346.

90. Moog F, Bangerter M, Kotzerke J, Guhlman A, Frickhofen N, Reske SN. 18-F-fluorodeoxyglucose-positron emision tomography as a new approach to detect lymphomatous bone marrow. *J Clin Oncol,* 1998:16:603-609.

91. Jerusalem G, Warland V, Najjar F, Paulus P, Fassotte MF, Fillet G, Rigo P. Whole-body 18F-FDG PET for the evaluation of patients with Hodgkin's disease and non-Hodgkin's lymphoma. *Nucl Med Commun,* 1999:20:13-20.

92. Krishnan A, Shirkhoda A, Tehranzadeh J, Armin AR, Irwin R, Les K. Primary Bone Lymphoma: Radiographic–MR Imaging Correlation. Radiographics. 2003;23:1371-1383

93. Bar-Shalom R, Yefremov N, Haim N, et al. Camera-based FDG PET and ^{67}Ga SPECT in Evaluation of Lymphoma: Comparative Study. *Radiology* 2003 227: 353-360

94. Bar-Shalom R, Mor M, Yefremov N, Goldsmith SJ. The value of Ga-67 scintigraphy and F-18 fluorodeoxyglucose positron emission tomography in staging and monitoring the response of lymphoma to treatment. *Semin Nucl Med* 2001; 31:177-190.

95. Kostakoglu L, Goldsmith SJ. Positron emission tomography in lymphoma: comparison with computed tomography and gallium-67 single photon emission computed tomography. Clin Lymphoma 2000; 1:67-74.

96. Wirth A, Seymour JF, Hicks RJ, et al. Fluorine-18 fluorodeoxyglucose positron emission tomography, gallium-67 scintigraphy, and conventional staging for Hodgkin's disease and non-Hodgkin's lymphoma. *Am J Med,* 2002:112:262-268.

97. Shen YY, Kao A, Yen RF. Comparison of 18F-fluoro-2-deoxyglucose positron emission tomography and gallium-67 citrate scintigraphy for detecting malignant lymphoma. *Oncol Rep* 2002: 9:321-325.

98. Brandt L, Kimby E, Nygren P, Glimelius B. A systematic overview of chemotherapy effects in Hodgkin's disease. *Acta Oncol.* 2001;40:185-197.

99. Coiffier B, Gisselbrecht C, Vose JM, et al. prognostic factors in aggressive malignant lymphomas. Description and validation of prognostic index that could identify patients requiring a more intensive therapy. *J Clin Oncol.* 1991;9:211-219.

100. Hueltenschmidt B, Sautter-Bihl ML, Lang O, Maul FD, Fischer J, Mergenthaler HG, Bihl H. Whole body positron emission tomography in the treatment of Hodgkin disease. *Cancer,* 2001: 91:302-310.

101. Cremerius U, Fabry U, Kroll U, Zimny M, Neuerburg J, Osieka R, Bull U. Clinical value of FDG PET for therapy monitoring of malignant lymphoma-results of a retrospective study in 72 patients. *Nuklearmedizin,* 1999, 38:24-30.

102. Chelson MS, Herman TG, Stomper PC, et al. Planning mantle radiation therapy in patients with hodgkin's disease:the role of gallium-67 scintigraphy. *AJR Am J Roentgenol,* 1988:151:1229-1232.

103. Surbone A, Longo DL, DeVita VT, et al. Residual abdominal masses in aggressive non-Hodgkin's lymphoma after combination chemotherapy:significance and management. *J Clin Oncol.* 1988;6:1832-1837.

104. Spaepen K, Stroobants S, Dupont P, et al. Prognostic value of positron emission tomography (PET) with fluorine-18 fluorodeoxyglucose ([18F]FDG after first line

chemotherapy in non-Hodgkins lymphoma: Is ([^{18}F]FDG PET a valid alternative to conventional diagnostic methods? *J Clin Oncol.* 2001;19:414-419.

105. Kostakoglu L, Coleman M, Leonard JP, Kuji I, Zoe H, Goldsmith SJ. Positron emission tomography predicts prognosis after one cycle of chemotherapy in aggressive lymphoma and Hodgkin's disease. *J Nucl Med*, 2002;43: 1018-1027.

106. Mikhaeel NG, Mainwaring P, Nunan T, Timothy AR. Prognostic value of interim and post treatment FDG-PET scanning in Hodgkin lymphoma [abstract]. *Ann Oncol* 2002; 13 (Suppl 2):21.

107. Spaepen K; Stroobants S; Dupont P; et al. Can positron emission tomography with [(18)F]-fluorodeoxyglucose after first-line treatment distinguish Hodgkin's disease patients who need additional therapy from others in whom additional therapy would mean avoidable toxicity? *Br J Haematol* 2001;115:272-278

108. Mikhaeel NG, Timothy AR, O'Doherty MJ,Hain S, Maisey T. 18-FDG PET as a prognostic indicator in the treatment of aggressive non-Hodgkin's lymphoma-comoparison with CT. *Leuk Lymphoma.* 2000;39: 543-553.

109. Zinzani PL, Magagnoli M, Chierichetti F, et al. The role of positron emission tomography (PET) in the management of lymphoma patients. *Ann Oncol*, 1999:10:1181-1184.

110. Ng AK, Bernardo MV, Weller E, et al: Second malignancy after Hodgkin disease treated with radiation therapy with or without chemotherapy: long-term risks and risk factors. *Blood* 2002;100:1989-1996.

111. de Wit M, Bohuslavizki KH, Buchert, Bumann D, Clausen M, Hossfeld DK. ^{18}FDG-PET following treatment as valid predictor for disease-free survival in Hodgkin's lymphoma. *Ann Oncol*, 2001:12:29-37.

112. Weihrauch MR, Re D, Scheidhauer K, et al. Thoracic positron emission tomography using ^{18}F-fluorodeoxyglucose for the evaluation of residual mediastinal Hodgkin disease. *Blood.* 2001;98:2930-2934.

113. Armitage JO, Weisenburger DD, Hutchins M, et al. Chemotherapy for diffuse large-cell lymphoma--rapidly responding patients have more durable remissions. *J Clin Oncol* 1986; 4:160-164.

114. Haw R, Sawka CA, Franssen E, Berinstein HL. Significance of a partial or slow response to front-line chemotherapy in the management of intermediate-grade or high-grade non-Hodgkin's lymphoma: a literature review. J Clin Oncol 1994;12:1074-1084

115. Romer W, Hanauske A-R, Ziegler S, et al. Positron emission tomography in non-Hodgkin's lymphoma:assesment o chemotherapy with fluorodeoxyglucose. *Blood*, 1998:91:4464-4471.

116. Jerusalem G, Beguin Y, Fassotte MF, et al. Persistent tumor 18F-FDG uptake after a few cycles of polychemotherapy is predictive of treatment failure in non-Hodgkin's lymphoma. *Haematologica.* 2000;85:613-618.

117. Spaepen K, Stroobants S, Dupont P, et al. Early restaging positron emission tomography with 18F-fluorodeoxyglucose predicts outcome in patients with aggressive non-Hodgkin's lymphoma. *Ann Oncol* 2002; 13:1356–1363

118. Kostakoglu L, Coleman M, Somrov S, Leonard JP, Verma S, Sherman CH,. Goldsmith SJ. FDG-PET after one cycle of chemotherapy accurately predicts response to therapy in large cell (aggressive) non-Hodgkin's lymphoma (NHL) and Hodgkin's disease (HD). *J Nucl Med*, 2004;45: 316P.

119. Becherer A, Mitterbauer M, Jaeger U et al. Positron emission tomography with [18F]2-fluoro-D-2-deoxyglucose (FDG-PET) predicts relapse of malignant lymphoma after high-dose therapy with stem cell transplantation. *Leukemia*, 2002;16:260-267.

120. Cremerius U, Fabry U, Wildberger JE, et al. Pre-transplant positron emission tomography using fluorine-18-fluoro-deoxyglucose predicts outcome in patients treated with high-dose chemotherapy and autologous stem cell transplantation for non-Hodgkin's lymphoma. *Bone Marrow Transplant* 2002; 30:103–111.

121. Hoekstra O, Ossenkoppele GJ, Golding R, et al. Early treatment   response in malignant lymphoma, as determined by planar fluorine-18-fluorodeoxyglucose scintigraphy. *J Nucl Med,* 1993;34:1706-1710.

122. Townsend DW and Beyer T. A combined PET/CT scanner: the path to true image fusion. *Br J Radiol,* 2002;75:S24-30.

123. Schaefer NG, Hany TF, Taverna C, Seifert B, Stumpe KD, Von Schulthess GK, Goerres GW. Non-Hodgkin Lymphoma and Hodgkin Disease: Coregistered FDG PET and CT at Staging and Restaging--Do We Need Contrast-enhanced CT? *Radiology.* 2004 Jul 23 [Epub ahead of print].

124. Larson SM; Rasey JS; Allen DR; Nelson NJ; Grunbaum Z; Harp GD; Williams DL Common pathway for tumor cell uptake of gallium-67 and iron-59 via a transferrin receptor. J Natl Cancer Inst 1980, 64:41-53

125. Vallabhajosula S; Goldsmith SJ; Lipszyc H; Chahinian AP; Ohnuma T. ^{67}Ga-transferrin and ^{67}Ga-lactoferrin binding to tumor cells: specific versus nonspecific glycoprotein-cell interaction. Eur J Nucl Med, 1983: 8354-357

126. Nejmeddine F, Caillat-Vigneron N, Escaig F, Moretti JL, Raphael M, Galle P. Mechanism involved in gallium-67 (Ga-67) uptake by human lymphoid cell lines. Cell Mol Biol (Noisy-le-grand). 1998;44:1215-20.

127. Gallamini A, Biggi A, Fruttero A, et al. Revisiting the prognostic role of gallium scintigraphy in low-grade non-Hodgkin's lymphoma. *Eur J Nucl Med,* 1997:24:1499-1506.

128. Kostakoglu L, Yeh SD, Portlock C, Heelan R, Yao TJ, Niedzwiecki D, Larson SM. Validation of gallium-67-citrate single-photon emission computed tomography in biopsy-confirmed residual Hodgkin's disease in the mediastinum. J Nucl Med. 1992;33:345-50

129. Front D, Israel O, Epelbaum R, et al. Ga-67 SPECT before and after treatment of lymphoma. Radiology 1990; 175:515-519.

130. Mansberg R, Wadhwa SS, Mansberg V. Tl-201 and Ga-67 scintigraphy in non-Hodgkin's lymphoma. Clin Nucl Med, 1999, 24:239-242

131. Johnston G, Benua RS, Teates CD, Edwards CL, Kniseley RM. ^{67}Ga-citrate imaging in untreated Hodgkin's disease: preliminary report of Cooperative Group. *J Nucl Med,* 1974, 15:399-403.

132. Cabanillas F,Zornoza J, Haynie TP. Comparison of lymphangiograms and gallium scans in the non-Hodgkin's lymphomas. *Cancer,* 1977: 39:85-88.

133. Setoin FJ, Pons F, Herranz R, et al. Ga-67 scintigraphy for the evaluation of recurrences and residual masses in patients with lymphoma. *Nuc Med Commun,* 1997:18:405-411.

134. Ben-Haim S, Bar-Shalom R, Israel O, et al. Utility of gallium-67 scintigraphy in low-grade non-Hodgkin's lymphoma. *J Clin Oncol,*1996, 14:1936-1942

135. Bastion Y, Berger F, Bryon PA, Felman P, Ffrench M, Coiffier B. Follicular lymphomas: assessment of prognostic factors in 127 patients followed for 10 years. *Ann Oncol,* 1991:2 Suppl 2:123-129.

136. Mclaughlin AF, Southee AE. Gallium scintigraphy in tumor diagnosis and management, in Murray IPC, Ell PJ (eds):Nuclear Medicine in clinical diagnosis and treatment. Vol1. New York, Churchill Livingstone, 1994:711-727.

137. Turner DA, Fordham EW, Ali A. Gallium-67 imaging in the management of Hodgkin's disease and other malignant lymphomas. *Semin Nucl Med,* 1978:8:205-218.

138. Devizzi L, Maffioli L, Bonfante V, et al. Comparison of gallium scan, computed tomography, and magnetic resonance in patients with mediastinal Hodgkin's disease. *Ann Oncol,* 1997, 8 Suppl 1 53-56.

139. Brascho DJ. Hodgkin's disease and non-Hodgkin's lymphoma. In: Abdominal ultrasound in the cancer patient. D.J. Brasco and T.H. Strawber (eds). Wiley, New York 1980. Hussain R, Christie DR, Gebski V, Barton MB, Gruenewald SM. The role of the gallium scan in primary extranodal lymphoma. *J Nucl Med,* 1998, 39:95-98

140. Hussain R, Christie DR, Gebski V, Barton MB, Gruenewald SM. The role of the gallium scan in primary extranodal lymphoma. *J Nucl Med*, 1998, 39:95-98

141. Zornoza J; Ginaldi S. Computed Tomography in hepatic lymphoma. Radiology, 1981;138:405-410.

142 . Ora Israel JNM 2002.
Front D, Bar-Shalom R, Israel O. The continuing clinical role of gallium 67 scintigraphy in the age of receptor imaging. *Semin Nucl Med*, 1997, 27:68-74.

143. Kostakoglu L, Goldsmith SJ. [F-18] Fluorodeoxyglucose positron emission tomography in staging and follow-up of lymphoma. Is it time to shift gears? *Eur J Nucl Med*, 2000;27:564-1578.

144. Stroszczynski C, Amthauer H, Hosten N, et al. Use of Ga-67 SPECT in patients with malignant lymphoma after primary chemotherapy for further treatment planning:comparison with spiral CT. *Rofo Fortschr Geb Rontgenstr Neuen Bildgeb Verfahr*, 1997:167:458-466.

145. Devizzi L, Maffioli L, Bonfante V, et al. Comparison of gallium scan, computed tomography, and magnetic resonance in patients with mediastinal Hodgkin's disease. *Ann Oncol*, 1997, 8 Suppl 1 53-56.

146. Ha CS, Choe JG, Kong JS, Allen PK, Oh YK, Cox JD, Edmund E. Agreement rates among single photon emission computed tomography using gallium-67, computed axial tomography and lymphangiography for Hodgkin's disease and correlation of image findings with clinical outcome. *Cancer*, 2000; 89:1371-1379.

147. Front D, Ben-Haim S, Israel O, Epelbaum R, Haim N, Even-Sapir E, Kolodny GM, Robinson E Lymphoma. predictive value of Ga-67 scintigraphy after treatment. *Radiology*, 1992, 182: 359-363.

148. Even-Sapir E, Bar-Shalom R, Israel O, et al. Single-photon emission computed tomography quantitation of gallium citrate uptake for the differentiation of lymphoma from benign hilar uptake. J Clin Oncol. 1995 Apr;13(4):942-6.

149. Ionescu I, Brice P, Simon D, et al. Restaging with gallium scan identifies chemosensitive patients and predicts survival of poor-prognosis mediastinal Hodgkin's disease patients. *Med Oncol*, 2000, 17:127-134.

150. Gasparini MD, Balzarini L, Castellani MR, et al. Current role of gallium scan and magnetic resonance imaging in the management of mediastinal Hodgkin lymphoma. *Cancer*, 1993, 72:577-582 .

151. Bogart JA, Chung CT, Mariados NF, Vermont AI, Lemke SM, Grethlein S, Graziano SL. The value of gallium imaging after therapy for Hodgkin's disease. *Cancer*, 15 1998, 82:754-759.

152. Vose JM, Bierman PJ, Anderson JR, Harrison KA, Dalrymple GV, Byar K, Kessinger A, Armitage JO. Single-photon emission computed tomography gallium imaging versus computed tomography: predictive value in patients undergoing high-dose chemotherapy and autologous stem-cell transplantation for non-Hodgkin's lymphoma. *J Clin Oncol*, 1996:14:2473-2479.

153. Kaplan WD; Jochelson MS; Herman T et al. Gallium-67 imaging: a predictor of residual tumor viability and clinical outcome in patients with diffuse large-cell lymphoma. *J Clin Oncol*, 1990, 8:1966-1070.

154. Shipp MA. Prognostic factors in aggressive non- Hodgkin's lymphoma: who has "high-risk" disease*? Blood* 1994; 83:1165-1173.

155. Israel O, Mor M, Epelbaum R, et al. Clinical pretreatment risk factors and Ga-67 scintigraphy early during treatment for prediction of outcome of patients with aggressive non-Hodgkin lymphoma. *Cancer*, 2002: 94:873-878.

156. Waxman AD. Thallium 201 in nuclear oncology. In: Freeman LM, ed. Nuclear Mediine Annual . New York:Raven , 1991:193

157. Abdel-Dayem HM, et al. Role of Tl-201 chloride and Tc-99m-sestamibi in tumor imaging. Nucl Med Annual 1994; 181-234.

158. Lin J, Leung WT, Ho SKW, et al. Quantitative evaluation of thallium-201 uptake in predicting chemotherapeutic response of osteosarcoma. *Eur J Nucl Med* 1995; 22: 553–555.

159. Elgazzar AH, Fernandes-Ulloa M, Silberstein EB. Tl-201 as a tumour-localizing agent: current status and future considerations. *Nucl Med Commun* 1993; 14: 96–103

160. Piwnica-Worms D; Rao VV; Kronauge JF; Croop JM Characterization of multidrug resistance P-glycoprotein transport function with an organotechnetium cation. Biochemistry, 26 1995, 34(38) p12210-20

161. Del-Vecchio S, et al. Fractional retention of Tc-99m-Sestamibi as an index of P-glycoprotein expression in untreated breast cancer patients. J Nucl Med 1997; 38: 1348-1351

162. Kostakoglu L, et al. Clinical validation of the influence of P-glycoprotein on Tc-99m-sestamibi uptake in malignant tumors. . J Nucl Med 1997; 38: 1003-1008

163. Roach P.J., Cooper R.A, Arthur C.K,. Ravich R.B, Comparison of thallium-201 and gallium-67 scintigraphy in the evaluation of non-Hodgkin's lymphoma. *Aust N Z J Med 1998;* **28:**33–38.

164. Haas RL, Valdes-Olmos RA, Hoefnagel CA, Verheij M, de Jong D, Hart AA, Bartelink H. Thallium-201-chloride scintigraphy in staging and monitoring radiotherapy response in follicular lymphoma patients. Radiother Oncol. 2003;69(:323-328.

165. Skiest DJ, Erdman W, Chang WE, Oz OK, Ware A, Fleckenstein J. SPECT thallium-201 combined with Toxoplasma serology for the presumptive diagnosis of focal central nervous system mass lesions in patients with AIDS. J Infect. 2000;40:274-81.

166. Kao CH,Tsai SC,Wang JJ, Ho YJ, Ho ST, Changlai SP. Technetium-99m-sestamethoxyisobutylisonitrile scan as a predictor of chemotherapy response in malignant lymphomas compared with P-glycoprotein expression, multidrug resistance-related protein expression and other prognosis factors. Br J Haematol 2001, 113:369-374

167. Liang JA; Shiau YC; Yang SN; Lin FJ; Kao A; Lee CC Prediction of chemotherapy response in untreated malignant lymphomas using technetium-99m methoxyisobutylisonitrile scan: comparison with P-glycoprotein expression and other prognostic factors. A preliminary report. Jpn J Clin Oncol 2002, 32(4) p140-5

168. Ohta M; Isobe K; Kuyama J et al. Clinical role of Tc-99m-MIBI scintigraphy in non-Hodgkin's lymphoma. Oncol Rep 2001, 8(4) :841-845.

169. Nadel HR. Thallium-201 for oncologic imaging in children. Semin Nucl Med 1993;23: 243-254.

170. Leners N, Jamar F, Fiasse R, Ferrant A, Pauwels S. Indium-111-pentetreotide uptake in endocrine tumors and lymphoma. J Nucl Med. 1996;37:916-22.

171. Van Hagen PM, Krenning EP, Reubi JC, et al. Somatostatin analogue scintigraphy of malignant lymphomas. Br J Haematol. 1993;83:75–79

172. Lipp RW, Silly H, Ranner G, et al. Radiolabeled octreotide for the demonstration of somatostatin receptors in malignant lymphoma and lymphadenopathy. J Nucl Med. 1995;36:13-18

173. Lugtenburg PJ, Krenning EP, Valkema R, Oei HY, Lamberts SW, Eijkemans MJ, van Putten WL, Lowenberg B. Somatostatin receptor scintigraphy useful in stage I-II Hodgkin's disease: more extended disease identified. Br J Haematol. 2001 Mar;112(4):936-44.

174. Dalm VA, Hofland LJ, Mooy CM et al, Somatostatin receptors in malignant lymphomas: targets for radiotherapy? J Nucl Med 2004: 45: 8

Chapter 14

NOVEL SMALL MOLECULES IN THE TREATMENT OF LYMPHOMAS

John Gerecitano, MD, PhD and Owen A. O'Connor, MD, PhD*

Memorial Sloan Kettering Cancer Center, Department of Medicine, Division of Hematologic Oncology, Lymphoma and Developmental Chemotherapy Services, New York, N.Y.

1. INTRODUCTION

Despite the enormous progress that has been made over the last decade in the treatment of many lymphomas, the prognosis for patients with relapsed disease, and particular sub-types of lymphoma like mantle cell and T-cell lymphoma, remain poor. While major advances in the use of combination chemotherapy, monoclonal antibodies, peripheral blood stem cell transplants, and radioimmunotherapy have provided new opportunities to affect cure and even manage more chronic forms of lymphoma, these traditional approaches have not benefited all patients or sub-types of lymphoma. In addition, the rapid pace of understanding the molecular basis for the discrete sub-types of lymphoma is affording new opportunities to both risk stratify patients and identify potentially "drugable" targets. These advances in understanding the major molecular defects in lymphoma have provided a new context in which we can consider the use of new and old drugs. The panoply of new targets and drugs now becoming available for the treatment of lymphoma is truly mind-boggling. A plethora of new small molecules that target Bcl-2, mTOR, histone deactylases, and NF-kB have shown promising preclinical activity, and now promising early phase clinical activity. In select cases, the empirical observations from early phase I clinical trials have provided invaluable clues to potentially valuable drugs like bortezomib, depsipeptide, and SAHA. These empirical observations, based on the inclusion of patients with lymphoma in these studies, have proven to be as or more valuable than any other 'rational' target based approach. In addition, beyond the novel small molecules affecting unique and heretofore unrecognized biological pathways, there continues to be a robust and important effort to identify new derivatives of older generation drugs with better activity and less toxicity. For example, new generation anthracenediones and anti-folates, and new formulations of older drugs like doxorubicin, irinotecan, and vincristine can favorably change the pharmacokinetic profile of these agents and improve their overall safety profile. While it would not be possible to address each and every new such drug, we hope to touch on some of the major new themes and agents emerging for the treatment of Hodgkin's Disease and non-Hodgkin's lymphoma.

2.   NOVEL AGENTS

2.1   Proteasome Inhibitors

2.1.1   Mechanism of Action

Targeting the proteasome is a very new strategy in cancer treatment. Until the 1990s, it was thought that the major mechanism for protein degradation within the cell was dependent on the lysosome. The discovery of the ubiquitin-proteasome mediated pathway and the clarification of its role in modulating protein turnover has turned out to be one of the more fruitful breakthroughs in our understanding of basic cellular and cancer biology. The ubiquitin-proteasome pathway is now known to play a major role in regulating everything from cell proliferation to apoptosis, and angiogenesis to metastasis. For their sentinel work in describing the role of ubiquitination in the degradation of intracellular protein, Ciechanover, Hersko and Rose were awarded the Nobel Prize in Chemistry in 2004. It is now widely recognized that the ubiquitin-proteasome pathway is the major extra-lysosomal pathway for the elimination of intracellular proteins [1]. At the heart of this degradative pathway is the 26S proteasome, which contains three different proteases responsible for cleaving the protein substrates. Among the key proteins that are known to be temporally degraded by the proteasome are the cyclins A, B, D and E and the cyclin-dependent kinase inhibitors p21 and p27 [Kip1] [2]. Both p21 and p27 can induce cell cycle arrest by inhibiting the cyclin D-, E- and A-dependent kinases [3]. Interfering with the temporal degradation of these regulatory proteins by inhibiting proteasome function provides a new mechanism for effecting cell cycle arrest in malignant cells.

Another potentially important mechanism of action for proteasome inhibitors pertains to its effects on nuclear factor-κB (NF-κB). NF-κB is an important transcription factor whose activation is regulated by proteasome-mediated degradation of its cognate inhibitor protein IκB [4]; [5]. NF-kB regulates innumerable biological pathways including cell proliferation, apoptosis, and cytokine release. In addition, cell adhesion molecules (CAMs) such as E-selectin, ICAM-1, and VCAM-1 are also regulated by NF-κB, and play a major role in tumor cell metastasis and angiogenesis *in vivo* [6,7]. During metastasis, these molecules direct the adhesion and extravasation of tumor cells to and from the vasculature to distant tissue sites. Inhibiting NF-κB activation through the stabilization of IκB protein can theoretically limit metastasis through the down-regulation of NF-κB-dependent cell adhesion molecules, and can mitigate the NF-kB induced stress response that follows exposure to noxious stimuli and cytotoxic agents, ultimately leading to apoptosis.

Collectively, these observations suggest that inhibitors of the proteasome can act through multiple mechanisms to arrest tumor growth, tumor spread and angiogenesis. Bortezomib, a dipeptidyl boronic acid inhibitor with high specificity for the chymotryptic moiety of the proteasome [8,9], is the first in its class of molecules to be approved by the U.S. Food and Drug Administration for the treatment of cancer. Preclinical studies have demonstrated its ability to prevent proteasome-mediated degradation of ubiquitinated proteins, including a host of cyclins, cdk inhibitors, p53, and IκB [10], leading to a number of effects that include cell cycle arrest and apoptosis.

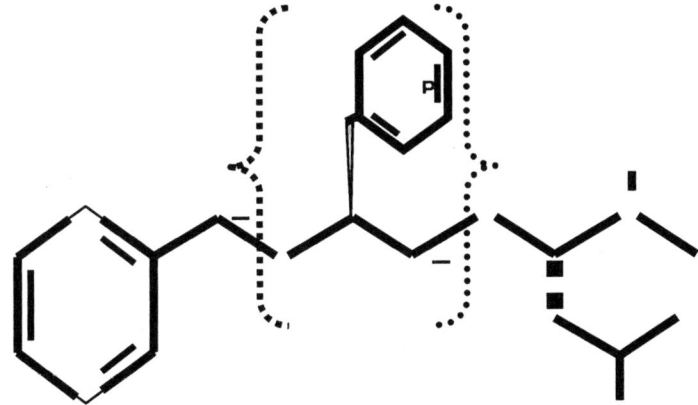

N-Pyrazinecarbonyl-L-phenylalanine-L-leucineboronic acid

2.1.2   Preclinical Data

Various dipeptide boronic acid proteasome inhibitors have been tested in the NIH panel of 60 human tumor cell lines to date [11]. Most of these compounds have demonstrated significant cytotoxic activities that appear to correlate with the effectiveness of proteasome blockade in all cell lines tested. What was unique to bortezomib was its selectivity for the chymotryptic protease in the 26S proteasome (see Figure 1). Of the available proteasome inhibitors that had been studied, PS-341 (bortezomib) was selected for further development based on its water solubility and favorable inhibition constants against the proteasome proteases. Using the NCI algorithm COMPARE, where a library of antineoplastic compounds is compared against the new compound being screened, the mechanism of bortezomib cytotoxicity was identified as truly unique, compared with over 60,000 other compounds in the NCI library. Bortezomib was shown to inhibit progression through the cell cycle, to induce apoptosis, and to cause the accumulation of the cdk inhibitor p21. Xenograft models of the PC-3 tumor line in mice showed major tumor regression in response to weekly intravenous and intratumoral injections of bortezomib [11]. Important pharmacodynamic studies demonstrated that this particular derivative specifically inhibited only the chymotryptic protease and not other intracellular proteases [11]. This effect reached a maximal level relatively quickly, typically within an hour of exposure, and persisted with a half-life of about 24 hours. The main adverse effects of bortezomib in these murine experiments were anorexia, emesis and diarrhea, all occurring in a dose-dependent manner. Very little myelosuppression was observed. Perhaps most interesting is the observation that transformed cell lines were more susceptible to proteasome inhibition than primary cell lines. While the precise mechanism for this has yet to be resolved, most attribute it to the greater dependence of transformed cells on NF-kB compared to normal cells [11].

2.1.3   Clinical Data

Bortezomib has been studied in three phase I trials in patients with both hematologic[12] and solid tumor [13,14] malignancies. Bortezomib was administered either twice a week for two weeks with a one week rest or twice a week for four weeks with a two week rest. In most cases, the drug was administered as an intravenous push in doses ranging from 0.13 to 1.56 mg/m^2. The major toxicities included secretory diarrhea, fatigue, fever, reversible thrombocytopenia and peripheral neuropathy. Objective responses were documented in one patient with multiple myeloma (MM) (though most MM patients had a reduction in the quantity of paraproteins), one patient with follicular lymphoma (FL), and one patient with mantle cell lymphoma (MCL).

Among the patients with solid tumors, a suggestion of activity was appreciated in patients with cancers of the prostate, kidney, head and neck, and lung. A large phase II study in myeloma has subsequently led to FDA approval of bortezomib in the treatment of relapsed or refractory multiple myeloma[15].

2.1.4   Phase II Trials in Lymphoma

Based on the activity seen in the Phase I studies, single agent Phase II trials of bortezomib in indolent and mantle cell lymphoma were initiated. An ongoing phase II study of bortezomib in patients with predominantly relapsed or refractory indolent non-Hodgkin's lymphoma (NHL) has recently been reported by our group[16,17]. To date, fifty-nine patients have been registered, representing all major sub-types of indolent and mantle cell NHL. Bortezomib was administered at a dose of 1.5 mg/m^2 on a day 1, 4, 8 and 11 schedule every 21 days. The patients were heavily pre-treated with a median of 3 prior therapies. Overall the drug was very well tolerated, with most patients experiencing toxicities well known to be associated with the drug, including thrombocytopenia, sensory neuropathy, diarrhea, and asthenia. Among the 15 assessable patients with FL, the overall response rate (ORR) was 60%, including 7 partial responses (PR) and two patients meeting criteria for complete remission (CR)/complete response unconfirmed (CRu). One of these complete responses lasted 9 months, which was significantly longer than that achieved with her prior therapy. Among 26 assessable patients with MCL, the ORR was 54%, including 9 PR and 5 CR/CRu. Interestingly, one patient who attained a PR maintained his first remission for over 19 months, after attaining only a 6 month remission from a rituximab-CHOP (cyclophosphamide, doxorubicin, vincristine and prednisone) based chemotherapy regimen. On relapse, this patient was re-treated on this protocol and attained a second major partial remission that has lasted approximately 7 to 8 months. Of 6 assessable patients with marginal zone lymphoma (MZL), 3 (50%) achieved a PR, while only 1 of the 5 patients (20%) with SLL showed any response to therapy (PR). Overall, the median progression free survival (PFS) for responding patients with MCL and all other non-MCL patients was 12 and 18 months respectively. The median time to response was also significantly different among the different sub-groups, with MCL and FL lymphoma patients demonstrating a median time to progression (TTR) of 5 and 11 weeks, respectively. This particular difference has potentially significant ramifications regarding how much therapy to give before one can adequately assess drug activity in follicular lymphoma.

Goy *et al.* at M.D. Anderson Cancer Center began a broader single-agent, single-institution study of bortezomib in patients with any B-cell neoplasm, regardless of their prior number of treatments[18]. Otherwise, this and the MSKCC studies are similar in design. Of 60 registered patients comprising a variety of different lymphomas, 33 had mantle cell lymphoma, 12 had diffuse large B-cell lymphoma, and the remainder had a variety of other subtypes, including small lymphocytic lymphoma, follicular lymphoma, Waldenstrom's Macroglobulinemia, and a transformed lymphoma. Overall, this population of patients was more heavily pretreated, with a median number of prior therapies of 3 in the MCL group and 4 in the other NHL patients. The overwhelming majority of patients had markedly elevated LDH and β_2-microglobulin prior to study enrollment. Of 29 assessable patients with mantle cell lymphoma, 12 (41%) achieved a major response, with 6 (20.5%) of them attaining a complete remission, and 6 (20.5%) attaining a partial remission. Overall, the duration of response was approximately 6 months. Among the patients with diffuse large B-cell lymphoma, only one of the 12 assessable patients achieved a partial remission, with the other patients demonstrating either stable or progressive disease. No activity was seen in patients with small lymphocytic lymphoma or in the one assessable patient with transformed lymphoma. While the numbers of patients with other sub-types of NHL were small, the collective experience suggests that there may be significant differences among the different sub-types of lymphoma. The minimal activity seen in large cell lymphoma has been curious, especially when put into the context of some gene expression array studies which seem to suggest that constitutive over-expression of NF-κB appears to define a select sub-set of diffuse large B-cell lymphoma known as post germinal center large cell lymphoma. These lymphomas are thought to derive from activated B-cells (ABC), and seem to be associated with more chemotherapy refractory disease and worse overall prognosis than patients with germinal center large cell lymphomas [19]. While this observation remains to be reconciled, it raises important questions about the use of prognostic markers identified in gene expression arrays as therapeutic targets. Alternatively, it may suggest that drugs like bortezomib and others that affect NF-κB may need to be used in combination with other drugs, and that merely affecting this singular mechanism may be insufficient in achieving the best therapeutic result. Nevertheless, studies are now beginning to address the merits of combining bortezomib with R-CHOP based chemotherapy in aggressive large B-cell lymphoma.

In addition to the above studies, two other phase II studies have treated patients with bortezomib at a dose of 1.3 mg/m², using the same treatment schedule outlined above. The National Cancer Institute of Canada (NCIC) reported on a study in patients with both treated and untreated mantle cell lymphoma [20]. A total of 30 patients were accrued, of whom 28 were assessable for response at the time of reporting. The number of prior treatments was limited to 2. Interestingly, there was no difference in ORR between chemonaïve and chemotherapy refractory patients. Among the 13 patients who had no prior therapy, 6 achieved a PR (ORR 46.2%), while among the 15 previously treated patients, 6 achieved PR and 1 achieved a CRu (ORR 46.7%). Most adverse events were grade 1 or 2, although there was an unusual vascular leak syndrome that occurred in some patients treated early in the study that may have been attributed to the fact that many of these patients had pre-existing effusions. Interestingly, this toxicity was not seen in other trials. Straus *et al.* [21] have enrolled 45 patients with NHL (21 MCL, 12 FL, 5 Waldenstrom's macroglobulinemia (WM), 4 Hodgkin's disease and 3 other). Responses were seen in 7 of 18 MCL patients (1 CR/CRu, 6 PR), 2 of 11 FL patients (both PR with late responses, 3 months after initiation of treatment), and 2 of 5 WM patients (both PR). No responses were seen in patients with aggressive lymphomas. Again, the most common toxicities were grade 3-4 thrombocytopenia, fatigue, and peripheral neuropathy (along with the additional toxicity of grade 3-4 anemia).

Collectively, these data demonstrate that bortezomib has meaningful activity in select sub-types of lymphoma, and perhaps more importantly, that the duration of response can be clinically significant (see Table 2). The future challenge, of course, is trying to figure out how best to integrate this promising new class of molecules into the present standards of care for lymphoma. Emerging preclinical data suggest a potential schedule-dependent synergy between bortezomib and a host of cytotoxic agents [22]. Future clinical trials will need to address these preclinical observations as we refine the use of this and other novel small molecules. In addition, a number of new generation proteasome inhibitors are being synthesized and are beginning to enter the clinic. These new agents will offer opportunities to improve on the efficacy and toxicity of bortezomib by targeting other proteins in the ubiquitin-proteasome pathway. Theoretically, these targets can include other proteases in the proteasome, and even the specific ubiquitin E3 ligases that catalyze the ubiquitination of very specific proteins or oncogenic substrates. To date, several small molecules have emerged which appear to inhibit the IkB kinases which phosphorylate IkB, initiating the cascade of events that will lead to its eventual proteolytic degradation. These drugs hold the promise of affecting the NF-κB pathway more directly. While the merits of targeting these new pathways remains to be seen, it is clear that our refined understanding of this novel pathway is beginning to afford innumerable opportunities to influence cancer cell biology at its core.

2.2   Targeting Bcl-2

2.2.1   Mechanism of Action

Bcl-2 is a well known anti-apoptotic protein involved in the intrinsic apoptosis pathway. The *bcl-2* gene is known to be over-expressed in many types of cancer, including NHL. For example, the juxtaposition of the *bcl-2* gene downstream from the immunoglobulin heavy chain gene promoter (t(11:14)) leads to the marked over-expression of Bcl-2 protein in follicular lymphoma. This molecular lesion is the sine qua non of the diagnosis. In addition to NHL, over-expression of Bcl-2 has been demonstrated in AML, CLL, MM, melanoma, prostate cancer, breast cancer, colorectal cancer and lung cancer [23], while it tumorigenicity as been demonstrated by the observation that transgenic mice that over-express Bcl-2 develop B cell malignancies [24,25]. Bcl-2 over-expression also confers marked resistance to chemotherapy, and contributes to cellular immortality. The stimuli required to induce apoptosis involve a shift in pro- and anti-apoptotic proteins in the mitochondrial membrane, the balance of which determines the likelihood cell death. A shift towards pro-apoptosis (i.e. an increase in pro-apoptotic proteins and a decrease in anti-apoptotic proteins) effects release of cytochrome c into the cytosol and the induction of programmed cell death. Once in the cytosol, cytochrome c activates apoptotic protease activating factor-1 (Apaf-1), which in turn activates the cascade of downstream caspase proteases. Bcl-2 stabilizes the mitochondrial membrane preventing cytochrome c release, thus blocking this intrinsic apoptotic pathway [23]. Through this mechanism, Bcl-2 can confer resistance to many different apoptotic stimuli, including cytotoxic drugs, radiation, hypoxia and antitumor antibodies[26]. The rational design of drugs against Bcl-2 affords unique opportunities to influence this critical biology. One such approach has involved the synthesis of antisense oligonucleotides to *bcl-2* which decrease the quantity of available messenger RNA capable of being translated into Bcl-2 protein. Other approaches have involved rational drug design to identify small molecules capable of inhibiting specific members of the Bcl-2 family, such as Bcl-xL.

Short sequences of single-stranded DNA complementary to known gene coding regions (antisense oligonucleotides) can lead to Watson-Crick base paring of the oligonucleotide with mRNA sequences. This specific hybridization prevents mRNA translation and targets the mRNA for cleavage by RNase H [27,28]. Antisense oligonucleotides can also activate non-specific immune mediated effects if they contain CpG motifs flanked by certain nucleic acid sequences [29]. Antisense oligonucleotides against *bcl-2* have demonstrated *in vitro* cell killing and cell cycle arrest in human leukemia cell lines, though potency in early studies was limited by poor transfection efficiency [30]. Second generation oligonucleotides with a sulfur atom substituted for an oxygen atom in the pohosphodiester backbone have conferred increased cellular uptake and decreased susceptibility to intracellular nucleases [31,32]. One of these products, oblimersen sodium, was identified as the most biologically active of over 40 such modified oligonucleotides and has been carried forward into clinical development [23].

2.2.2 Pre-Clinical Data

Bcl-2 antisense oligonucleotides have been shown to down regulate Bcl-2 protein and induce apoptosis in lymphoma cell lines [33,34]. Oblimersen, given as a continuous infusion to SCID and NOD/SCID mice inoculated with DoHH2 lymphoma cells to establish xenograft tumors, has shown significant activity compared with control non-sense oligodeoxynucleotides [35-37]. In the Klasa study, mice were treated with oblimersen, cyclophosphamide, or a combination of the two drugs. Treatment with oblimersen prolonged median survival and cured some animals in a dose- and schedule-dependent fashion. Of note, long term survival was achieved in this model even when sub-therapeutic doses of cyclophosphamide were used in conjunction with oblimersen, suggesting that oblimersen can potentiate the sensitivity of tumor cells to other chemotherapeutic agents without adding to toxicity.

In another such xenograft model, immortalized human lymphoblastoid B cells (a model of a post-transplant lymphoproliferative disorder) were injected intraperitoneally into SCID mice to establish tumors. Fifteen days later, the mice were treated with intraperitoneal oblimersen, rituximab, or a combination of these two agents. Among the animals in the single drug cohorts, the median survival was improved compared with control, though all animals still died with tumor. In contrast, 5 of the 7 animals treated with both agents were disease free at 150+ days. These data suggest that a Bcl-2 targeted drug can potentiate the activity of both cytotoxic and biological agents, and have given rise to a number of clinical trials addressing these questions specifically.

2.2.3 Clinical Data

The pharmacokinetic profile of oblimersen has been studied in patients with lymphoma, acute leukemia, melanoma, prostate cancer, colorectal cancer and other solid tumors [38-47]. Steady state concentrations above 1 µg/ml, which were found to be effective in animal studies [32], were achieved in all patients treated with greater than 2-3 mg/kg/day. Given the preclinical data, and the observations that lowering levels of Bcl-2 may sensitize tumor cells to chemotherapy, several clinical studies have been launched. These trials have focused on exploiting the potential synergistic interaction between Bcl-2-targeted treatment and conventional cytotoxic therapies.

A phase I study performed in 21 patients with advanced NHL administered oblimersen via a portable infusion pump, with continuous subcutaneous infusions over 14 days [38,48]. Dose levels ranged from 4.6 mg/m^2 to 195.8 mg/m^2/day, with pharmacokinetic analyses being obtained 48 hours after initiation of the infusion. These data confirmed linearity of the plasma concentrations as a function of dose, with plasma concentrations ranging from 0.4 μg/ml to 5.63 μg/ml, well within the concentration range required to effect cell kill based upon *in vitro* assays. The major dose limiting toxicities included thrombocytopenia, hypotension, fever and asthenia, and were seen predominantly at plasma concentrations greater than 4 μg/ml. A maximum tolerated dose (MTD) of 147 mg/m^2/day was established by this study. Among this selected population of patients with lymphoma, one CR and 2 minor responses were observed (all in patients with FL), with 9 patients experiencing stable disease. The one patient with CR remained free of disease for 5 years despite failing four prior therapies and progressing on his last prior treatment. All three patients with DLBCL progressed while on trial. This observation supports the underlying biology and potential merit of targeting Bcl-2 in follicular lymphoma.

Leonard *et al.* [49] reported on the safety and efficacy of oblimersen alone and with R-CHOP in patients with relapsed, refractory or chemotherapy naive mantle cell lymphoma. All patients were initially treated with oblimersen at a dose of 3 to 5 mg/kg/day for 7 days every 21 days for up to 6 cycles as long as there was no progression of disease. Chemotherapy naïve patients without a complete response were then treated with oblimersen + R-CHOP for up to 6 cycles, with R-CHOP starting on day 5 of the oblimersen infusion. Of 18 assessable relapsed/refractory patients treated with 3 mg/kg/day of oblimersen alone, there was 1 CR, 7 SD and 10 patients with progression of disease (POD) (of 3 assessable patients treated with 4-5 mg/kg/day, 2 had PR). In the chemotherapy naïve group, there were 5 patients with SD and 8 with POD. Of the 8 chemotherapy naïve patients who went on to receive 6 cycles of oblimersen plus R-CHOP, there were 2 CR, 4 PR and 2 SD. Oblimersen was well tolerated in this study, and did not appear to increase the toxicity of R-CHOP. Though the numbers are small, and a randomized study would be required to determine whether oblimersen actually improves the activity of R-CHOP, the study suggests that the drugs can be given together safely.

Based on findings that oblimersen enhances the anti-tumor activity of rituximab in NHL cell lines and lymphoma xenografts, Pro *et al.* [50] treated

21 patients with relapsed or refractory B-cell NHL with oblimersen (3 mg/kg/day for 7 days weeks 1, 3 and 5) in combination with concomitant rituximab (375 mg/m^2 weekly for 6 doses). The median number of prior treatments was 2, and most patients had indolent disease (8 with FL, 6 with SLL, 3 with MCL, 2 with MALT, 2 with large cell lymphoma (LCL)). Of 15 assessable patients, 5 responded (33% ORR): one patient with stage IV MALT had a CR, while 3 patients with FL and one with MCL achieved a PR. One patient with FL had a minor response, and 7 patients had stable disease. Adverse effects included grade 3 or 4 neutropenia, neutropenic fever, grade 3 thrombocytopenia along with anemia, hypotension, fatigue and chills. These data, obtained in a more relapsed or refractory population of patients, do not appear to suggest any dramatic synergy between rituximab and oblimersen. Future studies will likely address this question in a less heavily treated population of patients.

A randomized phase III trial compared fludarabine and cyclophosphamide with fludarabine, cyclophosphamide and oblimersen in patients with intermediate or high risk relapsed/refractory CLL [51]. Of 241 patients there were more than twice as many major responses with the addition of oblimersen (16% vs. 7%, p=0.039). Hematopoietic toxicities were similar in the two groups, with the exception of more grade 3 or 4 thrombocytopenia in the oblimersen arm (55% vs. 32%).

The promise of targeting Bcl-2 in many different forms of cancer, but especially in lymphoma, has given rise to a number of new generation small molecules that affect this target. Recently, Fesik *et al.* reported on the development of one such compound, ABT-737[52]. In an effort to rationally optimize the design and efficacy of their drug, this team used NMR-based screening, parallel synthesis and structure-based design to synthesize and purify a protein that was able to bind and interfere with the function of Bcl-2 without significant adsorption to albumin. Sixty-seven cell lines were then screened for cytotoxicity with ABT-737, with cell lines derived from lymphoid malignancies and small-cell lung cancer lines showing the most sensitivity to the compound. As expected from drugs that target Bcl-2, ABT-737 was also found to sensitize cells to the cytotoxic effects of chemotherapeutics and radiation. In addition to this and the antisense molecules, many other efforts are focusing on identifying new drugs that affect Bcl-2, including novel derivatives of the cotton seed extract based compound gossypol[53,54]. Stereoselective derivatives of gossypol interact with other important Bcl-2 family members, and together with a host of other agents will hopefully continue to validate this approach in the treatment of lymphoma.

2.3   Immunomodulatory Drugs

2.3.1   Mechanism of Action

During the mid-1950s, thalidomide (α-(N-phthalimido)glutarimide) was marketed as a sedative and antiemetic, and was widely used in Europe as a treatment for pregnancy-associated nausea. The teratogenic effects of thalidomide led to its rapid withdrawal from the market. In the 1960s, an Israeli dermatologist using thalidomide for its sedative effects coincidentally found that it reduced lesions, night sweats and fevers in patients with erythema nodosum leprosum (ENL), an inflammatory complication of lepromatous leprosy [55,56]. The anti-inflammatory effects of thalidomide can be explained in part by its inhibition of TNF-α production in monocytes [57]. The immunomodulatory effects of thalidomide have since found applications in the treatment of multiple myeloma and autoimmune diseases including various rheumatologic conditions.

In the 1970s, work in Judah Folkman's lab revealed that thalidomide could prevent basic fibroblast growth factor (bFGF)-induced angiogenesis [58]. This finding has prompted research into the use of thalidomide as an antineoplastic agent. Additional interest in thalidomide surfaced when it was discovered to have potentially important activity in patients with multiple myeloma, attributed to its impact on the 'cytokine milieu'. In multiple myeloma thalidomide was associated with a relatively high response rate of 30 to 40% in patients with advanced and refractory disease[59]. Thalidomide has also been tested in other microvessel-rich tumors, such as renal cell carcinoma, prostatic adenocarcinoma, glioma, and melanoma with less clear benefits [60-63].

Thalidomide is obviously not a drug with trivial side effects. In addition to being associated with severe teratogenic effects, it is also associated with a hypercoagulable state that increases the risk of deep venous thromboses, potentially significant peripheral sensory neuropathy and sedation. The development of thalidomide analogs was prompted by the desire to decrease these side effects – particularly the teratogenicity - while trying to improve on the efficacy of the parent compound [64]. The first generation of immunomodulatory drugs, or "IMiDs," were designed in the 1990s to increase the inhibitory effects against TNF-α. Many of these thalidomide analogs, most of which had an amino group added to the fourth carbon of the phthaloyl ring of thalidomide (see Figure 2), have been shown to have 50,000 times more potent anti-TNF-α activity than thalidomide itself [65]. One of these analogs, CC-5013 (lenalidomide, Revlimid) has also been shown to be non-teratogenic in New Zealand rabbits, the best animal model for screening teratogenic potential [55]. At present, two such derivatives have been identified as lead compounds for further pre-clinical and clinical development, including CC-5013 (Revlimid) and CC-4047 (Actimid) [55].

2.3.2   Preclinical Data

CC-5013 and CC-4047 have been shown to be even more potent anti-angiogenic drugs than thalidomide [66]. Although the mechanism of action for their antiangiogenic properties is not completely known, both CC-5013 and CC-4047 inhibit angiogenic sprouting in the rat aorta assay, and inhibit formation of tubules in a human angiogenesis system. CC-5013, the more potent anti-angiogenic analog, blocks migration of endothelial cells (EC) in a wound healing assay without inhibiting EC proliferation [55,66,67]. *In vitro* studies have shown that these molecules also inhibit NF-κB and induce growth arrest and caspase-mediated apoptosis in cultured tumor cells [68,69]. CC-5013 and CC-4047 have also been shown to potentiate the effects of dexamethasone and the proteasome inhibitor bortezomib on TNF-related apoptosis-induced ligand (TRAIL) activation [55], while CC-4047 acts as a co-stimulator of T cells *in vivo* [70]. Both compounds have been shown to be more potent than thalidomide in suppressing tumor growth *in vivo*, and in suppressing anti-angiogenic effects in murine models of B-cell malignancies [67].

2.3.3   Clinical Data

Phase I trials in multiple myeloma [71,72] and in solid tumors [73] have shown no serious side effects of CC-5013 [74]. In particular, the somnolence, constipation and neuropathy observed with thalidomide were not found to be dose-limiting toxicities with CC-5013. The first completed phase I clinical trial of CC-5013 was reported in 2002 [71]. In this study, five of seven patients with refractory multiple myeloma (MM) showed partial response (PR) with CC-5013. CC-5013 has now entered a phase III clinical trial for metastatic malignant melanoma and MM. In the MM trial (http://www.ecog.org/active_reports/Myeloma.html), patients will be randomized to treatment with CC-5013 and a high or low dose of dexamethasone. Patients who progress will be treated with thalidomide plus dexamethasone. The trial is designed to compare the effectiveness and relative toxicities of CC-5013 and thalidomide, and to define the efficacy of high- vs. low-dose dexamethasone in patients with relapsed/refractory MM. Phase I and II trials are now enrolling patients with relapsed and metastatic MM, recurrent high grade glioma, and refractory solid tumors. An NCI-sponsored phase I trial of CC-5013 in refractory solid tumors and lymphoma recently   began   enrollment   in   2003 (http://clinicalstudies.info.nih.gov/cgi/detail.cgi?A_2002-C-0083.html).

To date, CC-4047 has been studied in only one phase I trial[75]. Phase I/II trials are currently enrolling patients with advanced MM and metastatic hormone refractory prostate cancer.

The promise of immunomodulatory drugs in the treatment of lymphoma was recently highlighted in a phase II study in which patients with relapsed and refractory MCL were treated with rituximab plus thalidomide[76]. Of the 16 patients enrolled in this trial, all had received prior CHOP-like regimens, 3 had prior rituximab, and 3 had undergone prior peripheral blood stem cell transplants. All patients were treated with 4 weekly standard doses of rituximab plus an escalating dose of oral thalidomide (200 mg daily for 2 weeks, then 400 mg daily), with continued maintenance thalidomide until progression of disease.   Even in this historically refractory group of patients, 13 patients responded to treatment (ORR = 81%), including 4 CR and 1 CRu. The median progression free survival was an impressive 20.4 months, which was almost double the median PFS (12.7 months) after the prior treatment for these patients (see Figure 3). Of the 8 patients who relapsed or progressed on trial, 3 were "re-induced" with rituximab while continuing thalidomide treatment. Two of the three responded to re-treatment, with second remissions lasting 13 and over 18 months.   While these results seem very impressive, the overwhelming number of patients on study were rituximab naïve. Given the current standard of care in North America, where patients are unlikely to be rituximab naïve after their initial therapy, it is not clear how thalidomide and rituximab will impact those patients with primarily rituximab refractory disease. Clearly, there is a mechanistic rationale in support of the positive interaction between the IMiDs and rituximab. Future studies with new derivatives will need to target rituximab refractory patients in order to address the true potential of this drug-drug interaction.

2.4   Histone Deacetylase Inhibitors

2.4.1   Mechanism of Action

Nucleosomal histones play an important role in the regulation of genetic transcription. When histones are acetylated, chromatin assumes a relaxed configuration that allows easy access to transcription factors. Deacetylation causes condensation of the chromatin, reducing access to transcription factors and leading to decreased expression of certain genes. This form of epigenetic transcriptional regulation has been shown to play a complex role in many forms of cancer, including NHL. One example of this complex regulation is illustrated by the role of Bcl-6 in lymphoma (see Figure 4). Bcl-6 is selectively expressed only in mature B-cells within the germinal center [77,78], where it blocks apoptosis and differentiation by functioning as a potent transcriptional repressor of genes involved in these pathways[79,80]. Bcl-6 is overexpressed in the majority of diffuse large B-cell lymphomas, where it may aberrantly prevent apoptosis and differentiation. Several lines of evidence suggest that Bcl-6 down-regulation is dependent on its acetylation status[81]. The Bcl-6 protein itself is subject to acetylation by the histone acetyltransferase (HAT) p300, and deacetylation by a variety of histone deacetylases (HDACs). Acetylation of Bcl-6 inactivates the trans-repressor activity of the protein, allowing Bcl-6 to turn on a host of genes. Deacetylation of Bcl-6 restores the trans-repressor state of Bcl-6, thereby down-regulating a host of genes. For example, Bcl-6 is a repressor of p21^{WAF1} expression, which is typically expressed when Bcl-6 is acetylated. In order for cells to complete differentiation and exit the germinal center, Bcl-6 expression must be down-regulated [77]. Normally, this occurs when B-cells are stimulated by antigens or other T-cell signals.

Disrupting the normal balance between histone acetylation and deacetylation has been explored as a potential mechanism for changing the expression of genes involved in cell cycling and apoptosis. To date, several structural classes of HDAC inhibitors (HDACIs) (see Table 3) have been developed, including short-chain fatty acids (e.g., butyrates), hydroxamic acids (e.g., trichostatin A), suberoylanilide hydroxamic acid (SAHA), and oxamflatin), cyclic tetrapeptides (e.g., trapoxin A, FR901228 and apicidin) and benzamides (e.g., MS-27-275) [82]. For the purposes of this review, we will limit our discussion to two HDAC inhibitors which have been studied to some extent in lymphoma, including depsipeptide (NSC 6,30176, FR901228) and suberoylanalide hydroxamic acid (SAHA).

SAHA   Depsipeptide

2.4.2   Preclinical Data

Depsipeptide is a bicyclic peptide HDACI isolated from *Chromobacterim violaceu.* The drug was initially selected based on its ability to induce morphological reversion of H-*ras*-transformed NIH-3T3 cells *in vitro* [83,84]. Depsipeptide has been shown to cause cell cycle arrest and induce apoptosis, both of which were correlated with the degree of histone hyperacetylation in the M-8 cell line[85]. Depsipeptide has also shown excellent *in vitro* and *in vivo* antitumor activity against human tumor lines representing lung adenocarcinomas (A549 and MCF-7), breast adenocarcinoma (ZR-75-1) and melanoma (LOX IMVI) [83].

Similarly, SAHA has shown the ability to induce differentiation and /or apoptosis in a variety of cancer cell lines [82]. *In vitro*, treatment with SAHA inhibits the growth of hormone dependent LNCaP and hormone-independent PC-3 and TSU-Pr1 prostate cell lines at micromolar concentrations (2.5-7.5 μM) [86,87]. In addition, SAHA induces differentiation of murine erythroleukemia (MEL), human bladder transitional cell carcinoma (T24) and human breast adenocarcinoma (MCF-7), and induces apoptosis in human myeloma (ARP-1) and human neuroblastoma cells (KCN-69n)[88]. *In vivo*, established palpable CWR22 prostate cancer xenografts treated with SAHA showed significant tumor regression (up to 97% reduction compared to control animals) with no changes in weight or changes in normal organs at necropsy[87].

In separate studies, the chemopreventive effects of SAHA were assessed in the N-methylnitrosourea (NMU)-induced rat mammary tumor model [89]. Tumor development was monitored by palpation throughout the study, and at termination of the study, tumor incidence, number, multiplicity, latency and volume was determined. A dose of 900 ppm of SAHA in the diet reduced the incidence of NMU-induced mammary tumors by 40%, the total of number of tumors by 66%, and mean tumor volume by 78%, with no detectable toxic side effects. Similar experiments were performed in female A/J mice treated with nitrosamine 4-(methylnitro-amino)-1-butanone (NNK) in which treatment with SAHA inhibited lung tumor formation without apparent toxicity [90]. These very interesting studies suggested a potential role of SAHA in chemoprevention.

The mechanism of action of SAHA has been studied in detail. Eight HDACs have been identified in mammals, including the yeast RPD3 homologs HDAC1, HDAC2, HDAC3 and HDAC8[91-97], and the yeast HDA1 homologs HDAC4/HDAC-A, HDAC5/mHDA1, HDAC6/mHDA2 and HDAC7 [98-103]. SAHA inhibits HDAC by a direct interaction with the catalytic site[104]. A crystallographic study of the conserved deacetylase catalytic core reveals a narrow, tube-like pocket that has hydrophobic walls and a polar bottom. The pocket bottom contains a metal-cofactor binding site, two Asp-His charge relay systems and a tyrosine, all features of which appear to be conserved across the HDAC family. The structure of deacetylase-Zn^{2+}-SAHA complex shows that SAHA inserts its aliphatic chain into this pocket, coordinating the Zn^{2+} ion in a bidentate fashion with its hydroxamic acid. The residues that contact SAHA are conserved across the HDAC family, which accounts for the observation that SAHA is a general inhibitor of several members of the HDAC protein family[86].

2.4.3   Clinical Data

Given the theoretical background for the importance of HDACIs in NHL, along with promising *in vivo* data in human tumors, this new class of drugs has been brought into clinical trials in a variety of settings. In 2001, Piekarz *et al.* reported on 4 cases of patients with cutaneous T-cell lymphoma treated with depsipeptide in the context of a phase I study [105]. All four patients showed marked improvement of their skin lesions, including two patients with Sezary syndrome who had been refractory to prior therapies (including CHOP and CVP (cyclophosphamide, vincristine and prednisone)) who showed rapid clearing of peripheral Sezary cells. In the final report of this phase I study, the dose limiting toxicities included fatigue, nausea, vomiting and thrombocytopenia, with an MTD defined as 17.8 mg/m^2 given as an IV infusion over four hours on days one and five of a 21 day cycle [106]. Clinically significant cardiac toxicity, which had been of concern based on preclinical trials, was not observed.

This study was expanded to a phase II trial for patients with cutaneous T-cell lymphoma (CTCL), peripheral T-cell lymphoma (PTCL) and other mature T-cell lymphomas. Of 39 patients reported to date [107], 7 of 14 patients (50%) with CTCL treated with up to 2 prior regimens showed a complete (n=3) or partial (n=4) response. The duration of response has ranged from 6 to over 34 months. Of 17 patients with PTCL, 4 (24%) have achieved a partial response, and the duration of response in each of these patients has been approximately 9 months (n=1), 12 months (n=1), and over 4 months (n=2). The most common toxicities have included those observed in the phase I trial, with the addition of neutropenia and hypocalcemia.

SAHA has been studied in phase I trials as both an intravenous infusion [108] and as an oral formulation. To date, 12 patients have been treated on the IV trial and 23 on the oral trial [109]. Overall, all patients were very heavily pretreated, with a median number of prior treatments of 7 in the IV trial and 5 in the oral trial. Over half of the patients on the IV study, and about one-third of the patients on the oral study received prior stem cell transplantation. Interestingly, the dose limiting toxicities (DLTs) were slightly different for the two formulations. For patients receiving IV SAHA, the DLTs were predominantly hematologic (neutropenia and thrombocytopenia), and reversed with a median of 4 to 5 days after drug discontinuation. For patients receiving the oral formulation of SAHA, the DLTs were predominantly non-hematologic (dehydration, anorexia, diarrhea and fatigue) and were also rapidly reversed with a median of 3 days off treatment. These differences are likely related to major differences in the C_{max} and AUC obtained with the different formulations. Reduction in measurable tumor has been seen in 3 patients (all with Hodgkin's disease

(HD)) treated with IV SAHA, and in 4 patients treated with oral SAHA (1 with HD, 2 with DLBCL, and 1 with CTCL). One patient with transformed small lymphocytic lymphoma (SLL) had resolution of subcutaneous nodules, axillary adenopathy and a large gastrohepatic mass. One patient with refractory HD had stable disease on treatment for over 9 months. All responses were PRs, except for one CR in a patient with transformed large cell lymphoma treated with oral SAHA.

Clearly, the HDACIs will continue to be a potentially important group of drugs to be studied in the treatment of lymphoma. Whether they find niche uses in diseases like cutaneous T-cell lymphomas or find a broader application in the treatment of other B-cell malignancies remains to be seen. Certainly, based at least on the Bcl-6 rationale, it seems that B-cell lymphomas may be a very logical place to develop this class of drugs. One major area of investigation that remains largely speculative is how best to combine them with other more conventional drugs. For example, there may be genes turned on by HDACIs that can play an important role in potentiating the cytotoxicity of conventional agents. While gene expression array based data could provide important clues regarding which genes or gene products to target, empirical pre-clinical observations will remain an important venue for identifying these potential combinations. Alternatively, the cytostatic properties of SAHA and other HDACIs may confer the potential of maintaining stable disease in patients with otherwise rapidly progressive and incurable lymphoma. While thinking of these drugs as maintenance drugs to be used for extended periods of time to sustain major remissions may not be the first venue for development, turning some forms of aggressive lymphoma into a more chronic disease is a treatment strategy that deserves attention, especially in the post-transplant setting.

2.5   mTOR Inhibitors

2.5.1   Mechanism of Action

Rapamycin was initially isolated from a strain of *Streptomyces hygroscopicus* more than 20 years ago, and has been successfully employed as an antifungal agent. It has subsequently been found to have potent immunosuppressive and antineoplastic properties in mammalian cells [110]. The parallel development of rapamycin and FK506 as mammalian immunosuppressive agents led to the discovery of a family of intracellular binding proteins termed FK506 binding proteins (FKBP), which inhibit T-cell activation in the presence of immuonophilin proteins [111,112]. Of these, FKB12 is probably the most important rapamycin binding protein. In 1995, the protein kinase targeted by the FKBP12-Rapamycin complex was identified and named the "molecular target of rapamycin (mTOR)." When rapamycin binds to FKB12, the resulting complex binds to and inhibits the kinase action of mTOR, leading to G1 arrest in various cell types [113-115].

Although the full spectrum of biological effects of mTOR has not been fully clarified, mTOR is known to be a member of the phosphatidylinositol 3-kinase (PI3K) related family of protein kinases [116]. In its uninhibited state, mTOR is activated by a diverse set of inputs, including growth factors like insulin growth factor – 1 (IGF-1), which activates the PI3K/Akt signaling pathway [116]. While this pathway is inhibited by the tumor suppressor PTEN, inactivation of PTEN or constitutive activation of Akt can both lead to uncontrolled activation of mTOR and increased cellular proliferation [117]. Inhibition of mTOR, which leads to decreased cellular proliferation, occurs during times of nutritional deprivation in an Akt independent pathway [116], indicating that other upstream regulators are also likely to be important in mTOR regulation. Once phosphorylated, mTOR activates at least two downstream pathways (see Figure 5). The eukaryotic translation initiation factor 4E binding protein (4E-BP1), and the 40S ribosomal protein p70 S6 kinase both regulate translation of specific mRNAs that promote progression through the cell cycle. These proteins are both phosphorylated by activated mTOR, leading to cell cycle transition from G1 through S phase [118-120]. Other proteins regulated by mTOR include cyclin D3 and c-myc [120]. Hypoxia-inducible factor (HIF-1α) gene expression, which is important in the pathogenesis of renal cell carcinoma, is also influenced by mRNA translation and protein stabilization in which mTOR may play a role [121,122].

2.5.2   Preclinical Data

In preclinical studies, rapamycin and its derivatives have shown significant antitumor activity at low concentrations in a variety of NCI tumor cell lines, including breast cancer, prostate cancer, leukemia, melanoma, renal cell cancer, glioblastoma and pancreatic cancer lines [123]. Growth inhibition of xenografts in mice has also been noted, although tumor regression has been limited [117]. CCI-779 (Wyeth-Ayerst), an ester of rapamycin, has been shown to work at a threshold dose, and does not exhibit the classical linear increase in activity as a function of increasing dose [124]. Furthermore, intermittent dosing was shown to be effective, as a dosing schedule based on a 2-week interval appears to exhibit the best activity in a mouse xenograft study [124].

2.5.3   Clinical Data

CCI-779 has now been brought into phase I and phase II clinical trials. Two phase I studies have been conducted, using different dosing schedules of CCI-779 [125,126]. In one of these studies, CCI-779 was given intravenously weekly, with no dose-limiting toxicities at doses from 7.5 to 220 mg/m^2/wk (although grade 3 mucositis was seen) [125]. A partial response (PR) was seen in one patient each with renal cell cancer (RCC), breast cancer, and a neuroendocrine tumor. The second phase I study employed a daily intravenous infusion of CCI-779 for 5 days, repeated every 2 weeks [126]. The maximally-tolerated dose in this study was 15mg/m^2/day in heavily pretreated patients and 19 mg/m^2/day in minimally pretreated patients. One patient with non-small-cell lung cancer achieved a PR. Dose-limiting toxicities in this study included grade 3 hypocalcemia, grade 3 elevation in liver function tests, and grade 3 thrombocytopenia. Three phase I studies have begun to look at CCI-779 in combination with gemcitabine, 5-fluorouracil plus leucovorin [117], and IFN in patients with RCC [127].

Recently, very interesting results of a trial using CCI-779 in patients with MCL were reported [128]. Thirty-four patients with refractory MCL and a median of 3 prior therapies were treated with a starting dose of 250 mg CCI-779 IV weekly. Although 54% of the patients were refractory to their prior treatment, a promising ORR of 38% (13/34) was observed, with 1 CR and 12 PRs. The median duration of response was 5.7 months (95% CI: 5.2-13.2). Most patients (32/35) experienced a grade 3 or 4 toxicity, the most frequent of which was thrombocytopenia. These toxicities limited the treatment dose, resulting in a median treatment dose of 45 mg per week. This group is now evaluating CCI-779 at a dose of 25 mg per week.

3.   DERIVATIVES OF MORE TRADITIONAL AGENTS

3.1   Novel Anthracycline Derivatives - Pixantrone

3.1.1   Mechanism of Action

Anthracycline based combination chemotherapy regimens have been an important first-line treatment for aggressive NHL, as well as many other sub-types of cancer. The activity of anthracyclines relates to their ability to intercalate into helical DNA structures and to inhibit the function of topoisomerase II. Both of these actions can inhibit the replication of neoplastic cells, given their frequently higher rate of cell cycle progression and over-expression of topoisomerases [129]. The clinical use of anthracyclines however, is limited by their susceptibility to cell efflux mechanisms (p-glycoprotein and MDR), and to their cumulative cardiotoxicity. Modifications of the anthracenedione backbone and new potentially less toxic liposomal formulations of these important drugs have been developed in order overcome some of these toxicity barriers.

Pixantrone was developed as an analogue of mitoxantrone in a search for anthracyclines with decreased cardiotoxicity (see Figure 6). It is thought that the cardiotoxicity of mitoxantrone and doxorubicin is related to the shuttling of electrons through their aromatic structures and quinone moieties, the chemistry of which appears to be dependent on the 5,8-dihydroxy substitution groups on the anthracene ring [130,131]. Therefore, anthracenediones without these hydroxyl groups were developed in an effort to influence this chemistry. By introducing nitrogen atoms into the anthracinedione chromophore, creating an additional hydrogen bonding basic site, a planar structure could be achieved that also has increased affinity for DNA and topoisomerase II. Mono-aza derivatives bearing the nitrogen in position 2 have antitumor activity, which eventually led to the discovery and development of the drug pixantrone [132]. Pixantrone, like its parent compound mitoxantrone, intercalates into DNA and inhibits and topoisomerase II [132].

Pixantrone

3.1.2   Preclinical Data

In vitro, pixantrone is about 10 times less potent than mitoxantrone, and is cross resistant with both doxorubicin in MDR over-expressing cell lines and mitoxantrone in the HT29/Mitoxantrone cell line [132]. However, pixantrone is significantly less cardiotoxic at equally effective doses, is less myelosuppressive, and shows better *in vivo* activity in leukemia and lymphoma models [133-136]. Pixantrone has demonstrated significant cytotoxic activity in a variety of secondary cell lines, including the P388, L1210 and YC-8 murine hematologic tumor models, and even improved survival in a YC-8 murine lymphoma model [133,137]. Cardiac function assessed in two rodent models showed minimal cardiotoxicity in treatment-naïve rodents, and no worsening of pre-existing doxorubicin-induced cardiomyopathy in mice (unlike mitoxantrone and doxorubicin, which exacerbated pre-existing cardiomyopathy in this model) [137,138].

3.1.3   Clinical Data

In a phase I study of pixantrone in 26 patients with advanced or refractory NHL [132], the only dose limiting toxicity was myelosuppression. Other adverse effects included nausea and vomiting controlled by antiemetics, alopecia and temporary blue discoloration of the skin. No clinical evidence of cardiotoxicity was seen. Three complete remissions were noted at the MTD of 84 mg/m^2, including: (1) one that lasted 8 months in a patient with DLBCL in second relapse; (2) one that lasted 14+ months in a patient with aggressive B-cell NHL in second relapse, and; (3) one in a patient with primary refractory follicular lymphoma. Two partial responses were seen, including one in a patient with transformed aggressive NHL in third relapse, and one in a patient with mantle-cell lymphoma in third relapse. Both partial responses were seen in patients treated with doses of pixantrone well below the MTD. Four of the 5 responses occurred in patients who were considered anthracycline refractory.

In a multicenter phase II trial, 33 patients with relapsed aggressive NHL with a median of 2 prior chemotherapy regimens were enrolled [139]. Pixantrone was given at a dose of 85 mg/m^2 by intravenous infusion weekly for 3 weeks, followed by a one week rest each cycle for a planned total of 6 cycles. Complete remissions were seen in 5 patients, and PR in 4 (ORR = 27%), with a median progression-free survival of 106 days. Thirteen patients experienced progression of disease on study. The major toxicity was neutropenia, with 19 patients experiencing a grade 3 or 4 neutropenia lasting a median of about 7 days. All patients were followed with serial MUGA scans after every second cycle of treatment. Three patients, all of whom had been treated with prior anthracyclines, developed an absolute decrease of more than 10% of their left ventricular ejection fraction (LVEF), but two of these patients had started with a compromised LVEF (<45%). Other drug-related events included a mild increase in alkaline phosphatase, arthritis and asthenia (each occurring in one patient), alopecia in 3 patients, and mild to moderate nausea in 10 patients.

Another obvious strategy for drugs like pixantrone is to incorporate them directly into pre-existing regimens, either by substituting them for select drugs, or by adding them to pre-existing regimens. One such study substituted pixantrone for etoposide in the ESHAP regimen (methylprednisolone, cisplatin and cytosine arabinoside) in patients with relapsed or refractory aggressive NHL [140]. The MTD of pixantrone when administered with ESHAP was 80 mg/m^2. Of the 21 patients studied, 18 carried the diagnosis of DLBCL (86%), 2 had follicular large cell lymphoma, and 1 had transformed disease. The median number of prior therapies was one, and all patients were considered anthracycline refractory. The major dose limiting toxicities were grade 3 infection and febrile neutropenia, which defined the first dose level of 80 mg/m^2 as the MTD. Overall, the regimen was well tolerated, and included a variety of expected toxicities including grade 4 neutropenia (68%), febrile neutropenia (26%), thrombocytopenia (42%) and anemia (21%). Nonhematologic toxicities were also minor, and included grade 1 or 2 nausea, blue urine and fatigue. Interestingly, no clinically significant cardiac events were observed. Of 18 assessable patients, there were 7 (39%) CRs and 4 (22%) PRs.

Borchmann *et al.* [141] adopted a similar strategy, substituting pixantrone for doxorubicin in a CHOP regimen used to treat patients with relapsed aggressive NHL. Twelve of the 18 assessable patients had DLBCL, and all had received prior anthracycline-based therapies. Patients were treated with traditional doses of cyclophosphamide (750 mg/m^{2}day 1), vincristine (1.4 mg/m^2,capped at 2 mg day 1) and prednisone (100 mg/day, day 1-5), with pixantrone dosed at 100, 120 and 150 mg/m^2. The dose-limiting toxicity was neutropenia, occurring in 3 of the 6 patients at the 150 mg/m^2 dose. A pixantrone-related decrease in ejection fraction from 44% to 27% was noted in one patient after 6 cycles of therapy. Overall, the response rate was significant (13/18), with six patients meeting criteria for CR, 7 patients achieving PR, and 3 patients progressing on therapy. The remainder of patients were not assessable at the time of this report.

To address the issue of pixantrone cardiotoxicity, Borchmann *et al.* [142] have compiled data on adverse events in 79 patients treated thus far in 5 phase I and II trials. Pixantrone was used as a single agent in 33 patients and in combination regimens in 46 patients. Sixty-five of 79 patients had received prior anthracyclines, and three of these patients experienced treatment-related, non-lethal cardiac events (all 3 patients had a history of cardiovascular disease). No events were observed in anthracycline-naïve patients.

While more direct comparisons between pixantrone and doxorubicin in combination chemotherapy regimens will be necessary to fully understand the differences between these agents, it is clear that the improved toxicity profile of pixantrone, especially its cardiotoxicity, offers unique opportunities to improve the treatment of select sub-types of lymphoma. Anthracyclines are among the most important classes of drug used for the treatment of diffuse large B-cell lymphoma. Most patients with this disease receive between 6 to 8 cycles of standard R-CHOP based chemotherapy, giving them a cumulative dose of doxorubicin between 600 and 800 mg/m^2. Most cytoreduction regimens for patients with relapsed disease employ other non-cross resistant drugs like cytarabine, carboplatin, ifosfamide, etoposide and steroids. Because the risk of cardiotoxicity increases dramatically when the cumulative doxorubicin dose exceeds 800 mg/m^2, these drugs typically cannot be integrated into traditional cytoreductive regimens. Hence, one potentially useful application for new generation anthracyclines with minimal cardiotoxicity is to integrate them into the second-line chemotherapy programs prior to stem cell transplantation. Such approaches offer the chance to improve complete remission rates before high-dose chemotherapy, and could offer a promising new strategy for improving the outcome of patients undergoing stem cell transplantation.

3.2   Novel Multifunctional Alkylating Agents - Bendamustine

3.2.1   Mechanism of Action

Bendamustine is an alkylating agent that may also function as a purine analog. This bifunctional alkylator is structurally related to chlorambucil, and was first synthesized in Germany in 1963 [143]. In bendamustine, the benzene ring of chlorambucil is replaced by a 1-methyl-benzimidazole ring, which may also function as a purine analog. The nitrogen mustard group of bendamustine functions as a potent alkylating agent (i.e. strong electrophile), while the hydrochloride residue added to the butyric acid side chain confers increased water solubility. This structure was derived with the goal of producing an anticancer agent with both alkylating and antimetabolite properties, with the added benefit of improved oral bioavailability [144,145]. Like other alkylating agents, bendamustine produces intra-strand and interstrand cross-links between DNA bases, which inhibits DNA replication, repair and transcription. Bendamustine is only partially cross-resistance with other alkylating agents, perhaps because it creates more double-stranded breaks that are more difficult to repair [143,146]. Furthermore, the benzimidazole ring may function as a purine analog, based on the observation that bendamustine, like fludarabine, appears to be a potent modulator of ara-C metabolism in leukemia blasts [147]. This may give bendamustine potential antimetabolite activity that is lacking in other alkylating agents. These properties make bendamustine a particularly attractive agent for combination regimens in lymphoma.

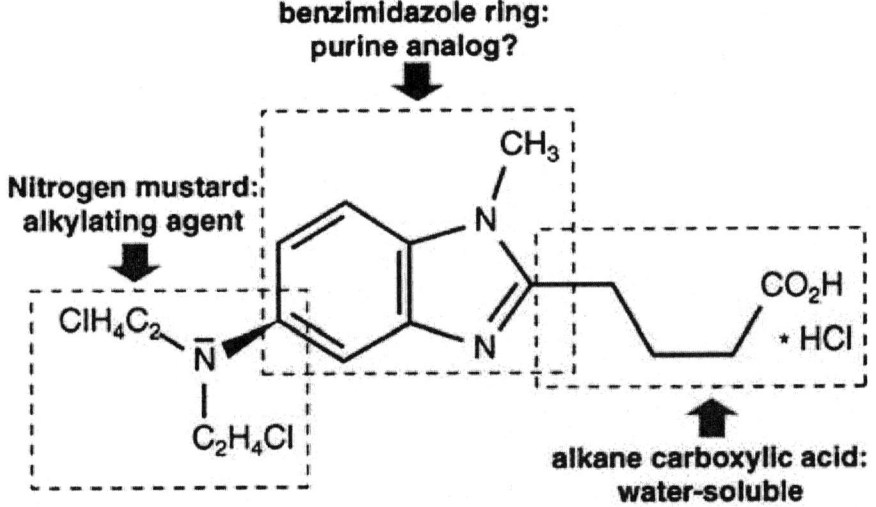

4 - {5 - [Bis (2-chloroethyl) amino] -1-
methyl-2-benzimidazolyl} butyric acid

14ₒ

3.2.2 Preclinical Data

Bendamustine has been shown to have variable effectiveness in different secondary human cell lines. Konstantinov *et al.* demonstrated that bendamustine induced apoptosis in leukemic cells of lymphoid origin, but not in myeloid or breast carcinoma lines [148]. Schwanen *et al.* have shown bendamustine to be a pro-apoptotic agent in peripheral lymphocytes harvested from 26 patients with CLL [149]. These authors also demonstrated a synergistic interaction between bendamustine and fludarabine in cells derived from these patients. Rummel *et al.* have shown a similar synergy between bendamustine and rituximab in cultured NHL and *ex vivo* CLL cells [150].

3.2.3   Clinical Data

Bendamustine has been studied in a wide range of doses and dosing schedules in the context of several phase I and II trials in different diseases [151]. In patients with relapsed indolent lymphomas, bendamustine has been administered at a dose of 120 mg/m^2/day over a one-hour infusion on days 1 and 2 every 3 weeks [152]. Of 52 assessable patients, CR was seen in 11% and PR in 62% of patients. In patients with CLL, bendamustine at a dose of 50 to 60 mg/m^2/day on days 1 through 5 repeated every 4 weeks effected complete and partial remissions in 6 and 9 of 23 patients respectively [153]. At a dose of 100 mg/m^2/d infused on days 1 and 2 every week, 5 of 14 patients with relapsed/refractory CLL achieved complete remission, while 4 patients met criteria for partial hematologic remissions [154]. In a very similar kind of study, Bremer and Gerda [155] treated 22 patients with indolent NHL and CLL with single-agent bendamustine at a dose of 60 mg/m^2. These authors reported an overall response rate of 78% in treatment naïve patients (CR = 11%, PR = 67%), and an ORR of 62% in relapsed patients (CR=15%, PR = 47%). Overall, the toxicities in these single agent studies were mild and included nausea and mild myelosuppression, with one study showing grade 3 or 4 leukopenia [153].

The promising activity seen in indolent lymphoma has also been seen in aggressive lymphomas. A single-agent phase II trial in patients with relapsed/refractory large B-cell lymphoma employed a dose of 120 mg/m^2 infused on 2 consecutive days every three weeks [156]. Of 18 assessable patients, the overall response rate was 44% (CR in 3/18, PR in 5/18), though in this study, dosing delays and dose reduction occurred in about 20% of the patients secondary to advanced grade hematologic toxicities.

To date, a number of studies have begun to explore the combination of bendamustine with other agents active in NHL. Koenigsmann *et al.* [157] studied bendamustine at a dose of 30 or 40 mg/m^2/day with fludarabine given at a dose of 30 mg/m^2/day, both on days 1 and 3 of a 4 week cycle. A total of 29 patients with relapsed or refractory indolent or mantle cell lymphoma were enrolled, of which 19 were assessable for response. An overall response rate of 77% was noted, which include a CR rate of 45% and a PR rate of 32% in an intent-to-treat analysis. Rummel *et al.* translated the preclinical synergy between bendamustine and rituximab discussed earlier into a phase II trial, enrolling 60 patients with relapsed indolent and mantle cell NHL [158]. The overall response rate in 49 assessable patients was 92%, with a CR rate of 65%. Weide *et al.* [159]found bendamustine (90 mg/m^2, day 1-2) to be well tolerated in combination with mitoxantrone (10 mg/m^2 on day 1) and rituximab (375 mg/m^2, weeks 2, 3, 4 and 5) in a group of 54 patients with relapsed or refractory indolent lymphoma who had received a median of 2 prior lines of chemotherapy. The overall response rate was 96% in 54 patients (41% CR, 55% PR), with meaningful durations of response in patients with indolent lymphoma (32 months) and CLL (13 months).

These data suggest that bendamustine may prove to be a valuable non-cross-resistant, orally bioavailable alkylating agent (with possible purine analog function) that can be used in combination with other cytotoxic agents. The many possible useful combinations of this drug are under active clinical investigation, the results of which will continue to emerge in the next few years.

3.3 Novel Antifolate Derivatives – 10-Propargyl-10-deazaaminopterin (PDX)

3.3.1 Mechanism of Action

The antifolate methotrexate is a traditional agent used in the treatment of many types of lymphoma, including diffuse large B-cell lymphoma, Burkitt's lymphoma, cutaneous T cell lymphoma, primary central nervous system lymphoma, and cerebrospinal lymphomatous metastases [160-163]. Due to its dose-limiting myelosuppression and mucositis, as well as the emergence of resistance in the clinical setting, alternatives to MTX have been developed on a routine basis over the past 30 to 40 years.

In the 1980s, it was found that alkyl substitution of the 10-deazaaminopterin at the C10 position markedly enhanced antifolate activity based on dihydrofolate reductase inhibition assays[164-166]. These deaza-aminopterins are more efficient permeants for the one-carbon, reduced folate transporter (RFC-1), leading to increased cellular uptake. They are also more effective substrates for the folylpolyglutamate synthetase (FPGS), which catalyzes the polyglutamylation of folate derivatives, which in turn serves to increase the intracellular retention of folates, and, coincidentally, antifolates. Together, these biochemical features of antifolate metabolism lead to markedly increased cellular concentrations of the 10-deazaaminopterins which appear to be associated with a significant improvement in antitumor activity in a variety of preclinical models [164-167](see Table 4). Edatrexate (EDX, 10-ethyl-10-deazaaminopterin) was shown in phase II clinical trials to yield major response rates significantly better than MTX in patients with metastatic non-small-cell lung cancer, breast cancer, and one form of soft issue sarcoma [168-170]. In the early 1990s, a propargyl group was substituted at position 10 to generate PDX (10-propargyl-10-deazaaminopterin), with the hopes of further improving the pharmacologic parameters and cytotoxic activity [171].

METHOTREXATE

10-Propargyl-10-
Deazaaminopterin (PDX)

3.3.2   Preclinical Data

PDX has shown encouraging activity compared with other antifolates in preclinical models. Sirotnak *et al.*[172] have shown that PDX, EDX and MTX are all potent inhibitors of dihydrofolate reductase (DHFR). PDX was the most efficient permeant of four folate analogues tested for the one-carbon, RFC-1. PDX was also found to have an affinity for FPGS similar to EDX, both being four times better substrates than MTX. A direct test of polyglutamate addition showed PDX to generate longer-chain polyglutamate tails than EDX and MTX, which may improve its affinity for DHFR. Given the potential to achieve greater intracellular concentrations, these data suggested greater cytotoxic activity for PDX. In fact, PDX showed cytotoxicity superior to EDX and ten- to twenty-fold higher than MTX in six different cell lines representing three different human malignancies (acute lymphocytic leukemia, breast carcinoma and non-small-cell lung cancer). *In vivo* activity against xenografts in nude mice showed increased partial and complete response rates in mice treated with PDX as compared to both EDX and MTX in transplanted mammary carcinoma and two different human non-small cell lung carcinomas.

Our group recently reported on the activity of PDX in a panel of human lymphoma cell lines and in three 3 lymphoma xenograft models [167]. All five human lymphoma cell lines, representing Hodgkin's disease (Hs445), diffuse large B cell lymphoma (HT and SKI-DLBCL), Burkitt's lymphoma (Raji), and transformed follicular lymphoma (RL) showed at least ten-fold greater sensitivity to PDX over MTX. Subcutaneous xenografts of the human lymphoma lines HT, SKI-DLBCL-1 and RL in NOD/SCID mice revealed that PDX was markedly superior to MTX (see Figure 7), effecting complete long term remissions in 30 to 40% of the treated animals. Results were even more dramatic in HT xenografted mice, where MTX led to only modest growth delay, while PDX induced complete regression in 89% of the mice treated. These preclinical data suggested a marked improvement in treatment response with PDX which was far superior to that seen with MTX. These data formed the basis of a clinical trial in very chemotherapy refractory lymphoma.

3.3.3   Clinical Data

To date, phase I data with PDX have been reported only in patients with non-small cell lung cancer (NSCLC)[173]. Mucositis was the dose limiting toxicity when PDX was given weekly for three consecutive weeks of a four-week cycle. When dosing was performed every two weeks, the maximum tolerated dose was 170 mg/m^2. The dose limiting toxicity was mucositis, with essentially no other toxicities. A phase I/II trial in patients with relapsed or refractory aggressive NHL and HD is now ongoing in our group. Early in this trial, treatment was started at a dose of 135 mg/m^2, administered on days 1 and 15 in a 28 day cycle. Higher rates of grade 2 to 4 stomatitis were seen in this patient population than in the prior population of NSCLC patients. Of the 5 patients who experienced grade 2 stomatitis, 4 had no further stomatitis with re-treatment after prophylactic folic acid and vitamin B12 supplementation. Based on these preliminary findings, ongoing therapy is incorporating prescreening for nutritional status, with B12 and folate supplementation given to patients with elevated homocysteine or methylmalonic acid levels. While only anecdotal at this point, the revision of the study to employ lower doses on a weekly schedule with requirements for adequate nutritional states has apparently abrogated the stomatitis risk thus far, with the observation that patients with relapsed or refractory T-cell lymphoma have been experiencing significant responses early in their treatment (unpublished data).

4.   FUTURE DIRECTIONS

There has never been a more exciting time to be engaged in the discovery and development of new drugs for the treatment cancer, and especially for the treatment of lymphoma. As our basic understanding of cancer biology continues to blossom, new targets, new rationales, and new strategies for treating this remarkably complex set of diseases will continue to emerge. With all the advances in our understanding of this biology, and now the ability to rapidly identify novel small molecules with activity against discrete targets through high-throughput screening, the rate limiting steps now become those which drive an understanding of the pre-clinical and clinical pharmacology of the new drug regimens.

The major challenges that will affect the development of new drugs today, as we see them, will revolve around 4 important issues: (1) Does the candidate drug have significant single agent activity and safety in lymphoma; (2) Can we establish the nature of the drug's activity in the context of the underlying molecular pathology; (3) Can we clarify the basic pre-clinical pharmacology of the candidate drugs and determine how best to integrate them with established therapeutics; and finally, (4) Can we demonstrate that the activity of novel combinations is better than the conventional standard of care. The faster we can determine the answers to the above questions, the faster we can take advantage of the promise of these new drugs. It will be necessary to strike a balance that moves from bench-to-bed and back to the bench for us to refine our understanding of these new agents. But, ultimately, the rate limiting step in this entire process will be our ability to accrue clinical trials in these often-times rare sub-types of lymphoma in as expeditious a manner as is possible. As our understanding of the lymphomas continues to emerge, and as our drugs become more and more specialized in terms of the signaling pathways that they influence, it is likely - in fact probable - that our target population of patients will continue to dwindle, making it harder to execute these trials in a timely fashion. It is for this reason that efficient multicenter collaborations will be required so one set of answers can be gained, allowing us to generate the next set of important questions. The best way to accomplishing this will be to enroll patients on clinical trials whenever possible, and to make sure that the pre-clinical models we use to evaluate the general pharmacology of these agents reasonably reflects the biology we hope to address in the clinic.

5. ACKNOWLEDGMENTS

OAO is the recipient of the Leukemia and Lymphoma Society Scholar in Research Award. OAO would also like to thank Mortimer J. Lacher and the generous support from the Werner and Elaine Dannheisser Fund for Research on the Biology of Aging of the Lymphoma Foundation.

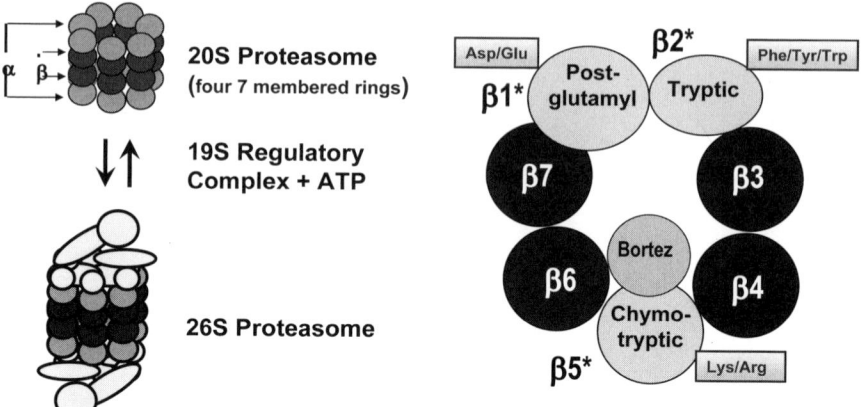

Figure 1. Schematic of the 26S proteasome, showing the binding site of bortezomib. The binding of bortezomib with the chymotriptic domain is a tight but reversible interaction.

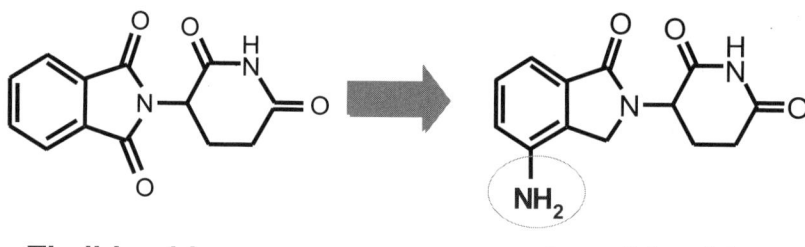

Thalidomide   **Lenalidomide**

- 4-amino-glutamyl analogue
- 10–1000 times more potent
- <u>Safety profile</u>: non-neurotoxic, non-teratogenic, non-sedating

Bartlett JB et al.[55] *Nat Rev Cancer.* 2004;4:314
Stirling D.[56] *Semin Oncol.* 2001;28:602

Figure 2. Chemical structure of the immunomodulatory agents thalidomide and lenalidomide (CC-5013). Bartlett JB et al.[55], *Nat Rev Cancer.* 2004;4:314 Stirling D.[56] *Semin Oncol.* 2001;28:602

THALIDOMIDE + RITUXIMAB IN MCL
Progression Free and Overall Survival

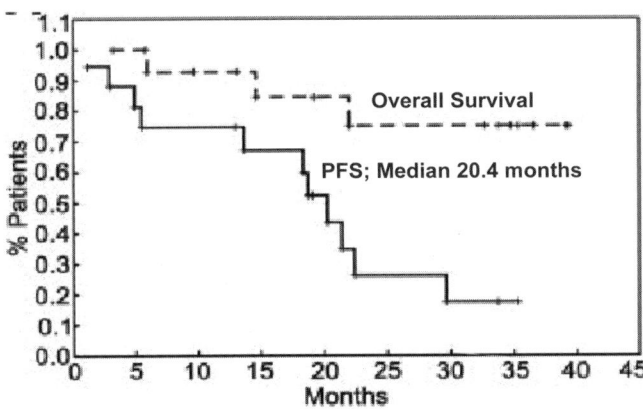

Kaufmann et al[76], Blood 104, 2004

Figure 3. Progression-free survival in patients with refractory mantle cell lymphoma treated with thalidomide plus rituximab. Kaufmann et al[76], *Blood 104*, 2004.

TARGETING BCL-6 IN LYMPHOMA

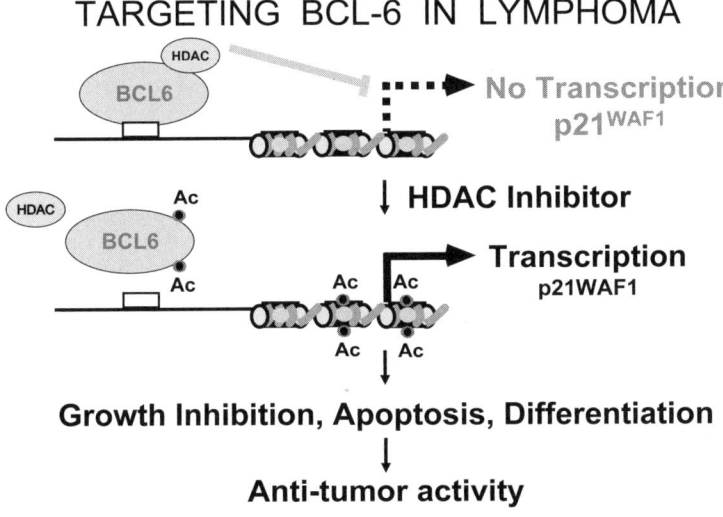

Figure 4. Effects of acetylation on Bcl-6 activity. In the de-acetylated form, Bcl-6 is acts as a transcriptional repressor, decreasing the expression of genes that lead to growth inhibition, apoptosis and differentiation. Histone deacetylase inhibitors displace histone deacetylase (HDAC) on Bcl-6, allowing for its acetylation. In the acetylated form, Bcl-6 no longer functions as a trans-repressor. Acetylation also loosens the chromatin structure around histones, further promoting transcription of the target genes.

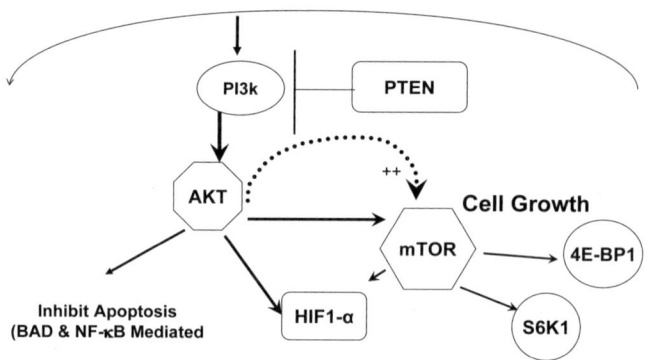

Figure 5. Schematic of mTOR signaling pathways.

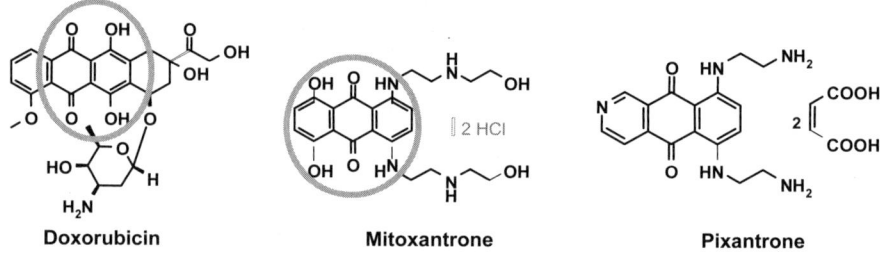

Figure 6. Chemical structure of the anthracenediones. Beggiolin et al.[137] *Tumori.* 2001;87:407-416. Krapcho et al.[133] *J Med Chem.* 1994;37:828-837

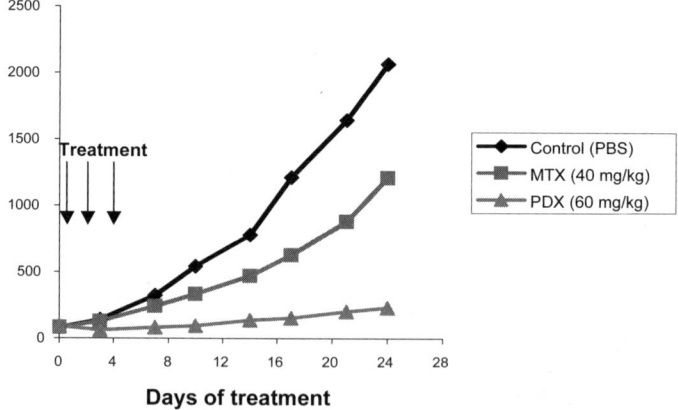

Figure 7. PDX is more effective against a transformed non-Hodgkin's lymphoma cell line than methotrexate in a NOD/SCID xenograft model.

Table 1: Summary of Clinical Data for New Small Molecules in the Treatment of Lymphoma

Agent	Mechanism	MTD	DLT	Activity	Comments	Refs
Bortezomib	Proteasome inhibition	1.5mg/m^2 days 1, 4, 8 and 11 every 21 days	thrombocytopenia neuropathy	Indolent NHLs		16, 17, 18, 20
Oblimersen	Bcl-2 Antisense Oligonucleotide	3 to 5 mg/kg/day for 7 days every 21days	myelosuppression hypotension, fatigue	MCL, MALT, FL, CLL	Has been combined with rituximab and R-CHOP New small molecule Bcl-2 inhibitors under development	49, 50, 51
CC-5013	Immunomodulator	25 mg/d	myelosuppression	MM, phase I lymphoma study currently enrolling		71, www.clinicaltrials.gov
Thalidomide	Immunomodulator	400 mg/day + rituximab weekly x4	fatigue, neurotoxicity	MCL		76
Depsipeptide	HDACI	17.8 mg/m^2 days 1 and 5 every 21 days	fatigue, nausea, vomiting and thrombocytopenia	CTCL, PTCL		106, 107
SAHA	HDACI	IV: 300 mg/m^2/day x 5 days x 3 weeks Oral: 200 mg BID	myelosuppression, dehydration, anorexia, diarrhea and fatigue	HD, indolent and aggressive NHL		108, unpublished data

CCI-779	mTOR inhibitor	250 mg IV weekly	thrombocytopenia	MCL		128
Pixantrone	Anthracycline	85 mg/m² IV weekly for 3 weeks, followed by a one week break	neutropenia	Aggressive NHL, indolent NHL	Has been substituted for etoposide in the ESHAP[140], and for doxorubicin in CHOP[141] No cardiotoxicity seen to date[142]	139, 140, 141, 174
Bendamustine	Alkylator/purine analog	120 mg/m²/day days 1 and 2 every 21 days	myelosuppression	Indolent NHL, CLL	Combinations with fludarabine[157], rituximab[158], and mitoxantrone plus rituximab[159]	152, 153, 155, 156, 157, 158, 159
PDX	Antifolate	<135 mg/m², on days 1 and 15 every 28 days	mucositis	Aggressive NHL, HD	Pretreatment with B12 and folate in appropriate patients may eliminate mucositis	173, unpublished data

Abbreviations: NHL = non-Hodgkin's lymphoma; MCL = mantle cell lymphoma; MALT = mucosa associated lymphoid tissue;

FL = follicular lymphoma; CLL = chronic lymphocytic leukemia; R-CHOP = rituximab, cyclophosphamide, doxorubicin, prednisone;

MM = multiple myeloma; HDACI = histone deacetylase inhibitor; CTCL = cutaneous T-cell lymphoma; PTCL = peripheral T-cell lymphoma;

HD = Hodgkin's disease; mTOR = molecular target of rapamycin; ESHAP = etoposide, methylprednisolone, cisplatin, and cytosine arabinoside;

PDX = 10-propargyl-10-deazaaminopterin

Table 2. Combined Clinical Experience with Bortezomib as a Single Agent in NHL

Disease	n	CR/CRu	PR	ORR	SD	POD
DLBCL	13/13	0	1	8%	1	8
MCL	101/114	13	33	46%	19	25
FL	34/38	2	10	35%	9	9
MZL	6/6	0	3	50%	2	1
SLL/CLL	9/10	1	1	22%	2	4
TOTAL	163/181	16	48	40%	20	19

O'Connor et al., ASH 2004[22]; Goy et al., JCO 2005[18]; Belch et al., ASH 2004[20]; Strauss et al., ASH 2004[21]

Table 3. Current Data on Histone Deacetylase Inhibitors (HDACIs)

Agent	Dosing	DLT	PK	Outcomes
PB-oral	TID	DLT=N/V; hypocalcemia, dyspesia, fatigue	BA: 78%; T ½ 1hr	7 pts with SD
Depsipeptide-IV	4hr infusion d1, 5 q21d	DLT-fatigue, N/V, thrombocytopenia, neutropenia	T ½α .42 hr. T ½β 8.1 hr	1 PR RCC; 1 CR PTCL, 2 PR Sezary; 1 CTCL
SAHA-IV	2 hr infusion 2-15 d	DLT-thrombo-cytopenia, neutropenia-hem pts.	T ½ .47 hr	1 PR Hodgkins ds.
SAHA-PO	Daily and BID	DLT-fatigue, N/V, dehydration	Apparent T ½ 1.4-2.1 hrs	1 CR DLBCL 5 PR
MS-275	PO twice weekly	DLT-?hypophosphatemia, asthenia, N/V	Apparent T ½ 100 hours	SD-Ewing's sarcoma, rectal, melanoma
LAQ824	3 hr infusion d 1-3 q21d	DLT-LFTs; thrombocytopenia, fatigue, A.Fib.	T ½ 8-14 hrs	---
LBH589A	½ hr infusion d1-3, d8-10 q21 or q 28 d	DLT- thrombo-cytopenia; ?neutropenia, hypoglycemia	T ½ 15-20 hrs	---

Table 4. Pharmacokinetic Properties of Folate Analogues

Drug	DHFR Inhib. K_i (pM)	Influx Km (mM)	Influx V_{max}	Vmax / K_m	FPGS K_m (mM)	FPGS V_{max}	V_{max}/K_m
AMT	4.9 ± 1	1.2 ± 0.2	3.6 ± 1.0	3.0	5.8 ± 1	117	20.2
MTX	5.4 ± 2	4.8 ± 1.0	4.1 ± 1.2	0.9	32.2 ± 5	70	2.2
EDX	5.8 ± 1	1.1 ± 0.1	3.9 ± 0.9	3.5	6.3 ± 1	65	10.3
PDX	13.4 ± 1	0.3 ± 0.1	3.8 ± 1.3	12.6	5.9 ± 1	137	23.2

Vmax = pmol/min/mg protein

6.   REFERENCES

1.   Myung J, Kim KB, Crews CM. The ubiquitin-proteasome pathway and proteasome inhibitors. Medicinal Research Reviews. 2001;21:245-273.

2.   King RW, Deshaies RJ, Peters JM, Kirschner MW. How proteolysis drives the cell cycle. Science. 1996;274:1652-1659.

3.   Sherr CJ. Cancer cell cycles. Science. 1996;274:1672-1677.

4.   Read MA, Neish AS, Luscinskas FW, Palombella VJ, Maniatis T, Collins T. The proteasome pathway is required for cytokine-induced endothelial-leukocyte adhesion molecule expression. Immunity. 1995;2:493-506.

5.   Palombella VJ, Rando OJ, Goldberg AL, Maniatis T. The ubiquitin-proteasome pathway is required for processing the NF-kappa B1 precursor protein and the activation of NF-kappa B. Cell. 1994;78:773-785.

6.   Karin M, Cao Y, Greten FR, Li ZW. NF-kappaB in cancer: from innocent bystander to major culprit. Nature Reviews Cancer. 2002;2:301-310.

7.   Zetter BR. Adhesion molecules in tumor metastasis. Semin Cancer Biol. 1993;4:219-229.

8.   Perez-Soler R, Ling YH, Ellitott PJ, Adams J, Liebes L. Effect of the proteasome inhibitor PS-341 on cell cycle progression and bcl-2: a potentially unique mechanism of action. Clinical Cancer Research. 2000;6:4549s.

9.   Lum RT, Nelson MG, Joly A, et al. Selective inhibition of the chymotrypsin-like activity of the 20S proteasome by 5-methoxy-1-indanone dipeptide benzamides. Bioorganic & Medicinal Chemistry Letters. 1998;8:209-214.

10.   An WG, Hwang SG, Trepel JB, Blagosklonny MV. Protease inhibitor-induced apoptosis: accumulation of wt p53, p21WAF1/CIP1, and induction of apoptosis are independent markers of proteasome inhibition. Leukemia. 2000;14:1276-1283.

11.   Adams J, Palombella VJ, Elliott PJ. Proteasome inhibition: a new strategy in cancer treatment. Invest New Drugs. 1999;18:109-121.

12.   Orlowski RZ, Stinchcombe TE, Mitchell BS, et al. Phase I trial of the proteasome inhibitor PS-341 in patients with refractory hematologic malignancies. J Clin Oncol. 2002;20:4420-4427.

13.   Aghajanian C, Soignet S, Dizon DS, et al. A phase I trial of the novel proteasome inhibitor PS341 in advanced solid tumor malignancies. Clin Cancer Res. 2002;8:2505-2511.

14.   Papandreou C, Daliani D, Millikan RE, et al. Phase I study of intravenous (I.V.) proteasome inhibitor PS-341 in patients (pts) with advanced malignancies. Proc Am Soc Clin Oncol. 2001:Abstract #340.

15.   Richardson PG, Barlogie B, Berenson J, et al. A phase 2 study of bortezomib in relapsed, refractory myeloma. N Engl J Med. 2003;348:2609-2617.

16.   O'Connor OA. Marked clinical activity of the novel proteasome inhibitor bortezomib in patients with relapsed follicular (RL) and mantle cell lymphoma (MCL). Journal of Clinical Oncology. 2004;22:6582.

17.   O'Connor OA, Wright, J., Moskowitz, C., Muzzy, J., MacGregor-Cortelli, B., Stubblefield, M., Straus, D., Portlock, C., Hamlin, P., Choi, E., Dumetrescu, O., Qin, J., Esseltine, D., Trehu, E., Adams, J., Schenkein, D, Zelenetz, A. Phase II clinical experience with the novel proteasome inhibitor bortezomib in patients with indolent non-Hodgkin's lymphoma and mantle cell lymphoma. Journal of Clinical Oncology. 2005;23:676-684.

18.   Goy A, Younes A, McLaughlin P, et al. Phase II study of proteasome inhibitor bortezomib in relapsed or refractory B-Cell non-Hodgkin's lymphoma. Journal of Clinical Oncology. 2005;23:667-675.

19.   Rosenwald A, Wright G, Chan WC, et al. The use of molecular profiling to predict survival after chemotherapy for diffuse large-B-cell lymphoma.[see comment]. New England Journal of Medicine. 2002;346:1937-1947.

20.   Belch A, Kouroukis CT, Crump M, et al. Phase II Trial of Bortezomib in Mantle Cell Lymphoma. Blood. 2004;104:Abstract #608.

21.   Strauss SJ, Maharaj L, Stec J, et al. Phase II Clinical Study of Bortezomib (VELCADE®) in Patients (pts) with Relapsed / Refractory Non-Hodgkin's Lymphoma (NHL) and Hodgkin's Disease (HD). Blood. 2004;104:Abstract #1386.

22.   O'Connor OA, Wright J, Moskowitz C, et al. A Multicenter Experience with Single Agent Bortezomib in Non-Hodgkin's Lymphoma Reveals Marked Differences in Sub-Type Sensitivity to Proteasome Inhibition. Blood. 2004;104:Abstract #607.

23.   Klasa RJ, Gillum AM, Klem RE, Frankel SR. Oblimersen Bcl-2 antisense: facilitating apoptosis in anticancer treatment. Antisense & Nucleic Acid Drug Development. 2002;12:193-213.

24.   Veis DJ, Sorenson CM, Shutter JR, Korsmeyer SJ. Bcl-2-deficient mice demonstrate fulminant lymphoid apoptosis, polycystic kidneys, and hypopigmented hair. Cell. 1993;75:229-240.

25.   McDonnell TJ, Korsmeyer SJ. Progression from lymphoid hyperplasia to high-grade malignant lymphoma in mice transgenic for the t(14; 18). Nature. 1991;349:254-256.

26.   Reed JC. Dysregulation of apoptosis in cancer. Journal of Clinical Oncology. 1999;17:2941-2953.

27.   Zamecnik PC, Stephenson ML. Inhibition of Rous sarcoma virus replication and cell transformation by a specific oligodeoxynucleotide. Proceedings of the National Academy of Sciences of the United States of America. 1978;75:280-284.

28.   Stephenson ML, Zamecnik PC. Inhibition of Rous sarcoma viral RNA translation by a specific oligodeoxyribonucleotide. Proceedings of the National Academy of Sciences of the United States of America. 1978;75:285-288.

29.   Krieg AM, Yi AK, Matson S, et al. CpG motifs in bacterial DNA trigger direct B-cell activation. Nature. 1995;374:546-549.

30.   Reed JC, Stein C, Subasinghe C, et al. Antisense-mediated inhibition of BCL2 protooncogene expression and leukemic cell growth and survival: comparisons of phosphodiester and phosphorothioate oligodeoxynucleotides. Cancer Research. 1990;50:6565-6570.

31.   Agrawal S, Temsamani J, Tang JY. Pharmacokinetics, biodistribution, and stability of oligodeoxynucleotide phosphorothioates in mice. Proceedings of the National Academy of Sciences of the United States of America. 1991;88:7595-7599.

32.   Raynaud FI, Orr RM, Goddard PM, et al. Pharmacokinetics of G3139, a phosphorothioate oligodeoxynucleotide antisense to bcl-2, after intravenous administration or continuous subcutaneous infusion to mice. Journal of Pharmacology & Experimental Therapeutics. 1997;281:420-427.

33.   Kitada S, Miyashita T, Tanaka S, Reed JC. Investigations of antisense oligonucleotides targeted against bcl-2 RNAs. Antisense Research & Development. 1993;3:157-169.

34.   Tormo M, Tari AM, McDonnell TJ, Cabanillas F, Garcia-Conde J, Lopez-Berestein G. Apoptotic induction in transformed follicular lymphoma cells by Bcl-2 downregulation. Leukemia & Lymphoma. 1998;30:367-379.

35.   Waters JS, Clarke PA, Cunningham D, et al. Bcl-2 antisense oligonucleotide (ODN) (G3139) therapy exerts it antitumor action through a sequence-specific antisense effect, and not a cell-mediated immune response. Proc Am Soc Clin Oncol. 2000;19:Abstract #48.

36.   Cotter FE, Waters J, Cunningham D. Human Bcl-2 antisense therapy for lymphomas. Biochimica et Biophysica Acta. 1999;1489:97-106.

37.   Klasa RJ, Bally MB, Ng R, Goldie JH, Gascoyne RD, Wong FM. Eradication of human non-Hodgkin's lymphoma in SCID mice by BCL-2 antisense oligonucleotides combined with low-dose cyclophosphamide. Clinical Cancer Research. 2000;6:2492-2500.

38.   Waters JS, Webb A, Cunningham D, et al. Phase I clinical and pharmacokinetic study of bcl-2 antisense oligonucleotide therapy in patients with non-Hodgkin's lymphoma.[see comment]. Journal of Clinical Oncology. 2000;18:1812-1823.

39.   Marcucci G, Byrd JC, Catalano SR, et al. Signficant disease response to Genesense™ (G3139, Genta), a Bcl-2 antisense, in combination with chemotherapy in refractory or relapsed acute leukemia: A phase I study. American Academy Cancer Research - National Cancer Institiute - European Organization for the Research and Treatment of Cancer International Conference. Miami Beach, FL; 2001.

40.   Jansen B, Schlagbauer-Wadl H, Brown BD, et al. Clinical, pharmacologic, and pharmacodynamic study of Genesense (G3139, Bcl-2 antisense oligonucleotide) and dacarbazine (DTIC) in patients with malignant melanoma. Proc Am Soc Clin Oncol. 2001;20:357a.

41.   De Bono JS, Rowinsky EK, Kuhn J, et al. Phase I pharmacokinetic (PK) and pharmacodynamic (PD) trial of bcl-2 antisense (Genasense) and docetaxel (D) in hormone refractory prostate cancer. Proc Am Soc Clin Oncol. 2001;20:119a.

42.   Morris MJ, Tong W, Osman I, et al. A phase I/IIA dose-escalating trial of *bcl-2* antisense (G3139) treatment by 14-day continuous intravenous infusion (CI) for patients with androgen-independent prostate cancer or other advanced solid tumor malignancies. Proc Am Soc Clin Oncol. 1999;18:323a.

43.   Morris MJ, Tong WP, Cordon-Cardo C, et al. Phase I trial of BCL-2 antisense oligonucleotide (G3139) administered by continuous intravenous infusion in patients with advanced cancer. Clinical Cancer Research. 2002;8:679-683.

44. Scher HI, Morris MJ, Tong WP, et al. A phase I trial of G3139 (Genta, Inc.), a BCL2 antisense drug, by continuous infusion (CI) as a single agent and with weekly Taxol (T). Proc Am Soc Clin Oncol. 2000;19:199a.

45. Ochoa L, Kuhn J, Salinas R, et al. A phase I, pharmacokinetic, and biologic correlative study of G3139 and irinotecan (CPT-11) in patients with metastatic colorectal cancer. Proc Am Soc Clin Oncol. 2001;20:75a.

46. Ochoa L, Kuhn J, Salinas R, et al. G3139 downregulates the expression of *bcl-2* in patients with metastatic colorectal cancer treated with irinotecan (CPT-11). Proc Am Soc Clin Oncol. 2001;42:848.

47. Chen HX, Marshall JL, Trocky N, et al. A phase I study of Bcl-2 antisense G3139 (Genta) and weekly docetaxel in patients with advanced breast cancer and other solid tumors. Proc Am Soc Clin Oncol. 2000;19:140-142.

48. Webb A, Cunningham D, Cotter F, et al. BCL-2 antisense therapy in patients with non-Hodgkin lymphoma. Lancet. 1997;349:1137-1141.

49. Leonard JP, Hainsworth J, Bernstein S, et al. Genasense™ (Oblimersen Sodium, G3139) Is Active and Well-Tolerated Both Alone and with R-CHOP in Mantle Cell Lymphoma (MCL). Blood. 2003;102:Abstract #490.

50. Pro B, Smith MR, Younes A, et al. Oblimersen sodium (Bcl-2 antisense) plus rituximab in patients with recurrent B-cell non-Hodgkin's lymphoma: Preliminary phase II results. Proc Am Soc Clin Oncol. 2004;22:6572.

51. Rai KR, Moore JO, Boyd TE, et al. Phase 3 Randomized Trial of Fludarabine/Cyclophosphamide Chemotherapy with or without Oblimersen Sodium (Bcl-2 Antisense; Genasense; G3139) for Patients with Relapsed or Refractory Chronic Lymphocytic Leukemia (CLL). Blood. 2004;104:Abstract #338.

52. Fesik SW. Discovery of Bcl-2/Bcl-xL Inhibitors for the Treatment of Cancer. ASH Annual Meeting. San Diego, CA; 2004.

53. Mohammad RM, Wang S, Aboukameel A, et al. Preclinical studies of a nonpeptidic small-molecule inhibitor of Bcl-2 and Bcl-X(L) [(-)-gossypol] against diffuse large cell lymphoma. Molecular Cancer Therapeutics. 2005;4:13-21.

54. Oliver CL, Miranda MB, Shangary S, Land S, Wang S, Johnson DE. (-)-Gossypol acts directly on the mitochondria to overcome Bcl-2- and Bcl-X(L)-mediated apoptosis resistance. Molecular Cancer Therapeutics. 2005;4:23-31.

55. Bartlett JB, Dredge K, Dalgleish AG. The evolution of thalidomide and its IMiD derivatives as anticancer agents. Nature Reviews Cancer. 2004;4:314-322.

56. Stirling D. Thalidomide: a novel template for anticancer drugs. Seminars in Oncology. 2001;28:602-606.

57. Sampaio EP, Sarno EN, Galilly R, Cohn ZA, Kaplan G. Thalidomide selectively inhibits tumor necrosis factor alpha production by stimulated human monocytes. Journal of Experimental Medicine. 1991;173:699-703.

58. D'Amato RJ, Loughnan MS, Flynn E, Folkman J. Thalidomide is an inhibitor of angiogenesis. Proc Natl Acad Sci U S A. 1994;91:4082-4085.

59. Singhal S, Mehta J, Desikan R, et al. Antitumor activity of thalidomide in refractory multiple myeloma.[see comment][erratum appears in N Engl J Med 2000 Feb 3;342(5):364]. New England Journal of Medicine. 1999;341:1565-1571.

60. Stebbing J, Benson C, Eisen T, et al. The treatment of advanced renal cell cancer with high-dose oral thalidomide. British Journal of Cancer. 2001;85:953-958.

61. Macpherson GR, Franks M, Tomoaia-Cotisel A, Ando Y, Price DK, Figg WD. Current status of thalidomide and its role in the treatment of metastatic prostate cancer. Critical Reviews in Oncology-Hematology. 2003;46 Suppl:S49-57.

62. Fine HA, Figg WD, Jaeckle K, et al. Phase II trial of the antiangiogenic agent thalidomide in patients with recurrent high-grade gliomas.[see comment]. Journal of Clinical Oncology. 2000;18:708-715.

63.   Eisen T, Boshoff C, Mak I, et al. Continuous low dose Thalidomide: a phase II study in advanced melanoma, renal cell, ovarian and breast cancer. British Journal of Cancer. 2000;82:812-817.

64.   Marriott JB, Muller G, Stirling D, Dalgleish AG. Immunotherapeutic and antitumour potential of thalidomide analogues. Expert Opinion on Biological Therapy. 2001;1:675-682.

65.   Muller GW, Chen R, Huang SY, et al. Amino-substituted thalidomide analogs: potent inhibitors of TNF-alpha production. Bioorganic & Medicinal Chemistry Letters. 1999;9:1625-1630.

66.   Dredge K, Marriott JB, Macdonald CD, et al. Novel thalidomide analogues display anti-angiogenic activity independently of immunomodulatory effects. British Journal of Cancer. 2002;87:1166-1172.

67.   Lentzsch S, Rogers MS, LeBlanc R, et al. S-3-Amino-phthalimido-glutarimide inhibits angiogenesis and growth of B-cell neoplasias in mice. Cancer Research. 2002;62:2300-2305.

68.   Hideshima T, Chauhan D, Shima Y, et al. Thalidomide and its analogs overcome drug resistance of human multiple myeloma cells to conventional therapy. Blood. 2000;96:2943-2950.

69.   Mitsiades N, Mitsiades CS, Poulaki V, et al. Apoptotic signaling induced by immunomodulatory thalidomide analogs in human multiple myeloma cells: therapeutic implications. Blood. 2002;99:4525-4530.

70.   Dredge K, Marriott JB, Todryk SM, et al. Protective antitumor immunity induced by a costimulatory thalidomide analog in conjunction with whole tumor cell vaccination is mediated by increased Th1-type immunity. Journal of Immunology. 2002;168:4914-4919.

71.   Richardson PG, Schlossman RL, Weller E, et al. Immunomodulatory drug CC-5013 overcomes drug resistance and is well tolerated in patients with relapsed multiple myeloma. Blood. 2002;100:3063-3067.

72.   Zangari M, Tricot G, Zeldis J, Eddlemon P, Saghafifar F, Barlogie B. Results of phase I study of CC-5013 for the treatment of multiple myeloma (MM) patients who relapse after high dose chemotherapy (HDCT). Blood. 2001;98:775a.

73.   Marriott JB, Clarke IA, Dredge K, et al. Thalidomide analogue CDC-5013 is safe and well tolerated by patients with end stage cancer and shows evidence of clinical responses and extensive immune activation. British Journal of Cancer. 2002;86:S26.

74.   Gupta D, Treon SP, Shima Y, et al. Adherence of multiple myeloma cells to bone marrow stromal cells upregulates vascular endothelial growth factor secretion: therapeutic applications. Leukemia. 2001;15:1950-1961.

75.   Schey SA, Jones RW, Raj K, Streetley M. A phase I study of an immunomodulatory drug (CC-4047), a structural analogue of thalidomide, in relapsed/refractory multiple myeloma. Proceedings of the 31st Annual Meeting of the International Society of Experimental Hematology. Montreal, Canada; 2002.

76.   Kaufmann H, Raderer M, Wohrer S, et al. Antitumor activity of rituximab plus thalidomide in patients with relapsed/refractory mantle cell lymphoma. Blood. 2004;104:2269-2271.

77.   Cattoretti G, Chang CC, Cechova K, et al. BCL-6 protein is expressed in germinal-center B cells. Blood. 1995;86:45-53.

78.   Onizuka T, Moriyama M, Yamochi T, et al. BCL-6 gene product, a 92- to 98-kD nuclear phosphoprotein, is highly expressed in germinal center B cells and their neoplastic counterparts. Blood. 1995;86:28-37.

79.   Shaffer AL, Yu X, He Y, Boldrick J, Chan EP, Staudt LM. BCL-6 represses genes that function in lymphocyte differentiation, inflammation, and cell cycle control. Immunity. 2000;13:199-212.

80. Reljic R, Wagner SD, Peakman LJ, Fearon DT. Suppression of signal transducer and activator of transcription 3-dependent B lymphocyte terminal differentiation by BCL-6. Journal of Experimental Medicine. 2000;192:1841-1848.

81. Pasqualucci L, Bereschenko O, Niu H, et al. Molecular pathogenesis of non-Hodgkin's lymphoma: the role of Bcl-6. Leukemia & Lymphoma. 2003;44 Suppl 3:S5-12.

82. Marks PA, Richon VM, Rifkind RA. Histone deacetylase inhibitors: inducers of differentiation or apoptosis of transformed cells. Journal of the National Cancer Institute. 2000;92:1210-1216.

83. Ueda H, Manda T, Matsumoto S, et al. FR901228, a novel antitumor bicyclic depsipeptide produced by *Chromobacterium violaceum* No. 968. III. Antitumor activities on experimental tumors in mice. Journal of Antibiotics. 1994;47:315-323.

84. Ueda H, Nakajima H, Hori Y, ct al. FR901228, a novel antitumor bicyclic depsipeptide produced by Chromobacterium violaceum No. 968. I. Taxonomy, fermentation, isolation, physico-chemical and biological properties, and antitumor activity. Journal of Antibiotics. 1994;47:301-310.

85. Nakajima H, Kim YB, Terano H, Yoshida M, Horinouchi S. FR901228, a potent antitumor antibiotic, is a novel histone deacetylase inhibitor. Experimental Cell Research. 1998;241:126-133.

86. Richon VM, Emiliani S, Verdin E, et al. A class of hybrid polar inducers of transformed cell differentiation inhibits histone deacetylases. Proc Natl Acad Sci U S A. 1998;95:3003-3007.

87. Butler LM, Agus DB, Scher HI, et al. Suberoylanilide hydroxamic acid, an inhibitor of histone deacetylase, suppresses the growth of prostate cancer cells in vitro and in vivo. Cancer Res. 2000;60:5165-5170.

88. Richon VM, Webb Y, Merger R, et al. Second generation hybrid polar compounds are potent inducers of transformed cell differentiation. Proceedings of the National Academy of Sciences of the United States of America. 1996;93:5705-5708.

89. Cohen LA, Amin S, Marks PA, Rifkind RA, Desai D, Richon VM. Chemoprevention of carcinogen-induced mammary tumorigenesis by the hybrid polar cytodifferentiation agent, suberanilohydroxamic acid (SAHA). Anticancer Research. 1999;19:4999-5005.

90. Desai D, El-Bayoumy K, Amin S. Chemoprevention efficacy of suberanilhydroxamic acid (SAHA), a cytodifferentiating agent, against tobacco-specific nitrosamine 4-(meth-ylnitros-amino)-1-(3-pyridyl)-1-butanone (NNK)-induced lung tumorgenesis in female A/J mice. Proc Amer Assoc Cancer Res. 1999;40:Abstract #2396.

91. Taunton J, Hassig CA, Schreiber SL. A mammalian histone deacetylase related to the yeast transcriptional regulator Rpd3p.[see comment]. Science. 1996;272:408-411.

92. Emiliani S, Fischle W, Van Lint C, Al-Abed Y, Verdin E. Characterization of a human RPD3 ortholog, HDAC3. Proceedings of the National Academy of Sciences of the United States of America. 1998;95:2795-2800.

93. Yang WM, Yao YL, Sun JM, Davie JR, Seto E. Isolation and characterization of cDNAs corresponding to an additional member of the human histone deacetylase gene family. Journal of Biological Chemistry. 1997;272:28001-28007.

94. Dangond F, Hafler DA, Tong JK, et al. Differential display cloning of a novel human histone deacetylase (HDAC3) cDNA from PHA-activated immune cells. Biochemical & Biophysical Research Communications. 1998;242:648-652.

95. Buggy JJ, Sideris ML, Mak P, Lorimer DD, McIntosh B, Clark JM. Cloning and characterization of a novel human histone deacetylase, HDAC8. Biochemical Journal. 2000;350 Pt 1:199-205.

96. Hu E, Chen Z, Fredrickson T, et al. Cloning and characterization of a novel human class I histone deacetylase that functions as a transcription repressor. Journal of Biological Chemistry. 2000;275:15254-15264.

97. Van den Wyngaert I, de Vries W, Kremer A, et al. Cloning and characterization of human histone deacetylase 8. FEBS Letters. 2000;478:77-83.
98. Grozinger CM, Hassig CA, Schreiber SL. Three proteins define a class of human histone deacetylases related to yeast Hda1p. Proceedings of the National Academy of Sciences of the United States of America. 1999;96:4868-4873.
99. Verdel A, Khochbin S. Identification of a new family of higher eukaryotic histone deacetylases. Coordinate expression of differentiation-dependent chromatin modifiers. Journal of Biological Chemistry. 1999;274:2440-2445.
100. Fischle W, Emiliani S, Hendzel MJ, et al. A new family of human histone deacetylases related to Saccharomyces cerevisiae HDA1p. Journal of Biological Chemistry. 1999;274:11713-11720.
101. Miska EA, Karlsson C, Langley E, Nielsen SJ, Pines J, Kouzarides T. HDAC4 deacetylase associates with and represses the MEF2 transcription factor. EMBO Journal. 1999;18:5099-5107.
102. Wang AH, Bertos NR, Vezmar M, et al. HDAC4, a human histone deacetylase related to yeast HDA1, is a transcriptional corepressor. Molecular & Cellular Biology. 1999;19:7816-7827.
103. Kao HY, Downes M, Ordentlich P, Evans RM. Isolation of a novel histone deacetylase reveals that class I and class II deacetylases promote SMRT-mediated repression. Genes & Development. 2000;14:55-66.
104. Finnin MS, Donigian JR, Cohen A, et al. Structures of a histone deacetylase homologue bound to the TSA and SAHA inhibitors. Nature. 1999;401:188-193.
105. Piekarz RL, Robey R, Sandor V, et al. Inhibitor of histone deacetylation, depsipeptide (FR901228), in the treatment of peripheral and cutaneous T-cell lymphoma: a case report. Blood. 2001;98:2865-2868.
106. Sandor V, Bakke S, Robey RW, et al. Phase I trial of the histone deacetylase inhibitor, depsipeptide (FR901228, NSC 630176), in patients with refractory neoplasms.[see comment]. Clinical Cancer Research. 2002;8:718-728.
107. Piekarz R, Frye R, Turner M, et al. Update on the phase II trial and correlative studies of depsipetptide in patients with cutaneous T-cell lymphoma and relapsed peripheral T-cell lymphoma. Journal of Clinical Oncology. 2004;22:3028.
108. Kelly WK, Richon VM, O'Connor O, et al. Phase I clinical trial of histone deacetylase inhibitor: suberoylanilide hydroxamic acid administered intravenously. Clinical Cancer Research. 2003;9:3578-3588.
109. Kelly WK, O'Connor OA, Krug L, et al. Phase I Study of the Oral Histone Deacetylase Inhibitor, Suberoylanilide Hydroxamic Acid (SAHA), in Patients with Advanced Cancer. Journal of Clinical Oncology. 2005;Submitted 1/05.
110. Mita MM, Mita A, Rowinsky EK. The molecular target of rapamycin (mTOR) as a therapeutic target against cancer. Cancer Biology & Therapy. 2003;2:S169-177.
111. Dumont FJ, Melino MR, Staruch MJ, Koprak SL, Fischer PA, Sigal NH. The immunosuppressive macrolides FK-506 and rapamycin act as reciprocal antagonists in murine T cells. Journal of Immunology. 1990;144:1418-1424.
112. Dumont FJ, Staruch MJ, Koprak SL, Melino MR, Sigal NH. Distinct mechanisms of suppression of murine T cell activation by the related macrolides FK-506 and rapamycin. Journal of Immunology. 1990;144:251-258.
113. Abraham RT. Identification of TOR signaling complexes: more TORC for the cell growth engine. Cell. 2002;111:9-12.
114. Schmelzle T, Hall MN. TOR, a central controller of cell growth.[see comment]. Cell. 2000;103:253-262.
115. Shamji AF, Kuruvilla FG, Schreiber SL. Partitioning the transcriptional program induced by rapamycin among the effectors of the Tor proteins. Current Biology. 2000;10:1574-1581.

116. Sawyers CL. Will mTOR inhibitors make it as cancer drugs? Cancer Cell. 2003;4:343-348.

117. Dutcher JP. Mammalian target of rapamycin (mTOR) Inhibitors. Current Oncology Reports. 2004;6:111-115.

118. Hidalgo M, Rowinsky EK. The rapamycin-sensitive signal transduction pathway as a target for cancer therapy. Oncogene. 2000;19:6680-6686.

119. Dudkin L, Dilling MB, Cheshire PJ, et al. Biochemical correlates of mTOR inhibition by the rapamycin ester CCI-779 and tumor growth inhibition. Clinical Cancer Research. 2001;7:1758-1764.

120. Yu K, Toral-Barza L, Discafani C, et al. mTOR, a novel target in breast cancer: the effect of CCI-779, an mTOR inhibitor, in preclinical models of breast cancer. Endocrine-Related Cancer. 2001;8:249-258.

121. Hudson CC, Liu M, Chiang GG, et al. Regulation of hypoxia-inducible factor 1alpha expression and function by the mammalian target of rapamycin. Molecular & Cellular Biology. 2002;22:7004-7014.

122. Hopfl G, Wenger RH, Ziegler U, et al. Rescue of hypoxia-inducible factor-1alpha-deficient tumor growth by wild-type cells is independent of vascular endothelial growth factor. Cancer Research. 2002;62:2962-2970.

123. Gibbons JJ, Discafani C, Peterson R, al et. The effect of CCI-779, a novel macrolide antitumor agent, on the growth of human tumor cells in vitro and in nude mouse xenograft in vivo. Proc Am Assoc Cancer Res. 2000;40:301.

124. Geoerger B, Kerr K, Tang CB, et al. Antitumor activity of the rapamycin analog CCI-779 in human primitive neuroectodermal tumor/medulloblastoma models as single agent and in combination chemotherapy. Cancer Research. 2001;61:1527-1532.

125. Raymond E, Alexander J, Depenbrock H, al. e. CCI-779, an ester analog of rapamycin that interacts with PTEN/PI3 kinase pathways: a phase I study utilizing a weekly intravenous schedule. 11th NCI-EORTC-AACR Symposium on New Drugs in Cancer Therapy. Amsterdam; 2000.

126. Hidalgo M, Rowinsky E, Erlichman C, al. e. Phase I and phramcaologic study of CCI-779, a cell cycle inhibitor. 11th NCI-EORTC-AACR Symposium on New Drugs in Cancer Therapy. Amsterdam; 2000.

127. Dutcher JP, Hudes G, Motzer R, et al. Preliminary report of a phase 1 study of intravenous (IV) CCI-779 given in combination with interferon-a (IFN) to patients with advanced renal cell carcinoma (RCC). Proc Am Soc Clin Oncol. 2003;21:36.

128. Witzig T, Geyer S, Ghobrial I, et al. Anti-Tumor Activity of Single-Agent CCI-779 for Relapsed Mantle Cell Lymphoma: A Phase II Trial in the North Central Cancer Treatment Group. Blood. 2004;104:Abstract #129.

129. Denny WA. Emerging DNA topoisomerase inhibitors as anticancer drugs. Expert Opinion in Emerging Drugs. 2004;9:105-132.

130. Lown JW, Morgan AR, Yen SF, Wang YH, Wilson WD. Characteristics of the binding of the anticancer agents mitoxantrone and ametantrone and related structures to deoxyribonucleic acids. Biochemistry. 1985;24:4028-4035.

131. Denny WA, Wakelin LP. Kinetics of the binding of mitoxantrone, ametantrone and analogues to DNA: relationship with binding mode and anti-tumour activity. Anti-Cancer Drug Design. 1990;5:189-200.

132. Borchmann P, Schnell R, Knippertz R, et al. Phase I study of BBR 2778, a new aza-anthracenedione, in advanced or refractory non-Hodgkin's lymphoma. Annals of Oncology. 2001;12:661-667.

133. Krapcho AP, Petry ME, Getahun Z, et al. 6,9-Bis[(aminoalkyl)amino]benzo[g]isoquinoline-5,10-diones. A novel class of chromophore-modified antitumor anthracene-9,10-diones: synthesis and antitumor evaluations. Journal of Medicinal Chemistry. 1994;37:828-837.

134. Cavalletti E, Crippa L, Melloni E, Bellini O, Tognella S, Giulini FC. BBR 2778, a novel aza-anthracenedione: preclinical toxicological evaluation. Proc Am Assoc Cancer Res. 1993;34:374.

135. De Isabella P, Palumbo M, Sissi C, et al. Topoisomerase II DNA cleavage stimulation, DNA binding activity, cytotoxicity, and physico-chemical properties of 2-aza- and 2-aza-oxide-anthracenedione derivatives. Molecular Pharmacology. 1995;48:30-38.

136. Hazlehurst LA, Krapcho AP, Hacker MP. Comparison of aza-anthracenedione-induced DNA damage and cytotoxicity in experimental tumor cells. Biochemical Pharmacology. 1995;50:1087-1094.

137. Beggiolin G, Crippa L, Menta E, et al. Bbr 2778, an aza-anthracenedione endowed with preclinical anticancer activity and lack of delayed cardiotoxicity. Tumori. 2001;87:407-416.

138. Crippa L, Franca S, Di Luccio E, Mainardi P, al. e. The aza-anthracenedione Pixantrone (BBR 2778) confirms its reduced cardiotoxic potential vs. reference standards also in mouse pre-treated with anthracyclines. AACR-NCI-EORTC International Conference on Molecular Targets and Cancer Therapeutics. Boston, MA; 2003.

139. Borchmann P, Morschhauser F, Parry A, et al. Phase-II study of the new aza-anthracenedione, BBR 2778, in patients with relapsed aggressive non-Hodgkin's lymphomas. Haematologica. 2003;88:888-894.

140. Camboni G, Fayad L, Tulpule A, et al. A phase I/II trial of BBR-2778 (pixantrone), methylprednisolone, cisplatin, and cytosine arabinoside (BSHAP) in relapsed/refractory aggressive non-Hodgkin's lymphoma (NHL). Proc Am Soc Clin Oncol. 2004;22:6590.

141. Borchmann P, Schnell R, Morschhauser F, et al. A Phase I Study of Pixantrone (BBR 2778) in Combination with Cyclophosphamide, Vincristine and Prednisone in Patients with Relapsed Aggressive Non-Hodgkins Lymphoma. Blood. 2003;102:Abstract # 2639.

142. Borchmann P, Engert A, Davite C, Camboni G. Evaluation of Cardiac Events in Patients Treated with Pixantrone, a Novel Anthracycline Derived Drug. Blood. 2003;102:Abstract #4887.

143. Gandhi V. Metabolism and mechanisms of action of bendamustine: rationales for combination therapies. Seminars in Oncology. 2002;29:4-11.

144. Ozegowski W, Krebs D. w-[bis-(beta-chlorethyl)-aminobenzimidazolyl-(2)]-propionic or butyric acids as potential cytostatic agents. Prakt Chem. 1963;20:178-186.

145. Ozegowski W, Krebs D. IMET 3393, gamma-[1-methyl-5-bis-(beta-chlorethyl)-amino-benzimiazolyl-(2)]-butyric acid hydrochloride, a new cytostatic agent from the benzimidazole mustard series. Zbl Pharm. 1971;110:1013-1019.

146. Strumberg D, Harstrick A, Doll K, Hoffmann B, Seeber S. Bendamustine hydrochloride activity against doxorubicin-resistant human breast carcinoma cell lines. Anti-Cancer Drugs. 1996;7:415-421.

147. Staib P, Schinkothe T, Dimski T, al et. In vitro modulation of ara-CTP accumulation in fresh AML cells by bendamustine in comparison with fludarabine, 2-CdA and gemcitabine. Blood. 1999;94:63a.

148. Konstantinov SM, Kostovski A, Topashka-Ancheva M, Genova M, Berger MR. Cytotoxic efficacy of bendamustine in human leukemia and breast cancer cell lines. Journal of Cancer Research & Clinical Oncology. 2002;128:271-278.

149. Schwanen C, Hecker T, Hubinger G, et al. In vitro evaluation of bendamustine induced apoptosis in B-chronic lymphocytic leukemia. Leukemia. 2002;16:2096-2105.

150. Rummel MJ, Chow KU, Hoelzer D, Mitrou PS, Weidmann E. In vitro studies with bendamustine: enhanced activity in combination with rituximab. Seminars in Oncology. 2002;29:12-14.

151. Schrijvers D, Vermorken JB. Phase I studies with bendamustine: an update. Seminars in Oncology. 2002;29:15-18.

152. Heider A, Niederle N. Efficacy and toxicity of bendamustine in patients with relapsed low-grade non-Hodgkin's lymphomas. Anti-Cancer Drugs. 2001;12:725-729.

153. Kath R, Blumenstengel K, Fricke HJ, Hoffken K. Bendamustine monotherapy in advanced and refractory chronic lymphocytic leukemia. Journal of Cancer Research & Clinical Oncology. 2001;127:48-54.

154. Aivado M, Becker K, Niese M, Strupp C, Losem C, Haas R. Bendamustine is an efficient and well-tolerated option in the palliation of pretreated B-cell chronic lymphocytic leukemias. Proceedings of the American Society of Clinical Oncology. 2001;20:306a.

155. Bremer D, Gerda B. Bendamustine weekly: An effective and well tolerated regimen for indolent NHL (non-Hodgkin's lymphoma) and B-CLL (chronic lymphocytic leukemia). Proc Am Soc Clin Oncol. 2003;22:599, Abstract 2410.

156. Weidmann E, Kim SZ, Rost A, et al. Bendamustine is effective in relapsed or refractory aggressive non-Hodgkin's lymphoma. Annals of Oncology. 2002;13:1285-1289.

157. Koenigsmann M, Knauf W, Herold M, et al. Fludarabine and bendamustine in refractory and relapsed indolent lymphoma - a multicenter phase I/II trial of the East German Society of Hematology and Oncology (OSHO). Leukemia & Lymphoma. 2004;45:1821-1827.

158. Rummel MJ, Kim SZ, Chow KU, et al. Bendamustine and rituximab act synergistically *in vitro* and are effective in the treatment of relapsed or refractory indolent and mantle-cell lymphomas. Blood. 2003;102.

159. Weide R, Heymanns J, Schneider A, Pandorf A, Koeppler H. Bendamustine / Mitoxantrone / Rituximab (BMR): A new effective treatment for refractory or relapsed indolent lymphomas. Final evaluation of a pilot study. Blood. 2003;102.

160. Dhaliwal HS, Rohatiner AZ, Gregory W, et al. Combination chemotherapy for intermediate and high grade non-Hodgkin's lymphoma. British Journal of Cancer. 1993;68:767-774.

161. Dorigo A, Mansberg R, Kwan YL. Lomustine, etoposide, methotrexate and prednisone (LEMP) therapy for relapsed and refractory non-Hodgkin's lymphoma. European Journal of Haematology. 1993;50:37-40.

162. Sarris AH, Phan A, Duvic M, et al. Trimetrexate in relapsed T-cell lymphoma with skin involvement. Journal of Clinical Oncology. 2002;20:2876-2880.

163. De Vita V, Hellman S, Rosenberg SA. Biologic Therapy of Cancer. Philadelphia: Lippincott Williams & Wilkins; 1995.

164. Sirotnak FM, Schmid FA, Samuels LL, DeGraw JI. 10-Ethyl-10-deaza-aminopterin: structural design and biochemical, pharmacologic, and antitumor properties. NCI Monographs. 1987:127-131.

165. Sirotnak FM, DeGraw JI, Moccio DM, Samuels LL, Goutas LJ. New folate analogs of the 10-deaza-aminopterin series. Basis for structural design and biochemical and pharmacologic properties. Cancer Chemotherapy & Pharmacology. 1984;12:18-25.

166. Sirotnak FM, DeGraw JI, Schmid FA, Goutas LJ, Moccio DM. New folate analogs of the 10-deaza-aminopterin series. Further evidence for markedly increased antitumor efficacy compared with methotrexate in ascitic and solid murine tumor models. Cancer Chemotherapy & Pharmacology. 1984;12:26-30.

167. Wang ES, O'Connor O, She Y, Zelenetz AD, Sirotnak FM, Moore MA. Activity of a novel anti-folate (PDX, 10-propargyl 10-deazaaminopterin) against human lymphoma is superior to methotrexate and correlates with tumor RFC-1 gene expression. Leukemia & Lymphoma. 2003;44:1027-1035.

168. Shum KY, Kris MG, Gralla RJ, Burke MT, Marks LD, Heelan RT. Phase II study of 10-ethyl-10-deaza-aminopterin in patients with stage III and IV non-small-cell lung cancer. Journal of Clinical Oncology. 1988;6:446-450.

169. Casper ES, Christman KL, Schwartz GK, Johnson B, Brennan MF, Bertino JR. Edatrexate in patients with soft tissue sarcoma. Activity in malignant fibrous histiocytoma. Cancer. 1993;72:766-770.

170. Vandenberg TA, Pritchard KI, Eisenhauer EA, et al. Phase II study of weekly edatrexate as first-line chemotherapy for metastatic breast cancer: a National Cancer Institute of Canada Clinical Trials Group study. Journal of Clinical Oncology. 1993;11:1241-1244.

171. DeGraw JI, Colwell WT, Piper JR, Sirotnak FM. Synthesis and antitumor activity of 10-propargyl-10-deazaaminopterin. Journal of Medicinal Chemistry. 1993;36:2228-2231.

172. Sirotnak FM, DeGraw JI, Colwell WT, Piper JR. A new analogue of 10-deazaaminopterin with markedly enhanced curative effects against human tumor xenografts in mice. Cancer Chemotherapy & Pharmacology. 1998;42:313-318.

173. Krug LM, Azzoli CG, Kris MG, et al. 10-propargyl-10-deazaaminopterin: an antifolate with activity in patients with previously treated non-small cell lung cancer. Clinical Cancer Research. 2003;9:2072-2078.

174. Fayad L, Liebmann J, Modiano M, et al. Preliminary Results of a Phase I/II Trial of BBR-2778 (Pixantrone) in Combination with Fludarabine, Dexamethasone, and Rituximab (FPD-R) in the Treatment of Patients with Relapsed/Refractory Indolent Non-Hodgkin's Lymphoma (NHL). Blood. 2004;104:Abstract #1324.

INDEX